MADE IN U. S. A.

PRESS OF
W. B. SAUNDERS COMPANY
PHILADELPHIA

YOUNG'S
PRACTICE OF UROLOG

BASED ON A STUDY OF 12,500 CASES

By

HUGH H. YOUNG

and

DAVID M. DAVIS

With the Collaboration of

FRANKLIN P. JOHNSON

WITH OVER 1000 ILLUSTRATIONS, 20 BEING COLOR PLATE

by

WILLIAM P. DIDUSCH

VOLUME I

PHILADELPHIA AND LONDON

W. B. SAUNDERS COMPANY

PREFACE

Why another "Urology"? Have we not the recent great treatises by Legueu, Marion in France, Thompson-Walker in England, Watson and Cunningham, Guiteras, Chetwood, Keyes, and Cabot in America. Certainly a veritable *embarras de richesse*.

In the urologic literature are to be found a number of books written long ago which are still of great interest, largely on account of the detailed recital of cases and personal experiences which they contain. We need only to refer here to such milestones as Sir Astley Cooper's Diseases of the Testis; John Hunter's volumes on The Venereal Disease, Syphilis, and Strictures of the Urethra; Sir Henry Thompson's Lithotomy, Tumors of the Bladder, Stricture of the Urethra, and Diseases of the Prostate; Jean Civiale's Lithotritie and Retention d'Urine; J. C. Guyon's Leçons Cliniques and Atlas; Joachin Albarran's Tumeurs de la Vessie, Tumeurs du Rein, and Médecine Opératoire des Voies Urinaires; Max Nitze's Lehrbuch der Kystoscopie; James Israel's Chirurgische Klinik der Nierenkrankheiten; Samuel Gross's Diseases of the Bladder, Prostate and Urethra, and Jacob Henry Bigelow's Litholapaxy. These classic tomes have inspired us to assemble a searching clinical study of our experiences in the practice of urology, and these two volumes are the final outcome of this effort, in the execution of which we realize we have fallen far short of our ideals. Nevertheless, we here present the results, based on a study of the cases we have individually worked over, with others that have been added by a public clinic, under our direction, aggregating in all some 12,500 histories now filed away at the James Buchanan Brady Urological Institute.

Before beginning a critical study of these records it became necessary to prepare elaborate indices, and to send out questionnaires, and requests to report in person, to thousands of patients. The clinical researches required to digest the information amassed have been staggering, but with the help of very willing assistants the work has gone on until almost all of the important subjects have been analytically studied in the light of our collected histories as well as from the facts gleaned in the formidable literature.

To a succession of splendid residents and house officers who have left behind them excellent clinical and laboratory records, and who have been responsible for much of the success of this clinic, we owe a great debt of gratitude, and we delight in naming them, and their university appointments, here:

W. E. Huger, Charleston Medical College (deceased); Joseph Hume, now of Tulane University; H. A. Fowler, Howard University; J. T. Geraghty, Johns Hopkins University (deceased); Louis C. Lehr, Georgetown University; Charles M. Remsen, New York City; A. R. Stevens, Bellevue Medical College; John W. Churchman, Cornell Medical School; Alexander Randall, University of Pennsylvania; John R. Caulk, Washington University; M. L. Boyd, Emory University; H. W. Plaggemeyer, Detroit College of Medicine; Arthur B. Cecil, Los Angeles, California; Frank Hinman, University of California; William A. Frontz, Johns Hopkins

University; J. A. C. Colston, Johns Hopkins University; William C. Quinby, Harvard University; J. E. Burns, Kansas City, Mo.; E. G. Davis, University of Nebraska; B. E. Harrell, Norfolk, Va.; W. O. Wilder, Springfield, Mass.; R. F. Hain, Seattle, Wash.; Howard L. Cecil, Dallas, Texas; William D. Jack, Chicago, Ill.; C. L. Deming, Yale University; David M. Davis, University of Rochester; F. P. Johnson, Portland, Ore.; C. Y. Bidgood, Hartford, Conn.; E. C. Shaw, Miami, Fla.

The achievements of these men, and the distinguished urologic positions now occupied by them in the medical schools indicated above, are a great delight to us who were associated with them in their residence here.

It has seemed incumbent upon us to justify the various procedures, mechanical devices, and original researches which have had their inception with us. On this account we have given much space and detailed study to the following conditions:

The physiology of micturition and demonstration of the function of the trigone to open the prostatic orifice; acute and chronic cystitis, pyonephrosis, and general peritonitis due to the gonococcus; chronic cystitis, pyonephrosis, and renal calculus due to the bacillus typhosus; stricture of the lower end of the ureter due to seminal vesiculitis; the symptom complex in calculus of the lower end of the ureter; vesical diverticula containing cancer; preliminary treatment before prostatectomy; the diagnosis and cure of congenital valves of the prostatic urethra; a proven case of lateral hermaphroditism; and cases of obstructive hypertrophy of the trigone and of ulcerative detachment of the trigone.

The following operative procedures: A special Bottini technic for middle lobe cases; cystoscopic removal of calculus from the lower end of ureter; conservative perineal prostatectomy; a radical operation for carcinoma of the prostate; the relief of obstruction in carcinoma of the prostate by conservative perineal prostatectomy; the punch operation for contracture of the vesical orifice; a plastic operation on urethral and vesical sphincters for the cure of incontinence; intravesical diverticulectomy; a retrograde perineal operation for impermeable stricture of the urethra; a combined vesical and perineal operation for cure of recto-urethral fistulæ; heminephrectomy in double kidney with calculus; resection of the kidney in nephrolithiasis; an operation for epispadias; an operation for the cure of incontinence associated with epispadias and exstrophy of the bladder; the radical removal of the entire seminal tract for tuberculosis; the removal of cysts at the prostatic orifice with a cystoscopic rongeur or destruction with fulguration; operations for hypospadias; a more radical operation for cancer of the penis; a transperitoneal technic for kidney tumors with removal of the peritoneal covering.

The following urologic instruments: A Bottini cautery incisor with interchangeable blades; the prostatic tractor; the long urethral prostatic tractor; the cystoscopic rongeur; the prostatic bar excisor or punch; the evacuating cystoscopic lithotrite; the tubular urethroscope with a freely movable lamp carrier; various cystoscopic radium applicators for the treatment of vesical and prostatic carcinoma; the "boomerang" needle-holder; a urethrotomy staff; the combined x-ray and cystoscopic table; the automatic perineal elevator; a special kidney elevator; the phthaleinometer; a decompressing manometer and automatic bladder irrigator.

The following products of our laboratories: Presentation of new germicides, mercurochrome and meroxyl, and a new antisyphilitic drug, flumerin; the intravenous attack upon local and general infections and infectious diseases with intravenous injections of mercurochrome and of gentian-violet; an extensive series of cases demonstrating the possibility of a therapia sterilisans magna.

We perhaps should apologize for having devoted so much space to this personal work, but, as mentioned before, our interpretation of the reason for the lasting value of many old medical books, that are still full of interest after a lapse of many years, is their individual character and their detailed description of personal experiences and inventions. "By their fruits ye shall know them."

Hence our plan and its present execution. We have tried, however, to see that all subjects were adequately and fairly presented and have given due consideration to the best to be found in the literature, which has been deeply studied and profusely quoted.

The arrangement of the subject matter has been made almost entirely on the basis of the pathology. We have treated separately in the early part of the book all lesions due to obstruction of the urinary tract, which are the same regardless of the cause of the obstruction. The pathology in each instance has been extensively considered, as we feel that this is absolutely essential to a proper knowledge of urologic disease. Operative treatment is taken up separately, which avoids the necessity of describing the same operation repeatedly under different headings.

Nearly all of the illustrations are original and are the result of years of patient work and enthusiasm for artistic ideals on the part of Mr. William P. Didusch. Some of his illustrations, prepared for other members of the staff, have been used, and the original articles from which they are taken are generally referred to in footnotes.

We wish to thank especially for much assistance Dr. John T. Geraghty, who helped us in the study of vesical tumors. Dr. Geraghty's recent death, when in his prime, has been a great blow to the Institute and, indeed, to Urology. Dr. Franklin P. Johnson has collaborated with us in the chapter on Malformations and Abnormalities of the Urogenital Tract, which is very largely his work. Without his splendid knowledge of embryology this chapter could not have been written. We wish to acknowledge our gratitude to Dr. William A. Frontz and Dr. J. A. C. Colston for their help, and to Miss Mary Gover for her statistical study of 1000 cases of perineal prostatectomy. Miss Margaret Boise has made a thorough study of anesthesia in our cases, which we have incorporated.

Our thanks are also due to W. L. Denny, C. Y. Bidgood, E. C. Shaw, W. W. Scott, Everett Sanner, R. Glenn Craig, Robert McKay, Charles Levy, Vincent Vermooten, E. C. James, W. L. Mallard, Kenneth Legge, W. L. Sherman, LeRoy Fleming, Henry Browne, M. S. Mathis, and George Char.

Our special thanks are due to Dr. E. G. Davis, who was largely responsible for the inception and early discoveries in the search for a urinary antiseptic with compounds with phenolsulphonephthalein and for many subsequent excellent papers on germicidal dyes; Dr. E. C. White, who collaborated with Dr. Davis and prepared many new compounds of dyes and other antiseptics; to Dr. E. O. Swartz, Dr. J. A. C. Colston, and others who collaborated and added splendid papers on this important series in our search for the ideal antiseptic; and to Justina H. Hill, for her exhaustive studies on the bacteriology of the urinary tract and her bacteriologic and animal researches with germicides.

We are indebted to Dr. Miley B. Wesson for his work on the anatomy of the bladder and trigone while an assistant in our Clinic, and for his subsequent work on cysts of the prostate, which we have quoted at length.

To Dr. D. S. Macht for the section on Organotherapy, to Dr. C. A. Waters and Miss Mary Goldthwaite for their splendid radiographic work and their assistance in the selection of x-ray plates to illustrate this book, as also to C. F. Elvers, who has prepared the microphotographs, and to E. H. Slade, Dorothy Schad, Lawrence Lanahan, Clara Rapp, and particularly to Bertha M. Trott, and Minnie Blogg, librarian, we offer our sincere thanks.

Dr. M. C. Winternitz, of Yale, and Mr. Henry Wade, of Edinburgh, have furnished us with splendid illustrations of pathologic material.

But especially do we wish to express our deep sense of gratitude to that keen man of affairs and remarkable sportsman who presented us with two-thirds of a million to build to his memory the James Buchanan Brady Urological Institute. Its possibilities of usefulness for research, however, would have been far less had it not been that many thousands for investigation have been furnished by such splendid friends as Hobart J. Park, Robert W. Kelley, Henry K. McHarg, W. S. Kilmer, August Heckscher, Francis P. Garvan, Edward W. Orrin, and others.

Without the assistance of these, one and all, these volumes could hardly have been written.

THE AUTHORS.

BALTIMORE, MD.

CONTENTS—VOLUMES I AND II

VOLUME I

VOLUME II

PRACTICE OF UROLOGY

CHAPTER I

THE PHYSIOLOGY AND PATHOLOGY OF MICTURITION

THE URETER

THE urine passes down through the *ureter* from the kidney as the result of peristaltic waves which originate in the musculature of the pelvis, and extend to the ureterovesical orifice. Observed cystoscopically, the normal ureters eject urine into the bladder every fourteen to thirty-eight seconds. The two ureters may contract at different times and at different rates[1] and independently of bladder contractions. In experimental animals approximately the same rates have been observed. Henderson[2] notes that the rhythm may be not quite regular. Sokoloff and Luchsinger[3] and others, by perfusing the ureters, have determined that the rate and vigor of contraction increase as the quantity of urine increases, so that the urine is removed whatever the rate of renal secretion. The peristaltic wave (in rabbits) advances at the rate of 18.3 mm. per second in the upper ureter, 15.4 mm. per second in the middle ureter, and 13.3 mm. per second in the lower ureter.[4] The pelvis contracts more rapidly than the ureter, though less vigorously, and acts as the "pace-maker" for the normal peristaltic wave.[5] Ringleb[6] described a pump-like or sucking action of the renal calices dependent upon rings of muscle about their narrow portions, but this has not been confirmed.

The ureter contains nerve-fibers, and ganglia in the adventitia. According to Disse[7] there are also small ganglia in the muscularis. The nerve supply is from the renal, spermatic, and hypogastric plexuses, all of which supply sympathetic fibers to the upper, middle, and lower segments respectively. Pharmacologically there is definite evidence[8] of the presence of sympathetic and autonomic fibers and of ganglia. Satani[9] found the response to sympathetic stimulating drugs most marked at the upper end, and to autonomic-stimulating drugs most marked at the lower end. Some pelvic autonomics, therefore, coming by the nervus erigens to the vesical plexus, may run to the lower ureter. Stimulation of these nerve trunks produces comparatively little effect on the ureter, that of the hypogastric being the most marked. This fact caused Engelmann[10] in 1869 to suggest that the

---

[1] Sampson: Johns Hopkins Hospital Bulletin, 1903, xiv, 334–352.

[2] Journal of Physiology, 1905–06, xxxiii, 175–188.

[3] Archiv für die Gesamte Physiologie, 1881, xxvi, 464–469.

[4] Graves and Davidoff: Journal of Urology, 1923, x, 185–231.

[5] Lucas: American Journal of Physiology, 1906–07, xvii, 392–407; 1907–08, xxii, 245–278.

[6] Zeitschrift für Urologie, 1923 (3), 154, 155.

[7] Bardeleben's Handbuch der Anatomie, 1902, vii, 105–112.

[8] Macht: Journal of Urology, 1917, i, 97–111.

[9] American Journal of Physiology, 1919, xlix, 474–495; 1920, l, 342–351.

[10] Archiv für die Gesamte Physiologie, 1869, ii, 243–293.

peristaltic wave is myogenic, and propagated without the intermediary of nerves. Penfield[1] found that dog ureters, normal or dilated, showed normal peristaltic waves when entirely isolated and suspended in Locke's solution. Ureteral peristalsis continues after transverse cord lesions.

We[2] in 1898 noted that the ureters cease discharging urine into the bladder after the intravesical pressure rises above a certain point. Sampson[3] and others find that any increase of the pressure against which the ureters work causes an increase in the rate, amplitude, and vigor of the contractions. Henderson[4] notes that when this pressure rises above 26 to 32 mm. of mercury in the dog, ureteral peristalsis ceases. Individual ureteral contractions, however, may produce a pressure of 36 mm. mercury (dog, Henderson) or 92 cm. water (isolated dog ureter, Lucas[5]). This is less than the pressure the bladder can produce, which may be 200 cm. water (dog, Mosso[6]). It is to be distinguished from the secretion pressure of the urine, which, of course, varies with the blood-pressure and is not developed except in the presence of back pressure in the pelvis itself.

Reverse peristalsis has not been noted in the intact ureter, except possibly as the result of electric stimulation of the hypogastrics.[7]

Obstruction to the ureteral flow causes increased peristalsis, muscular hypertrophy, later dilatation, and finally cessation of peristalsis. When the ureter is dilated the waves cannot propel the urine, since the lumen is not obliterated between waves, but exercise merely a compressive effect, like the heart or bladder. A point of irritation, trauma, or inflammation, as, for example, a stone in the ureter, may interrupt the wave, in which case independent waves may arise below the point of block. Experiments on animals show that when this occurs, especially if part of the fluid be removed from the dilated portion above, violent, irregular, and in part reverse peristaltic motions take place above the block. Wislocki and O'Conor[8] consider that such waves probably occur in renal colic, and that the reversed waves, causing sudden rises in the pelvic pressure, may well explain the intense and sudden renal pain, as well as the not infrequent "radiation."

Hinman has noted, upon section in dogs, active ureteral peristalsis above the point of obstruction, of ureters doubly ligated and divided for two or more years, by which time the kidney had undergone complete hydronephrotic atrophy. The dilated ureter by its own peristalsis was able to pump off the pelvic contents, even though the open ureteral end was at a slightly higher level than the kidney, thus preventing gravity syphonage, the secretory pressure in this case, of course, being nil.

Experimental work in repair hydronephrosis in dogs, cats, rabbits, and rats demonstrates that relief of obstruction does not cause shrinkage of the dilated ureter to near normal, as occurs with the dilated pelvis, which shrinks even in complete hydronephrotic atrophy, except in those cases in which relief of the obstruction produces renal repair and progressive increase of function. Then the ureter contracts with loss of its marked tortuosity and dilatation, the inference

---

[1] American Journal of the Medical Sciences, 1920, clx, 36–46.
[2] Young: Johns Hopkins Hospital Bulletin, 1898, ix, 100–113.
[3] Johns Hopkins Hospital Bulletin, 1903, xiv, 334–352.
[4] Journal of Physiology, xxxii, 1905–06, 175–188.
[5] American Journal of Physiology, 1908, xxii, 245–278.
[6] Archives Italiennes de Biologie, 1882, i, 97–128; 291–324.
[7] Elliott: Journal of Physiology, 1907, xxxv, 367–445.
[8] Johns Hopkins Hospital Bulletin, 1920, xxxi, 197–202.

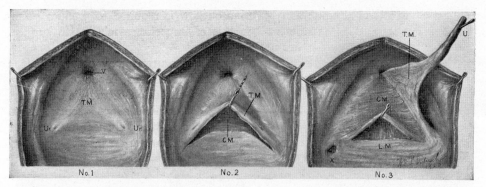

FIG. 1.—Successive stages in the dissection of the trigone after maceration: *V*, Vesical orifice; *TM*, trigonal muscle; *Ur*, ureteral orifice; *CM*, circular muscle of the bladder; *LM*, longitudinal muscle of the bladder; *U*, ureter; *X*, opening from which ureter has been removed. No. 1, Normal trigone; No. 2, the mucosa is incised behind the interureteric bar and the trigonal muscle raised from the circular muscle, carrying the ureteral orifices with it; No. 3, the trigonal muscle is completely separated from the circular muscle and lifted, taking the ureter along with it. Note the converging fibers of the trigonal muscle entering the vesical orifice. After incising the circular muscle it in its turn can be dissected away from the longitudinal or outermost layer.

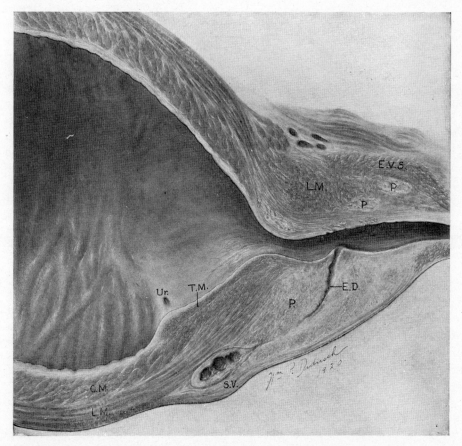

FIG. 2.—Sagittal section of bladder and prostate: *C.M.*, Circular muscle; *L.M.*, longitudinal muscle; *T.M.*, trigonal muscle, shown superimposed upon bladder muscle; *Ur*, ureter; *E.D.*, ejaculatory duct; *S.V.*, seminal vesicle; *P*, prostatic gland tissue; *E.V.S.*, external vesical sphincter. The arc-like course of the trigonal muscle which passes down the floor of the urethra is shown.

being that functional stimulation by urine outflow is required to produce structural restoration.   This experimental fact is of importance relative to surgical
repair or transplantation of hydro-ureters.

In infravesical obstructions reflux of urine in the ureter may occur with the
increased intravesical pressure.   (See Urogenital Infections, Mode of Infection,
where the question of reflux is considered at length, and also Obstructive Uropathy,
Pathology.)   The powerful ureteral contractions, which adapt themselves so
well to increased pressure or quantity of urine, protect the kidney from increased
pressure very efficiently until the effects of obstruction are very marked.

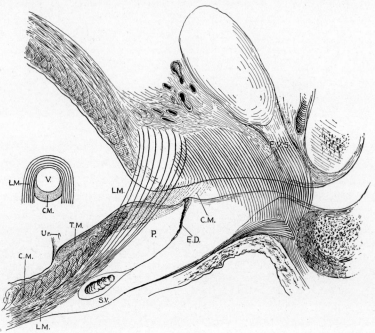

Fig. 3.—Sagittal section of bladder; diagram of Fig. 2.   The external longitudinal layer of the
base sweeps up over the vesical orifice, making a loop.   Within this loop the circular layer forms a
wedge below the orifice and flows down the urethra in an oblique direction, surrounding the canal as
a thin layer.   The result is a double loop and not a sphincter.   The small insert is a cross-section of
the vesical orifice, showing the upward pull of the loop from the circular muscle and the opposing action
of the longitudinal muscle loop.   V., Vesical orifice; L.M., longitudinal muscle; C.M., circular muscle;
T.M., trigonal muscle; E.V.S., external vesical sphincter (striated muscle); Ur., ureteral orifice; S.V.,
seminal vesicle; E.D., ejaculatory duct; P., prostate.   Wesson.

THE BLADDER

The neuromuscular mechanism by which the *bladder* receives and stores urine,
and discharges its contents completely at any desired time, is not only of great
scientific interest, but of great practical importance, since these functions must
always be preserved if an individual is to be able to enjoy life.   In discussing it
we may well include a few remarks about erection and ejaculation, since the nerves
and muscles involved are so largely in common.

The bladder is best considered as a hollow sac surrounded by a muscular coat,
which by its contractions can cause complete evacuation.   The anatomical division into layers is indistinct, and the whole musculature always contracts together,
so that it is best considered as one muscle, and is called the "detrusor" of the

bladder. In the base of the bladder is, however, an entirely separate layer of muscle, lying on the internal surface of the detrusor. This is known as the trigonal muscle. It develops in the embryo from the muscle layers surrounding the lower ends of the Wolffian ducts and ureters, as shown by Wesson.[1] As a result of expansion of the bladder in fetal life these muscles come to lie in the bladder, and their main bundles run from the ureteral orifices to the vesical orifice, where the bundles from the two sides join and run down, just beneath the urethral mucosa on the posterior aspect, to and beyond the verumontanum. In many animals, for example, the dog, this is the arrangement; in others, including man, certain bundles diverge toward the midline immediately after leaving the ureters, and interlace with similar bundles from the other side. The upper margin of these bundles passes straight across the bladder and forms Mercier's interureteric bar. The mass of muscle passing over the posterior edge of the vesical orifice forms Lieutaud's uvula (Fig. 1).

Here at the orifice, the division of the detrusor muscle into layers is more distinct (Figs. 2 and 3). From each of the two layers, just posterior and lateral to the vesical orifice, is sent a strong band of muscle-fibers, which runs down and forward into the prostatic mass to form a loop around the front of the urethra. The bundle from the external ("longitudinal") layer is thicker and external, while that from the internal ("circular") layer is thinner, and passes inside the external loop, but extends farther down the urethra, reaching the level of the verumontanum. These two arcuate muscle bands form the "internal sphincter." They distinctly are not a circular sphincter, like the sphincter ani.

The *urethra* has circular and longitudinal coats of smooth muscle, extending down as far as the membranous urethra. The upper part of these muscles, invaded in fetal life by prostatic tubules, make up a part of the prostatic mass, and no doubt, by their contraction, empty the prostate.

The ejaculatory ducts, vesicles, ampullæ, and vasa deferentia are surrounded by coats of smooth muscle.

The striated muscle of the urethra begins as a sheet on the anterior surface of the prostate, but does not surround the urethra above the level of the apex of the prostate. It covers the entire membranous urethra, where it is sometimes called the "compressor urethræ," and thickens at the level of the triangular ligament to form the "external sphincter." Certain fibers pass out laterally here in the substance of the ligament, and blend with other adjacent muscles, including the levator ani. The ischiocavernosus and bulbocavernosus muscles surround, respectively, the roots of the corpora cavernosa and the bulb of the corpus spongiosum.

Nerve Supply of the Urinary Tract

All these muscles derive their innervation from three sources: 1. True sympathetic fibers, arising from the third and fourth, sometimes the first or fifth, lumbar segments, and passing by way of the ganglia, lumbar splanchnics, inferior mesenteric plexus, and hypogastric nerves to the vesical plexus (Fig. 4). Developmentally, this system is related to the Wolffian body, which arises in the lumbar region, and the fibers go especially to the ureters, trigonal muscle, verumontanum, prostate, vesicles, and vasa deferentia. 2. Autonomic or parasympathetic fibers, arising from the first, second, and third sacral segments, leaving the sacral plexus low

[1] Journal of Urology, 1920, iv, 279–315.

down in the pelvis by the pelvic visceral nerve, or nervus erigens, and passing through the hemorrhoidal (or pelvic) plexus, on each side of the rectum, to the vesical plexus. These provide the principal innervation for the detrusor muscle, and also send branches to the posterior urethra. The fibers from these first two

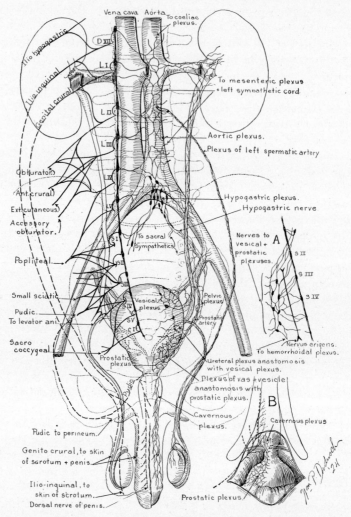

Fig. 4.—Diagram showing the nerve supply, both peripheral and sympathetic, of the male uro-genital system: A, The connections between the sympathetic cord and the pelvic plexus in the sacral region cannot be shown in the main diagram; they are indicated at the right in the small diagram. Note that the pelvic plexus receives fibers from the sacral sympathetic cord and also from the hypogastric nerves. This diagram has been compiled from a number of works on anatomy. B, Perineal view of prostate and urethra.

systems mingle in the vesical plexus, where there are some ganglion-cells, and pass directly by a multitude of small trunks to the ureters, bladder, vesicles, and pros-tate. Both include vasomotor fibers, but there are more in the nervus erigens, which contains the main vasodilators for the erectile tissue of the penis. 3. Periph-eral and autonomic fibers from the sacral segments, separating directly from the sacral plexus to form the pudic nerve (nervus pudendus) which runs through the perineum, giving off branches to the membranous urethra, external sphincter, corpora cavernosa, ischiocavernosus and bulbocavernosus muscles, and skin of the penis. This nerve innervates the striated muscle of the urethra and provides part of the sensory path from the penis. The spinal centers which maintain the tone of these muscles are at or just below the fifth lumbar segment. The nervus erigens contains the principal sensory fibers from the bladder, while there is little evidence to show sensory elements in the hypogastric.

Experiments on animals show that the mechanism by which these muscles and nerves act varies tremendously in different species. In each, therefore, there is a special adaptation, and we are not permitted to draw free analogies between one species and another from experiments or developmental studies. Certain definite facts are, however, known.

Hypogastric Nerves.—Stimulation causes contraction only in the base of the bladder and seminal vesicles.[1] In some animals the detrusor relaxes, in only a few does it contract strongly. The involuntary muscle of the urethra and prostate usually contracts. This nerve, therefore, does not control the mechanism leading to micturition, but there is reason to think it contains contractor fibers for the internal sphincter. When the hypogastrics are sectioned no change of importance is seen in function or sensation.

Nervi Erigentes (Pelvic Nerves).—Stimulation causes strong contraction of the detrusor, producing a pressure, in dogs, as high as 150 cm. of water. The smooth muscle of the urethra relaxes. The arteries of the erectile tissues dilate, causing erection. (This shows well how, in normal functioning, only a part of the fibers in a nerve trunk are active, since the bladder is emptied without an erection, or if present it rapidly disappears during urination. This should be remembered in interpreting stimulation experiments.) When the nervi erigentes are sectioned, the bladder dilates, although it still retains some slight tone, and loses its sensation. There is retention, due to contraction of some of the urethral muscles.

Pudic Nerves.—Stimulation causes vasoconstriction in the erectile tissue, the penis becoming small and flaccid. The striated urethral muscles contract. When the nerve is sectioned, however, erection does not occur. Sensation is lost in the penis, and, therefore, mechanical stimulation does not cause erection and ejaculation. There is a tendency to incontinence and dribbling, even if the other nerves are intact. If, however, the nervi erigentes have been previously sectioned, the retention with paradoxic or overflow incontinence is replaced by a true incontinence when the pudic is thrown out of action.

If the *spinal cord* is cut in the lumbar region, the bladder, while retaining some tone, cannot empty itself. Centers in the cauda equina portion of the spinal cord, below the site of the transection, keep up a slight but much reduced tonus in the detrusor, and apparently give rise to an automatic voiding reflex when the bladder becomes distended. This reflex, much weaker than the normal voiding reflex, may be strengthened by stimulating any sensory nerve which reaches the cord below the transection (stroking the leg, swabbing the penis, etc.). This automatic voiding is well observed in animals, but was thought not to occur in man until demonstrated by Riddock[2] and Head.[3] Automaticity may begin as

[1] Elliott: Journal of Physiology, 1907, xxxv, 367–445.

[2] Brain, 1917, xl, 264.

[3] Studies in Neurology, 1920, ii, 470.

early as two weeks after injury. The weakness of the contraction makes it easy to miss if studied by means of a manometer attached to a catheter, since slight pressure will dilate the bladder even during its contraction. While automatic voiding in humans is often incomplete, it may empty the bladder completely (Head), and in any case is most important, as it enables many of these unfortunate patients to get along without catheterization, thus diminishing the danger from infection.

THE ACT OF URINATION

Ordinarily, the *internal sphincter* exercises excellent control over micturition. The experiments of Rehfisch[1] show that when a metal catheter is inserted right up to the internal sphincter, the patient is still able to control voiding perfectly. In addition, his observation that voiding may begin when the intravesical pressure is nowhere near its height shows that the sphincter is actively opened more or less independently of the contraction of the detrusor.

The sensation of desire to void depends on the intravesical pressure, not on the volume contained. (The threshold of pressure, of course, depends on the degree of irritability present). This is shown by the well-known fact that if a desire to void be resisted the desire may pass away for a long time. The tone of the detrusor is constantly changing, since it reacts to a multitude of stimuli, psychogenic or reflex. Strong stimulation of any sensory peripheral nerve will cause the bladder to contract, while a desire to void may be produced by the sound of running water or even by the thought of voiding.

As to the *external sphincter*, x-ray pictures of animals, with artificially induced bladder paralyses, or of men in whom the internal sphincter has been destroyed or paralyzed by nerve lesions, show that the posterior urethra is filled with urine, and that the external sphincter is retaining the urine perfectly. Men with perineal fistulæ leading into the prostatic urethra may have perfect control of urination through the fistula. In other cases the urine flows constantly through the perineum, showing that the internal sphincter is out of action, yet as soon as the fistula closes, micturition through the penis is under normal control, and the patient is unaware that his internal sphincter is inactive. In an experiment of our own, designed to supplement that of Rehfisch in which the external sphincter was thrown out of action by inserting a metal catheter, we used a small metal tube, about $1\frac{3}{4}$ inches long, so mounted on a slender curved rod that it could be inserted into the vesical orifice, thus throwing the internal sphincter out of action. With this device in place, normal individuals were not only able to retain their urine, but to start and stop the flow with exactly the same ease as usual. It is clear, therefore, that either set of muscles can perform the function if necessary.

In normal voiding it is evident that the striated muscles are relaxed, since by a violent voluntary contraction of them, the stream can be cut off. It is also evident that the detrusor is contracting strongly, either as a result of stimulation from internal pressure or from an impulse originating voluntarily, since the pressure of the stream will be as high sometimes as 2 meters of water. The sphincter must also be relaxed. Fibers in the nervus erigens can cause this. In man at least the mechanism by which the free opening is produced is interesting.

[1] Virchow's Archiv für Pathologischen Anatomie, 1897, cl, 111–151.

PLATE I

URETHROSCOPIC VIEWS

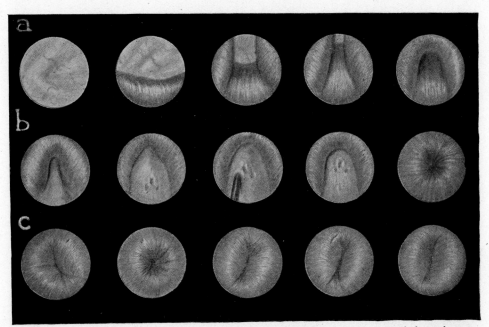

A. Successive views from bladder to pendulous portion of urethra with Young's tubular endoscope, magnified 2½ times. *a*, Normal case: (1) normal bladder; (2) median portion of prostate; (3) with lateral muscles shown; (4) same, orifices almost closed; (5) orifice closed. *b*, (1 to 4) Progressive views of verumontanum, utricle, and ejaculatory ducts; (5) membranous urethra. *c*, (1) Bulbous urethra; (2) penoscrotal juncture showing glands of Littré; (3, 4, 5), pendulous urethra near glans.

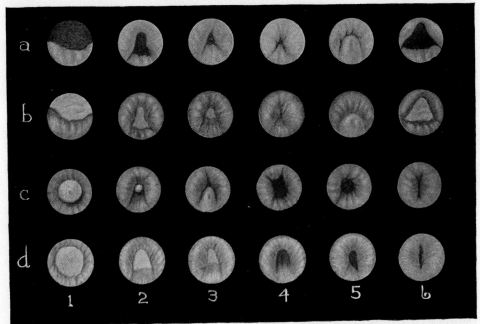

B. Rows *a* and *b*: Endoscopic views of the vesical orifice and posterior urethra of 2 normal cases. *a*, With the Greenberg water endoscope. *b*, With the Young endoscope (air). The instrument is gradually withdrawn showing (1) the median portion, (2 and 3) median portion and lateral muscles, (4 and 5) the verumontanum, (6) the tube was pushed backward so as to view the vesical orifice and the patient attempted to void. The contraction of the trigonal muscle pulled open the vesical orifice, giving the view shown here (6). *c* and *d*, Incontinence of urine in 2 cases of suprapubic prostatectomy (B. U. I. 11,534 and 11,971). (1) Dilated internal orifice, (2) incomplete closure, (3) verumontanum, (4) apex of prostate, (5) external sphincter relaxed, (6) bulbous urethra.

We[1] had noticed that in cases where there was urinary obstruction, the trigonal muscle was tremendously hypertrophied. Later, we observed, during cystoscopy, in the case of a man who was suddenly seized with an imperative desire to urinate, that the trigone became much shortened and thickened. The posterior margin of the orifice was flattened out and disappeared, and the verumontanum rose up almost into the bladder, where it could be viewed. Our studies have shown that the trigone always contracts during micturition, and have furnished the first clear explanation of the act of urination. Our first published statement was as follows:

This brings up the question of the part taken by the trigone in the act of urination. It seems to me to indicate that one function of the trigone is to pull open the internal sphincter of the bladder. I have long held to this view, as I have frequently observed during cystoscopy, that if violent desire to urinate came on, the trigone would contract greatly and the prostatic orifice would open widely, the median (posterior) portion being apparently drawn backward by the muscle-fibers which run from the trigone down into the posterior urethra, and which were seen to contract violently. The opening of the internal sphincter during urination will have to be viewed, therefore, not as an inhibitory action, as heretofore, but as the result of the contraction of the powerful trigonal muscle which passes in the form of an arc through a weaker muscle of circular shape (the vesical sphincter) and pulls it open when it contracts.

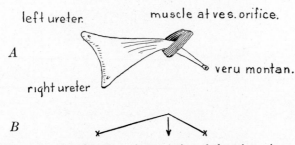

FIG. 5.—Diagrams to show the effect of contraction of the trigone in opening internal vesical sphincter: *A*, Trigonal muscles are shown passing through lateral muscles of the sphincter and over the uvula vesicæ. *B* shows the effect of contraction of the arc-shaped trigonal muscle, viz., to pull down the uvula vesicæ and open the sphincter.

The trigonal muscle, running down into the urethra, forms an arc, the contraction of which straightens it and results in depressing the "uvula vesicæ" and opening the vesical orifice. This is shown diagrammatically in Fig. 5. The opening of the sphincter is then positive—and not a relaxation due to "inhibition of the internal sphincter." This has been confirmed anatomically by Wesson, who has shown that the trigonal muscle pulls upon the orifice in the open side of the two sphincteric loops, and endoscopic views prepared by us in conjunction with Wesson[2] show the orifice being pulled, by the backward and outward impulse of the trigonal muscle, into a triangular, widely open hole. In the few cases where the trigone, dissected free by tuberculous ulceration, had been removed surgically, there was difficulty of urination.

The development of the trigonal muscle is different from that of the detrusor, and its innervation is by the true sympathetics through the hypogastric nerves.

[1] Young: Changes in the Trigone Due to Tuberculosis, etc., Surgery, Gynecology, and Obstetrics, 1918, 608–615; Young and Macht; The Physiology of Micturition, Journal of Pharmacology, 1923, xii, 329–354.

[2] Young and Wesson: The Anatomy and Surgery of the Trigone, Archives of Surgery, 1921, iii, 1–39.

That this is true for man is shown by the *in vitro* experiments of Macht, who finds that trigonal muscle contracts only with drugs acting on true sympathetic endings, while detrusor fibers contract with drugs acting on parasympathetic endings, as well.[1]

From these remarks it will be seen that the retention occurring in spinal cord disease ("spinal" or "paretic" bladder) is due first to a paralysis, partial or complete, of the detrusor, and second to a disturbance of the normal micturition complex. In this we may include the absence of the normal active opening of the internal sphincter (Fig. 5), and also a spastic condition of the striated sphincters, with inability to relax them normally. Section of the pudics would, no doubt, help to convert the condition into a true incontinence, but it is doubtful if this would be justified, as so many other effects would also be produced. Where the entire cord is involved, as in late multiple sclerosis or tabes, true incontinence may occur.

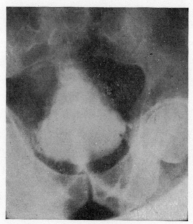

Fig. 6.—Cystogram in a case of cerebrospinal syphilis, showing unusual pyriform shape, marked trabeculation, but no dilatation of the internal sphincter. Symptoms were great frequency and difficulty. R. U., 60 c.c. B. C., 450 c.c. B. U. I., *x*-Ray 9896.

DESTRUCTION OF URINARY CONTROL BY SURGICAL MEANS

In operations in the pelvis, all of the above described structures should be preserved. There is no danger of injuring the hypogastrics, the nervi erigentes, or the vesical plexus in men—they lie well out of the way. They should be considered in extensive operations on the uterus and adnexa. In the bladder, the important muscular bands of the trigone run from ureter to vesical orifice—therefore, if anything is to be done, the trigone should be split in the midline, and subsequently restored as nearly as possible to normal. The internal sphincter is, of course, always preserved when possible. Its nerve supply is diffuse, and not likely to be entirely destroyed. Incisions in the prostate should be as small as possible, and directed so as best to spare the course of the many fibers which run diagonally down and forward through it to the urethra and erectile tissues. It is to be presumed that the autonomic vasodilators from the nervus erigens course downward through the prostate or in its vicinity. The striated (external) sphincter is also to be

[1] Young and Macht: Loc. cit.

spared carefully—often the fibers can be split and separated without dividing them. If they are divided, one should be sure that they do not remain separated so far that union cannot occur. More important, however, are the pudic nerves and their branches. Section of these nerves impairs sexual ability by anesthetising the penis and breaking the reflex arc on its sensory side. It also paralyzes the external sphincter. Perineal incisions, therefore, should always slope down posteriorly, to run parallel with the branches of the pudic, not too distant from the midline, and extensive dissection in an anteroposterior direction should be avoided, as this will cross the course of the nerves. If it is necessary to injure one pudic, extra efforts should be made to preserve the other.

We[1] have shown that it is possible to excise the entire carcinomatous prostate with its capsule and urethra, a cuff of the bladder adjacent, most of the trigone and both seminal vesicles in one piece, then anastomose the open bladder with the stump of the membranous urethra, and still have perfect urinary control. It is necessary, however, to preserve carefully the blood-vessels and pudic nerves which run along the sides and anterior aspect of the prostate to supply the triangular ligament, external sphincter, etc. If this is not done incontinence results from this radical operation. (See Cancer of Prostate, Radical Operation.) This restoration of normal urination after excision of the prostate and vesical neck shows the power of the external sphincter to function alone.

NEUROLOGIC LESIONS OF THE BLADDER

The various *functional changes* occurring in the urinary tract as results of obstruction, infection, and neoplastic growth will be taken up under the appropriate headings. We shall consider at this point the clinical aspects only of those resulting from *nervous lesions*.

The most important nervous disease affecting the bladder is tabes dorsalis, or locomotor ataxia. The percentage of cases in which bladder symptoms of greater or less severity are present at some time during the course is very high, usually estimated at 80 per cent. or over. The character of the involvement varies greatly, according to the nature and extent of the cord lesions. Both sensory and motor paths are usually involved, and the detrusor muscle is the first to be affected. This results in difficulty of urination, necessitating violent voluntary efforts, and the stream may be small and forceless, and slow in starting. Later lesions vary, and may be apparently in part irritative. Thus the sphincter may be spastic, which in combination with the weakness of the detrusor, produces inability to empty the bladder completely. Later overflow incontinence may be established, and occasionally there may be complete sphincteric paralysis with true incontinence, but this is exceptional. Sensation is usually impaired, so that often the patient has no desire to urinate, and the distended bladder is painless. The symptom complex, however, is very inconstant, and any combination may be expected. It is noteworthy that if cystotomy is performed on a tabetic bladder, the fistula will close promptly in spite of the distended bladder, in contrast with the failure to close if the distention is due to obstruction.

It is important to remember that in many cases the bladder symptoms are the initial symptoms of tabes, so that the urologist must constantly be on the watch

[1] Young: Journal of the American Medical Association, 1917, lxix, 1591–1597.

for this condition. Tabes may come on at any age, even in children who have congenital syphilis. It often begins in later life, during the "prostatic age," when the urinary symptoms must be distinguished from those due to prostatic obstructions. In the late stages the bladder is enormously distended, overflow incontinence is present, and infection has usually occurred, either spontaneously or from catheterization. Incontinence of feces is a frequent complication. The infection is a serious matter, and often terminates the process fatally when pyelonephritis supervenes. Calculi, single or multiple, may form in the urinary tract, usually following infection. In about 16 per cent. of cases of tabes there is complete loss of sexual power, which is often preceded by a period of increased sexual desire.

The diagnosis of tabetic bladder may be difficult if other characteristic symptoms cannot be elicited. Some cases will be missed unless a routine neurologic examination (pupils, reflexes, Wassermann) is done in every case with urinary symptoms. In the majority of cases the stigmata of tabes will be present and the diagnosis easy. If doubt is present, spinal puncture should be done, with cytologic study of the fluid, the test for globulin, and the Wassermann and colloidal gold or colloidal mastic tests.

If a definite diagnosis of tabes can be made, and the urine is sterile, it is well, in order to avoid infection, not to introduce any instruments into the bladder if the urinary symptoms are mild enough so that the patient is not greatly inconvenienced. In many cases, however, intervention will be necessary. This is especially true when the bladder is not entirely insensitive, and the distention causes pain. Other reasons include marked renal insufficiency, and hematuria. If the urine is already infected, there is less reason for avoiding cystoscopy, but special pains should be taken not to introduce new organisms into the bladder. If, for example, a colon group cystitis is changed into an alkaline cystitis, the patient is harmed, and stone formation is made more likely.

If cystoscopy is to be done, the residual urine and bladder capacity are measured. The outflow tube should then be attached to a manometer, and the intravesical pressure noted while the patient tries to void without the assistance of his abdominal muscles. The detrusor of the normal bladder should be able to produce a pressure of over 100 cm. (3 feet) of water, while when the bladder is paralyzed, the pressure will be much below this. (The bladder of obstruction may be very atonic, but its expulsive power will return rapidly if drainage is provided.)

Study of the vesical orifice, supplemented by rectal examination with the cystoscope in place, discloses prostatic hypertrophy, prostatic carcinoma, contracture of the vesical orifice, or median bar, if present. If the vesical sphincter is relaxed, as it often is in the later cases, its edge is seen to be indefinite, and one can often see the funnel-shaped prostatic urethra, and sometimes the verumontanum, by withdrawing the cystoscope a little way. This funnel-shaped dilatation of the vesical orifice may also be seen in a cystogram (Fig. 6), but it is an inconstant finding, since the internal sphincter, even if weakened, may retain sufficient power to contract at the time the cystogram is taken.[1]

The bladder wall has a characteristic appearance, due to the absence of any muscular hypertrophy. It may be smooth and pale, or may show a very fine trabeculation, very different from the trabeculation of obstruction, where the thickening of the muscle bundles can easily be seen (Plate V).

[1] Burns: Surgery, Gynecology, and Obstetrics, 1917, xxiv, 659–668.

There may be shreds of pus, reddening, or ulceration from infection. In some cases, especially where there has been infection, there may be a median bar or contracture of the orifice, which accentuates the retention. In a few cases the nerve supply of the trigone is preserved sufficiently to allow it to hypertrophy as a result of the efforts to void. Confusion may arise when a complicating lesion, such as the above, or a moderate prostatic hypertrophy, is present. If the attention is distracted by such a lesion, the bladder paralysis may be missed as an element in the clinical picture. The neurologic examination will usually prevent this mistake.

The treatment, locally, should be as little as possible. Antisyphilitic treatment is, of course, given to arrest the disease and prevent further damage to the cord if possible. If discomfort is great, or the residual urine large (over 400 c.c.), regular catheterization may be unavoidable.

If an obstructive lesion is present at the vesical orifice, systematic dilation, or a punch operation, may give great relief. In some cases it increases the incontinence, but has a good effect in sparing the kidneys. Where infection is severe, irrigations with potassium permanganate, 1 : 4000, or meroxyl, 1 : 1000, are useful. Instillations of mercurochrome, 1 per cent., or argyrol, 15 per cent., may be given. The Young-Shaw bladder decompressing apparatus may be used (see page 75), placing the overflow tube at a level only a few centimeters above that of the bladder. This device will keep an effective concentration of a germicide in the bladder at all times and in two recent cases has prevented infection. The primary object of all treatment is to avoid infection, since, once installed in the atonic urinary tract, it is almost impossible to eradicate it.

Complications are treated as they arise. Stones may be removed with the lithotrite.

Oppenheim[1] reports cases of incontinence treated with success by wrapping a strip of rectus abdominalis muscle, still attached at its upper end to preserve the nerve supply, about the vesical orifice to make a new sphincter. Deming has utilized the gracilis muscle for the same purpose, and has given us a personal report of a case in an individual of twenty-one years, with a very good result.

Other nervous diseases in which the bladder may be involved include cerebrospinal syphilis, transverse myelitis, toxic sclerosis in pernicious anemia, diabetes, etc., spina bifida and meningocele, multiple sclerosis, and ataxic paraplegia (Gowers). The bladder is usually not involved in the following conditions: epidemic cerebrospinal meningitis, acute poliomyelitis, encephalitis lethargica, chorea, epilepsy (except incontinence during attacks), the muscular dystrophies, lateral sclerosis or progressive muscular atrophy, paralysis agitans, syringomyelia, and Landry's paralysis. It has been suggested that the bladder may be affected in some cases of multiple neuritis, but this is not certain.

Concerning syphilis, it is scarcely necessary to mention that the bladder is involved in the same way in the so-called taboparesis, and in some cases of paresis, as in tabes. Other specific lesions are chronic syphilitic meningitis, syphilitic meningomyelitis, syphilitic myelitis (often secondary to syphilitic vascular disease), chronic syphilitic spinal paralysis (Erb's disease; this may be identical with the meningomyelitis), gumma of the cord, gumma of the meninges, gumma of the vertebræ, gumma of the cauda equina, and anomalous forms ("pseudotabes," etc.). In any of these forms the bladder may be involved. Other manifestations are

[1] Zentralblatt für Chirurgie, 1922, xlix (i), 221–223.

practically always present and help greatly in the diagnosis. The spinal puncture is positive in practically all these cases. The symptoms of the meningitic and myelitic involvements depend on the location of the lesions, while gummata resemble other spinal cord tumors. The bladder symptoms are less constant than in tabes and vary extremely according to the situation and extent of the lesion.

Transverse myelitis may be due to infection, either syphilitic or other, to hemorrhage, from vascular disease or other causes, to trauma, with either direct injury to the cord or pressure from fractured vertebræ, or to tumors, either involving the cord itself, or pressing upon it. Among the tumors are glioma, endothelioma, etc., of the cord, gumma, tuberculoma, etc., of the cord or vertebræ, and aneurysms which erode the vertebræ.

If the transverse lesion is complete, there is absolute loss of sexual power and of vesical sensation. At first there is retention, but later automatic voiding, as described above, may be established. Many such cases were seen during the late war,[1] when it was conclusively shown that it is much better to avoid catheterization and instructions to this effect were issued to the medical department of the American Expeditionary Forces. Sensation being entirely absent, there is little discomfort, although the bladder may become alarmingly distended. Suppression of urine from back pressure is not to be feared, nor is there danger of rupture of the bladder unless the patient accidentally receives a blow. If the program of non-intervention is resolutely carried out, urine eventually begins to escape through the urethra, the distention gradually diminishes, and we may see the patient at the end of, say, three weeks with effective automatic voiding, which empties or almost empties his bladder every hour or so, and with uninfected urine. The distention in the primary stage may be avoided by the use of the Young-Shaw decompressing apparatus, which is the only method of so doing in which infection is not sure to occur. After two weeks one should remove the apparatus cautiously to watch for the beginning of automatic voiding. The prospects, when infection is prevented, both for life and comfort, are tremendously bettered. If catheterization is resorted to, infection is inevitable, and this infection is permanent. It eventually leads to pyelonephritis, uremia, and death, and there is often stone formation as well. In some cases, unfortunately, infection will occur spontaneously even if no instruments are used. Some observers state that in rare instances dribbling does not begin, even after extreme distention. This is surely very exceptional, and since it is so easy to detect, by blood examination, the beginning of nitrogenous retention due to renal insufficiency, the mere presence of a distended bladder should not stampede the physician into catheterizing until at least several days have elapsed.

We have seen the autopsy specimen from the case of a young officer whose cord was divided by a machine-gun bullet. Unfortunately, catheterization was instituted at once on account of retention. The patient survived, with complete paraplegia, for nearly four years. Bed sores were combated by keeping him in a warm tub most of the time, where he enjoyed comparative comfort. Urinary infection was treated by irrigations, and instillations of argyrol. Death was due to uremia, and the kidneys were represented at this time by shells about 1 cm. thick, while the pelves, ureters, and bladder were almost filled by a multitude of moderate-sized

[1] Besley: Journal of the American Medical Association, 1917, lxix, 638–639; Young: Manual of Military Urology, Paris, 1918, 188–193; Plaggemeyer: Journal of Urology, 1919, iii, 367–406; 1921, vi, 183–193.

stones.   The mucosa everywhere, and the renal parenchyma, showed the effects of chronic infection.

Case: A broken needle in lumbar spine.   Urinary retention.

The following interesting case (B. U. I. 12,172) may be cited: The patient, aged fifty-two, had had several ulcers on the penis at the age of nineteen (thirty-three years previously). One year before admission, there had been an attack of what was called "dengue fever." Following this some weakness of the left arm was noticed.   Later the left leg was involved, and it was discovered that there was a pyuria.   Malarial plasmodia were found in the blood.   Treatment was by irrigations and quinin until five months before admission, when a Wassermann test proved positive.   Five intraspinous treatments were given, but the condition instead of improving, became worse, the right leg being involved.   Walking was now impossible.   Two months later, 7 more intraspinous treatments were given.   Following the last, there was a very severe reaction, the paralysis became worse, urinary retention occurred, and petechiæ appeared on the arms and legs.   On admission to the hospital, a broken lumbar puncture needle projecting into the spinal canal was discovered by means of the x-ray.   The spinal fluid and blood Wassermann tests were negative, while the colloidal gold test showed a meningitic curve.   Neurologic signs indicated an extensive encephalomyelopathy involving the cerebellar tracts and the posterior and lateral columns of the cord, but not the pyramidal tracts.   The needle was removed under local anesthesia and a small amount of general antisyphilitic treatment given.   A retention catheter was used on account of the bladder paralysis and severe urinary infection.   There was also incontinence of feces.   No improvement was noted, and the patient died five months after admission.   Autopsy showed a combined degeneration of the afferent and efferent tracts of the spinal cord, lymphocytic infiltration of the meninges, and bilateral acute pyelonephritis. It seems probable, from the serologic findings after admission, that the treatment had arrested the syphilitic process, but that the trauma and possibly infection from the broken needle had accounted for the later accentuation of the disease process, including the bladder paralysis.

Case: Injury to cord in spinal anesthesia.

In another case (B. U. I. 6504) the patient, aged fifty-six, had been well until four years before entering our clinic.   At that time he was given a spinal anesthetic (tropocain) for the excision of a fistula in ano.   The insertion of the needle was painful, the patient saying he felt as if he had received a blow in the back.   Retention of urine ensued immediately, and catheterization was instituted.   There were also partial incontinence of feces, and several attacks of pain in the back.   Sexual power was lost, but returned gradually after one year.   Two months before entering the clinic some weakness of the legs, causing difficulty in walking, was noted. On admission, there was 120 c.c. of residual urine, phthalein appearance time fifty minutes, a trace only in two hours.   The cystoscopic picture was typical for bladder paralysis.   The urine contained pus and bacilli.   A retention catheter was used, and water forced, resulting in a rise of the phthalein to 46 per cent. in two hours.   Later the residual rose to from 200 to 600 c.c. and cystoscopy disclosed a contracted vesical orifice, due to the chronic cystitis.   A punch operation was done, which made voiding easier and diminished the residual, but frequency and pyuria continued.   At the time of the last report, four years after the first admission, the residual was still 200 c.c., and the patient was using a catheter twice daily.   In this unfortunate case we were able to do no more than assist the renal function by assuring the emptying of the bladder.

Myelitis or toxic degeneration of the cord is rather common in the later stages of pernicious anemia, and is sometimes seen in diabetes.   The bladder symptoms resemble those of tabes, and often present difficult problems since, the lesion not being complete, sensation is retained, and distention of the bladder gives great discomfort.   Catheterization must, therefore, be resorted to, and we can only take every precaution to avoid or mitigate infection.

In spina bifida or meningocele the bladder is affected only if the defect includes the nerves supplying it.   The seat of the lesion is often low enough to avoid the upper roots of the sacral plexus, but includes enough of the nerves supplying the bladder so that there will be incontinence without paraplegia. A word of warning should be said concerning operations on these deformities. Since the nerve roots are sometimes spread out in the walls of the sac, they are easily injured at the time of operation. The operation is usually done at an early age, before voluntary control of urine and feces are established, so that the damage caused by the operation may not become apparent until some time afterward. Sacrifice of any nervous tissue must be avoided at all costs.

We have seen a case in which a spina bifida had been repaired shortly after birth (B. U. I. 9665) in which the detrusor was paralyzed, but the sphincters retained their tone. After a suprapubic fistula, which had existed for four years, had been closed, there was at first retention, but the patient soon learned to overcome the sphincteric tone by voluntary contraction of the abdominal muscles, and voided satisfactorily every two or three hours. There was complete anesthesia of the perineal region and genitalia, but no paraplegia.

In case retention or incontinence complicate spina bifida, the bladder must be treated according to the principles outlined above, avoiding instrumentation if possible.

Bladder symptoms, often anomalous, may result from spina bifida occulta. Persistent nocturnal enuresis may be due to this cause. This diagnosis will always be missed unless an x-ray of the spine is taken. The symptoms do not necessarily come on in infancy, but may begin at any time in childhood or early adult life. Operation on the spine is seldom to be recommended, as it is easy to do more harm than good. Occasionally a very skilful surgeon may be able to relieve successfully pressure caused by abnormal bony prominences of the deformed vertebræ.

In a certain number of cases, bladder paralysis, due to myelitis or toxic sclerosis, occurs in comparatively mild infectious diseases, such as influenza or septic sore throat. Sometimes this infection is noted only as a slight cold, and these cases may account for some of the anomalous conditions, apparently due to tabes, where syphilitic disease can never be demonstrated.

Case: Bladder paralysis following pharyngitis.

We have seen a case (B. U. I. 10,706) in which complete retention occurred in a young physician ten days after the onset of a "sore throat" or "tonsillitis" of only moderate severity. Retention was preceded for twenty-four hours by great difficulty in urination. On catheterization, which was necessitated by extreme discomfort, 1800 c.c. of urine was withdrawn. The same day marked weakness of the legs was first noted, which went on to almost complete paralysis, while sensory changes were noted as high as the nipples. In three days, the condition started to improve, but there was no voluntary voiding for three weeks. In spite of the greatest care, a colon bacillus infection finally appeared. The legs returned to normal, but three months after onset there was residual urine of 900 c.c. and three attacks of acute pyelitis had occurred. Shortly afterward there was an epididymitis. At the last report, seven months after the onset, there was still a residual of 300 c.c., and infection was still present, although the general health was excellent, and the patient was able to be about his work as usual.

In older patients these cases, when not detected, are undoubtedly responsible for some of the poor results following prostatectomy.

CHAPTER II

THE OBSTRUCTIVE UROPATHY

Definition.—Under this heading are grouped all the changes in the kidney, pelvis, ureter, bladder, and urethra resulting from obstruction to the free outflow of urine through the urinary tract. They include the purely *functional disorders*, and the *anatomic changes*, namely, the various degrees of hydronephrosis, hydroureter, dilated bladder, etc., and combinations of them.

Classification may be made along two lines: first, according to the *location* and *character* of the obstruction; and second, according to the presence or absence of *infection* as a complication.

PATHOLOGY

Kidney and Ureter.—An essential fact is that the results of obstruction upon the kidney are fundamentally exactly the same regardless of the point at which the obstruction occurs. There are variations, however, in the course of the lesion, and in the relative importance of the functional and anatomic changes, according to the distance at which the obstruction is located from the kidney.

The accompanying diagram (Fig. 7) shows graphically the sites of obstruction, and gives the nature of those occurring at all commonly.

Obstructions occurring distal to the bladder are modified in their effect on the kidney by the interposition of the bladder, which is a muscular organ, and which hypertrophies and increases its expulsive efforts as the obstruction below increases. As long as it is able to empty itself fairly normally, the valve-like arrangement at the ureterovesical orifice functions, and the kidney is able to discharge its urine freely into the bladder between voidings. The bladder, therefore, serves to protect the kidneys during this period. Later the bladder fails to empty itself, in spite of violent, frequent, and prolonged contractions, and the pressure within it, therefore, is constantly elevated above normal. When this pressure approaches, during a considerable part of the time, the normal intra-ureteric pressure (during a peristaltic wave) the outflow of urine from the ureter is no longer free. The ureter now increases the force of its contractions, and takes up the task of protecting the kidney. Eventually it, too, is overpowered, and dilates like the bladder. It must be remembered that the conditions at the ureterovesical orifice are the resultant of two sets of forces, namely the expulsive force of the bladder and that of the ureter, and that these two forces do not operate together nor in the same rhythm. When the ureter is unable to expel urine into the bladder, its expulsive force must operate only to stretch open the ureterovesical orifice. It is obvious from a consideration of simple physical principles that the force which first dilates this orifice must come from within the ureter; once dilated, however, the ureter, pelvis, and bladder become one freely communicating system, and muscular contractions anywhere in this system will increase the pressure equally throughout. It is of interest in this connection that one occasionally sees only the lowermost portion of the ureter dilated. This finding is not common probably because it represents only a transitory stage.

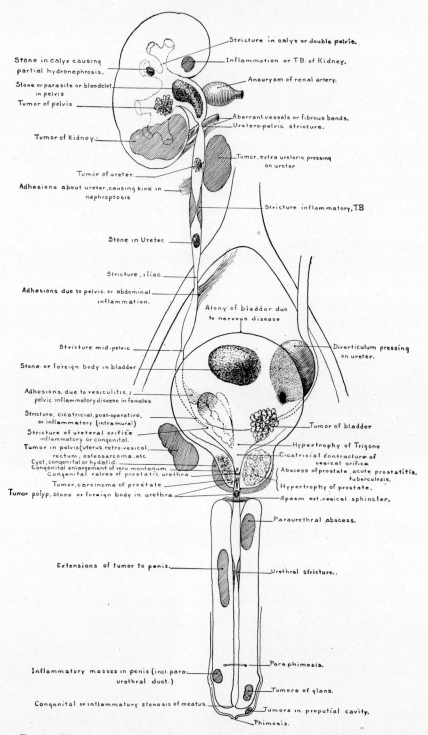

Stricture in calyx or double pelvis.

Inflammation or T.B. of Kidney.

Aneurysm of renal artery.

Stone in calyx causing partial hydronephrosis.

Stone or parasite or bloodclot in pelvis

Tumor of pelvis

Aberrant vessels or fibrous bands.
Uretero-pelvic stricture.

Tumor of Kidney.

Tumor, extra ureteric pressing on ureter

Tumor of ureter.

Adhesions about ureter, causing kink in nephroptosis

Stricture inflammatory, T.B.

Stone in Ureter.

Stricture, iliac.

Adhesions due to pelvic or abdominal inflammation.

Atony of bladder due to nervous disease

Stricture mid-pelvic.

Diverticulum pressing on ureter

Stone or foreign body in bladder

Adhesions, due to vesiculitis, pelvic inflammatory disease in females

Stricture, cicatricial, post-operative, or inflammatory (intramural)

Tumor of bladder

Stricture of ureteral orifice inflammatory or congenital.

Hypertrophy of Trigone

Tumor in pelvis(uterus retro-vesical, rectum, osteosarcoma, etc.

Cicatricial contracture of vesical orifice

Cyst, congenital or hydatid.

Congenital enlargement of veru montanum.

Congenital valves of prostatic urethra.

Abscess of prostate, acute prostatitis, tuberculosis.

Tumor, carcinoma of prostate.

Hypertrophy of prostate.

Tumor polyp, stone or foreign body in urethra.

Spasm ext. vesical sphincter.

Paraurethral abscess.

Extensions of tumor to penis.

Urethral stricture.

Inflammatory masses in penis (incl. para-urethral duct.)

Paraphimosis.

Tumors of glans.

Congenital or inflammatory stenosis of meatus.

Tumors in preputial cavity.

Phimosis.

FIG. 7.—Diagram showing the principal causes of obstruction in the urinary tract.

Recent experiments of Wislocki and O'Conor[1] have shown that ureteral reflux may occur in normal ureters, but it is doubtful if this plays an important part in the formation of hydro-ureter, since it occurs only infrequently.

It is after the bladder becomes decompensated, *i. e.*, unable to empty itself, that outflow of urine from the kidney is no longer free, and, in spite of the efforts of the ureter, the intrapelvic pressure frequently rises above the normal. While it may not be high enough, at any rate constantly, to cause a total suppression of renal function, the urinary secretion is interfered with, and eventually becomes insufficient. Since the period between this beginning of renal functional impairment and the development of hydroureter and hydronephrosis in this class of cases may be quite long, the *functional aspect* of the obstructive nephropathy is usually in the foreground when the obstruction is distal to the bladder.

When the obstruction is between the bladder and the kidney, the *anatomic* changes are in the foreground, for two reasons: first, the pressure effects come on more acutely, in the absence of the protective action of the bladder; and, second, the functional impairment usually causes no symptoms, since the excretory needs of the body are taken care of by a compensatory increase in the activity of the opposite kidney.

Clinically a reflex vesical inhibition of renal function is recognized, commonly in cases of prostatic obstruction with renal insufficiency from back pressure, at the period before back pressure has become active at the kidney level, that is, before there has been any decompensation of the ureters or ureterovesical valves.

We have classified *hydronephrosis* as (1) bilateral, due to infravesical obstruction; (2) bilateral, due to double supravesical obstruction, and (3) unilateral, due to one-sided supravesical obstruction.

It must be remembered, however, that combinations of obstructions may occur, for example, if a prostatic obstruction causes a diverticulum on one side of the bladder, the diverticulum may in its turn press upon the ureter of the same side and cause a unilateral hydronephrosis, due indirectly to the infravesical obstruction, but directly to the supravesical obstruction. It is also true that where bilateral hydronephrosis is due to an infravesical obstruction, one side may be larger than the other. Obstructions may be described as partial or complete, and either kind may be constant or intermittent.

It has been frequently stated that hydronephrosis does not occur if the ureter be suddenly and completely blocked. The experiments of Keith[2] show that this is not true in the dog since such a procedure produces hydronephrosis of moderate size. We must assume that the epithelium of the kidney retains enough activity to maintain in the pelvis the pressure at which secretion ceased—and that this pressure is sufficient, aided by the rhythmic contraction of the pelvic muscles, to dilate the pelvis to a certain extent.

Recent experiments by Hinman and Lee-Brown[3] show that when the intrapelvic pressure is raised, even to a slight degree, part of the pelvic contents passes into the venous circulation of the kidney by means of anastomoses which develop, by a means not yet fully explained, in the terminal sulci of the calices. While the

[1] Johns Hopkins Hospital Bulletin, 1920, xxxi, 197–202.

[2] Keith and Snowden: Archives of Internal Medicine, 1915, xv, 239–264; Keith and Pulford: Archives of Internal Medicine, 1917, xx, 853–878.

[3] Journal of the American Medical Association, 1924, lxxxii, 607–612.

amount of urine escaping into the blood-stream in this way is not sufficient to prevent the development of hydronephrosis, it does constitute a partial safety valve action, and allows the kidney to go on secreting a certain amount of urine even in the presence of obstruction. The flow of urine into the blood-stream is of little importance, since, except for those few substances which undergo metabolism in the kidney, the situation is the same as though the urine had not been secreted, and the substances composing it are removed by the other kidney, if it is functionally efficient.

Experimental work by Hinman has demonstrated that the effect of complete occlusion of the ureter is either (1) primary atrophy or (2) hydronephrotic atrophy. Primary atrophy is possible only with sudden and complete anuria which has not been seen in experimental work in rats or rabbits. It has been very exceptionally observed in dogs and most frequently (about once in 20) in cats. The incidence of an acute pyelonephritis or other infection seems a definite factor in the causation of the anuria and the subsequent primary atrophy, which is a degenerative atrophy without tubular or pelvic dilatation. Complete occlusion that would be analogous to these experimental conditions is rare in man, but in those cases observed, as after accidental ligature at the time of operation, hydronephrotic atrophy is the rule just as in all animal experimentation.[1]

Relative to intrapelvic pressure there are two types of pressure to be considered: (1) Static pressure or the existing pressure in an hydronephrosis, and (2) secretory pressure or the height to which active secretion after relief of obstruction can raise the fluid in a manometer. Experiments on rabbits or dogs show that static pressures fall rapidly in the early stages of progressive hydronephrosis with complete obstruction, so that in a dog the ordinary renal secretory pressure of 70 to 90 mm. mercury of a healthy kidney, after a few weeks complete ureteral block shows an existing pelvic or ureteral pressure, that is, a static pressure, of only 5 to 10 mm. mercury, and within a few months nothing measurable, although a period of about two years is required for complete hydronephrotic atrophy to occur. Curiously enough, as shown by Hinman and Lee-Brown, the degree of intrapelvic pressure necessary to cause back-flow of pelvic contents into the venous circulation falls more or less proportionately to the fall in static pressures with progressive hydronephrosis, but tubular reabsorption undoubtedly also occurs as a factor in permitting continued renal activity with complete ureteral occlusion. In proof of this experiments were done by Hinman in collaboration with T. E. Gibson, in which the collecting tubules alone (Bellini) in the single papillæ of rabbits were obstructed without obstructing the ureter, thus removing completely any pyelovenous back-flow as a factor. Still there resulted pronounced tubular dilatation without, of course, any pelvic dilatation. The secretory pressure, on the other hand, of a hydronephrosis is related to the reparability of that kidney and the problem of renal counterbalance, being practically the same as the static pressure when measured immediately upon relief of obstruction, but rising or falling, in the periods following, according to the respective degree of restitution or of secondary atrophy then present. A practical method of measuring secretory pressure would be a good test of renal function, but with the inherent defect of all functional tests of not indicating potentiality or past ability.

These same authors go on to show how the dilatation of the pelvis in hydro-

[1] Herman: Journal of Urology, 1923, ix, 151–179.

nephrosis is accompanied by a dilatation of the secreting tubules, the result of which is compression and partial occlusion of the peritubular venous network. Since all of the blood must pass through the peritubular networks after leaving the glomeruli, the renal circulation is thus impeded, and the resulting ischemia hastens and furthers the atrophy of the renal parenchyma.

The study of the vascular changes with progressive hydronephrosis in man by injection methods[1] has demonstrated the importance of disturbances of blood-supply by urinary back pressure in relation to the tissue changes of ordinary hydronephrotic atrophy, and the great significance of these circulatory changes both in the development of large sacs (dilatation) and in the thinning out by group atrophy of the tubular system (degeneration) has also been shown by a series of animal experiments.[2] They consisted of, first, partial obstruction of the renal artery and, second, of the renal vein with complete ureteral obstruction both (a) with, and (b) without, complete destruction of the perirenal or capsular blood-supply. The intrapelvic pressure is commonly regarded as the primary and principal factor in pelvic dilatation and renal atrophy (hydronephrotic atrophy), therefore increasing this should hasten its rate of development. Lindemann[3] early contended that the type and change of the collateral circulation present determined whether the result in ureteral obstruction would be primary (without pelvic or tubular dilatation) or hydronephrotic atrophy. Primary atrophy followed ureteral obstruction when the capsular circulation was poorly developed and failed to form a collateral system. In rabbits this has been found to be quite inconstant and, although the rabbit has quite a well-marked capsular circulation, complete ligature of all perirenal or capsular vessels fails to prevent, with but few exceptions, the development of hydronephrosis as is ordinarily seen with simple complete ligature. When a band is so placed on a renal vein as only partially to occlude it, the intrarenal pressure obviously is raised and should hasten the development of a hydronephrotic atrophy. Hinman has found experimentally that it does have a definite hastening effect, but for the first three or four weeks only, after which a progressive rate comparable to the normal is established, the explanation being that it takes three to four weeks for a good collateral venous outflow to form and compensate for the venous occlusion. If the capsular vessels are all ligated at the time of ureteral ligature, there is a more uniform increase in the progressive atrophy.

Partial obstruction of the renal artery lowers intrarenal pressure, and should, therefore, according to the older ideas, slow the rate of development of hydronephrosis, but, provided the degree of occlusion is not too great, it is found that a very marked increase in the rate of development follows, so that within two or three weeks a kidney with ureteral ligature and partial obstruction of its artery will show a hydronephrotic atrophy comparable to one of one to three months' duration with simple ureteral ligature. More striking even is the result that follows complete ligature of an anterior or posterior branch of the renal artery with

[1] Hinman and Morison: Comparative Study of Circulatory Changes in Hydronephrosis, Caseocavernous Tuberculosis, and Polycystic Kidney, Journal of Urology, 1924, xi, 131–141. Ibid.: Experimental Study of Circulatory Changes in Hydronephrosis; Preliminary Report Relating to Unilobed Kidney as Instanced in the Rabbit, Journal of Urology, 1924, xi, 435–452.

[2] Hinman and Hepler: In press (Surgery, Gynecology, and Obstetrics).

[3] Sur le Mode d'Action de Certains Poisons Rénaux, Annales de l'Institut Pasteur, 1900, xiv, 49.

complete ureteral obstruction—a huge renal diverticulum quickly develops, replacing the half of the kidney which the ligated branch supplied.

These experiments establish the fundamental relationship of urinary back pressure, the primary factor, to the blood-supply, the secondary and by far more important factor producing the dilatation and atrophy. Renal atrophy from direct pressure, that is, pressure degeneration, is probably of very minor importance. Those areas first deprived of blood by pressure, which are the peritubular venous capillaries, degenerate first and the less injured areas which have a more direct blood-supply maintain secretion and thus the atrophy progresses. Those tubules supplied by main trunks survive longest, as their blood-supply is least affected, and these seem to be the straight terminal branches as a rule, so that in unilobed kidneys a very definite median sagittal strip of parenchyma persists after there has been complete fibrosis and atrophy of the parenchymal tissues in the lateral and polar areas, and in the final stages, when all tubular groups on the two terminal trunks even have disappeared, many glomeruli, some remarkably well preserved, persist to the last stages.

The largest hydronephroses occur in cases where the obstruction is partial, as in incomplete strictures, slowly growing tumors pressing upon the ureter, movable stones, etc. The kidney may attain an enormous size. In the Musée Dupuytren at Paris is a specimen of hydronephrotic kidney said to have contained 25 liters. In such cases the pressure within the sac varies from time to time, as may be proved by noting the increase in the size of the tumor, in its tenseness, and in the discomfort of the patient following the ingestion of large quantities of water. In addition, it is sometimes possible to catheterize such a kidney, and a small proportion of phenolsuphonephthalein may be excreted from it. When the ureter is completely blocked, as by a stone, early atrophy and fibrosis may occur, producing the condition spoken of as "autonephrectomy." This is graphically shown in one of our autopsy specimens (Fig. 192). This may even occur without noteworthy symptoms. Clinically, the completely blocked kidney is called "closed" hydronephrosis, while that where the obstruction is partial or transitory is "open."

The relative frequency of occurrence of the different classes of hydronephrosis is shown in Table 1 together with the causative factors, in a series of 165 cases studied at the Brady Institute. It must be understood that the figures for Class I are very incomplete, since moderate hydronephrosis occurs in very many cases of infravesical obstruction where the condition cannot be verified, owing to the complete recovery of the patient, as for example, after prostatectomy.

The exact relations between the degree of hydronephrosis and the degree of functional impairment vary somewhat in different cases. In obstructions in the lower urinary tract well-marked functional impairment is sometimes seen when no hydronephrosis is demonstrable. On the other hand, a kidney with a considerably dilated pelvis may show a normal function. These differences are more apparent than real, and depend almost entirely upon conditions at the time of examination. Functional impairment, with a gradually increasing obstruction, practically always appears before dilatation is evident, but, even after the pelvis has been increased to as much as two or three times its normal size, or even more, the function may return to normal within a very short time after the obstruction is relieved. The repeated comparative relief of intrarenal pressure occurring in an "open"

TABLE 1
Cause of Hydronephrosis—Series of 165 Cases

Class I. Bilateral infravesical obstruction.		Class II. Bilateral double supravesical obstruction.			Class III. Unilateral single supravesical obstruction.	
			Kidneys.	Cases.		
Prostatic hypertrophy.......	12	Renal calculus, one side.......	5		Ureteral calculus............	15
		Ureteral calculus, opposite side	5	5		
Carcinoma of bladder........	10	Stricture of ureter, with pyelitis, both sides..............	8	4	Stricture of ureter, undifferentiated...................	14
Congenital valve of urethra..	5	Stricture of ureter, both sides..	8	4	Renal calculus, undifferentiated....................	11
Urethral stricture..........	4	Stricture of ureter, tuberculous, both sides.............	6	3	Stricture of ureteropelvic junction.......................	10
Unknown.................	3	Renal calculus, both sides.....	4	2	Renal calculus, single........	9
Contracture of vesical orifice.	3	Stricture at ureteropelvic junction, both sides	2	1	Unknown..................	9
Carcinoma of prostate......	2	Stricture at ureterovesical orifice, both sides	2	1	Stricture (?) of ureter with pyelitis...................	5
Prostatic abscess...........	1	Ureteral calculus, one side.....	1		Stricture of ureter, tuberculous......................	4
		Ureteral stricture, opposite side	1	1		
Vesical calculi..............	1	Nephroptosis with aberrant vessels, both sides...........	2	1	Stricture of ureter, aberrant vessels...................	4
Urethral calculus...........	1	Total......................	44	22	Renal calculi, multiple.......	4
Retrovesical sarcoma.......	1				Stricture of ureter, carcinoma, metastasis...............	3
Total....................	43				Carcinoma, prostate ....2 Carcinoma, bladder.....1	
					Ectopic kidney.............	3
					Stricture of ureter, carcinoma, extension intramural........	2
					Carcinoma, prostate ....1 Carcinoma, bladder 1	
					Stricture in pelvis, inflammatory, partial hydronephrosis.	1
					Stricture of ureter, pressure of abdominal tumor...........	1
					Stricture of ureter, postoperative....................	1
					Nephroptosis with aberrant vessels....................	1
					Stricture at ureterovesical meatus...................	1
					Total......................	98
					Prostatic hypertrophy in patients having only a single kidney....................	2

Summary of Table 1

II. Bilateral, double supravesical obstruction:

Kidneys considered individually:		Cases.	Per cent.
Renal calculus........... 9 ⎫ Calculi.................		15	34
Ureteral calculus......... 6 ⎭			
Ureteral strictures, all types.........................		27	58
Nephroptosis with aberrant vessels....................		2	7
Total..		44	

III. Unilateral, single supravesical obstruction:

		Cases.	Per cent.
Renal calculus........... 24 ⎫ Calculi.................		39	39
Ureteral calculus........ 15 ⎭			
Ureteral strictures, all.............................		45	45
Stricture of pelvis.................................		1	1
Unknown..		9	9
Ectopic kidney....................................		3	3
Nephroptosis with aberrant vessels....................		1	1
Total..		98	

hydronephrosis, characterized by recurrent attacks of pain and swelling, with inter-missions, tends to preserve renal function beyond what it would be if the obstruction were more constant. One should, therefore, always take into consideration any condition which may have relieved the obstruction prior to the examination.

The *microscopic pathology of the kidney* in the obstructive nephropathy when the *functional changes* are in the foreground has not been sufficiently studied, but enough is known to enable us to say that visible changes are not great. When infection is absent, the kidney remains in abeyance, as it were, and is ready to take up its function when the obstruction is removed. In most of the specimens available for

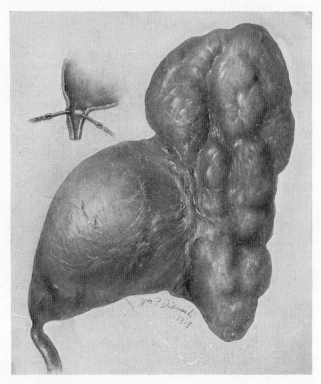

Fig. 8.—Autopsy specimen of hydronephrosis due to congenital stricture at the ureteropelvic juncture. The pelvis is extrarenal in type. No evidence of inflammatory thickening, bands of adhesions, or aberrant blood-vessels at the site of the stricture.

study, pyelonephritis or chronic diffuse nephritis is present in varying degree, masking changes due purely to obstruction. In parts of the organ not involved in these changes, the structures, with the possible exception of slight tubular dilatation, appear to be approximately normal. The compression of the peri-tubular capillary plexuses can be demonstrated in injected and cleared specimens.

As the process goes on, *dilatation* of the pelvis commences. If it is extrarenal, the pelvis proper enlarges more rapidly than the calices, which are surrounded by the more resistant kidney tissue. In the later stages the kidney is represented by a nodule on one side of a large sac (Figs. 8, 9). If, on the contrary, the pelvis is intrarenal, the enlargement takes place radially, and the kidney tissue is spread out over the surface of the sac (Fig. 10). The calices are, of course, in direct communication with the pelvis at all times, and subject to the same pressures, so that their enlargement is not long delayed. It is marked at first by an obliteration of the cupping due to the protrusion into the calix of the tip of the pyramid (see pyelograms in section on Diagnosis). Later the calices become quite globular. The foramina connecting the calices with the pelvis may be greatly dilated (Fig. 9), or remain small (Fig. 10). The latter is especially apt to be true in the extrarenal type of pelvis. Beneath the mucosa of the pelvis ecchymoses may occur, probably related to changes in the pressure, and this is one of the sources of the hematuria of

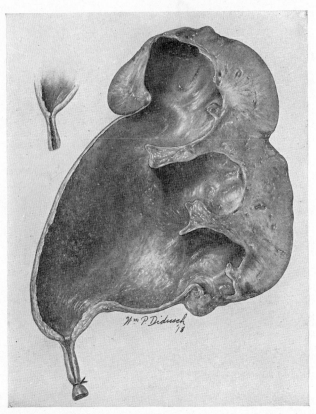

Fig. 9.—Longitudinal section of hydronephrotic kidney removed at operation. Destruction was caused by inflammatory stricture of the ureteropelvic juncture. The pelvis is extrarenal. The foramina of the calices are widely dilated. B. U. I. 5558.

hydronephrosis. Other changes in the pelvis are usually due to inflammation, which will be discussed later.

Within the kidney proper, the first change to appear is a dilatation of the collecting tubules. According to Kelly, this is most marked in the central part of the papilla, while toward the periphery, in the region of the vascular columns, the tubules are compressed and occluded. This change occurs coincidentally with the beginning of pelvic enlargement. Hinman and Lee-Brown[1] have shown that substances introduced into a hydronephrotic pelvis ascend but a short distance in the

[1] Journal of the American Medical Association, 1924, lxxxii, 607–612.

tubules. The dilatation later includes all portions of the kidney tubules. **If** venous injections are made at this stage, it will be seen that the peritubular capillary plexuses are compressed and occluded. As the process advances, this vascular occlusion becomes more and more pronounced, so that eventually the circulation of the kidney is reduced to only a few small vessels. This is thought to play a large part in the parenchymal atrophy of hydronephrosis. The glomeruli do not

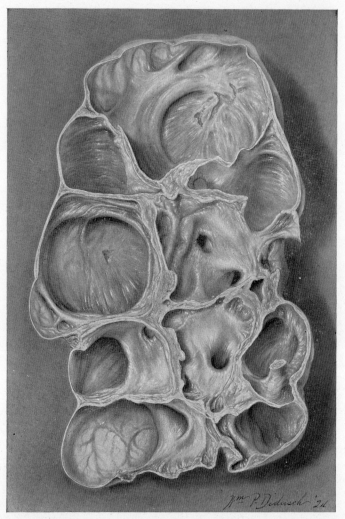

Fig. 10.—Nephrectomy specimen. Very large hydronephrosis, the result of obstruction by a small calculus. This is the intrarenal type. B. U. I. Path. 1041.

dilate, but, on the contrary, they show capsular, and later general fibrosis, with eventual hyalinization. The tubular epithelium undergoes degeneration and eventually a fibrotic change replaces a great part of the entire kidney structure. This is in the late stages of the condition when there is marked thinning of the renal tissue (Fig. 12). Cortex and medulla together may be stretched out into a layer only 10, 5, or even 1 mm. thick. These changes explain why, after a certain degree of hydronephrosis has been reached, restitution of kidney function is impossible. A small hydronephrosis can return completely to normal, as in one of our cases (Figs. 13 and 14).

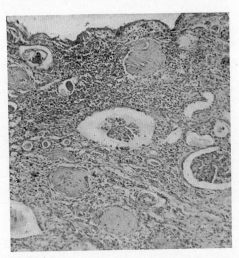

FIG. 11.—Section from the wall of a large hydronephrotic sac. The total thickness of this wall was only about twice what is shown in the picture. The picture represents the outer or cortical portion. Note the fibrosis, round-cell infiltration, many hyaline glomeruli, and very great destruction of tubules. B. U. I. Path. 4886.

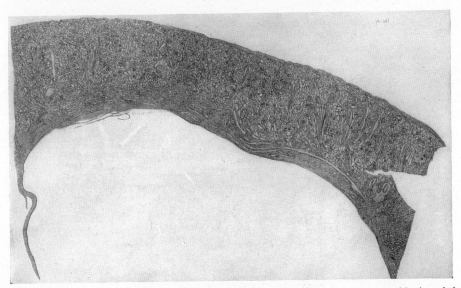

FIG. 12.—Section from the wall of a large hydronephrotic sac. Note the extreme thinning of the kidney substance, more at the expense of the medulla than of the cortex. The tubules are dilated, but the glomeruli are, for the most part, in good condition. By courtesy of Dr. M. C. Winternitz.

Hinman[1] has shown that a kidney damaged by hydronephrosis may atrophy after the obstruction is relieved, the other kidney taking over the entire function,

[1] Journal of Urology, 1923, ix, 289–314.

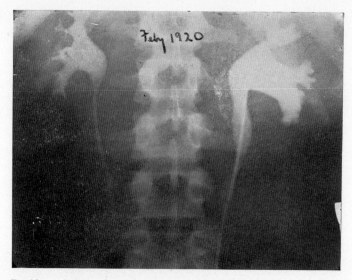

Fig. 13.—Double pyelogram, showing left hydronephrosis and dilatation of the upper ureter due to a stone impacted opposite the third lumbar vertebra. The stone, being soft, was broken up and dislodged by the ureteral catheter and passed spontaneously. B. U. I. x-Ray 2236.

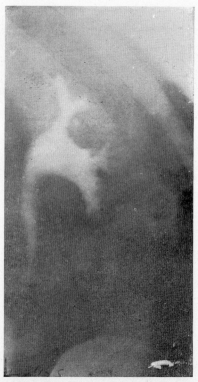

Fig. 14.—Same case as preceding picture. Pyelogram, showing complete return of hydronephrotic pelvis to normal six months after passage of stone. B. U. I. x-Ray 2396.

and the damaged kidney being unable to compete with it. On the other hand, secretion is going on continually—otherwise the hydronephrosis would cease to grow. Small areas of comparatively normal tissue can be found here and there in almost any hydronephrotic sac. Patients with congenital obstruction of the posterior urethra, giving rise to large bilateral hydronephrosis, may live in comparatively good health for many years, and studies of the blood and urine show that renal function is at least a fair percentage of normal. Hydronephrotic kidneys return more promptly and completely to normal if the other kidney is removed or insufficient. It is, therefore, frequently a question of nice surgical and pathologic judgment whether a dilated kidney should be removed or not, in cases where the obstruction can be relieved. Even if the function does not return to normal

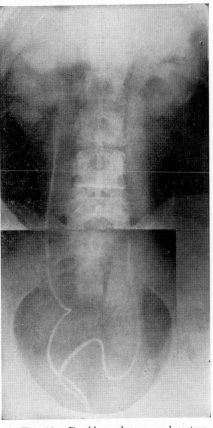

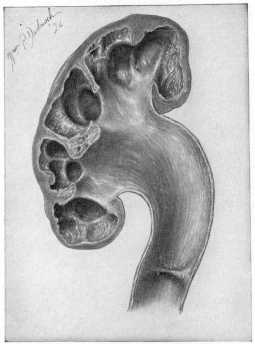

FIG. 15.—Operative specimen. Nephro-ureterectomy. Ureter and pelvis greatly dilated, kidney sacculated and thin. B. U. I.

FIG. 16.—Double pyelogram and ureterogram showing very great bilateral hydronephrosis and hydro-ureter due to ureteral strictures (?) in the intramural portion. The strictures were divided at suprapubic operation, but the convalescence was complicated by thrombophlebitis and the patient finally died, probably of pyelonephritis. B. U. I. 5168.

(Donati) it may improve enough so that the kidney may be a very useful, or in certain events, an invaluable organ. The presence of a marked infection of the kidney would make the indication for nephrectomy more positive.

In cases where the obstruction occurs at the ureteropelvic junction or in the *upper part of the ureter*, the enlargement of the kidney itself has a profound effect on the obstruction. The organ is bounded by firm structures dorsally and above, and, therefore, it must enlarge laterally and downward. The pedicle, however, is

TABLE 2

FREQUENCE OF INFECTION AND OF PYONEPHROSIS—SERIES OF 150 CASES OF HYDRONEPHROSIS

Character of hydronephrosis: Location of obstruction.	Total number of cases.	Both infected. / Infected, with opposite side infected.	One side infected, opposite side sterile. / Infected, with opposite side sterile.	Sterile, with opposite side infected.	Both sterile. / Sterile, with opposite side sterile.	Infected, with opposite kidney absent.	Sterile, with opposite kidney absent.
I. Bilateral infravesical obstruction.	35	32 cases, 91% of class, 22% of total.	0		3 cases, 8.5% of class, 2% of total.		
Pyonephrosis, one side.	2	2 cases, 6% of class, 1.3% of total.	0				
Pyonephrosis, both sides.	14	14 cases, 40% of class, 9% of total.	0				
II. Bilateral; double supravesical obstruction.	21	15 cases, 71% of class, 10% of total.	1 case, 5% of class, 0.6% of total.		5 cases, 24% of class, 3.3% of total.		
Pyonephrosis, one side.	4	4 cases, 19% of class, 2.6% of total.	0				
Pyonephrosis, both sides.	1	1 case, 5% of class, 0.6% of total.	0				
III. Unilateral supravesical obstruction.	94	25 cases, 26.5% of class, 17% of total.	30 cases, 32% of class, 20% of total.	0	37 cases, 39% of class, 25% of total	2 cases, 2% of class, 1.3% of total.	0
Pyonephrosis.	22	10 cases, 10.5% of class, 6.6% of total.	12 cases, 13% of class, 8% of total.	0	0	0	

Summary of Table 2

	Cases.	Per cent.
Total cases, Class I, bilateral, infravesical obstruction...........	35	
Infected...	32	91.5
Pyonephrosis in...	16	46
Of infected cases, pyonephrosis in 50 per cent.		
Total cases, Class II, bilateral, double supravesical obstruction ..	21	
Of the 42 kidneys, there were infected.....................	31	73.8
Of the 21 cases, there was infection in.....................	16	76
Pyonephrosis in...	5	24
Of infected cases, pyonephrosis in 34 per cent.		
Total cases, Class III, unilateral, single supravesical obstruction .	94	
Infection in...	57	60.5
Pyonephrosis in...	22	23.5
Of infected cases, pyonephrosis in 40 per cent.		

Grand total, 150 cases, of which 105, or 70 per cent., were infected.

Bilateral cases 56 = 112 kidneys ⎰Grand total, 206 kidneys, of which 130,
Unilateral cases 94 = 94 kidneys ⎱ or 63 per cent., were infected.

Of cases due to supravesical obstruction, average infection = 65 per cent.

Pyonephrosis in 24 per cent. of total cases, or 37 per cent. of infected cases.

fixed, and the convex surface of the kidney for this reason must rotate downward and a little forward. This causes the kidney to press upon the ureter. In addition, the ureteropelvic junction, being near the pedicle, is comparatively fixed, so that as the enlargement and rotation of the kidney continue, the ureter is drawn out and compressed along its medial border. This relation must be borne in mind at operation, and it frequently makes the plastic procedure for the repair of the obstruction more extensive than it would otherwise be.

Table 2 shows the frequence of infection, and of pyonephrosis, in our cases of hydronephrosis. Complete discussion is deferred to the section on Infections of the Urinary Tract.

Great *bilateral dilatation of the kidneys and ureters,* or ureters alone (megalo-ureter) without discoverable obstruction or other cause has been the subject of interesting discussion.[1] We have had a case in a woman (B. U. I. 5168) in which the ureters were at least 3 cm. in diameter and the kidney pelves also dilated, in which at cystoscopy and suprapubic cystotomy no obstruction could be found in the urethra, at the vesical orifice, or in the bladder or ureters. Nevertheless it is probable that some obstruction—perhaps only spasmodic—was present in the intramural portion of the ureter. The pyelogram of this case is shown in Fig. 16.

Bladder.—The function of the bladder in the early stages of infravesical obstruction has already been considered. The change in the bladder wall itself begins with a *muscular hypertrophy* following the increased effort necessary to empty the bladder. Cystoscopic study shows that *hypertrophy of the trigone* is one of the first changes to occur (Plate II, Fig. 18). As we[2] have shown in studies upon the anatomy and physiology of the trigone, the principal function of the trigone is not, as described by Bell and others since, to close the ureteral orifices, but to open the prostatic urethra and allow the bladder muscle to expel its contents. This feature is discussed at greater length in the section on the Physiology and Pathology of

[1] Caulk: Journal of Urology, 1923, ix, 315–330.

[2] Young: Surgery, Gynecology, and Obstetrics, 1918, xxvi, 608–615; Young and Macht: Journal of Pharmacology, 1923, xxii, 329–354.

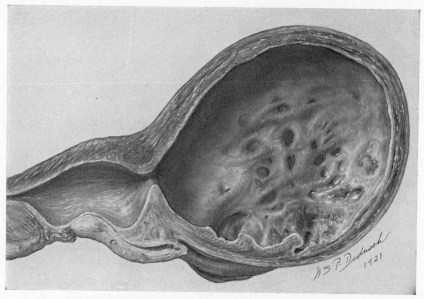

FIG. 17.—Autopsy specimen showing trabeculation of the bladder and hypertrophy of the trigone. In this case there were two obstructions—a contracture of the vesical orifice and a stricture of the urethra, the latter accounting for the dilatation of the prostatic urethra. The trabeculation is so extreme that some of the depressions really constitute cellules.

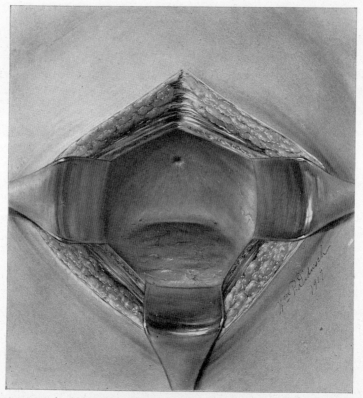

FIG. 18.—Contracture of vesical orifice, obstruction to urination, hypertrophied trigone with pouch behind, and trabeculation of bladder wall.

PLATE II

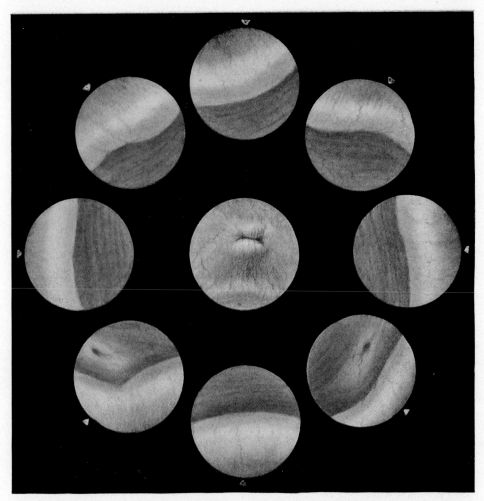

A. Cystoscopic views of prostatic orifice showing a small rounded anterior bar and a small rounded posterior median bar. The prostatic margin is shown external and bladder internal in the series of pictures. The central portion of trigone is obscured around median bar, but ureteral orifices are visible. In the center is shown the orifice as it appears when the bladder is opened suprapubically (B. U. I. 13,168).

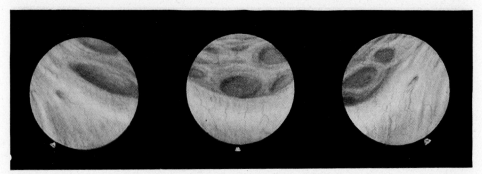

B. Hypertrophied trigone with pouch behind it, trabeculated bladder with cellules. Ureteral orifices negative.

Micturition. The enlargement of the trigone comes as a result of the unusual work which falls upon it as a result of the development of prostatic adenoma in the median portion of the prostate and often gives the first definite cystoscopic evidence of obstruction.

When seen at autopsy or operation at this stage the bladder wall is found to be in the contracted condition, markedly thicker than normal, sometimes reaching 2 cm. (See Fig. 19.) Microscopic examination shows the muscle bundles thickened and a slight increase only in the fibrous tissue. When viewed cysto-scopically, under varying conditions of pressure, one notes that this individual enlargement of the muscle bundles brings them into prominent relief, separated by polyhedral depressions when the bladder becomes filled. This condition is known as *trabeculation* of the bladder (Fig. 17), and the size of the muscle bundles themselves is important in connection with obstruction, since the depressions between them are seen in certain neurogenic conditions where the bundles are not hypertrophied.

With the onset of hypertrophy, the *irritability* of the bladder is usually increased, even when infection is absent, so that it tends to empty itself more frequently, and for a time the capacity is less than normal.

As the obstruction increases, a point is finally reached at which the bladder is unable to empty itself completely. This follows from the fact that the muscle fibers contract most efficiently when moderately extended, and as the bladder becomes smaller, its expulsive force diminishes. Consequently, a certain amount of urine remains constantly in the bladder, and this is known as *residual urine*. Infection is now more apt to occur, and if it does so, it is rebellious to treatment, as the residual urine provides a constantly present culture-medium for the organisms. The bladder is still able, however, to expel the urine, as it is formed, usually in frequent voidings. Rarely, residual urine may be present without frequency. This equilibrium may continue for a long time, but as practically all obstructions tend to increase, the residual urine usually increases in quantity. This increase may be slow, or acute retention may suddenly occur as the result of infection with edema, overexertion, fatigue, overindulgence in food or drink, etc. In either case the mechanical results are fundamentally the same. The bladder is unable to expel the urine as fast as it forms, and consequently becomes *distended*. The muscle-fibers in its walls are now overstretched to a point where they are no longer able to contract efficiently, and can, therefore, expel no urine, or only very small quantities. The situation is exactly comparable to that in a dilated heart, and we may quite properly speak of such a bladder as being *decompensated*. The effects on the ureters and kidneys have already been discussed, but it should be stated that dilatation of the ureteral orifice may occur before the bladder is decompensated, since the pressures developed in obstructed, hypertrophied bladders may be very great, often reaching 8 feet or more of water, or 250 mm. or more of mercury. Figure 19 shows a sectional view taken from an autopsied case. As seen here the trigone is greatly hypertrophied and the bladder trabeculated.

Cellules and Diverticula.—As the bladder dilates, the muscle bundles or trabeculæ are stretched apart, increasing the size of the polyhedral spaces between them. These spaces are covered only by the mucosa and a bit of fibrous and elastic tissue connecting the widely separated muscle bundles. Occasionally a few isolated muscle-fibers are seen in sections. If the pressure increases further, the mucosa herniates through the opening, and the sac so formed, no longer restricted by a muscular coat, is free to dilate to any size. When such a sac is small, it is a *cellule*, and when larger, a *diverticulum*.[1]

The mechanism of the formation of diverticula was beautifully illustrated in a case observed by us. In this patient the ordinary sensitiveness of the bladder was diminished, so that it was possible to introduce large quantities of fluid. The muscle bundles, while not hypertrophied, could be outlined under these conditions. After about 850 c.c. of water had been run in, the cystoscopist suddenly saw a cellule develop before his eyes in the base of the bladder behind the trigone (Plate IX). The fluid was now allowed to run out, and after about 150 c.c. had done so, the mucosa popped back into place again, the cellule being obliterated as suddenly

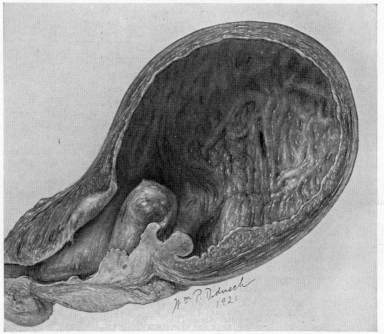

Fig. 19.—Autopsy specimen from sixty-five-year-old patient. Median sagittal section. Obstruction due to enlarged prostate, median lobe large, lateral lobes also hypertrophied. Trigone greatly hypertrophied. Bladder trabeculated. Prostatic urethra shows great slit-like widening.

as it had formed. This phenomenon could be repeated at will. It is a clear indication that even defects in the muscular coat are not enough to cause diverticulum formation in the absence of obstruction and great rise in intravesical pressure.

Since there is no muscle, or very little, in the walls of a diverticulum, it has no expulsive force, and after reaching a size where the elasticity of the mucosa will not obliterate it, or if it has become adherent to surrounding tissues, it will not empty even if the obstruction is relieved. It is, therefore, an ideal place for the development of infection, or of a calculus, and both of these are of common occurrence. The orifice may be small or large. If small, the diverticulum may be practically

[1] Young: Vesical Diverticula, Johns Hopkins Hospital Reports, 1906, xiii, 401–446; Gayet and Gauthier: Les Diverticules de la Vessie; Rapport à l'Association Française d'Urologie, Paris, 1922 (Lit.).

In a series of 41 cases studied by us, the number of diverticula present was: one diverticulum, 21 cases; two diverticula, 10 cases; three diverticula, 4 cases; four diverticula, 2 cases; six diverticula, 1 case; seven diverticula, 1 case; "several" diverticula, 2 cases.

Diverticula are especially due to slowly developing obstructions; of these the most conspicuous is contracture of the vesical orifice, though prostatic hypertrophy runs a close second. Some interesting points are shown by the age table of our 41 cases as shown in the following table:

TABLE 3

Age, years.	Total cases.	Cases due to contracture.	Cases due to prostatic hypertrophy.	Congenital (urachus).	?
1–10........	1	0	0	0	1
11–20........	0	0	0	0	0
21–30........	2	1	0	0	1
31–40........	3	2	0	1	0
41–50........	11	6	3	0	1
51–60........	12	7	6	0	0
61–70........	10	2	8	0	0
71–80........	2	1	1	0	0
Total.......	41	19	18	1	3

The total cases are most numerous at fifty to fifty-five years (corresponding to Hinman's figures[1]), the cases due to hypertrophy, however, are most numerous at sixty to sixty-five, while if these are excluded, the cases due to contracture of the vesical orifice fall mostly at forty-five to fifty-five. They are exceedingly rare in women.

The question of *congenital diverticula* is not altogether settled.[2] It is probable, however, that the majority, so-called, are due to congenital obstructions of the urethra in infants and children, as they usually show other signs of obstruction. The sites of predilection are where the ureters and the urachus enter the bladder. It may well be, however, that congenital defects in the bladder musculature predispose to the development of diverticula. Solitary diverticula are not infrequently seen in the region of the urachus following obstruction. *Congenitally patent urachus* is rare, but we had one such case in an infant which became infected and led to an extensive prevesical abscess. For further discussion, see the section on Embryology and Congenital Malformations of the Urogenital Tract.

If the obstruction is relieved the dilated, and even the decompensated, bladder will return to normal, provided no diverticula are present. The muscular hypertrophy eventually disappears and cellules often flatten out completely. In general, the restitution will be slower the more long standing and pronounced the dilatation. Large diverticula, on the other hand, show no tendency to disappear, and

[1] Journal of Urology, 1919, iii, 207–245.
[2] Ibid.

are serious obstacles to health in that they harbor infection and encourage stone formation, even when obstruction no longer exists.

In general, a bladder may be said to be fairly compensated as long as the residual urine remains below 250 c.c., though this is no indication to defer treatment, as we have seen. Above 400 c.c. the progress usually becomes more rapid. As in the heart, an indefinite "quality" in the muscle seems to have much to do with the course, as some bladders resist dilation much more strongly than others. When extreme dilatation supervenes, the bladder may hold 2000, 3000, or even 4500 c.c. In such cases small amounts of urine may be voided at intervals, mostly by straining with the abdominal muscles. In one of our cases, however, with 2100 c.c. residual urine, the bladder compensation was perfect and the patient voided at normal intervals. His only complaint was that his abdomen was getting constantly larger, requiring more frequent purchase of new trousers.

In women, who seldom have diverticula, residual urine is very frequent during and after pregnancy. We may assume from this that a hypotonic condition of the bladder plays a more important rôle in this condition than obstruction. Stevens and Arthurs[1] state that residual urine is present in 80 per cent. of postpartum cases. Cystoceles, due to injuries to the pelvic floor during labor, are frequently unaccompanied by residual urine. According to the principle of hydrostatics, this should be so, provided the muscular apparatus of the bladder is uninjured, entirely independent of the dependent position of any part of it.

Urethra.—The effects of obstruction are principally a simple dilatation. Even the prostatic urethra may be markedly dilated. The sulci at either side of the verumontanum are deepened and broadened, and the posterior portion of the sphincter vesicæ may project over their upper portions like a shelf (Fig. 17). The sphincter itself, when its nervous mechanism is not affected, continues to close even when the urethra is greatly dilated.

If the wall of the urethra is weakened by inflammation or neoplastic growth above a stricture or other obstruction, spontaneous rupture may occur, with consequent extravasation of urine.

Diverticula of the urethra are usually not caused by intra-urethral pressure, but arise from abscesses opening into the urethra, or are in the nature of congenital cysts.[2] In a recent case a diverticulum, the size of a small pear, formed in the sinus after perineal prostatectomy.

The diameter of the urethra above a tight stricture may attain 3 cm.

While obstructions in the urinary tract are very frequently complicated by infectious processes, discussion of this phase is deferred to the section on Infections of the Urinary Tract.

In this section we have grouped all of the lesions due purely to the mechanical effects of obstruction, since we feel that it is important to keep the effects of obstruction clearly separated in the mind from those of infection, especially as they are so often associated in the same patient.

SYMPTOMS

Kidney.—*The symptomatology of the obstructive nephropathy* will depend, in the first place, on whether the obstruction lies *above the vesical orifice of the*

---

[1] Journal of the American Medical Association, 1924, lxxxiii, 1656–1662.

[2] Watts: Johns Hopkins Hospital Reports, 1906, xiii, 49–90.

ureter (supravesical), in which case only one kidney will usually be affected, or *at the prostatic orifice or below* it (infravesical), in which case both kidneys will usually be affected equally. There are also a third group of cases, those in which two separate obstructions in the upper urinary tract affect both kidneys simultaneously and a fourth, in which the general symptoms from a unilateral obstruction are the same as from a bilateral, owing to the absence, atrophy, or previous functional destruction of the opposite kidney.

The essential fact, common to all cases, is that the damage done to the kidney is always of the same kind. Where the lesion is unilateral, and the opposite kidney sound, hypertrophy of the healthy organ occurs, which may reach as high as 140 per cent. of the original volume and weight. There is hyperplasia of the epithelium of the convoluted tubules. New tubules and glomeruli probably do not develop, though this is still a disputed question, but regardless of that, the function increases to such a degree that an individual having but one kidney seems to be in every way normal and possessed of the same factors of safety and expectation of life as a normal individual. Exception must be made for the possible second occurrence of local destructive kidney disease, but it does not appear clearly that the one-kidneyed person is more susceptible to Bright's disease than if he had two kidneys. The various tests of the functional capacity of the kidney give normal figures.

It may be said, therefore, that symptoms due to the functional renal disturbance when the obstructive nephropathy is *unilateral* ordinarily do not exist. It is the symptoms dependent upon *anatomic changes* which generally bring the patient to the doctor, and it is on these symptoms alone that the urologist must rely for aid in making his diagnosis. The determination of the existence of a hydronephrosis or of a pyonephrosis is not sufficient; it is the duty of the urologist to discover the cause and extent of the changes in the kidney, and also to determine the condition of the other kidney.

When the obstruction is *bilateral*, a considerable degree of hydronephrosis may come to exist in both kidneys, but, as a rule, the *renal functional disturbances* cause the patient to be ill before these anatomic changes become marked.

We hasten to say at the outset that the complex of general systemic symptoms accompanying the *obstructive nephropathy* cannot be distinguished by any laboratory or clinical procedure from that resulting from *chronic nephritis*, or Bright's disease. It is only by local examination that the true cause of the condition can be found. The reason for the above-mentioned fact, which is of prime importance, not only to the urologist but to every internist and general practitioner, is that in both cases the symptoms are due to an impairment of the normal excretory powers of the kidney, and are, therefore, those classed under the head of *uremia*. Bright's disease may exist at the same time as urinary obstruction. The second point of prime importance, which we desire to make at this time, is that the only possible method by which the obstructive nephropathy can be distinguished from Bright's disease is to observe the course of the patient after a *continually free exit has been provided for the urine*. It is in this manner also that one determines what proportion of the renal impairment is due to obstruction, and what to permanent structural damage of the kidney. The reason for this is that the *purely functional disturbance* of the kidney due to urinary obstruction undergoes *complete restitution to normal* when the obstruction is removed, provided no permanent structural change in the kidney, from infection, or in the nature of hydronephrosis, has occurred. In all cases with uremia and especially in men over forty-five years of age, the possibility of urinary obstruction should be considered.

The symptom complex of *uremia* is so well known that it is unnecessary to detail it here. Suffice it to say that the principal features are thirst, headache, loss of memory, dizziness, drowsiness, edema, dyspnea, a foul breath, hypertension, hiccup, anorexia and vomiting, diarrhea, and polyuria. In all patients with urinary obstruction, however, whether they have any such symptoms or not, it is incumbent on the urologist to use every means to estimate the functional capacity of the kidney. Equally, it is incumbent on the internist to keep in mind the obstructive nephropathy, especially in elderly men, who are very apt to have enlargement of the prostate. We have seen such cases treated for months on a mistaken diagnosis of chronic nephritis (Bright's disease).

The occurrence of gross *anatomic changes* in the kidneys brings an entirely different train of symptoms into the picture. This usually occurs in the unilateral type of obstruction where, owing to the assumption of the excretory function by the sound kidney, general symptoms do not ensue, and the diseased kidney has time to undergo the more advanced alterations. More rarely, hydronephrosis of varying degree may occur bilaterally in incomplete obstructions below the bladder. In this case, the local renal symptoms are secondary to general symptoms of the uremic type, but do not differ otherwise in any fundamental way from the unilateral cases. A special type of obstructive lesion, which may have both local and general symptoms, is congenital cystic kidney (polycystic kidney). In this disease, the obstruction occurs within the parenchyma of the kidney itself. It is for this reason so much distinguished from the other forms of obstructive nephropathy that a closer consideration of its features will be deferred to the subsequent section on this subject under Malformations of the Urogenital Tract.

Since *hydronephrosis* may occur as the result of so many different obstructive lesions, the symptomatology and diagnosis can best be considered at this point, while the treatment, which always has as its object the removal of the obstruction, will be taken up under the headings of various types of obstructions.

The principal symptoms of hydronephrosis, due directly to the local condition, are *pain* and *tumor*. *Hematuria* is usually associated with calculus and *pyuria* with infection. Those of less importance are urgency and frequency of urination and transient polyuria, while sometimes diarrhea, constipation, intestinal obstruction, nausea, and vomiting, due indirectly to the kidney condition, are seen. In bilateral hydronephrosis the larger sacs are usually incompatible with life, so that they are seen only rarely, and usually early in life in congenital obstructions of the urethra.[1]

Pain is the most characteristic symptom, although it may frequently be absent altogether. It is usually colicky and recurrent in type. In such cases it may be associated with increased ingestion of fluids. Posture usually has little effect. The pain is usually in the loin, and may *radiate* downward along the course of the ureter, though this varies with the nature of the obstruction. When hydronephrosis is associated with stone in the ureter, there may be typical ureteral colic, but when the obstruction is in the pelvis or at the ureteropelvic junction, the downward radiation of pain is less frequent and less well defined. When the pain occurs in definite colicky spasms, it may be associated with nausea, vomiting, and suppression of urine. The cessation of pain may be accompanied by the passage of abnormally

[1] Young, Frontz, and Baldwin: Journal of Urology, 1919, iii, 289–365.

large quantities of urine, with a decrease in the size of the tumor. It has further been shown that this polyuria is not always due to an emptying of the sac, but may be a polyuria from the sound kidney, following suppression during the acute stages of the pain. In certain cases the pain may be a dull, constant, aching pain, in the lumbar region, or referred to the umbilical region or elsewhere in the areas innervated by the lower thoracic and upper lumbar fibers.

Tumor is an inconstant sign. Pain may become severe before any mass is palpable. In stout individuals it may be impossible to feel a large hydronephrosis. On the other hand, a large mass may appear before any other symptoms make themselves felt. The patient may note that the mass varies in size from time to time, and may observe the transient polyuria mentioned above. The pressure of the mass when large may cause dyspnea, palpitation and various gastro-intestinal symptoms, including complete intestinal obstruction.

Hematuria in the absence of stone occurs somewhat rarely, but may be the first symptom noted. It may be constant or transitory. In cases due to calculi hematuria is common.

When a hydronephrosis becomes infected a large number of other important symptoms are found in addition to those already cited. These are fully treated in the section on Infections of the Kidney.

Tables 4 and 5 show the age incidence and the frequence with which the principal symptoms occurred in a series of 162 cases studied at the Brady Institute.

Ureter.—Dilatation of the ureters is accompanied by symptoms which are indistinguishable from those of obstructive nephropathy, unless there be a definite obstruction within the ureter itself (stone, stricture, pressure from extraneous objects) when characteristic symptoms may be present.

Bladder.—The first symptom of bladder obstruction is usually *frequency of urination*. The hypertrophied trigone and vesical muscle empty the bladder without giving the patient any sensation of difficulty in voiding. *Hesitation* and *stoppage* before the completion of the act of micturition are also early symptoms (the "miction en deux temps" of the French). In strictures, however, the first symptoms may be a *decrease in size of the stream* and *straining* to void. When the obstruction is below the vesical orifice, the filling of the urethra increases the sensory phenomena. In sudden obstructions, as from a stone or blood-clot in the urethra, *difficulty* and *straining* are, of course, the first manifestation.

As the residual urine increases, so does the frequency, and diminished amounts are voided on each occasion. Bladder *pain* ensues from the irritation and spasmodic efforts of the vesical muscle. These symptoms are usually all increased when infection sets in, and to them is added *pyuria*. If the cystitis is acute and severe, *hematuria* may also be present.

It was noted as early as 1864 by Traube that infection in such cases usually came on after the first catheterization, but it may sometimes appear spontaneously. In such cases the path is undoubtedly from the blood by way of the kidney.

Acute retention may occur at any time, and is especially apt to follow overindulgence in food or drink, overexertion, fatigue, mental strain and worry, jarring, as from a long carriage or automobile ride, exposure to cold, prostatic massage, or instrumentation. The patient, who has usually noticed a pre-existent frequency, suddenly becomes totally unable to void. The pain is very great, and usually a palpable *tumor*, due to the distended bladder, soon appears. If relief is not given

TABLE 4

Symptoms of Hydronephrosis in 160 Cases

	Diffuse pain.	Colic.	Radiation (typical).	Atypical radiation.	No radiation.	Tumor.	Hematuria.	Pyuria.	Total cases.
I. Bilateral: Infravesical obstruction...........	7	4	3	1	0	3	16	35	41
II. Bilateral: Supravesical obstruction: Calculus { Ureteral..........	1	2	1	1	0	0	1	2	2
Calculus { Renal..........	1	2	1	0	0	1	2	3	4
Other causes...........	7	4	1	1	2	3	9	12	15
III. Unilateral: Supravesical obstruction: Calculus { Ureteral..........	12	15	14	0	1	6	11	13	19
Calculus { Renal..........	9	12	8	3	1	4	11	16	24
Other causes...........	19	19	10	2	7	14	22	37	55
Bilateral: Infravesical obstruction...........	7 (17%)	4 (10%)	3 (7%)	1 (2.5%)	0	3 (7%)	16 (40%)	35 (85%)	41
Bilateral: Supravesical obstruction...........	9 (43%)	8 (38%)	3 (14.5%)	2 (9.5%)	2 (9.5%)	4 (19%)	12 (57%)	17 (81%)	21
Unilateral: Supravesical obstruction...........	40 (40%)	46 (47%)	32 (32%)	5 (5%)	9 (9%)	24 (24%)	44 (44%)	66 (61%)	98

TABLE 5

AGE AT WHICH HYDRONEPHROSIS OCCURS—A SERIES OF 162 CASES

	0-9.	10-19.	20-29.	30-39.	40-49.	50-59.	60-69.	70-79.	80-89.	90-99.	No record.	Total.
I. Bilateral; infravesical...............	1	4	1	2	2	7	13	10	0	0	2	42
II. Bilateral; Supravesical due to: Calculus......................	0	0	0	1	1	2	1	0	0	0	0	5
Other causes...................	0	1	4	2	4	2	2	0	0	0	0	15
III. Unilateral; supravesical due to: Calculus......................	1	3	10	9	10	8	2	1	0	0	0	44
Other causes...................	1	3	12	17	12	3	5	1	0	0	2	56
Total....................	3	11	27	31	29	22	23	12	0	0	4	162

by catheterization or otherwise, a *paradoxical incontinence*, with constant dribbling, may appear, although if the obstruction is really complete, death may eventually occur from uremia. On the other hand, where the retention is due to inflammatory or edematous swellings, these may subside, aided by hypnotics and local applications, and voiding be again established.

The dilated bladder never ruptures spontaneously, but may easily do so as the result of a fall or blow. In that case, the symptoms of urinary extravasation, pain, swelling, prostration, fever, etc., appear, supplemented by those of acute peritonitis when the rupture has opened into the peritoneal cavity.

If retention does not occur, the frequency may grow so great that it is practically a constant dribbling. When the residual is more than 350 c.c. the distended bladder will usually be palpable, and enlargement of the abdomen may be noticed by the patient.

If pyelitis occurs, either from the blood or by extension through dilated ureters from the bladder, the localized symptoms of this disease, with, in addition, fever, sweats, prostration, and pain may occur.

Associated with these marked degrees of infravesical obstruction, there is usually present *impairment of renal function*, with its *uremic* symptoms, as described above.

Diverticula do not produce any characteristic symptoms unless they are very large. When this is true, an asymmetric or midline *tumor* may appear in the lower abdomen. Sometimes the tumor persists after catheterization, in which case it must be distinguished from neoplasm. In other cases the tumor appears and disappears from time to time. Pressure on the rectum by a diverticulum may cause constipation, difficulty and pain at stool. Pressure on the ureter may give the symptoms of hydronephrosis. Retrovesical diverticula may elevate the base of the bladder or reduce its capacity and lead to frequency of urination and sometimes dysuria.

Ordinarily symptoms due to the diverticulum are obscured by those due to the obstruction causing it. In some cases, after removal of the obstruction, purely diverticular symptoms are well seen; they are usually difficult urination, and persistent infection, with a very dirty urine. In 2 of our cases the patients were able to empty their bladders only after massaging and pressing the lower abdomen, which presumably forced the urine out of the diverticulum into the bladder proper.

The symptoms, therefore, which are most nearly characteristic for diverticulum are difficulty of urination, practically always accompanied by frequency, and sometimes by a small weak stream, over a long period. The duration of symptoms in our 41 cases is shown in the following table:

TABLE 6

DURATION OF SYMPTOMS IN CASES OF DIVERTICULA

	Total cases.	Cases due to contracture.	Cases due to prostatic hyper-trophy.	Congenital (urachus).	?
0– 1 yr..............	5	3	2	0	0
1– 2 yrs............	6	2	3	0	1
2– 3 yrs............	2	1	1	0	1
3– 5 yrs............	3	1	1	1	0
5–10 yrs............	9	5	4	0	0
10–15 yrs............	9	4	4	0	1
15–20 yrs............	3	1	2	0	0
20–30 yrs............	2	1	1	0	0
30–40 yrs............	1	1	0	0	0
Total.............	41				

Over 5 years.............. 24 (58.5%)
Over 10 years.............. 15 (36.6%)

Urethra.—Obstruction in the urethra below the prostate is characterized by *difficulty in urination, small stream*, which may be forked or irregular, and *dribbling* after voiding. In slowly developing obstructions of long standing the symptoms of bladder stasis may also appear. A stage may be reached in which urine can only be voided in drops, or acute retention may occur.

It is interesting that the symptoms of stricture should differ as much as they do from those of prostatic obstruction. The filling of the posterior urethra undoubtedly increases the sensory phenomena, and the dribbling after urination is caused by the gradual emptying of this dilated portion of the urethra. The stricture is inelastic, and while the urine can escape freely, until the last stages, it must do so through a reduced aperture. The prostatic obstruction, on the other hand, is usually elastic, and while urine may escape in a good stream, much increased pressure is necessary to expel it. The peri-urethral infiltration in stricture prevents the complete contraction of the muscle of the bulb and some of the urine remains in the bulbous urethra and dribbles out later. In some cases, however, a distinction between these two conditions from symptoms alone is not possible.

Congenital obstructions of the urethra, usually in the prostatic region, give rise to a symptom complex in children which is characteristic. There is a general dilatation of the urinary tract with such great enlargement of the ureters that they may be seen through the child's emaciated abdominal wall. The kidneys and bladder are often greatly dilated also. In some of these cases the chief complaint is incontinence of urine, but difficulty of urination, pain, dysuria, and at times complete retention of urine occur. In 12 cases which we reported in 1919, the symptoms were as follows[1]:

[1] Young, Frontz, and Baldwin: Journal of Urology, 1919, iii, 289–365.

TABLE 7

SYMPTOMS ACCOMPANYING CONGENITAL VALVES OF THE PROSTATIC URETHRA

	Our cases.	Cases from the literature.	Total.
Abdominal distention	2	3	5
Vomiting......................	3	1	4
Loss of weight.................	2	2	4
Urinary: Difficulty...................	4	6	10
Pain.......................	4	2	6
Incontinence.................	1	4	5
Retention......	3	1	4
Frequency...................	3	0	3
Pyuria......................	1	1	2
Hematuria...................	0	2	2

The congenital urethral obstructions are usually due to valves or diaphragms running from the verumontanum to the urethral wall. When boy babies or infants are brought in with distended abdomens, incontinence, symptoms of chronic uremia, etc., valves of the prostate should be thought of. Bugbee and Wollstein[1] recently reported 3 cases of fatal obstruction to urination due to congenital enlargement of the verumontanum in infants. The mechanical effects and complications are the same as those of congenital valves above described. Spina bifida is often accompanied by a clinical picture not unlike congenital valves; viz., incontinence.

DIAGNOSIS

Kidney and Ureter.—Various tests for *kidney function* have been proposed, many of which, as the methylene-blue, lactose, freezing-point, and phloridzin tests, having become obsolete in America, will not be further mentioned here.

Nitrogen retention in the blood occurs at a fairly early stage of renal insufficiency and may be determined by measuring the non-protein nitrogen or the urea in the blood. The values of these two methods are about equal, although the relations between them vary. The difference between the total non-protein nitrogen and the urea nitrogen of the blood, called the "rest-nitrogen" has been made the object of much study, but up to the present time no rules have been deduced which enable us to draw from it any conclusions of value. Since the various modifications of Marshall's[2] urease method have made the determination of *blood urea* so simple and so accurate, it is recommended.[3] The normal figure is usually given as 0.20 to 0.35 gram per liter of urea, not urea nitrogen, but in older persons and in those

[1] Journal of Urology, 1923, x, 477–490.

[2] Journal of Biological Chemistry, 1913, xv, 487–494.

[3] *Method of determining blood urea:*

1. Place 5 c.c. citrated blood in a test-tube.

2. Add urease (1 c.c. 5 per cent. jack bean emulsion, or 2 urease tablets in 1 c.c. of water).

3. Add 5 c.c. of phosphate buffer solution (5 gm. KH_2PO_4 and 1 gm. Na_2HPO_4 per liter, using CO_2-free water; this step may be omitted).

4. Incubate at 50° C. by immersing in a cup of water for twenty to thirty minutes.

5. An aërating apparatus with a wash bottle containing concentrated H_2SO_4 (to remove ammonia vapor from the air), 2 aërating tubes in series, and a suction pump, is arranged. In the second aërating tube (nearest the pump) is placed 20 c.c. N/50 HCl, colored with a few drops of alizarin sodium sulphonate solution, and diluted up to a suitable quantity (about 40

on a diet rich in proteids 0.6 may not be pathological, as may be shown by reducing the proteid intake.

The *urea constant* of Ambard and its modification by McLean are intended to express the relation between the urea concentration in the blood and the quantitative excretion of urea in the urine in a given period. Careful studies in this country and also in France have cast doubt on the accuracy of Ambard's conclusions, and since the test consumes much time and labor, is open to many sources of error, and gives no information not to be obtained from a simultaneous determination of the blood urea and the phenolsulphonephthalein excretion, it may well be omitted.

The work of Addis[1] is of interest in connection with functional studies of the kidney. He has criticised and apparently disproved Ambard's hypothesis, and believes that in order to obtain an accurate idea of the functional power of the kidney by means of comparing the concentration of urea in the urine with that in the blood, it is necessary to stimulate all of the functioning renal tissue present to its maximum activity by giving a dose of urea.

Creatinin is the most easily excretable constituent of the urine, and therefore, the last to become retained in the blood. The study of blood creatinin becomes, therefore, of important prognostic value in the graver cases of advanced renal insufficiency. The normal figure is about 2 mgm. per 100 c.c. of blood, and a retention of 7 mgm. or higher practically always presages a fatal outcome.[2]

---

c.c.) with neutral water. Two drops of octyl alcohol are added to prevent foaming, and the air tube and stopper inserted.

6. The incubated blood is poured into the first aërating tube, using as little wash water as possible (2 or 3 c.c.). Ten c.c. of alcohol and 2 drops of octyl alcohol are then added.

7. With the apparatus completely connected, the stopper of the tube containing the blood is lifted just sufficiently to admit a small spoonful of powdered sodium or potassium carbonate, and quickly replaced. The air current is at once turned on.

8. Aërate slowly for five minutes then as rapidly as the apparatus will stand without splashing for forty-five minutes.

9. The acid is now titrated with N/50 NaOH to neutrality, the alizarin sodium sulphonate acting as indicator.

Calculation: Subtract the number of cubic centimeters of N/50 NaOH required to reach the end point from 20 (the number of cubic centimeters of N/50 HCl used). Multiply the figure obtained by this subtraction by 0.12, which gives the result in grams of urea per liter of blood.

[1] The Rate of Urea Excretion: A Criticism of Ambard and Weill's Laws of Urea Excretion, Journal of Biological Chemistry, 1916, xxiv, 203–222. Renal Function and the Amount of Functioning Tissue, Archives of Internal Medicine, 1922, xxx, 378–385. The Rate of Urea Excretion, Journal of Biological Chemistry, 1923, lv, 105–111, 629–638. The Regulation of Renal Activity. The Relation Between the Rate of Urea Excretion and the Size of the Kidneys, American Journal of Physiology, 1923, lxv, 55–61. The Regulation of Renal Activity. The Effect of Unilateral Nephrectomy on the Function and Structure of the Remaining Kidney, Archives of Internal Medicine, 1924, xxxiv, 243–257.

[2] *Method for Blood Creatinin.*—A specimen of pure creatinin must be at hand. This may be prepared by the method of Benedict, Journal of Biological Chemistry, 1914, xviii, 183–194. A solution containing 1 mgm. per cubic centimeter is kept in the laboratory.

1. Place 6 c.c. of this solution in a liter flask.
2. Add 10 c.c. normal HCl.
3. Dilute to the liter mark.
4. Transfer to a bottle and add 4 or 5 drops of toluene or xylene. Five c.c. of this solution contains 0.03 mgm. of creatinin. This diluted with 15 c.c. of water is the standard needed for most human bloods, i. e., about 1 to 2 mgm. per 100 c.c. of blood. If the blood contains excessive amounts take 10 c.c. of the standard solution plus 10 c.c. of water, giving a range of 2 to 4 mgm. per 100 c.c. of blood. In the same way, 15 c.c. of standard plus 5 c.c. of water = 4

The value of *blood uric acid* determination is still under experimental investigation.

The retention of hydrogen ions gives rise first to a reduction in the "alkali reserve" of the body, and later to uncompensated *acidosis*. This is best measured by the "CO_2 combining power" of the plasma (see page 54).

The various *polyuria* tests are for the purpose of determining to what point the kidney can increase the concentration of the urine under given circumstances. The procedure may be facilitated by giving the patient a dose of urea (5 gm.) by mouth. They often give the first indication of renal damage, but are of minimal value to the urologist, since he is concerned usually with gross lesions.[1]

---

to 6 mgm. per 100 c.c. of blood, and 20 c.c. of standard = 6 to 8 mgm. per 100 c.c. of blood.

Determination.—To 20 c.c. of distilled water in a 50 (or 25) c.c. centrifuge tube are added 5 c.c. of the well-mixed oxalated blood (or oxalated plasma). This is then stirred with a glass rod until the blood is hemolyzed completely, after which about 1 gram of dry picric acid (sufficient to precipitate the proteins and render the solution saturated) is added. The mixture is thoroughly stirred until it is uniformly yellow and then at intervals for twenty to thirty minutes, after which it is centrifuged and filtered. (There are advantages in stoppering these tubes and placing them in a shaking machine after the preliminary stirring.) Sufficient filtrate is obtained for the estimation of both the creatinin and the sugar. To 10 c.c. of this filtrate is added 0.5 c.c. of 10 per cent. sodium hydroxid and a similar amount of alkali is added to each of three standards (10 c.c. of standard creatinin in saturated picric acid, containing 0.3, 0.5, and 1.0 mgm. creatinin to 100 c.c. of picric acid). A standard is selected which approximates the color intensity of the unknown, and set at the 15 mm. mark. With blood showing much over 5 mgm. creatinin it is desirable to make a 1 to 10 or 15 dilution of the blood so that when the color is developed in the filtrate it will closely match the standard (1.0 mgm.), *i. e.*, read between 12 and 18 mm. with the standard at 15 mm. (In an emergency where sufficient blood is not available for a second dilution, it may be allowable to secure the added dilution by further diluting the 1 to 5 picric acid filtrate. However, with blood creatinin figures of over 5 mgm. the 1 to 5 dilution is not entirely adequate for a complete extraction of the creatinin.) The colors are compared after they have been allowed to develop for eight minutes.

Calculation.—For the calculation the following formula may be used: $\frac{S}{R} \times S_1 \times D = mgm.$ creatinin to 100 c.c. of blood, in which "S" represents the depth of the standard (15 mm.), "R" the reading of the unknown, "S_1" the strength of the standard, and "D" the dilution of the blood. For example, with a reading of 15, a standard of 0.3 mg. and a blood dilution of 5 the formula would work out: $\frac{15}{15} \times 0.3 \times 5 = 1.5$ mgm. creatinin to 100 c.c.

For literature and full discussion, see Myers, Practical Analysis of Blood, 2d ed. (Mosby), 1924.

[1] *The Polyuria Test.*—The night urine is collected at 10 P. M., the morning urine at 5 A. M. After this a light, dry breakfast is given with 600 c.c. of water. Urine is collected hourly for five or more hours, and nothing is taken by mouth until the end of the test period. The specimens may be analyzed for urea, sodium chlorid, freezing-point, etc., but simple determination of the specific gravity is satisfactory. In normal individuals the later specimens will show a regularly increasing specific gravity, while if the kidneys are damaged, they may be able to secrete only a dilute urine.

It has been suggested that 5 gm. of urea may be given by mouth during the test when we desire to ascertain the maximum possible concentration. This would scarcely be justifiable if there were any nitrogen retention in the blood.

The night urine (that secreted during the resting hours) is normally more concentrated than the day urine. In renal involvement this difference may disappear. Along with the drop in concentration, the night urine may become more profuse. This nocturnal polyuria of early nephritis may sometimes be mistaken at first for the nocturnal frequency of obstruction, and vice versa.

Of foreign substances used for kidney tests, only indigocarmin and phenol-sulphonephthalein have survived.

Indigocarmin may be used for tests of the combined function of the two kidneys, but is not as reliable as phenolsuphonephthalein and its quantitative determination in the voided urine has serious technical difficulties. Its principal use is as an aid to ureteral meatoscopy, in which rôle it is frequently invaluable for the location of a ureter in a much distorted bladder, or for determining which kidney is affected in a case where there are no localizing symptoms and where the ureters cannot be catheterized (chromocystoscopy).

Phenolsulphonephthalein was discovered by Remsen. Abel found that it was excreted practically exclusively by the kidney in healthy animals. Rowntree and Geraghty,[1] in an exhaustive experimental and clinical report, showed its great value in clinical use.[2] Numerous studies since that time have only served to confirm the extraordinary value of this test. McLean, Mosenthal, and others have published studies of cases in which both the phthalein and Ambard constant have been carefully estimated, and have concluded that the phthalein test is a more accurate indication of the exact condition of renal impairment.

[1] Archives of Internal Medicine, 1912, ix, 284–338.

[2] B. U. I. 1932. This case is very interesting in that it was the first human being upon which the phthalein test was employed.

A few days previously Dr. Rowntree had presented to the Interurban Surgical Society experimental work on a dog in which he had ligated one ureter and brought it out in the loin. Following this he had introduced uranium nitrate into the renal artery to produce an experimental nephritis. Phenolsulphonephthalein was subsequently injected into the dog and a study of the divided urines showed that more of the dye was excreted through the kidney which had been operated on than through the unoperated kidney. From this Dr. Rowntree deduced that phenol-sulphonephthalein was eliminated more rapidly by a diseased kidney than by a healthy kidney. He asserted that he thought he produced an experimental nephritis by the injection of uranium nitrate. This kidney had excreted more of the phenolsulphonephthalein than the other side, presumably normal.

Following his demonstration I talked to Dr. Rowntree. I told him I had on the ward a patient who presented exactly the same condition as his operated dog, *i. e.*, the right ureter was blocked and all the urine was coming out through the right loin following this operation upon the right kidney. I, therefore, proposed that phenolsulphonephthalein be injected in this case. Dr. Rowntree came to Ward C, first floor, and gave the patient in my presence an injection into the right arm of 1 c.c. of 6/10 per cent. solution of phenolsulphonephthalein. Urine was collected from the fistula in the right side and by catheter from the bladder. I do not remember for what length of time it was collected, but on the following day Dr. Rowntree informed me that this case confirmed absolutely his experimental work on the dog, *i. e.*, more phthalein was excreted from the fistula in the right side than through the left ureter which opened into the bladder from which the urine was collected by a catheter. Within a few days after this experiment the patient developed a fever and marked pain and swelling in the left side. A large mass was easily palpable in the region of the left kidney and patient became rapidly uremic. With a hasty operation I exposed the left kidney and found it was a mere shell and filled with pus. It is evident, therefore, that at the time the experiment with phthalein was carried out by Dr. Rowntree the left kidney was really the bad kidney and the phthalein test simply showed that a bad kidney excretes less than a comparatively good kidney. Other cases in which the test was tried after this confirmed our findings in this case and it was promptly demonstrated that phthalein was eliminated more rapidly by a good kidney than a bad kidney, and in a larger amount.

The deduction which one draws is that the intra-arterial injection of uranium which Dr. Rowntree carried out produced congestion and probably hyperemia of the kidney with increase in its functional capacity. Perhaps nephritis with impairment of function might have come on later or it is quite possible that the dosage of uranium nitrate used was too low to produce nephritis at the time Dr. Rowntree made the phthalein test (Young).

Recently, phthalein has replaced the Ambard constant in a number of the foremost French clinics, both urologic and medical, where results similar to the above were obtained, and where the technical simplicity of the phthalein test is appreciated.

The *phenolsulphonephthalein test* (hereafter called the phthalein test) consists of an injection of a watery solution of the dye into muscle or vein, watching for its appearance in the catheterized urine, and then estimating colorimetrically the amount secreted in a given time (generally one and two hours).

While the phthalein test is simple in its technic, it must, like all other tests of precision, be performed carefully and by competent individuals. The quantity used is 1 c.c. of a 0.6 per cent. solution, containing 0.006 gm. This quantity is, however, in no way essential, since what we wish to observe is the *proportion*, of that which is injected, which is eliminated by the kidneys in a given time. The results, therefore, are always given as percentages. The injection may be made intramuscularly or intravenously. In the past reactions were observed following intravenous injection, with chills, fever, and vomiting. These were due to certain impurities in the drug as supplied commercially. The manufacturers have now successfully eliminated these impurities, and no such reactions have been observed in our clinic for over two years.

Braasch and Kendall[1] of the Mayo Clinic have noted in certain cases differences between the results following intravenous and intramuscular injections in the same individual which they take to indicate a retention of waste products in the tissues themselves, and which may occur even in the absence of frank edema. This retention of phthalein in the tissues is increased by acidosis. The figures approach each other as the condition returns to normal. For routine use the intravenous method is recommended, since it reduces the sources of error. The path of introduction should always be noted, however, as the appearance time is less with the intravenous route. The patient should be made to drink water freely, both during the test and for twenty minutes before it, since an excess of water does not alter the results, and, if the urine is dilute, the errors resulting from the loss of a few drops, or from small quantities remaining in the bladder, are minimized.

The *appearance time* is important. Normally, with intravenous injections, it is from two to three minutes; with intramuscular injection, from five to eight minutes. In case there is residual urine, or in case the patient is unable to void freely when called upon, a catheter should always be inserted. The urine is allowed to drip into a vessel containing 5 to 10 drops of a 15 per cent. sodium hydroxid solution, and the first pink tinge noted. In case the urine does not drip freely from the catheter, an irrigation of sterile water should be at hand, from which a small quantity is allowed to run in, and then out, of the catheter. This will bring with it urine from the bladder, and if these precautions are observed, there need never be any doubt about the appearance time. If an obstruction exists above the bladder, ureteral catheters must be introduced. This is, of course, also true where the respective functional capacities of the two kidneys are to be investigated. In this case errors cannot always be avoided, since it is sometimes impossible to empty a hydronephrotic sac completely or promptly through a ureteral catheter. If the mechanical situation is kept in mind, however, one will avoid falling into errors of interpretation.

[1] Journal of Urology, 1921, v, 127–132.

The appearance time once determined accurately, the elimination of the phthalein is observed during *two hourly periods*, beginning with the moment of appearance. Here again one must be sure that the bladder is completely emptied at the end of each period. In case there is any doubt, a catheter and an irrigation of sterile water should be employed. The unsuspected existence of residual urine is frequently the cause of gross errors in the phthalein test.

The amount of phthalein in the specimens obtained is now estimated by means of a *colorimeter*.

Comparators, colorimeters, and other instruments used for colorimetric determination fall roughly into two groups—plunger and dilution types. The plunger type is represented by that class in which we match the intensity of the color by varying the relative depth of the solution. The dilution type is that in which the color is compared with an equal volume of known standard. The apparatus herein described was designed in the laboratories of the Brady Urological Institute to facilitate the accurate and rapid reading of phenolsulphonephthalein output. It is of the dilution type.

In the early work on the phenolsulphonephthalein test in this department the Duboscq plunger-type colorimeter was employed, and studies which standardized the phthalein test were made here with this instrument by Rowntree and Geraghty. A little later the Hellige colorimeter, which is a somewhat simpler and cheaper apparatus, was employed, but with both of these instruments the preparation of the specimen and the standards was tedious and time consuming. Shortly afterward Dunning devised his simple colorimeter which consists of a series of tubes which contain known dilutions of the dye and which are used as standards to compare with the phthalein excreted in a given test. This simple cheap apparatus has given satisfactory results and has been widely used all over the world.

In a large clinic where great numbers of phthalein tests are done, all these methods have been, in our opinion, too time consuming and the apparatus has been too prone to breakage. We, therefore, set about to design an apparatus which would be free from these defects and would, if possible, give more accurate readings with greater range of fixed standards[1] for comparison. The instrument, which we call *the phthaleinometer*, consists of a wheel $6\frac{1}{2}$ inches in diameter and $\frac{5}{8}$ inch in thickness, which is made of solid aluminum alloy. From the convex surface of this, holes are drilled radially to accommodate 14 glass tubes with standards of varying strength, which are thus buried equidistant from each other in the substance of the wheel. The dilutions here represented are 5, 10, 15, 20, 25, 30, 35, 40, 45, 50, 60, 70, 80, 90 per cent. Holes of equal diameter are also drilled from one side to the other of the wheel through which observation of the unknown is made in comparing it with the standard. These tubes are cemented in place and a thin metal band is fitted around the perimeter of the wheel to cover the openings. Directly beneath each hole figures are stamped on the face of the wheel corresponding with the percentage of dye in each glass tube. For the unknown specimen a very simple device has been made. It consists simply of a small rubber bulb syringe made of the same glass tubing used for the standards, and pointed at the lower end with an orifice sufficiently small so that no fluid escapes when the tube is held in a vertical position. A receptacle for holding the tube is provided and placed just back of the wheel at its upper margin and in direct line with the standards. Back

[1] Young and Elvers, C. F.: Journal of Urology, 1925, xiii, 79–83.

of this is a window through which the light penetrates both the unknown solution and the known standards. Daylight may thus be used for making estimation or, if preferred on account of insufficient light, the window can be closed and artificial indirect illumination upon the whitened surface of the shutter employed. The mechanical details of the instrument are shown in the accompanying illustration (Fig. 22, A and B).

In place of phenolsulphonephthalein a new dyestuff which is of exactly the same color and absolutely permanent is now employed in preparing the standard tubes. The color is perfectly matched with freshly prepared phenolsulphonephthalein of the given strength and has now been observed for a year and a half without showing any deterioration or fading.

The advantages of this instrument[1] are self-evident, especially the avoidance of handling of standards and receptacles, and the fact that the matching of the unknown

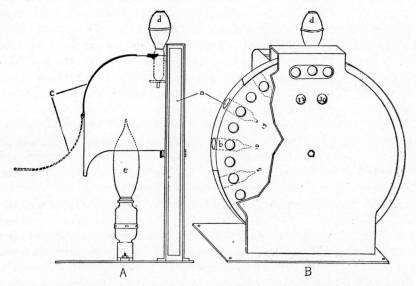

FIG. 22.—The Young-Elvers phthaleinometer: A, Side view of the phthaleinometer showing (c) window open as used when daylight is employed and also closed with curved surface giving indirect illumination when artificial light is used; d, syringe used for collecting unknown specimens. Same is here shown in position for reading. B, Sectional front view, the aluminum wheel here represented by a, and the ampules (b) embedded in the substance of the wheel.

with the standards and reading of the percentages of dye present is done simultaneously in one operation.

If the urine is highly colored, a tube containing the patient's urine, obtained before the test and appropriately diluted, should be placed behind the standard tube so as to add the urinary color. This enables one to compare the colors accurately. If the amount of phthalein in the urine is very small, the specimen should be diluted to less than 1000 c.c. and the proper calculation made later. In case the specimen, owing to polyuria or the use of quantities of irrigation fluid, exceeds 1000 c.c., it is compared at once with the standard after alkalinization, and the result multiplied by the volume of the specimen, expressed as liters and fractions

[1] This instrument, originally made in our shop, may now be obtained from Hynson, Westcott & Dunning, Charles and Chase Sts., Baltimore, Md.

thereof. When divided function through the ureteral catheters is studied, it is most important to empty the bladder at the end of the test period, to determine from this *transvesical urine* how much, if any, phthalein has escaped outside the catheters into the bladder. Serious errors are avoided in this way.

In interpreting the results, the appearance time is of great value. In many cases, improvement in the kidney function is indicated by a drop in the appearance time long before there is any increase in the percentage excretion. If the appearance time is greatly prolonged, operation should be delayed, even in the presence of fair percentage excretion.

We have been of the impression for a long time that the whole subject of renal function estimation should be investigated anew and, at our suggestion, a restudy of the phthalein test has been recently made by Shaw in this clinic.[1] It was found that the test will yield more accurate information when the urine collections are made at more frequent intervals. The normal curve of phthalein elimination was determined by a series of forty-four tests on 23 normal individuals in which the urine was collected at fifteen-minute intervals for two hours. The curve was characterized by an average output of 40 per cent. during the first fifteen-minute period, 17 per cent. during the second, 8 per cent. during the third, 4 per cent, during the fourth, and a gradual decrease to 0.5 per cent. during the eighth fifteen-minute period. The range of variation in normal cases is not great and in no case did it exceed 10 per cent. for the entire two hours.

There were one or more tests performed in the same manner in 56 cases with known renal lesions. There were included in this group practically all types of renal disease. All of these cases in which renal insufficiency was demonstrated by any other test showed definite abnormalities in the curve of phthalein elimination, and in several instances the presence of an abnormal curve indicated impending renal failure, while the other tests, including the Mosenthal test, gave normal results.

A majority of the cases studied were those with renal damage from back-pressure and infection. In this group a striking feature was an increase in appearance time and a delay in the peak of elimination that often was not reached until the third or fourth fifteen-minute period. In cases followed with repeated tests while retention catheter drainage and other therapeutic measures were being carried out, improvement of kidney function was much more accurately followed by plotting the curves of elimination than by the collection of the specimens at hourly intervals. Not infrequently the curve improved, while the total two-hour output remained unchanged (see Chart I).

Cases of parenchymatous nephritis and cardiovascular hypertensive renal disease that gave a normal two-hour output of phthalein showed striking variations from the normal curve of phthalein elimination when the specimens were collected at fifteen-minute intervals. In these cases the appearance time was normal or only slightly delayed, but the output during the first fifteen-minute period was lower than normal, while the output during the second and third period was often above the normal curve.

While the collection of urine specimens at fifteen-minute intervals is not necessary as a routine procedure, yet in cases in which the exact information concerning the kidney's ability to eliminate phthalein is desired, such a modification of the

[1] Journal of Urology, xiii, June, 1925.

test may be useful. For routine purposes collections may be made at thirty-minute intervals, and although some of the finer points shown by fifteen-minute collections are lost the information obtained is much greater than when the collections are made at one-hour intervals. It was also suggested that the collection be dated from the time of administration of the phthalein rather than from the time of appearance in the urine. The advantage claimed for the latter modification is that it incorporates the appearance time in the percentage figure rather than allowing it to exist as a separate entity, therby making comparison simpler.

When divided function is studied, various tests, by nature less accurate than the above, may be employed to show relative differences in the functional capacities of the two kidneys. Such are cryoscopy, electrical conductivity, specific gravity,

CHART I

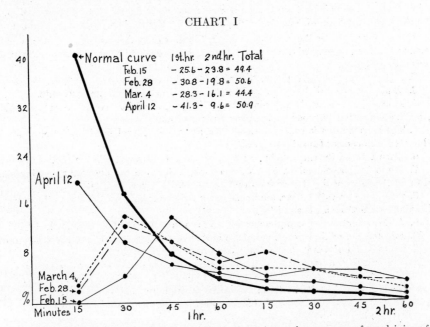

Chart showing curves of phthalein elimination made at intervals on a case of renal injury from back-pressure as a result of benign prostatic hypertrophy. The normal curve is also given for comparison. The tests were made during the period of retention catheter drainage. Note that the curve first taken on February 15th showed peak of elimination during the third fifteen-minute period and on February 28th and March 4th the peak occurred during the second fifteen-minute period. Operation was performed on March 8th. The test made on April 12th showed peak of elimination occurring during the first fifteen-minute period and a curve that closely approached the lower limits of normal, yet the total two-hour output at this time was practically the same as it was at the first test when the patient was on the verge of uremia. B. U. I. 13,197.

the hypobromite test, etc. Of these the most useful are the *specific gravity* test and the *hypobromite* test. They allow us to draw conclusions even where there has been leakage past the catheters and the relative volumes from the two sides are unknown. The hypobromite test, as commonly performed with the Doremus "Ureometer" is frequently called a urea test, but not properly, since a number of other constituents of urine decompose sodium hypobromite besides urea. These tests have their significance in disclosing variations in the concentration in the urine of various substances. Marked difference between the concentrations of the urine from the two sides usually indicates a unilateral lesion, and the diseased kidney usually secretes a more dilute urine than the normal one.

When uremia has set in, determination of the *acidosis* often accompanying it is of value for prognosis and as an indication for treatment aimed directly at the acidosis, such as intravenous injection of glucose and alkalies.[1]

If renal function is poor, and does not improve after free drainage has been instituted, it is certain that permanent damage has been done to the kidney. Improvement may be quite slow, but usually the point at which improvement ceases is fairly definite. We have seen improvement sufficient to permit operation delayed until four months after drainage was instituted. The permanent damage will be due, as a rule, to Bright's disease, to destruction following infection of the kidney (pyelonephritis) or to hydronephrosis. An exact knowledge of this irre-

---

[1] *Method of Determining Carbon Dioxid Combining Power of the Blood Plasma* (D. D. Van Slyke, Journal of Biological Chemistry, 1917, xxx, 347). Use the Van Slyke special apparatus.

1. Test apparatus for the presence of gas in the glass or rubber tubing, or leaks, by making a vacuum and then refilling with mercury. If no gas is present to act as a cushion, the mercury clicks on the stoppers.

2. Apparatus, including capillary tubes, is filled with mercury.

3. Wash the cup with 1 per cent. ammonia water which is free from carbonate.

4. Place 0.5 c.c. ammonia water in the cup (it should be slightly colored with phenolphthalein, which assures that there is no acid remaining in the cup.

5. Three c.c. plasma is shaken in a 300 c.c. separatory funnel filled with expired air from the lungs of the operator (to saturate it with CO_2).

6. Place 1 c.c. of the saturated plasma under the ammonia water in the cup.

7. Admit the plasma and part of the ammonia water into the apparatus, leaving enough fluid to fill the tubes of the stop-cock so that no bubbles of air can get in.

8. Wash the cup with 0.5 c.c. ammonia water twice, allowing it to flow into the apparatus, and taking care that no air is admitted.

9. Add several drops of caprylic alcohol, and run into the capillary tube of the apparatus.

10. Add 0.5 c.c. of 5 per cent. sulphuric acid, and run into the 50 c.c. chamber (if whole blood is used instead of plasma, substitute 20 per cent. tartaric acid).

11. Run in acid solution until the top of the mercury is exactly at the 2.5 c.c. mark.

12. Place a drop of mercury in the cup, and allow it to run down the capillary as far as the stop-cock to seal the latter. Wash the excess of sulphuric acid out of the cup.

13. Lower the mercury bulb, and allow the mercury (not the water) to fall exactly to the 50 c.c. mark, when the stop-cock is closed.

14. Shake the whole apparatus for several minutes.

15. Allow all the watery solution to flow into the collecting bulb below the 50 c.c. bulb by turning the stop-cock, but do not allow any air to follow it.

16. Turn stop-cock (lower) through 180 degrees, so that mercury is readmitted to the 50 c.c. bulb.

17. Raise mercury holder until the mercury level in it is the same as that in the measuring tube of the apparatus, *i. e.*, the gas inside is at atmospheric pressure.

18. The reading is made from the top level of the fluid in the measuring tube.

19. Make a barometer reading.

20. Calculate CO_2 combining power of plasma by tables of Van Slyke and Cullen, correcting for barometric pressure.

Myers (Practical Chemical Analysis of Blood, 2d ed., Mosby, 1924) gives the normal range of CO_2 combining power of the blood as from 53 to 77 volumes per cent. Figures above 77 indicate alkalosis, and are seldom present except after the excessive administration of alkali (sodium bicarbonate). Figures below 53 indicate acidosis. If 30 or below the acidosis is uncompensated (*i. e.*, the PH of the blood is no longer kept normal) and therapeutic measures are indicated. Unless the reaction of the blood can be speedily altered for the better, a fatal outcome may be expected. The lowest figure Myers has observed with recovery is 16. In uremia, acidosis is usually associated with nitrogen retention, but may occasionally occur separately. In such cases, the blood urea or N. P. N. figures will give no clue as to why the patient is so ill.

ducible minimum of permanent impairment is indispensable for the intelligent treatment of a case.

The laboratory tests of renal function have given rise to endless discussion, which we feel is largely due to misunderstanding.   The facts are that (1) laboratory tests *supplement* but do not replace direct observation of the patient; (2) the additional information gained from laboratory tests is *indispensable*, and (3) no single laboratory test proves anything; it is merely another element in the complete clinical picture of the patient we are trying to construct.

In urologic practice, the results of our tests and the information gained from direct observation should all fit together into a logical and understandable whole, from which the diagnosis, prognosis, and treatment can be deduced.   If there is a discrepancy anywhere, it means that we are still in ignorance of some important feature of the case, and further investigation is in order.

In all cases where laboratory tests are indicated, they should be repeated at frequent intervals, for two reasons: First, because it is much more important to know how much progress the patient is capable of, and is making, than to know his condition at any one time.   We are also able in this way to know what effect our treatment is having.   Second, in a series of tests, the effects of any technical errors, which might mislead if only one test is done, are eliminated.

In the particular matter of renal function in cases of urinary obstruction, it is often much more important, as we had occasion to remark more than twelve years ago,[1] to obtain a *stabilized* function than it is to attain any particular level of function as indicated by the various tests.   The time at which this stabilization of function is reached can only be shown by a series of frequently repeated tests.

Differential Diagnosis of Hydronephrosis.—Although hydronephrosis is the result of the same causes as those producing functional impairment of the kidney, its symptoms are essentially *local*, while those of the latter are *general*.   These two groups of symptoms must be kept distinct from each other in our minds.

Hydronephrosis must be distinguished, first, from extrarenal lesions and, second, from other pathologic conditions of the kidney.   In the first group come especially enlargements of the gall-bladder, of the spleen, tumors of the pancreas and stomach, retroperitoneal tumors, ovarian tumors, tumors of the intestine, especially the colon, tumors of the adrenal and aneurysm of the renal or other abdominal artery.   In the second group are new growths of the kidney, renal tuberculosis, polycystic kidney, perinephric abscess, movable kidney, hypertrophy of the kidney, diverticulum of the ureter, solitary cyst or hydatid cyst of the kidney, and other rare conditions.   Of these the first five are important.

Until the ureteral catheter was introduced, these distinctions were difficult and often impossible; now they should usually be made with accuracy.

The character and radiation of the *pain* are helpful in distinguishing extrarenal conditions.   It is especially characteristic of hydronephrosis that the symptoms occur in definite *attacks*, between which the health may appear perfect.

The *tumor* should be carefully examined, if present, and its condition in various postures and at different times noted.   The hydronephrotic sac is usually fluctuant, but may be quite tense and apparently hard.   It usually moves with respiration, a distinguishing mark from retroperitoneal tumors, and can often be pushed about

---

[1] Young: Transactions of the Section on Genito-urinary Diseases, American Medical Association, 1912, 69–70 (Disc.).

to a certain extent with the hand. The percussion note in the flank is flat, while in front the colonic tympany overlies it, and often serves to separate it from the liver edge. Pelvic examination in women will serve to disclose the lower portions of an ovarian or other tumor simulating a hydronephrosis.

A hydronephrosis usually descends somewhat when the patient stands erect, and this change of position is accompanied by a rotation downward and medially, due to the fixation of the pedicle. A diminution in size, due to partial emptying of the sac, will usually be perceptible on the lateral and upper borders of the tumor for the following reasons. As the sac enlarges, it rotates downward and inward as described above. This causes the pedicle to be at the upper and median angle of the tumor. When the sac empties, it allows the pedicle to lengthen somewhat. Therefore, any diminution in size on the lower border will often be compensated for by the dropping of the sac due to this lengthening and the lower border of the partially emptied sac may be actually lower than that of the tense sac. As a matter of fact, the palpation of renal enlargements is very unsatisfactory, and more dependence must be placed on cystoscopic studies.

A careful examination of the *urine* should be made in every urologic case. In hydronephrosis, however, it is not very helpful. In the typical case, it will be normal and uninfected. Where infection has occurred, pus and organisms will be present. Blood will sometimes be found, even when there is no stone, tuberculosis, or tumor, but is in no way characteristic. In case pus is present, careful study should be made for tubercle bacilli, since hydronephrosis is often present in tuberculosis of the kidney and ureter.

A carefully taken *history* and a thorough *general examination* will be very helpful where there is a question of hydronephrosis, but will often leave us in doubt, at the best. The diagnosis had frequently to be made by exploratory operation before the introduction of modern accurate methods of examining the urinary tract, but now all this has given place to a series of measures which are almost infallible.

In this list of modern procedures are x-ray examination, with and without ureteral catheterization, ureteral catheterization, with and without x-ray, and functional tests of the kidneys.

A *plain x-ray* is of use to show the size and position of the kidney and to disclose a stone which may be the cause of the hydronephrosis. When the diagnosis lies between hydronephrosis and kidney neoplasm, the plain x-ray will sometimes be helpful in showing a dense, heavy shadow in the kidney region in tumor, while the hydronephrotic sac does not impede the rays so much. Rowntree and his associates have lately shown that sodium iodid, when given by mouth, or better intravenously, will be excreted in the urine and make it possible to take a pyelogram without catheterizing the ureter. This procedure should prove very helpful in cases of hydronephrosis where catheterization is impossible or for any reason contraindicated. The dose is 5 grams by mouth or 250 c.c. of a 1 per cent. solution intravenously. The exposure should be made four hours after ingestion by mouth, or one to two hours after intravenous injection. This method, however, is not always successful.

The procedure of choice is *cystoscopy* with *ureteral catheterization*. In the the typical "open" hydronephrosis, this can usually be carried out without obstacle. In a "closed" hydronephrosis, catheterization of the affected side will be impossible, and no urinary secretion whatever will be observed. In certain "open" hydronephroses catheterization will be impossible owing to abnormalities in the course or narrowing of the lumen of the ureter. In these cases, if a catheter can be introduced far enough into the ureter to obtain secretion and inject a pyelographic medium, valuable information can still be obtained.

Observation of the *bladder* and *ureteral meatus* should also be carefully carried out. Obstructions at or near the orifice can usually be recognized in this manner, of which may be mentioned stones in the intramural portion of the ureter (*q. v.*), tuberculosis of the lower ureter (*q. v.*), tumor of the lower ureter (*q. v.*), stones or tumors of the bladder pressing on the ureter, and strictures at the vesico-ureteral orifice (bilateral hydronephrosis). One can also note a continuous flow of urine from the ureter, which occurs when the ureter too is dilated and the normal ureteral peristalsis absent. As an aid to this meatoscopy, it is sometimes useful to inject intravenously 10 c.c. of a 0.5 per cent. solution of indigocarmin.[1] This dye is secreted in the urine, appears in about ten minutes after injection, and the color is visible through the cystoscope. Its presence facilitates the location of a ureteral orifice when this is obscure, serves to make definite the character of the ureteral flow, and gives a rough idea of the relative functional capacities of the two kidneys. Its use as a precise functional test is not recommended.

When the ureter is catheterized, the catheter may or may not ascend into the hydronephrotic pelvis. Even when the catheter is in the normal pelvis, the flow through it will be interrupted, since the peristaltic wave has origin in the pelvis. The first characteristic of hydronephrosis, therefore, will be an *uninterrupted dripping of urine* from the catheter. This may be hastened, in some cases, by pressure on the kidney region. This second sign, when present, is absolutely diagnostic. A procedure which can now be followed is to *distend the pelvis*, presumably emptied. Sterile water or physiologic salt solution may be used. It is customary in many clinics to use a syringe for this purpose, but it is better done by gravity, using a head of not over 30 inches of water, for the reason that grave injury may be done to the kidney by too great pressure. Fluid should be run in until the patient complains of pain, or until no more will be run in without undue pressure. Often the patient will state that this pain is identical with that which he has previously experienced. If it is distinctly different, suspicion should be at once aroused that the source of the symptomatic pain is extrarenal. If it is, however, identified with the symptomatic pain, less reliance can be placed on it, since many patients are unable to distinguish accurately internal pains. The amount of fluid necessary to fill the pelvis is carefully noted. While the usual capacity of the pelvis is 7 c.c., pelves, to all intents and purposes normal, are found having capacities as great as 30 c.c., so that no definite conclusions can be drawn below this figure. Above it, however, one can be sure a hydronephrosis exists—always remembering that escape of urine around the catheter must be eliminated. For this reason the largest catheters possible should be used, since they diminish the possibility of leakage, and allow the fluid to flow in and out more rapidly. A No. 7 catheter is preferable as it usually completely plugs the ureter, but a No. 6 will often suffice. Where escape of urine around the catheter is suspected, the use of a Garceau conical catheter will completely fill the ureter. Colored fluids may

---

[1] This solution should be made fresh from the powdered dye and distilled water, and may be boiled in order to sterilize it.

be used to rule out leakage, but should be avoided when it is intended to do a phenolsulphonephthalein test later.   When they are used, one is able to be sure, from the absence of dye in the bladder urine, that no fluid has escaped down outside the catheter.   The fluid may also be measured as it escapes from the catheter after filling is complete.   If the quantity injected is recovered, one may be sure that there is no mistake.

In case doubt still remains, a *pyelogram* must be made.   This is especially true if the pelvis holds from 7 to 30 c.c., in which case we are unable to decide whether the pelvis is hydronephrotic or only a large normal until we see its outlines.

Collargol[1] was the opaque medium first used, but owing to its toxicity, its staining properties, and its cost, it has been superseded by other substances. Thorium nitrate, discovered by Burns[2] in this clinic in 1915, 15 per cent. solution, sodium iodid,[3] 15 per cent. solution, and sodium bromid, 25 per cent. solution,[4] are now the media of choice, and with any of them safe and satisfactory pyelograms can be made.   Cunningham, Graves, and Davis[5] have devised an antiseptic medium which does not require sterilization.

It has long been known that pyelographic media could find their way into the circulation when too forcibly injected, but the work of Hinman and Lee-Brown has demonstrated that this occurs by means of direct communications between the pelvis and the venæ rectæ.   It is, therefore, obvious that we are not justified in using any medium which is toxic on intravenous injection.   The passage of the pelvic contents into the circulation begins at a pressure of about 30 mm. of mercury.   This pressure should, therefore, not be exceeded during the procedure of pyelography.   Media remaining in the obstructed pelvis may eventually reach the circulation.   Every effort should be made to empty the pelvis after the picture is taken.

The following, then, are the principal *precautions* to be observed in pyelography: 1, The least toxic pyelographic medium should be used.   2, Injection should be made by the gravity method, the pressure never rising above 30 mm. of mercury. 3, The radiogram should be taken as soon as possible after the injection.   4, One should make sure, in a case where there is any obstruction of the ureter, that the injection fluid escapes completely.   Where this is not possible, it will usually be in a case where operation is indicated, and this operation should be performed at the earliest possible moment to avoid a secondary absorption of the pyelographic medium.

Small burets holding 50 c.c. are best for holding the pyelographic medium. With the buret, the upper level of the fluid is easily kept at the proper height, and one can quickly tell at all times just how much fluid has run into the pelvis.   All syringes are to be condemned for this purpose.

The medium is allowed to flow into the pelvis until no more will enter, or until the patient complains of pain.   The exposure is then made.   At the end of the procedure, the buret is depressed, and the medium should flow back into it.   If a

[1] Papin: Rapports de la Premiere Congres de la Société Internationale d'Urologie, 1921, i, 230–264; Young and Waters, 267–287.

[2] Journal of the American Medical Association, 1915, lxiv, 2126–2127.

[3] Cameron and Grandy: Journal of the American Medical Association, 1918, lxx, 1516–1517.

[4] Weld: Journal of the American Medical Association, 1918, lxxi, 1111–1112.

[5] Journal of Urology, 1923, x, 255–260.   Dissolve 1 gram of mercuric iodid in 3000 c.c. of 12 per cent. sodium iodid; this produces potassium mercuric iodid in an excess of potassium iodid.

quantity equal or superior to that introduced is recovered, one can be sure that no great amount of the medium remains in the pelvis.

Since the ureteral catheter tends to straighten the ureter while in place, it is sometimes desirable, especially where the ureter itself is the object of close study, to obtain a pyelo-ureterogram with no catheter in the ureter. In this case the catheter is withdrawn until only 8 cm. remains in the ureter. The rest of the procedure is the same. Since spasmodic contractions of the ureter may defeat the object of this method by obliterating its lumen and preventing the medium from reaching the upper ureter and pelvis, the maneuver must be carried out with the greatest gentleness. Joseph[1] recommends small catheters (Nos. 4 or 5, French) since they irritate the ureter less. A preliminary dose of morphin may be of

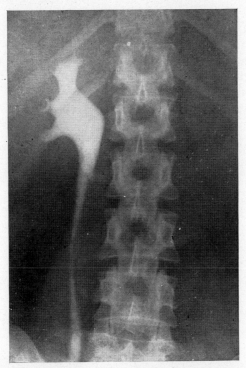

Fig. 23.—Pyelogram showing normal pelvis with a very simple arrangement of the calices, there being apparently only four minor calices. The pelvis is extrarenal. B. U. I. x-Ray 2707.

assistance. Ordinary pyelograms sometimes fail, possibly because of spasms of the renal pelvis. The same measures apply here.

Combined x-Ray and Cystoscopic Table.—Since the medium may escape from the pelvis and ureter quickly, it is important that there be no delay during pyelography. For this reason, a combined cystoscopic and x-ray table should be used. The model designed by us,[2] the first combined x-ray cystoscopic table, and which provided for stereoscopic pictures, has proved very successful. With this table, one has every convenience for cystoscopy and catheterization (Figs. 638, 639) and the x-ray can be taken immediately. In the latest

[1] Kystoskopische Technique, Berlin, 1923, 141–146.
[2] Young: Journal of Urology, 1921, v, 391–404.

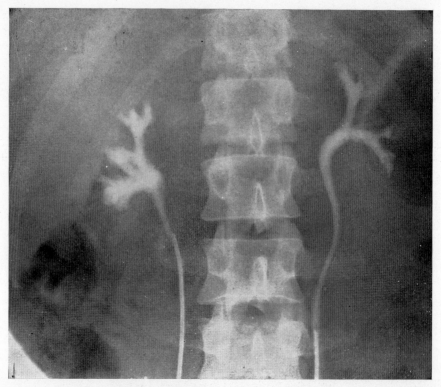

Fig. 24.—Bilateral pyelogram showing normal pelves and ureters. Note the extreme delicacy of the shadows of the tips of the minor calices. The two pelves differ considerably in shape, although the general type of each is the same. B. U. I. x-Ray 2758.

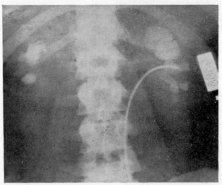

Fig. 25.—Pyelogram showing partial hydronephrosis of the left kidney. The upper calyx is very markedly dilated; the lower calices showing only slight blunting. This condition is due to a stone in the pelvis. The shadow seen in the right kidney region is caused by thorium which has partially run out and indicates moderate hydronephrosis due to a stone in the lower right ureter which does not appear in the picture. All stones were removed at two successive operations and the patient recovered completely. B. U. I. x-Ray 4566.

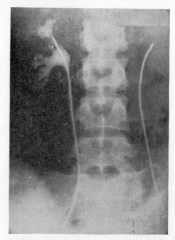

Fig. 26.—Pyelogram showing pelvis which is bifid but otherwise normal. Note the very delicate minor calices. B. U. I. x-Ray 2699.

model a special flat Bucky diaphragm has been provided, which greatly simplifies the mechanism of the combined table. The patient and plateholder are so arranged that the lower as well as the upper urinary tract can be included in the picture. There is the further advantage that the patient's head can be brought up through almost 90 degrees, so that pyelograms can be taken in both the recumbent and upright positions (Fig. 639)—the only way of determining exactly the degree of mobility of the kidney.

(This table, with the addition of kidney and perineal elevators, can be also used for any urologic operation.[1])

Stereoscopic pyelograms should be taken whenever possible. The third dimension is often of the greatest assistance in interpretation.

The *interpretation of pyelograms* requires a trained eye, and no instruction can take the place of experience. Every urologist, therefore, should take many pyelograms, and study them himself, in collaboration with someone more experienced. Where doubt exists, the subsequent course of the case will often elucidate it, and this the professional radiologist is usually unable to follow closely. The following important points in the diagnosis of hydronephrosis may be mentioned.

The earliest pyelographic sign of hydronephrosis is a *blunting of the sharp outlines of the calices* (Fig. 25). This means that the sulcus between the pyramid and the walls of the calix has been widened. Later the umbilication made in the tip of the calix by the tip of the pyramid itself is destroyed, and the calix becomes rounded or *globular*. A single normal calix, therefore, rules out a general hydronephrosis. On the other hand, there is the possibility of localized hydronephrosis resulting from obstruction of one calix from any cause, and the rather frequent occurrence of double kidney and pelvis (Fig. 25). Even where the pelvis is not frankly double, it may be elongated with a constriction at the midpoint (Fig. 26). Obstruction may occur at this midpoint, from stone or other cause, giving rise to localized hydronephrosis of approximately one-half the kidney.

Other irregularities in the contour of the pelvis are more apt to indicate neoplasm or inflammatory change, especially tuberculosis, under which headings they will be described in detail. Congenital cystic kidney (*q. v.*) has a long spidery pelvis which is almost pathognomonic (Figs. 511–513, page 28, Vol. II).

The great value of pyelography in connection with hydronephrosis is in the ability which it confers to recognize early hydronephrosis, that is, roughly speaking, below 30 c.c. This enables us to treat surgically such cases, with removal of the obstruction, before irreparable damage has been done to the secretory portion of the kidney. It is, of course, true that extensive or complete destruction of the kidney is sometimes seen in cases when the pelvic capacity lies in this range. It is usually the result of a complete obstruction, or where severe infection has been a complication. Observation of the kidney outline, as compared with that of the pelvis, and an estimation of the function, will usually clear up such cases. On certain occasions, when there is doubt about the size of the kidney, the procedure of injecting a gas, preferably oxygen, as proposed by Carelli,[2] into the perirenal tissues preliminary to a roentgenogram, may be of assistance.[3] The pictures

---

[1] Made by the Max Wocher Co. and the Liebel-Flarsheim Co., Cincinnati, Ohio.

[2] Carelli and Sordelli: Revue de l'Association Medicale, Argentina, 1921, xxxiv, 424.

[3] *Technic of Perirenal Insufflation.*—A lumbar puncture needle is inserted into the loin, with the patient lying on his side. The point is directed upward and inward toward the lower pole of the kidney. The distance to which the needle must be introduced varies, according to the thickness of the abdominal wall, from 4 to 6 cm. The path of the needle is along the outer border of the erector spinæ group of muscles, through the latissimus dorsi muscle, transversalis

obtained not only show the contour of the kidney but indicate, by the irregularities of the shadow, the presence of chronic inflammatory changes and adhesions about the kidney.

Quinby[1] has studied and utilized this method, and feels that it is of no advantage except in the occasional case where for any reason it is not possible to make a good stereoscopic pyelogram.

Pneumoperitoneum may be of assistance in taking x-rays of the kidney.[2] It may be combined with pyelography. Study of the kidney regions is greatly facilitated by placing the patient face down with supports under the symphysis and the chest.[3] This allows the intestines and abdominal wall to fall away from

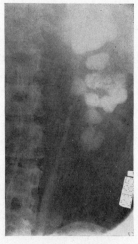

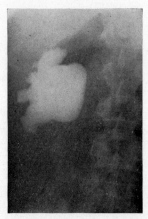

FIG. 28.—Pyelogram showing marked extrarenal hydronephrosis, evidently caused by a stricture at the ureteropelvic junction. It is possible that this may be in part congenital, since the left kidney was atrophic and secreted no phthalein, while the kidney shown was able to secrete 40 per cent. of phthalein in one-half hour. No operation was performed. B. U. I. x-Ray 1977.

FIG. 27.—Pyelogram showing very extensive intrarenal hydronephrosis due to a small stone in the pelvis. B. U. I. x-Ray 2158.

the spine, leaving a "prevertebral clear space" in which the kidney can be seen with great distinctness.

Large hydronephroses present no difficulties in the interpretation of the pyelogram. One caution, however, is to be observed. When for any reason the sac is not completely emptied at the time of catheterization, the pyelographic medium, mixing with the urine already present, may be so diluted that no visible shadow is

fascia, etc. The tip should just enter the perirenal fat, but should not touch the kidney. The gas (oxygen or carbon dioxid) is collected in a bottle, and is forced through the needle by allowing water to flow slowly into the bottle. The gas should be made to pass through a layer of sterile absorbent cotton to filter it. The pressure used should not exceed 2 feet of water. Five hundred c.c. of gas is injected. If oxygen is used, the best pictures are obtained twelve to fourteen hours after injection, with carbon dioxid somewhat sooner. When dense adhesions about the kidney are present, it is better to use smaller quantities, or perhaps omit the procedure (Quinby).

[1] Journal of Urology, 1923, ix, 13–20 (Lit.).

[2] The gas is introduced through a needle inserted in the midline below the umbilicus as in ordinary abdominal paracentesis or tapping. Complete distention is essential. The most complete aseptic precautions must be observed. The exposure is made from side to side.

[3] Sante: American Journal of Roentgenology, 1921, viii, 129–134.

thrown. Such an occurrence may lead to the mistaken diagnosis of an obliterated pelvis due to some such lesion as tumor. The ingestion or intravenous injection of sodium bromid, as recommended by Rowntree, might be of help in clearing up such a case.

The estimation of the *respective functional capacities* of the *two kidneys*, both relative and absolute, has become routine and indispensable in all cases in which the lesion is, or is suspected of being unilateral, or unequal in its effects on the two kidneys. *Phenolsuphonephthalein* is held by us to excel all other test substances for this purpose, since it gives not only the relative capacities of the two kidneys, but also an absolute indication of the capacity of each as compared to the normal. The details of the performance of this test have been described in the foregoing paragraphs on the diagnosis of the functional effects of obstruction. It is usually necessary to limit the period of collection to twenty or thirty minutes, but this may often be extended, to an hour if necessary, by withdrawing the cystoscope and leaving the catheters in place. If the patient is placed on a comfortable bed, the small catheters seldom cause annoyance. One must be sure that leakage outside the catheters does not occur, and that the flow through them is free. Here again inability to insert the catheter actually into the pelvis or incomplete emptying thereof from any cause may rise to complications. The first traces of pthalein which appear may be so diluted by the urine present, or the outflow so delayed that the appearance time as observed will be much longer than in fact. A very important quantity of phthalein-containing urine may remain in the pelvis at the end of the period of observation. Sometimes these errors cannot be eliminated, and then a knowledge of the exact or even approximate capacity of the sac will enable one to draw correct conclusions. In those rare cases where no idea of the size of the sac can be gained by any means, one must remember that the functional capacity of the kidney may be considerably greater, but never less, than that indicated by the test.

The *function of the presumably sound kidney* must be determined to make sure that it will be able to support life in case removal or further injury of the diseased kidney occurs. The compensatory hypertrophy and functional exaltation of the sound kidney are indicated by the phenolsulphonephthalein test—indeed this increase of 30 to 60 per cent. in the percentage output from the contralateral organ is very strong evidence that is is not diseased. If, on the contrary, it too shows diminished function, we are in a position, after learning the cause of this diminished function, and considering the total phthalein output,[1] to decide whether the patient is able to endure any operative procedure, and if so, whether radical or palliative measures should be adopted. When general renal functional impairment has occurred in this way, blood studies, etc., as described previously should be made. It is by careful study of such interrelations that we can avoid becoming the executioners of our very ill patients, and, by employing suitable preliminary treatment, whether operative or not, increase our percentage of cures.

The urine from a hydronephrotic kidney may often be, while abundant, considerably less concentrated than that from the other side. It is therefore of

---

[1] It is well, during the total phthalein test, to estimate also the excretion for a period, after the appearance time, equal to that employed in the divided functional test. We are then able to compare directly the excretion of each kidney with the total excretion for an identical length of time. The total should check with the sum of the divided phthaleins for an equal period.

value to compare the urines from the two sides by determination of *specific gravity* and by the *hypobromite* test. The hypobromite test has the advantages that it requires only a small quantity of urine, and is not affected by any leakage which may have occurred outside the ureteral catheter. Conclusions of value as to the function compared with normal cannot be drawn from it.

Certain further complications are introduced when it is impossible to make the catheter enter the pelvis of the kidney. This may be due to strictures at any point in the ureter, to kinks or bends, especially those produced by the growth and rotation of the hydronephrosis itself, or to impacted stones. Rotation of the sac may cause the ureter to be markedly lengthened. These cases may be further subdivided into those where the catheter will not enter the ureter at all, and those where it will ascend far enough to allow a collection of urine. The use of a wire stilet may help, but demands care to avoid wounding the ureter.

The former group of cases is one of great difficulty. A rough idea of the respective conditions of the two sides may be gained by means of meatoscopy with indigocarmin (10 c.c. of a 0.5 per cent. sol. intravenously). Functional study of the opposite kidney, especially when compared with the total, will throw light on the functional activity of the diseased side. These, with a study of the symptoms, the history, and the general physical examination, have to be relied on in such cases.

It is rare, however, that with perseverance, a catheter cannot be introduced at least part way up the ureter. In such cases, if care is taken to see that the ureteral meatus is completely occluded, to prevent backflow, preferably by a conical (the so-called "Garceau") catheter, practically all of the diagnostic measures which have been described can be carried out. It will not be necessary to repeat the descriptions of them, but the considerations concerning retention of phenol-sulphonephthalein in the sac apply with even greater force. One should be prepared moreover for difficulties arising from the fact that fluids, especially pyelographic media, introduced in such cases, may escape with difficulty or not at all. When this happens, pain is much increased, and while there is little likelihood of general intoxication with thorium nitrate, sodium bromid, or sodium iodid, it was occasionally seen with the older media, especially collargol. It is, therefore, well not to carry out these procedures in any place where operation cannot be performed promptly should it become necessary. Some authorities indeed go so far as to say that pyelograms should not be made in hydronephrosis cases until a few hours before it is planned to perform the operation. This, however, is an extreme view.

Should a pyelogram be made of the opposite kidney at the same sitting? The majority of urologists think not. Occasional attacks of severe pain and great prostration make it necessary to proceed with much caution. The importance of having pictures of both renal pelves may, however, be so great as to make simultaneous bilateral pyelography very desirable, and by taking great care not to overdistend, and to evacuate the pelvis completely, the double procedure can usually be carried out without danger. Such cases should be hospitalized if possible, or be under close observation for several hours after injection.

The further complications in the diagnosis of hydronephrosis when infection is present are fully discussed under the heading Infections of the Kidney.

Bladder.—If there is a question of bladder obstruction, the first problem is to determine the presence or absence of *infection*, and then, unless there are contraindications, the presence or absence of *residual urine*, and, if present, its quantity. If the symptoms suggest a *very large residual*, careful palpation and percussion of the suprapubic region should be made to discover an *overdistended bladder*. If such is present, it *should not be emptied by catheter*, lest complete suppression

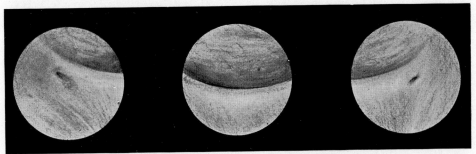

Fig. 29.—Cystoscopic views of a case of hypertrophied trigone with moderately deep pouch behind it. Ureteral orifices normal.

of urine and other serious symptoms come on. See preoperative treatment of cases of prostatic hypertrophy, and the use of the Young-Shaw *decompression apparatus*. If the bladder does not extend above the symphysis, one proceeds as follows: After the patient has voided as much as he can, a catheter is inserted, and

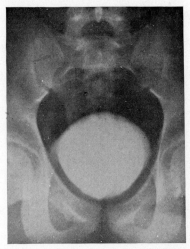

Fig. 30.—Cystogram with normal bladder. B. U. I. x-Ray 4970.

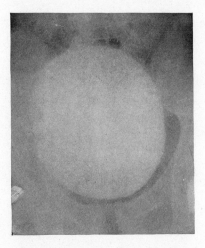

Fig. 31.—Cystogram shows the extent to which an apparently normal bladder may be distended. There is very slight irregularity of the edge of the shadow indicating a little herniation of the mucosa between the muscle bundles. Bladder function in this case was normal and the urine was clear and sterile, although the patient had previously suffered from tonsillitis and attacks of pyelitis. B. U. I. x-Ray 3531.

the residual urine removed and measured. The urine obtained is examined for infection. Since, as we have seen, the bladder capacity may be diminished in early obstructions, and much increased in the later stages, the *bladder capacity* should be determined by filling it with fluid through the catheter. The *expulsive force* is noted as the fluid flows out. These two figures give an excellent idea of the extent to which the bladder has been altered by the obstruction. If large diverticula are present, the bladder may be pushed to one side, in which case the catheter may

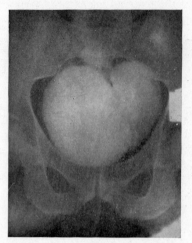

FIG. 32.—A cystogram in a case of multiple diverticula of bladder. Four diverticula can be counted in this picture. B. U. I. x-Ray 2445.

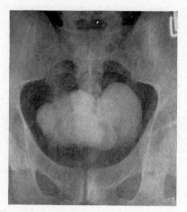

FIG. 33.—Cystogram of multiple diverticula of the bladder. Same case as previous picture. The thorium has been allowed to flow out, emptying bladder, but leaving diverticula filled   At least 6 diverticula can now be counted. B. U. I. x-Ray 2445.

be seen to deviate to the right or left of the midline. The diverticulum may not be emptied by the catheter, in which case a palpable tumor in the bladder region

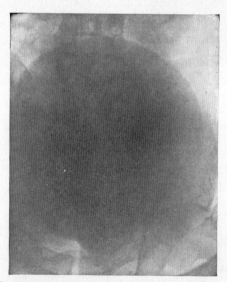

FIG. 34.—Huge single diverticulum of bladder; cystogram. This patient was unable to void; urine came out very slowly through a retention catheter on account of small and muscular diverticular orifice. B. U. I. x-Ray 3321.

will remain. Sometimes, if the catheter remains in place, the urine from the diverticulum will gradually find its way out, with disappearance of the tumor.

Certain well-founded generalizations may be made at this point. If the residual urine is not over 300 c.c., the bladder capacity 450 c.c. or less, and the expulsive force good, the bladder is still compensated, and no special measures are necessary

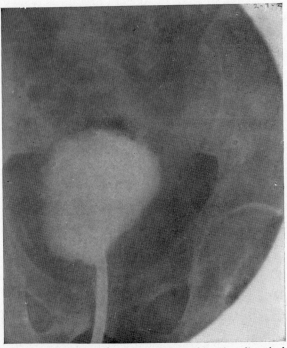

FIG. 35.—Same case as preceding picture. Cystogram taken after diverticulectomy. Trabeculation is still present, but the bladder is completely restored at the site of the diverticulum. Symptoms entirely relieved. B. U. I. x-Ray 4393.

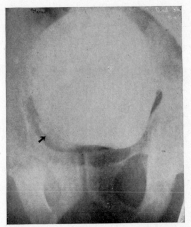

FIG. 36.—Cystogram of a large single diverticulum of the bladder. The bladder having emptied its urine into the diverticulum is collapsed and represented by the small irregular shadow indicated by the arrow. B. U. I. x-Ray 3383.

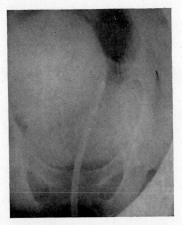

FIG. 37.—Same case as the preceding picture. Cystogram taken with both diverticulum and bladder distended with thorium. The catheter lies in the bladder proper. (This picture has been reversed in reproduction. The catheter should lie to the right side.) B. U. I. x-Ray 3387.

to fit it for its rôle after operation. A period of drainage, however, may be indicated in all cases with residual urine of 80 c.c. or over, as we have seen that in such bladders the kidneys are sometimes seriously affected. If, on the contrary, the bladder capacity is increased, the residual large, and the expulsive force poor, bladder drainage is essential to allow the organ to regain its tone before operation. Atonic bladders are easy prey to infection, and this is especially true if the urine is quite sterile with a large residual present. The course of postoperative infections in such cases is rapid and unfavorable, and they need oftentimes a prolonged

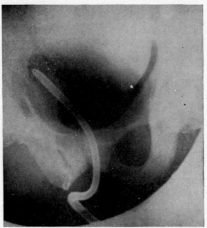

Fig. 38.—Diverticulum of the bladder. Same case as the preceding picture. The thorium has been allowed to run out of the bladder, which has then been inflated with air. The diverticulum remains full of thorium. B. U. I. x-Ray 3387.

period of drainage before they can function normally. These desiderata concerning the bladder are, of course, in addition to conclusions reached as to the state of kidney function.

The residual urine may be estimated roughly when catheterization is impossible or contraindicated by giving sodium iodid by mouth (5 gm.) and taking a roentgenogram of the bladder about four hours later, immediately after voiding.

Fig. 39.—Stereoscopic x-ray pictures of cystogram in a case of multiple vesical diverticula. B. U. I. x-Ray 5599.

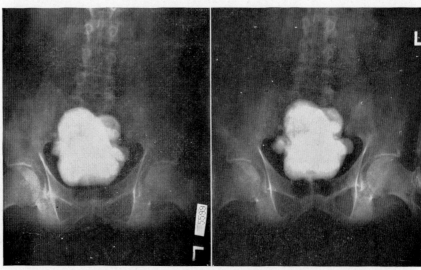

As shown in the following section on treatment, it is often advisable not to empty the bladder completely, but to decompress it gradually by means of suitable apparatus. In these cases, selected according to the presence of a palpable bladder or increased vesical flatness to percussion above the symphysis, the measurement

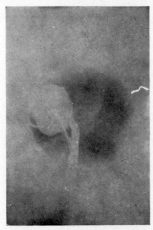

FIG. 40.—Diverticulogram obtained by filling a single diverticulum independently by a catheter placed in its orifice. A second catheter can be seen in the right ureter. B. U. I. x-Ray 2081.

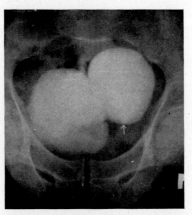

FIG. 41.—Cystogram of diverticulum of the bladder. The bladder is pushed to the right side by the diverticulum. The arrow points to the shadow of a stone in the lower end of the left ureter which was only disclosed after operation. (See Fig. 42.) B. U. I. 9808.

of the residual is omitted, and cystoscopy and phthalein tests deferred until after decompression is accomplished.

Cystoscopy, which is necessary also in determining the nature of the obstructing lesion, is utilized to confirm the conclusions already drawn after catheteriza-

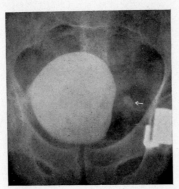

FIG. 42.—Same case as the preceding picture. Cystogram taken after complete excision of the diverticulum. The stone indicated by the arrow and lying in the lower end of the left ureter was not suspected until this picture was taken. The clean-cut bladder shadow shows a perfect result after diverticulectomy. B. U. I. x-Ray 3195.

tion, and to determine trabeculation, diverticula, cystitis, etc. One notes the thickness of the muscle bundles and the size and depth of the depressions between them. *Trabeculation* often gives early evidence of obstruction, and may be seen when there is no residual urine. It may not involve the entire bladder, and usually begins and is most conspicuous on the posterior wall immediately behind the inter-

ureteric ligament.   The irrigating channel of the cystoscope should be attached to a
reservoir about 4 feet above the patient, so that the quantity of fluid in the
bladder can be varied as desired.   This often serves to bring out trabeculation and

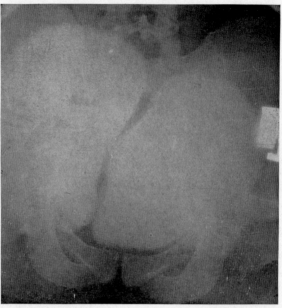

FIG. 43.—Cystogram showing two enormous diverticula of the bladder.   These were successfully removed at operation.   B. U. I. x-Ray 2759.

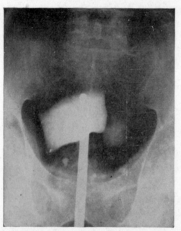

FIG. 44.—x-Ray taken in a case of multiple
vesical diverticula.   The bladder is filled with
thorium and its distortion by the diverticula
which lie around it is well shown.   To the left
side of the bladder a cloud of thorium can be seen
just beginning to enter one of the large diverticula
and mix with its contents.   B. U. I. x-Ray 2409.

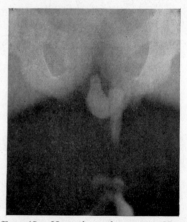

FIG. 45.—Normal urethrogram.   Note the
considerable distention of which the bulbous
urethra is capable and the sharp line of demarcation at the closed external sphincter or cut-off
muscle.   B. U. I. x-Ray 4183.

other lesions to the best advantage, and should not be omitted.   It is easy to mis-
interpret cystoscopic pictures if the bladder is improperly filled.

Hypertrophy of the trigone is another important sign of obstruction.   Since the

PLATE III

VESICAL TRABECULATION, CELLULES, AND DIVERTICULUM FORMATION

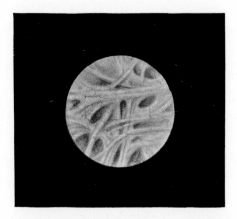

A. Marked trabeculation of bladder caused by prostatic obstruction. Numerous small cellules. B. U. I. 12,806.

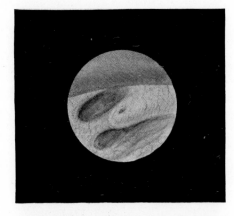

B. Cellules external to ureter in hypertrophied ridge behind median bar (inverted view). B. U. I. 12,806.

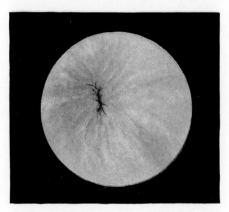

C. Very small orifice of a large vesical diverticulum. B. U. I. 7613.

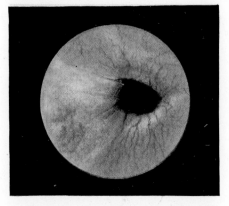

D. Large diverticulum into which the ureteral ridge, ureter, and left corner of trigone have been drawn. B. U. I. 1261.

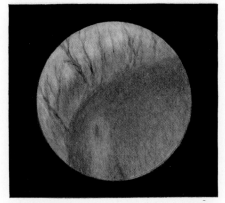

E. Interior of diverticulum D, ureteral ridge and orifice seen in diverticular cavity, edge of which is shown.

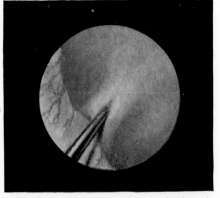

F. Same case (D and E). Catheterization of ureteral orifice within the diverticulum.

trigonal muscle is a firm pad and is not composed of interlacing bundles, it is never trabeculated. This hypertrophy (Fig. 29) is, as we pointed out, due to the increased work which the trigonal muscle is required to do when the median portion of the prostate becomes enlarged, and thus renders the orifice more difficult to pull open. If the mucosa of the trigone is inflamed, edema may account for part of the enlargement observed.

Small *diverticula* and cellules can be discovered only by cystoscopic examination. The orifices may be open and the interior visible or they may appear as round or oval black spots, since the light does not illuminate the interior. Blood-clots may simulate this picture, and investigation with a ureteral catheter or bougie will clear up any uncertainty, as well as enable one to gage the depth of the diverticulum.

It is often possible, by manipulating the cystoscope, to introduce its beak into larger diverticula. One can then see the size of the diverticulum, estimate the degree of infection present, discover stones or neoplasms lying within it, or find whether a ureteral orifice opens into it. In certain cases of large diverticula with comparatively small orifices in which the bladder is contracted and irritable, it may not be possible to discover the diverticular orifice.

The entire bladder should be studied and notes or diagrams made of the location of each diverticulum.

x-Ray cystograms made by filling the bladder with an opaque medium are valuable aids. The outline of a trabeculated bladder is characteristically irregular and shaggy (Fig. 35). Diverticula and cellules are seen as rounded projections (Fig. 32 *et seq.*). If the diverticulum is large and the bladder contracted, an opaque instrument passed into the bladder will help greatly in identifying the bladder proper (Figs. 37, 38), and the value of all these pictures is enhanced if they are taken stereoscopically (Fig. 39). Individual diverticula may be filled separately by introducing a ureteral catheter in the orifice. If the opaque medium is colored with a dye, one can by watching through the cystoscope determine the exact moment at which the diverticulum is completely filled, and the fluid starts to run out into the bladder. Beautiful pictures of single diverticula may be made in this way (Fig. 40). One may also allow the medium to flow out of the bladder, and then refill it with air. If the diverticula do not empty, beautiful "contrast" pictures result (Fig. 38). Cystography is particularly useful in women.

The presence of encysted calculi will be shown by the *x*-ray.

General physical examination will disclose the tumors due to distended bladders or large diverticula, and tense bladders may often be palpated by rectal examination. If catheterization is impossible, we must rely on these examinations, together with the general condition and studies of the blood. In such cases cystostomy or perineal urethrotomy will usually be in order, and the condition of the bladder can be determined at that time.

Urethra.—*Dilatation of the urethra* from obstruction is of great importance in cases of valves or diaphragms of the prostatic urethra. A cystogram in these cases shows a short thick projection of the shadow for a short distance into the prostatic urethra (Fig. 569). Other pouches or diverticula may be diagnosed by endoscopic or urethroscopic examination after passing the obstruction, or by filling the urethra with opaque medium and taking a urethrogram (Fig. 45).

The lesions producing obstructive uropathy, stones, strictures, tumors, prostatic hypertrophy, etc., are discussed at length under appropriate chapters.

TREATMENT

It will be seen that urinary obstructions, regardless of their nature, have certain well-defined and important injurious effects on all portions of the urinary tract lying above them. The treatment of the obstructive uropathy, therefore, has two aims in view: first, by proper permanent drainage, to allow all affected parts of the urinary tract to return as nearly as possible to normal before embarking upon serious operative measures, and, second, the removal of the obstruction. The exception to this rule is where the obstruction is unilateral and supravesical, and there is conclusive evidence that the opposite kidney has assumed, or is capable of assuming, the entire function. One may then proceed at once to operative treatment.

Kidney.—The treatment is always based on two simple principles: first, *relief of the obstruction*, which should be, if possible, *non-operative* until the renal function has reached its optimum level; and second, assistance of kidney function by the copious *administration of fluids*.

The routine study during treatment of cases of functional impairment of the kidney due to urinary obstruction is best carried out by repeated determination of the *blood urea* and of the *phenolsulphonephthalein* excretion, reserving the other tests for extreme or atypical cases.

Where the damage to the kidneys is entirely of the transitory kind due to obstruction, the function as shown by the two above-mentioned tests will promptly return to normal after drainage is established. Where permanent damage to the kidney has occurred, as the result of infection, hydronephrosis, or from a concurrent Bright's disease, the function will often improve to a certain *optimum point*, beyond which there will be no further change. This point can only be determined by frequently repeated tests (our routine is twice a week) since it may be reached in a few days or delayed for periods up to four or five months.

Where obtructions have existed for some time, the phthalein excretion may be reduced to zero, and the blood urea raised to four or five times the normal figure. With free drainage and the generous exhibition of water, a rapid change for the better is usually seen, with rise of the phthalein and fall of the blood urea. The blood urea usually reaches normal before the phthalein, and it is quite usual to see a patient with a permanently reduced phthalein, such as for example 30 per cent. in two hours, with a normal blood urea. On the other hand, an elevated blood urea in a patient with normal phthalein is rare, and usually leads one to suspect the accuracy of the tests. It may occur just after an obstruction has been relieved, but is transitory.

We are accustomed to feel that when, in an individual over fifty years of age, the blood urea has fallen below 0.45 gm. per liter, the phthalein appearance time is not over ten minutes, and the total excretion for two hours not under 45 per cent., with the greater part appearing in the first hour, the condition is good, and the operative risk, cæteris paribus, excellent. If, however, renal function reaches its optimum level before these figures are attained, operation is by no means contraindicated. It is undoubtedly true that free drainage and ingestion of water do much to stabilize the kidney function even when restitution to normal, in terms of laboratory findings, is impossible. It is, therefore, always wise, in case of doubt, to drain a few days longer. We have never seen harm follow this procedure, whereas tragic results often follow in cases operated on too precipitately. It has occurred, however, that patients who, after a long period of drainage, have shown blood urea still slightly elevated (for example 0.65 gm. per liter) and a phthalein excretion of only 15 per cent. in two hours, with appearance time of twenty-five or more minutes, have been operated upon with splendid results. Strangely enough such cases sometimes show further functional improvement after surgical removal of the obstruction, to points which were unattainable with catheter or suprapubic drainage. It is probable that this has to do with the subsidence of infection in the absence of foreign bodies or wounds in the bladder. This class of cases, however, cannot be called free of risk, and the surgeon should hesitate unless the condition is such that life without the operation offers no prospect of comfort. With a prolonged preoperative period of drainage in these cases of prostatic hypertrophy with impaired renal function, a very fair chance of success can be offered them, and, in fact, practically every such case at the Brady Institute comes, eventually, to prostatectomy.

The following case is an excellent illustration of recovery of renal function under continuous drainage:

B. U. I. 10,541, age fifty-nine, March 15, 1922. History essentially negative, denies venereal disease. Frequency for three years. Difficulty for six weeks. "Incontinence" while asleep. No hematuria. Weakness, fatigue and mental haziness for one month. Examination showed moderate prostatic hypertrophy, with residual urine of 800 c.c. The urine was infected, containing bacilli and cocci. The phthalein was only a trace in two hours, the blood urea 1.35 gm. per liter, non-protein nitrogen 86.4 mgm. per 100 c.c., creatinin 7.9 mgm. per 100 c.c., blood-pressure 168/98. Constant drainage and force water were continued until May 8, 1922 (seven weeks). The laboratory findings were:

TABLE 8

		March 17th.	March 18th.	March 21st.	March 25th.	March 30th.	April 5th.	April 10th.	April 18th.	April 24th.	April 28th.	May 2d.	May 5th.	May 8th.
Phthalein	App. min......	....	....	....	....	....	....	85	....	115				
	First hour.....	....	....	....	....	....	....	6	....	8				Operation.
	Second hour...	....	....	....	....	....	....	4	....	7				
	Total.........	Trace.	....	Trace.	3%	Trace.	Trace.	10%	....	15%				
Blood urea........		1.38	1.20	....	0.86	0.75	0.58	0.45	0.53	0.56				
Blood N. P. N.....		86.4	....	66.7	61.2	74.9	60.0	48.8	....	57.2	45.4	50.8	48.8	
Blood creatinin....		7.9	....	3.3	3.5	3.1	....	2.2	....	2.5	2.6	3.1	2.8	
Blood CO$_2$........		....	....	....	46.4	39.9	44.8							

During this time the patient had three severe febrile attacks, undoubtedly due to renal infection. In view of the extremely poor renal function, efforts were made to accustom the patient to a catheter life, but these efforts precipitated the attacks. Since it was apparently impossible for the patient to have the slightest comfort, it was finally decided to operate, with the full approbation of the patient, in spite of the risks. Perineal prostatectomy May 8, 1922. The operation and convalescence were rapid and uneventful. The fistula closed in nine days. At the time of discharge the patient felt well, and voided freely and without pain every three hours in the day, and every four hours at night. Most noteworthy of all, the renal function showed a further improvement which it had not been possible to attain with artificial drainage; namely, phthalein, appearance forty minutes, first hour 13, second hour 8, total 21 per cent.; blood urea 0.62. The urine was infected, but the number of organisms and the amount of pus were very small.

In certain cases usually characterized by *dilated bladder* and *large residual urine*, with a certain degree of hydro-ureter there are grounds to believe that the kidney,

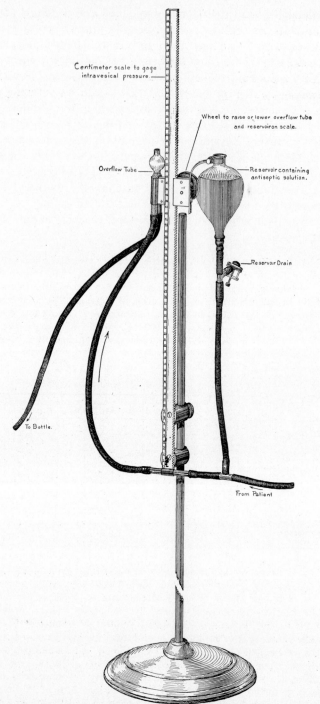

Centimeter scale to gage
intravesical pressure

Wheel to raise or lower overflow tube
and reservoir on scale.

Overflow Tube

Reservoir containing
antiseptic solution.

Reservoir Drain

To Bottle.

From Patient

FIG. 46.—Young-Shaw irrigating decompressor for bladder drainage.   Tube from patient is placed on a level with base of bladder.   Vesical tension is obtained by raising overflow tube until urine ceases to escape.   Height noted on centimeter scale.   Subsequent gradual lowering as described in text.

having functioned for some time against constantly increased pressure, is unfavorably influenced by a *too sudden release* of this pressure.   This question has been recently thoroughly studied by Shaw and Young,[1] with observations of normal and pathologic intravesical pressure and kidney function, with and without gradual diminution in the pressure. They feel that in such cases it is undoubtedly safer to reduce the pressure slowly, that renal function improves more rapidly, and in addition that acute ascending infections are less liable to occur. Certain unfavorable results of sudden release of urinary pressure are avoided, as shown in the following excerpt from the conclusions of their article:

In the majority of cases of chronic urinary obstruction with a residual urine of over 400 c.c., immediate and continuous bladder drainage is followed by a more or less severe reaction.

The reaction may be predominantly *renal, circulatory,* or *nervous,* but usually there are symptoms referable to all three systems.

The reaction in the *urinary tract* is the most constant, and is shown by bleeding from the bladder and kidneys; the appearance of albumin and casts in the urine, and frequently by an abrupt fall in the renal function as shown by the phthalein test and blood chemistry studies. All these symptoms may be present without any change in the blood-pressure.

The *circulatory* reaction consists mostly of a fall in blood-pressure.

Mild *nervous* and mental symptoms frequently follow sudden drainage of the overdistended bladder. These consist of irritability, lethargy, memory disturbance, and a tendency toward flighty speech. A few cases become violently delirious. These symptoms may occur without any changes in the blood chemistry.

By gradually reducing the bladder pressure the reaction can be avoided in most cases.

The apparatus which we now use is illustrated in Fig. 46. It includes an overflow tube which can easily be set, by means of a rack and pinion, at any desired height above the level of the bladder, and a reservoir arranged so that it moves up and down always on the same level as the overflow tube. An equally efficient but less convenient apparatus can be improvised with an irrigation bottle, two Y-tubes, a glass connecting tube, a few feet of rubber tubing, and an ordinary pole standard.

The method of procedure is as follows: The apparatus, after being sterilized by boiling and attached to the metal stand, is filled with a mild antiseptic solution. The intake tube and the tube leading from the reservoir are then clamped. The base line of the scale is set at the level of the base of the bladder and the cross-bar raised well above the anticipated bladder pressure. A soft-rubber catheter is passed into the bladder and connected with the intake tube without allowing any urine to escape. The clamp on the intake tube is then removed and after allowing several minutes for the bladder to become accustomed to the catheter, the intravesical pressure is read by lowering the cross-bar to a point where overflow occurs. Following this the clamp is removed from the tube leading from the reservoir.

The reservoir serves a double purpose. Primarily, it prevents fluctuations in the intravesical tension. The unco-operative and irrational patient is frequently changing posture and making straining movements that cause the overflow of a large quantity of urine. If no reservoir is attached, the relaxation following straining may be accompanied by a considerable sudden fall in pressure. The presence of a reservoir renders this impossible, as the slightest fall below the overflow level is accompanied by a flow of fluid from the reservoir into the bladder. The next bladder contraction must refill the reservoir before overflow occurs.

It has been found that with a catheter in place, the bladder undergoes periodic, automatic contractions, which are not perceptible to the patient, every thirty

[1] Journal of Urology, 1924, xi, 373–394.

minutes or so.   Unless the reservoir is present, so that its contents can flow back into the bladder when it relaxes, the pressure will fall markedly at that time.   The reservoir, therefore, not only maintains a constant pressure, but makes possible an automatic irrigation of the bladder, which occurs every time there is a periodic bladder contraction, and every time a little urine is squeezed out of the bladder by direct pressure or by the movements of the patient.   The reservoir should be drained and refilled—clamping its outflow tube during the process—about every six hours with meroxyl solution, 1:1000.   This keeps an effective concentration constantly in the bladder, and the effect thereof in preventing or controlling infection is most gratifying.   In 2 cases it has actually been possible to eliminate

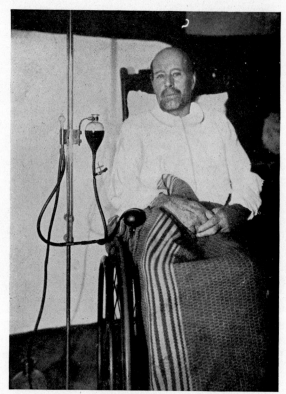

FIG. 47.—Young-Shaw irrigating decompression apparatus. Connected with catheter in urethra, reservoir filled with 1:200 meroxyl.

infection present at the time of admission, while in others which were not cured the bacterial count of the urine was markedly reduced.   Of 10 patients admitted with sterile urine, 7 were brought through the preparatory period to operation without any infection—an average of thirteen days each with a retained catheter.   This is an achievement which, we believe, is without precedent.

The rapidity with which the bladder pressure can be safely reduced depends in part upon the tone of the bladder musculature.   When the apparatus is first attached and the overflow level set at the initial intravesical pressure, the bladder will usually contract down to two-thirds its original size within twenty-four hours. The overflow level should not be lowered as long as the bladder continues to decrease in size, as shown by palpation and percussion.   In most cases it is safe to begin lowering the pressure at the end of twenty-four hours. Unless the patient is unusually obese, the outlines of the distended bladder can be fairly accurately determined by palpation and percussion. After the first twenty-four hours, the overflow can be lowered 2.5 cm. during each twelve-hour period. Should the urine at any time become blood-stained, the pressure should not be changed until it again becomes clear. When the pressure has been reduced to 15 cm. the bladder usually contains less than 200 c.c. and the danger of a reaction is past; but by continuing the use of the apparatus with the overflow set at this low level, the complications from urinary infection are materially reduced.

The patient is not confined to bed, but is urged to get up in a wheel chair. The apparatus can be moved about with him, and after adjustment to the new position, stands on the floor beside the chair (Fig. 47).

Along with free drainage, *water* should be given in *large amounts*. The only precautions to be observed are in regard to circulatory complications and edema. In persons with marked myocardial insufficiency or valvular disease, one must avoid overloading the vascular system with water.

The heart must be watched for signs of fibrillation, beginning dilatation, etc. Modern standards in the treatment of cardiac disease do not allow the indiscriminate digitalization formerly practised. The urologist should not treat cardiac complications unless he has made himself thoroughly competent in this field, and has preferably an electrocardiographic apparatus at his disposal. Certain forms of irregularity and the so-called "essential hypertension" require no treatment, while quinidine in fibrillation, or properly given digitalis in myocardial failure, are often essential to success, and may enable one to carry through preliminary and operative treatment in apparently desperate cases. If the circulation is embarrassed, or the excretion of water insufficient, as in kidneys with much permanent damage, edema will occur if much water is given. In these cases the circulation is to be helped, if possible, by appropriate treatment. Otherwise it is unavoidable that the water be cut down to a quantity which can be handled, although the existence of a moderate edema is in itself not harmful, provided it does not increase. With these few precautions in mind, one gives *as much water as possible*. Often much tact and diplomacy are necessary to prevail upon the patients to drink the requisite quantity, and there should be no hesitation, in case the patient cannot, for any reason, drink enough, to administer fluid by *subcutaneous infusion*. Where rapid effects are desired, *intravenous infusions* of salt solution may be given, and it has recently been suggested that, especially in cases with vomiting, the duodenal tube may be used for administration of fluid. Physiologic experiments show that the excretion of water requires no additional oxidation in the kidney, and throws no strain upon it, while the secretion of a dilute urine enables the kidney to excrete actually greater quantities of urinary constituents, in a given time, than when the urine is concentrated. In addition, recent researches show the prime importance of a plentiful supply of water for all the metabolic processes of the body, and one should remember that patients with urinary obstruction are often dehydrated when first seen on account of drinking as little as possible, to avoid frequent urination. By giving water, therefore, the kidney is greatly aided in its work of excretion. The ideal daily intake of fluid in these cases is considered to be *5000 c.c.*, but we always try to exceed this if possible. The absolute minimum, except in cases of circulatory complications, should be

4000 c.c. per day, while surprising and dramatic improvements have not infrequently been seen in uremic cases, where 10, 12, or even 15 liters have been given, by all routes, in twenty-four hours.

The most important advances in modern urology, which have changed its death rate from very high to very low, have been made possible by the recognition and proper treatment of the obstructive nephropathy. When the embarrassed kidney is enabled, by the intelligent application of rational diagnostic and therapeutic principles, which are now available, and which have been outlined above, to regain its optimum excretory power, extensive operative procedures may be carried out with an almost complete assurance of success. The urologist, to attain the highest standard in his work, must give the closest attention to these phases of his specialty. The fate of the patient is decided much more, at the present time, by the care and skill displayed in the ward before operation, than it is in the operating room itself.

The treatment of great hydronephrosis is usually eventually operative. It has one of two objects: (1) The removal of the obstruction; or (2) in case the kidney is so extensively destroyed that it is of no further value, or in case it is impossible to remove the obstruction, the removal of the kidney.

OPERATIVE TREATMENT.—The relief of obstruction often requires operations which vary according to the site and character of the lesion. Among the infravesical obstructions, the most common are for stricture of the urethra, prostatic obstruction, abscesses, and calculi.

Stricture of the urethra may respond to gradual dilatation with filiforms, followers, or sounds, but may also require urethrotomy, either the open or perineal, or the internal performed with a urethrotome. These procedures are described elsewhere. (See Chapter III on Infections for non-operative treatment.)

Prostatic obstruction may be of several types. The most common is that due to prostatic hypertrophy which is best treated (eventually) by "prostatectomy," either perineal (which we prefer) or suprapubic. Next in frequency come contractures or bars at the vesical orifice which may be cured by operative excision with our "punch," or division with the Bottini electrocautery. These instruments operate through the urethra. Open operations, suprapubic cystostomy through which the bar may be excised or divided, or perineal urethrotomy with division of the prostatic bar either with a Chetwood cautery incisor, or simple division with a knife may also be carried out. Our preference is the "punch operation," with or without the cautery blade. (See Chapter VII, where all prostatic obstructions except carcinoma are discussed.)

Congenital valves or *diaphragms* which may lead to tremendous dilatation of the ureters and kidneys, and are particularly seen in infancy, may be removed either by a small punch instrument, by open operation, suprapubic or perineal, or by fulguration.

Impacted calculi of the urethra, if only partially obstructing, may remain for years and lead to great dilatation and destruction above, which may be cured by their removal. (See Chapter VI on Urolithiasis.)

Intravesical obstruction to the ureters may be produced by a large vesical calculus, tumors, ulcers, inflammatory cicatrices, intramural stricture of the ureter, impacted calculus, and vesical diverticula. Each of these conditions requires individual operative treatment, described elsewhere.

Supravesical obstruction, due to stricture of the ureter, may sometimes be cured by dilation with ureteral bougies through a cystoscope. When due to adhesions to surrounding structures (e. g., seminal vesicle or vas, or ovary or tube) open operative relief with freeing of the inflammatory adhesions or excision of the inflamed organ (tube, ovary) may be sufficient. Not infrequently such cases are best treated by nephrectomy—especially if the kidney is badly impaired or infected.

Removal of *tumors* pressing upon the ureters is, of course, indicated.

Obstruction of the ureter due to kinking or torsion is generally relieved by fixation of the movable kidney, which usually accompanies it. One usually finds bands of fascia, adhesions or blood-vessels, over which the ureter is hooked or kinked, which can be easily divided, with a cure of the condition. In our own series of hydronephroses, there is no case due to nephroptosis alone; the condition is complicated by aberrant vessels or bands of adhesions in every case.

Numerous operations have been recommended for the various abnormalities of the ureter at its juncture with the renal pelvis, the object of which is to provide free drainage from the lowermost part of the pelvis. These plastics will be described elsewhere.

In hydronephrosis, not infrequently the destruction of the kidney substance, especially in the presence of infection, demands nephrectomy. This can best be determined by a careful study of the functional efficiency of the kidney, and comparing it with that of its sound fellow.

Pyelotomy or nephrolithotomy will remove an obstructive calculus of the pelvis or calix and allow regeneration of the kidney. In some cases resection of a concomitant badly diseased pole of the kidney may be preferable as insuring against recurrences, as advised by us.[1]

Localized cystic processes in the kidney, due to duct obstruction, may be excised, but the destruction of the kidney has generally been great, or the cyst so large that nephrectomy has usually been carried out.

In the case of *double kidney* with bifid pelvis and ureter accompanied by dilation of one-half of the kidney, excision of the diseased portion may be carried out. This is particularly true where a large calculus with abscess is present, as in our reported case.[2]

Résumé.—In the obstructive uropathy, wherever manifested, the problem is to remove the obstruction and restore the urinary organs above to normal. As pointed out the kidneys may be so greatly impaired by long-continued back-pressure as to make immediate operative removal of the obstruction dangerous (uremia, suppression, or complete anuria not infrequently ensuing). Some form of gradual decompression is, therefore, necessary, active urinary secretion being at the same time encouraged by taking large amounts of water, When semiweekly phthalein tests, accompanied, if low, by blood-urea estimations, show sufficient improvement and stabilization of the renal function, operation to remove the obstruction, whether prostate, stricture, valve, bar, or stone may be safely carried out.

Infection is most often a serious complication and requires careful attention before and after operation. The urologist should not be satisfied with the result or consider the patient cured until all the urinary organs are restored as nearly as possible to normal. This goal may require most careful treatment for a prolonged postoperative period.

[1] Young: Surgery, Gynecology, and Obstetrics, 1924, xxxviii, 107–111.
[2] Young and Davis, E. G.: Journal of Urology, 1917, i, 17–57.

The following table indicates the results obtained in our series of cases of hydronephrosis, according to the operation employed. Note how much more serious the condition is when bilateral.

TABLE 9

HYDRONEPHROSIS: RESULTS OF TREATMENT

Form of treatment.	Total.	Well.	Im-proved.	Unim-proved.	Died.	No record.
II. Bilateral; supravesical obstruction:						
Nephrectomy.............................	2		1		1	
Nephro- and ureterolithotomy.............	5		4		1	
Plastic operations........................	1		1			
Dilation of ureter........................	6		4	2		
Nephropexy..............................	1	1				
No treatment............................	4			1	2	1
Nephrostomy.............................	2		1		1	
Total, bilateral; supravesical obstruction..	21	1	11	3	5	1
III. Unilateral; supravesical obstruction:						
Nephrectomy.............................	45	27	13		3	2
Division of adhesions.....................	2	1	1			
Nephro- and ureterolithotomy.............	11	6	5			
Plastic operations........................	2	1	1			
Dilation of ureter........................	5		4	1		
Nephropexy..............................	1	1				
Nephrostomy.............................	2				2	
No treatment............................	8	2[1]		1	5	
Total, unilateral; supravesical obstruction.	76	38	24	2	10	2

Of the 97 cases due to supravesical obstruction, 74 were treated by operation, of which 37 are well, 27 improved, 1 unimproved, 8 dead, 1 no report.

II. Death rate in treated cases, bilateral; supravesical obstruction, 17.6 per cent.

III. Death rate in treated cases, unilateral; supravesical obstruction, 7.4 per cent.

The following analysis of the 8 cases with fatal result after operation listed in Table 9 is of interest:

II. Bilateral; supravesical obstruction.

B. U. I. 4375. Ureteral calculus on one side, ureteral stricture on other side; nephrectomy; died in hospital; autopsy showed extensive carcinoma of intestine.

B. U. I. 8471. Renal calculus on one side, ureteral stricture on other side; first operation, plastic on ureter, which failed to relieve obstruction. Second operation nephrolithotomy, which removed the renal calculus, but following which ureteral obstruction developed on this side also; third operation nephrostomy; died in hospital of uremia. This patient was in very bad condition before treatment was started.

B. U. I. 10,579. Renal calculus on one side, ureteral calculus on other side; ureterolithotomy; died in hospital; autopsy showed carcinoma of adrenal with metastases.

III. Unilateral; supravesical obstruction.

B. U. I. 352. Renal tuberculosis with tuberculous stricture of ureter; nephro-ureterectomy; good operative result; died some time later of tuberculosis.

B. U. I. 8331. Obstruction of ureter due to tumor, probably of pancreas; nephrectomy; died in hospital about a month later from effects of tumor, no autopsy.

B. U. I. 9699. Renal calculus, pyonephrosis; nephrectomy; died in hospital three hours after operation, cause not stated, no autopsy.

[1] Passed ureteral calculi spontaneously.

B. U. I. 9779. Ureteral stricture; nephrostomy; died in hospital, postoperative hemorrhage and septicemia, autopsy.

B. U. I. 10,767. Ectopic kidney, stricture of ureter, pyonephrosis, other kidney also infected; nephrostomy; died in hospital of uremia, autopsy.

Of the 3 cases of bilateral hydronephrosis it will be noted that 2 had malignant tumors of other organs, which were important factors in the fatal outcome. The third was a very difficult case, in bad condition from infection and impaired renal function before treatment began. Of the cases of unilateral hydronephrosis, 1 died of a malignant tumor of another organ, and 1 of tuberculosis. Of the 3 remaining cases, 1 apparently died of operative shock, while the other 2 succumbed to the effects of intercurrent infection. Of the 12 cases in the table which received no operative treatment, 7, or 58 per cent., are known to be dead.

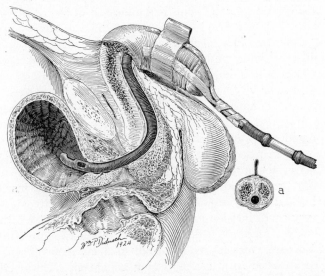

Fig. 48.—Diagram of retention catheter in place. A second fenestra is cut at the tip. The catheter is fastened closely to the glans with adhesive plaster strips. The strips are retained on the penis by a circular band. The expansion "pleat" allows for erections, thus preventing constriction. With redundant prepuce it is strongly drawn down over glans before placing adhesive strips.

Bladder.—The treatment of the bladder of obstruction is usually secondary to that directed at the kidneys. By the time permanent drainage has restored the kidney function to its optimum, the bladder will usually have regained its tone. With large residual urine and dilated bladder, a lengthy period of drainage is necessary, even if the renal function is fairly good. Since such bladders when uninfected usually become the seat of severe infections after operation, often with pyelitis or pyelonephritis consequent upon the dilated and presumably atonic ureters, it was formerly believed by many that the infection following the use of a retained catheter was an advantage. This was ascribed to the development of an immunity. It has been shown, however, that if the intravesical pressure be lowered gradually in such cases by the use of suitable apparatus, which allows also the frequent introduction of germicides, such as meroxyl, the bladder can contract to normal dimensions without becoming infected. Subsequent operation is then quite as safe as in cases without decompensated bladders. This gradual deflation of the bladder is accomplished by the apparatus already described on page 74, where it is fully discussed.

The restoration of the functions of the bladder and ureters to normal before operation is almost or quite as important as that of the kidney function from the point of view of the patient's general welfare. If it can be done without infection, many dangers are avoided, both immediate, to the patient's life, and remote, to the integrity of his kidneys.

The secret of the successful use of the *retained catheter* are: 1, Selection of the proper size catheter; 2, skilful introduction; 3, careful adjustment so that the flow is free at all times; 4, irrigation twice daily; and 5, change of catheter every three or four days. The accompanying diagram (Fig. 48) illustrates the method of attaching the catheter, the proper depth of insertion, and the second window, which should always be cut in the end. The application of adhesive directly to the glans is usually well tolerated, and is the method of choice, since the catheter may slip in and out if attached to the prepuce. The possibility of the accurate regulation in this manner of bladder pressure, and the greater comfort to the patient, make the retained catheter the best method for permanent drainage. In certain cases, however, where it is impossible or very difficult to catheterize, where the catheter causes pain, or where intractable infections, leading to pyelitis, epididymitis, or peri-urethral inflammations, are present, it may become necessary to perform *cystostomy* for drainage. This may be done in several ways. Some surgeons puncture the bladder suprapubically, inserting a small catheter through the cannula and leaving it in place. The more common method is to perform a simple open suprapubic cystostomy and at the same time examine the interior of the bladder and the prostatic enlargement. A drainage-tube is inserted and the bladder wound closed tightly around it. A second method is to expose the bladder wall, make a very small incision and quickly insert a de Pezzer catheter without allowing the bladder to become deflated. The latter two procedures have the advantage that the intravesical pressure is not suddenly removed and the drainage catheter can be attached to a decompressing apparatus. The operative technic is described elsewhere. We have personally always employed the open operation, as it is safer to see what you are doing.

OPERATIVE TREATMENT.—If important *anatomic changes* have occurred (hypertrophied trigone, diverticulum), it may be necessary to intervene surgically. The guiding principle is, however, to remove the obstruction first and operate on the bladder lesions only when necessary, as they may disappear after the obstruction is removed.

Hypertrophy of the trigone requires no treatment unless it has reached such size that it constitutes itself an obstruction, which will continue to operate as such after the primary obstruction is removed. It may then be divided with a punch instrument (dangerous—extravasation), or, preferably, with the scalpel after opening the bladder from above. These operations are described in Chapter XVI.

Diverticula, unless very small, will not disappear spontaneously after removal of the obstruction. If they cause no serious symptoms, and if they do not keep up a troublesome cystitis, they may be left alone. Usually, however, operation is necessary. It should include complete excision of the diverticula. It is often done subsequent to the removal of the obstruction (prostatic hypertrophy, stricture, etc.), but if the patient is in good condition, diverticulectomy may be done at the same time the obstruction is removed. This is more often possible in younger individuals with diverticula resulting from contracture of the vesical orifice, which is excised with scalpel or punch at the same time. Occasionally diverticula may be excised, in cases due to prostatic hypertrophy, leaving the prostatectomy for a second-stage operation, through the fistula (which, of course, will not close until the obstruction is removed).

Urethra.—Beyond the removal of the obstruction itself, no treatment is usually required to correct its effects in the urethra.

CHAPTER III

UROGENITAL INFECTIONS AND INFESTATIONS: GENERAL

MODES OF INFECTION

INFECTION may reach the urogenital tract through the blood-stream, from foci elsewhere in the body, or, directly from the outside, by introduction through the natural channels, by extension or ulceration from neighboring organs, or by a traumatic opening, as a surgical incision or a wound. Within the tract itself, however, infection may spread from one region to another by the lymphatics, through the intermediary of the general blood circulation, by direct extension, or through the lumina of the various ducts.

PATH OF INFECTION IN REACHING THE UROGENITAL TRACT

Direct Implantation.—*By Contact.*—Contact infection may occur without instrumentation, and this is the source of most veneral infections and of other spontaneous urogenital infections not arriving through the blood. The character and extent of the lesion, and its tendency to spread vary with the causative organism.

Urethral Implantation.—In this form of infection the organisms are introduced directly through the urethra into the bladder, usually by an instrument. Experience shows that it is almost impossible to carry out repeated catheterization more than a few times without urinary infection even with thorough aseptic and antiseptic precautions. Organisms exist in the outer portion of the urethra in normal individuals, and are carried into the bladder by the catheter. The most common bacteria of the anterior urethra are colon bacillus, Staphylococcus albus, various diplococci, and smegma bacillus. The posterior urethra is sterile in normal cases, and Young and Churchman[1] have shown that the smegma bacillus can always be removed by irrigation of the anterior urethra. Repeated catheterization, however, is done only when some retention is present, and this retention is a factor in the development of the infection. Experiments with dogs show that when colon bacilli or staphylococci are introduced into the healthy, unobstructed bladder, no infection occurs. In man, it has been found possible to prevent infection for as much as two weeks in obstructed bladders with retention catheter in place with the employment of germicides (see page 74). In the absence of effective drainage, even the frequent use of germicides is unsuccessful. Where infection has followed a temporary retention, as in persons catheterized after abdominal operations, the infection, as a rule (though unfortunately not always) quickly disappears, without treatment, as soon as normal bladder emptying is resumed. In simple cases of bladder infection of this kind, the bladder lesions, as seen by cystoscope or microscope, are sometimes so slight that it has been doubted if there is a real infection, rather than a simple proliferation of organisms in the urine (bacteriuria).

The extent of the lesions varies from those which are almost invisible to the extremes of pathologic change to be described later.

Ureteral Implantation.—Infection may be introduced directly in the ureters or

---

[1] American Journal of Medical Sciences, 1905, cxxx, 52–75.

renal pelvis by ureteral catheters. Here it is evident that in the absence of retention or pre-existing lesions infection does not usually occur.

Introduction through wounds is accidental or as a result of surgical operation.
New types of organisms may be added to pre-existent infections. The results are
determined by other conditions, already present, or caused by the trauma, as
stones, foreign bodies, obstruction, hematoma, extravasation, anemia, uremia,
cachexia, etc.

Direct extension from neighboring organs provides a focus which determines the
course of the infection. Occasionally the extension will permit an escape for pus
which may allow the infection to heal spontaneously.

Hematogenous Infection.—Urogenital infections frequently occur spontaneously, and it is then a question whether the organisms have come from the blood-
stream, or whether a pre-existent but quiescent infection, usually in the lower
urinary tract, and usually gonorrheal, has undergone extension. There is no
doubt that in many cases the blood-stream is responsible. The organisms must
enter the blood through a primary focus elsewhere in the body. In infectious
diseases, the organisms causing the disease have been found in the urine in 28 of
32 cases by A. G. Nichols,[1] usually with signs of kidney infection. Staphylococci
and streptococci have been found in the urine of cases of acute endocarditis,[2]
typhoid bacilli in cases of typhoid fever,[3] and pneumococci in cases of pneumonia.
Grawitz[4] showed that mould spores appeared in the urine after intravenous injection, and Wyssokowitsch[5] did the same for streptococcus, staphylococcus, and
Bacillus anthracis; Biedl and Kraus[6] noted that staphylococci appeared in rabbit
urine within twelve minutes of injection. Rosenow and his co-workers[7] have
reported the production of various urogenital infections in animals by the intravenous injection of organisms obtained from dental abscesses, tonsils, nasal sinuses,
etc., of patients with urogenital infections. Hinman,[8] after injecting a rabbit
intravenously with streptococci grown from an excised area of interstitial cystitis,
observed a similar lesion in the rabbit's bladder. Tubercle bacilli are found in the
urine in miliary tuberculosis. Heitz-Boyer[9] finds showers of colon bacilli in the
urine of certain patients from time to time, often without pus, and believes that
they enter the circulation from slight lesions in the intestinal mucosa, usually
associated with diminished motility. Furniss[10] states that pyelitis occurs more
frequently after intestinal operations than after others.

David and McGill[11] have produced urinary infections in dogs by damaging or
obstructing the intestine, and find the colon bacillus in the blood in some of these

[1] Montreal Medical Journal, 1899, xxviii, 161–183.

[2] Young: Johns Hopkins Hospital Reports, viii, 99–100; 401–420.

[3] McCrae: In Osler and McCrae's Modern Medicine, 2d ed., 1912, i; Lemierre and Abrami:
Journal d'Urologie, Medicine, et Chirurgie, 1912, ii, 21–32; Patrick: Journal of Pathology and
Bacteriology, 1913, xviii, 365–378.

[4] Virchow's Archiv, 1877, lxx, 546–598.

[5] Zeitschrift für Hygiene, 1886, i, 3–46.

[6] Ibid., 1897, xxvi, 353–376.

[7] Journal of Laboratory and Clinical Medicine, 1922, vii, 707–722; Journal of Urology,
1921, vi, 285–298.

[8] Journal of Urology, 1921, vi (discussion), 299–301.

[9] Journal Medical Français, 1922, xi, 178–212.

[10] Journal of the American Medical Association, 1913, lxi, 957–961.

[11] Journal of Urology, 1923, x, 233–254 (Lit.).

cases. Many cases have now been observed when renal infections clear up after tonsillectomy. Warthin[1] finds Treponema pallidum excreted by the kidney in syphilis.

The bacteria may float individually in the blood in diffuse hemic infections (bacteremia), or they may be in small masses which act as emboli. The latter condition usually arises from lesions which produce a localized thrombophlebitis, and the emboli are really bits of infected blood-clot. The infection in these cases, if in the kidney, may be accompanied and furthered by infarct information.

Infection Through the Lymphatics.—Some lymphatic channels from the intestine enter the same retroperitoneal lumbar lymph-nodes as certain of the channels from the kidney. Infection is possible by this path, but has never been proved. In the female there is some communication between the lymphatics of the uterus and those of the bladder, which may determine the path of infections extending directly from the internal genitalia to the bladder.

PATH OF INFECTION IN EXTENSION WITHIN THE UROGENITAL TRACT

As an infection spreads from its point of origin in the urogenital tract, it may proceed in the same direction as the secretory stream, or in the opposite direction. Thus an infection progressing in the direction kidney-to-ureteral meatus or testis-to-verumontanum is a *"descending" infection*, while if in the opposite direction, it is an *"ascending" infection*.[2]

Descending Infections.—Since the secretory stream carries the products of inflammation to parts at a distance, descending infections are the rule. Any point below the original lesion may be affected, local predisposition playing a part. For example, in cases of pyelitis, the trigone and prostatic urethra may be inflamed, while the fundus of the bladder and anterior urethra are normal; in tuberculosis the urethra may resist the infection for a long time, even while the bladder is extensively ulcerated.

The propagation of an infection by the secretory stream may be prevented when the duct is occluded. This often occurs in the duct of the epididymis, in the vas deferens, and in the seminal vesicle. Sometimes the ureter may be completely occluded, so that even if a pyonephrosis exists above, the urine may be clear and the bladder healthy.

In addition, infections may progress in a descending direction by contiguity, either along the mucosal surface, or by the lymphatics, entirely independent of the direction of secretory flow.

Ascending Infections.—Controversy has raged for decades over the mechanism of ascending infections. Many hematogenous infections were formerly supposed to be ascending. Ruling these out, it has been shown that infections may spread in a direction opposed by that of the secretory stream in three ways: (*a*) By the lumen; (*b*) by the lymphatics; (*c*) by the blood-stream, probably through the general circulation.

Helmholz[3] has studied rabbits by injecting the same strain of colon bacillus, intravenously in some animals, and intravesically in others. He frequently ob-

---

[1] Journal of Infectious Diseases, 1922, xxx, 569–591.

[2] Infections spreading from the seminal vesicles to the testes are sometimes spoken of as "descending" infections. This is incorrect, since they are progressing against the secretory stream.

[3] Journal of Urology, 1922, viii, 301–306.

tained cystitis in the latter group, even without obstruction, and renal infection was the rule. The lesions showed a tendency to be more pronounced in the cortex and pyramid when the injection was intravenous, and in the parietal portion of the pelvis, when the injection was intravesical. In the older lesions, however, the origin of the infection could not be determined by examining the kidney, since the pelvic inflammation could spread into the cortex, and vice versa. The spread seemed to be by way of the tubules. Many others, both in man and animals, have shown similarly that the old idea that hematogenous infections be can distinguished from ascending infections by the distribution of the lesions in the kidney is incorrect. Lesions limited almost entirely to the pelvis may be hematogenous.

By the Lumen.—Both ureter and vas deferens propel their contents onward by peristaltic waves, between which the lumen is obliterated by muscular contraction. Infection then cannot travel up the lumen unless there is reverse peristalsis, unless the current is obstructed and stagnates, or unless an increase of pressure below forces the contents back passively. The last alternative is spoken of as a reflux (Fig. 49), and is to be distinguished from reversed peristalsis.

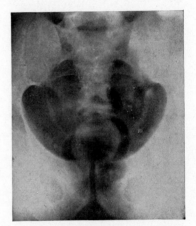

Reverse peristalsis may occur in the rabbit and cat,[1] but has not been observed directly in man. Cabot and Crabtree[2] have, however, seen a stone pass from the kidney pelvis into the ureter, and then rapidly back again, by means of the fluoroscope. In animals, reverse peristalsis has been seen above an obstruction. Since the pelvis, if normal, has little tendency to become infected by a momentary contact with bacteria, we feel that reverse peristalsis of the ureter plays a small rôle in the ordinary transmission of infection; however, when obstruction is present, it may be of some importance.

Fig. 49.—Cystogram showing a very small contracted bladder and bilateral ureteral reflux in a case of severe cystitis, probably tuberculous. B. U. I. x-Ray 2012.

Reverse peristalsis has been observed in the vasa deferentia of animals, and bacteria placed in the urethra have been found in the epididymis afterward.[3] This phenomenon is undoubtedly of more importance in the genital tract than in the urinary, especially since the infective agents are not nearly so quickly removed again by the normal peristalsis of the vas.

Young[4] and Sampson[5] studied ureteral reflux very thoroughly, and found that undilated ureters in the human cadaver do not permit fluid to be forced into them from the bladder unless inflamed. Sampson describes the valve mechanism, which consists of the thin-edged, wedge-shaped portion of bladder wall between the ureter

[1] Elliott: Journal of Physiology, 1907, xxxv, 367–445; Lewin and Goldschmidt: Virchow's Archiv, 1893, cxxxiv, 33–70.

[2] Surgery, Gynecology, and Obstetrics, 1916, xxii, 495–537

[3] Oppenheim and Löw: Virchow's Archiv, 1905, clxxxii, 39–64; Delli Santi: Riforma Medica, 1903, xix, 925–928; Walker and Hawes: St. Bartholomew's Hospital Reports (1911), 1912, xlvii, 135–147.

[4] Johns Hopkins Hospital Bulletin, 1898, ix, 100–113.

[5] Ibid., 1903, xiv, 334–352.

and bladder, and two lateral labia, which extend down beyond the actual orifice. In addition, the intramural portion of the ureter is flattened cross-ways when empty, so that any increase in the distention of the bladder closes it more firmly. If the intramural portion is involved in an inflammatory process, its walls may become stiffened, so that reflux is possible. This condition has been seen by numerous observers in patients with abdominal ureteral fistulæ, at autopsy, by the x-ray, and in other ways. Such a condition would no doubt aid in the spread of infection, especially in the presence of obstruction.

Reflux occurs very commonly in the rabbit, and sometimes in the dog, and has been studied by many observers. Graves and Davidoff[1] have lately reviewed the literature thoroughly and added many experiments of their own. It appears that in the rabbit, reflux is determined by increased intravesical pressure. This increase of pressure, however, is powerless to cause reflux unless the muscular tone of the bladder is good. Reflux will not occur from a flaccid, distended bladder no matter how much the pressure is raised. The effective intravesical pressure in rabbits is about 15 mm. of mercury, though Graves and Davidoff have observed reflux at various points from 9 to 50 mm. Hg. They observed bilateral reflux in 78.6 per cent. of their experiments, and in the others the two sides were involved with equal frequence. They state that in some cases the bladder contents mounted suddenly to the pelvis, and that this could occur even in the ureter on the side where a nephrectomy had previously been done. In other cases, the reflux was slower, and associated with ureteral peristalsis. The column of urine brought down the ureter found difficulty in entering the bladder as the pressure increased; it would "waver" back and forth at the orifice, and finally the ureter would be filled completely. The description of Wislocki and O'Conor[2] is similar. From these statements, it seems to us that reflux should be further subdivided into (1) that which occurs suddenly, as above described, which evidently occurs by a special mechanism in which the orifice is opened from within the bladder, and which has been demonstrated only in the rabbit; and (2) the gradual sort, in which the orifice is opened by pressure from within the ureter, and kept open as a result of increased intravesical pressure until the whole ureter and bladder become communicating cavities. This latter is the mechanism which leads to hydronephrosis and hydroureter in intravesical obstructions.

Kretschmer[3] has shown ureteral reflux with the x-ray in 3 of 10 normal children under ether anesthesia. It is occasionally seen in adult cystograms, and Quinby[4] states that he has observed it by the fluoroscope in patients essentially normal.

It seems, therefore, that reverse peristalsis occurs rarely if at all in man in the absence of obstruction, but that reflux may occur and may be the means of extension upward of an infection, especially if infravesical obstruction or inflammatory involvement of the lower ureter be present.

That reflux does not ordinarily occur in the vas deferens is shown by the absence of urine or vesicle contents from the wound after epididymectomy. If its wall is stiffened by inflammation, however, reflux may occur, as we have seen inguinal

[1] Journal of Urology, 1923, x, 185–231.
[2] Johns Hopkins Hospital Bulletin, 1920, xxxi, 197–202.
[3] Journal of the American Medical Association, 1918, lxxi, 1355–1359.
[4] New York Medical Journal and Medical Record, 1922, cxv, 520–523.

urinary fistulæ after epididymectomy in both tuberculous and simple chronic inflammations of the genital tract.

By the Lymphatics.—Lymphatics of the bladder, posterior urethra, and lower ureter pass into the hypogastric nodes. From the middle portion of the ureter trunks go to the lumbar nodes situated along the vena cava and aorta just above the bifurcation. From the upper portion of the ureter, the hilus of the kidney, and the fatty capsule, the drainage is into the aortic nodes both above and below the renal vessels. Ureter and bladder have each abundant networks of lymphatics in both muscularis and submucosa, which anastomose with each other and with the lymphatics of the kidney. The kidney is abundantly supplied with lymphatics, which surround all the tubules and glomeruli, and drain both through the hilic lymphatics and through the fibrous capsule into the lymphatics of the fatty capsule. The flow through these vessels is slow, and its direction has less influence on the progress of an infection than in the case of the blood-vessels. The existence of these open spaces is of importance in connection with the spread of infection from bladder to ureter and kidney, and from kidney to perirenal tissues.[1]

Lymphatics from the testis or ovary pass along the spermatic or ovarian vessels to the retroperitoneal region, where they enter aortic nodes of the same groups as those draining the kidney, and as high up as the renal vessels and as low down as the bifurcation of the aorta. The vas deferens is well supplied with lymphatics which anastomose with those of the epididymis, and also with those of the bladder, vesicles, prostate and posterior urethra. The channels about the prostatic urethra and vesical orifice are especially wide, and often conspicuous in sections.

Sweet and Stewart[2] performed a number of ingenious experiments to show the rôle of the lymphatics in ascending infections of the kidney. When the outside of the ureter was exposed to infection, without opening its lumen, diffuse infection of the kidney resulted, with little or no inflammation of the ureteral mucosa. When a piece of rubber tubing was substituted for the midportion of the ureter, thus interrupting the lymphatic channels but not the lumen, infection did not ascend to the kidney. When the pelvis was put in direct communication with the intestinal lumen, the infection was confined to the portion of the kidney in contact with the intestine, and was not carried through the pelvis to the more distant portions. Microscopic sections of the ureter showed the lymphatic channels distended with leukocytes. According to these authors, ascending infection of the ureters does not occur unless the bladder wall itself is invaded in the neighborhood of the ureteral orifice. Eisendrath[3] reports similar findings.

These interstitial involvements of ureter and vas would tend to cause obstruction, which would favor the development of infection above. If in the lower segment of the ureter, reflux would be favored. One often sees the wall of ureter or vas in cross-sections heavily infiltrated, with the mucosa practically normal.

[1] Bauereisen: Zeitschrift für Gynäkologische Urologie, 1911, ii, 132–153; 235–250; 276–284. Sugimura: Virchow's Archiv, 1911, ccvi, 20–36. Kumita: Archiv für Anatomie und Physiologie, Anatomische Abteilung, 1909, 49–58; 99–109. Stahr: Archiv für Anatomie und Physiologie, Anatomische Abteilung, 1900, 41–84. Sakata: Archiv für Anatomie und Physiologie, Anatomische Abteilung, 1903, 1–12. Satani: Journal of Urology, 1919, iii, 247–267; American Journal of Physiology, 1919, 1, 342–351. Quinby: Journal of Urology, 1922, vii, 259–270.

[2] Surgery, Gynecology, and Obstetrics, 1914, xviii, 460–469.

[3] Eisendrath and Schultz: Journal of Medical Research, 1916–17, xxxv, 295–335. Boston Medical and Surgical Journal, 1917, clxxvii, 10–13.

By the Blood-vessels.—There are numerous anastomoses between the blood-vessels of the various urogenital organs, but the currents do not run along the tract longitudinally.[1] For instance, while there are blood-channels all the way from bladder to kidney, yet none of the blood from the bladder goes to the kidney before entering the vena cava. It is, therefore, probable that the blood-vessels do not carry infection directly from one part of the urogenital tract to another, but one focus in the tract may perfectly well be the source of a blood-stream infection which could cause secondary hemogenic infection in another portion of the tract.

To summarize, descending infection is common, and, indeed, to be expected. Ascending infection by the lumen probably does not often occur unless there is obstruction, dilatation, and reflux. The rôle of reverse peristalsis is not certain, but probably very slight in the ureter, and somewhat more important in the vas deferens. There is good reason to believe that infection can ascend by the lymphatics, but only by extension through them, not by carriage of bacteria. In many cases it is difficult to determine where the earliest lesion was, and an infection may be incorrectly interpreted as ascending, if the lowermost lesions of a descending infection are discovered before the uppermost.

BACTERIOLOGY

This subject is one of extreme complexity, and little satisfaction can be gained from a study of the literature. In the older writings, the methods of differentiation, and the nomenclature, are so foreign to us now that often we do not even know what organism is being discussed; for example, the "Micrococcus ureæ." More recently, the only thorough studies have been on isolated species, the identifications in large series being made on simple and conservative lines. Since many of the strains isolated do not correspond exactly with common organisms, it is obvious that more careful investigations should be made, and now that the Society of American Bacteriologists has introduced a comprehensive scheme of classification, it should be followed for the sake of uniformity.[2]

COLON-TYPHOID BACILLI.—Excepting the gonococcus, *bacilli of the colon group* are among the most frequent invaders of the urinary tract, whether from the blood or by direct implantation, for self-evident reasons. This group is a large one, however, including numerous organisms which differ markedly in their characteristics, and a diagnosis of "Bacillus coli" is insufficient. Reference to Table 10, giving the results of 364 urine cultures made on our service, shows that four very definite varieties of this group occur in urine, while in a fifth heading, containing the largest number of cases, the organisms do not correspond exactly with any described strains. Most of these are closely related to Bacillus coli communis (Bacterium coli communis, Escherich, S. A. B.) and Bacillus coli communior (Bacterium coli communior, Durham, S. A. B.), but differ in some slight way. They all ferment lactose, with the production of acid and gas. In addition, the group which includes typhoid and related forms would often be included in the "colon group." This group all ferment carbohydrates with the production of acid, but no gas. In none of our cases were the organisms those of typhoid. Further studies must be made as to the identity of all these forms with those in

---

[1] Satani: Journal of Urology, 1919, iii, 247–267. Sampson: Johns Hopkins Hospital Bulletin, 1903, xiv, 334–352.

[2] Journal of Bacteriology, 1917, ii, 505, and 1920, v, 191.

the intestinal flora, and also as to specific pathogenicity. Bacterium fecalis alcaligenes has not appeared in our series, but has been found by others in the urine.[1]

TABLE 10

SUMMARY OF THE ORGANISMS OBTAINED BY CULTURE FROM 356 CASES OF UROGENITAL INFECTION

Group I. Gram-negative Bacilli, Including Organisms of the Colon Group and Related Forms.
  A. Organisms Fermenting Carbohydrates With the Production of Acid and Gas.
    1. Bacilli of the Bact. coli communior group:
        (a) Isolated in pure culture.................................. 24
        (b) Isolated with Staph. aureus only.......................... 2
        (c) Isolated with Staph. albus only........................... 3
        (d) Isolated with undifferentiated Staph. only................. 4
        (e) Isolated with Streptococcus only.......................... 1
        (f) Isolated with Staph. aureus and Streptococcus............. 1
        (g) Isolated with Pseudomonas pyocyanea only................. 1

                           Total pure................ 24 (66 per cent.)
                           Total mixed............... 12 (33 per cent.)

                           Combined total........... 36

    2. Bacilli of the Bact. coli communis group:
        (a) Isolated in pure culture.................................. 9
        (b) Isolated with Staph. albus only........................... 2

                           Total.................... 11

    3. Bacilli of the Bact. aërogenes group:
        (a) Isolated in pure culture.................................. 11
        (b) Isolated with Staph. albus only........................... 1
        (c) Isolated with Streptococcus only.......................... 1

                           Total.................... 13

    4. Bacilli of the Bact. mucosum capsulatum group:
        (a) Isolated in pure culture.................................. 2
    5. Undifferentiated bacilli fermenting carbohydrates, including lactose, with the production of acid and gas:
        (a) Isolated in pure culture.................................. 76
        (b) Isolated with Staph. aureus only.......................... 4
        (c) Isolated with Staph. albus only........................... 14
        (d) Isolated with undifferentiated Staph...................... 9
        (e) Isolated with Streptococcus only.......................... 10
        (f) Isolated with Streptococcus and Staph. albus.............. 2
        (g) Isolated with Streptococcus and undifferentiated Staph...... 1
        (h) Isolated with Pseduomonas pyocyanea only................. 2
        (i) Isolated with Pseudomonas pyocyanea and undifferentiated Staph... 1
        (j) Isolated with Streptococcus and Proteus 1
        (k) Isolated with Streptococcus and undifferentiated Staph. and Pseudomonas pyocyanea.............................. 1
        (l) Isolated with Streptococcus and undifferentiated Staph. and tetragenus....................................... 1

                           Total pure............... 76
                           Total mixed.............. 46

                           Combined total........... 122

[1] David: Surgery, Gynecology, and Obstetrics, 1914, xviii, 432–437.

TABLE 10—*Continued*

B. Organisms Fermenting Carbohydrates with the Production of Acid Without Gas (Typhoid Group):

  (*a*) Isolated in pure culture............................... 6
  (*b*) Isolated with Staph. aureus only......................... 1
  (*c*) Isolated with acid-fast bacilli only....................... 1

             Total................... 8

Group I Summary:

Total number of cases..................... 192 (53.9 per cent. of total series)
Number isolated in pure culture............ 128 (66.6 per cent. of all Group I cultures)
Number isolated in mixed culture.......... 64 (33.3 per cent. of all Group I cultures)
Mixed with Staph. only................... 40 (20.8 per cent. of all Group I cultures)
                 (62.5 per cent. of mixed Group I cultures)
Mixed with Streptococcus only.............. 12 (6.2 per cent. of all Group I cultures)
                 (18.7 per cent. of mixed Group I cultures)
Mixed with Pseudomonas pyocyanea only.... 3 (1.0 per cent. of all Group I cultures)
                 (4.6 per cent. of mixed Group I cultures)
Mixed with 2 or more organisms............ 8 (4.1 per cent. of all Group I cultures)
                 (12.6 per cent. of mixed Group I cultures)

Group II. Gram-positive Cocci.
 A. Staphylococci:
  1. Staphylococcus aureus:
   (*a*) Isolated in pure culture................................ 26
   (*b*) Isolated with undifferentiated colon group bacilli only....... 4
   (*c*) Isolated with bacilli of Bact. coli communior group only...... 2
   (*d*) Isolated with bacilli of typhoid group only................. 1
   (*e*) Isolated with Staph. albus only......................... 2
   (*f*) Isolated with Streptococci only.......................... 1
   (*g*) Isolated with acid-fast bacilli only....................... 1
   (*h*) Isolated with bacillus of Bact. coli communior group and Streptococcus... 1
   (*i*) Isolated with Proteus and Streptococcus................... 1
   (*j*) Isolated with Proteus and Diphtheroid.................... 1

        Total pure................ 26
        Total mixed.............. 14

        Combined total.......... 40

  2. Staphylococcus albus:
   (*a*) Isolated in pure culture................................ 56
   (*b*) Isolated with undifferentiated colon group bacilli only........ 14
   (*c*) Isolated with bacilli of Bact. coli communior group only..... 3
   (*d*) Isolated with bacilli of Bact. coli communis group only...... 2
   (*e*) Isolated with bacillus of Bact. aërogenes group only......... 1
   (*f*) Isolated with Streptococci only.................. 3
   (*g*) Isolated with Staph. aureus only......................... 2
   (*h*) Isolated with Pseudomonas pyocyanea only................. 2
   (*i*) Isolated with Proteus only.............................. 1
   (*j*) Isolated with Bacilli of colon group and Streptococci......... 2
   (*k*) Isolated with Gonococcus only........................... 5
   (*l*) Isolated with Gram-negative Diplococcus only (not gonococcus) 1

        Total pure................ 56
        Total mixed.............. 36

        Combined total.......... 92

TABLE 10—*Continued*

3. Undifferentiated Staphylococcus:
   (*a*) Isolated in pure culture................................. 16
   (*b*) Isolated with colon group bacilli only..................... 9
   (*c*) Isolated with bacilli of Bact. coli communior group only..... 4
   (*d*) Isolated with Streptococci only.......................... 5
   (*e*) Isolated with Proteus only.............................. 1
   (*f*) Isolated with Pseudomonas pyocyanea only................ 1
   (*g*) Isolated with Gonococcus only.......................... 2
   (*h*) Isolated with Gram-negative diplococcus only (not gonococcus) 1
   (*i*) Isolated with colon group bacillus and Streptococcus........ 1
   (*j*) Isolated with colon group bacillus and Streptococcus and
         Pseudomeonas pyocyanea and Staph. tetragenus.......... 1
   (*k*) Isolated with colon group bacillus and Streptococcus and
         Pseudomeonas pyocyanea............................. 1
   (*l*) Isolated with colon group bacillus and Ps. pyocyanea........ 1

                              Total pure............... 16
                              Total mixed............. 27
                              Combined total.......... 43

Staphylococcus Summary:

Total number of cases............................. 175 (49.1 per cent. of total series)
Number isolated in pure culture.................... 98 (56 per cent. of Staph.)
Number isolated in mixed culture................... 77 (44 per cent. of Staph.)

   (*a*) Isolated with undifferentiated colon group bacilli
         only..................................... 27 (15.4 per cent. of total Staph.)
                                                      (35   per cent. of mixed Staph.)

   (*b*) Isolated with bacilli of Bact. coli communior group
         only..................................... 9 (5.1 per cent. of total Staph.)
                                                      (11.6 per cent. of mixed Staph.)

   (*c*) Isolated with bacilli of Bact. coli communis group
         only..................................... 2 (1.1 per cent. of total Staph.)
                                                      (2.5 per cent. of mixed Staph.)

   (*d*) Isolated with bacillus of Bact. aërogenes group only 1 (0.5 per cent. of total Staph.)
                                                      (1.2 per cent. of mixed Staph.)

   (*e*) Isolated with bacillus of typhoid group only.... 1 (0.5 per cent. of total Staph.)
                                                      (1.2 per cent. of mixed Staph.)

   (*f*) Total number isolated with Group I bacilli only.. 40 (22.8 per cent. of total Staph.)
                                                      (51.9 per cent. of mixed Staph.)

   (*g*) Isolated with another Staph. only.............. 2 (1.1 per cent. of total Staph.)
                                                      (2.5 per cent. of mixed Staph.)

   (*h*) Isolated with Streptococcus only............... 9 (5.1 per cent. of total Staph.)
                                                      (11.6 per cent. of mixed Staph.)

   (*i*) Isolated with Pseudomonas pyocyanea only...... 3 (1.7 per cent. of total Staph.)
                                                      (3.8 per cent. of mixed Staph.)

   (*j*) Isolated with Proteus only.................... 2 (1.1 per cent. of total Staph.)
                                                      (2.5 per cent. of mixed Staph.)

   (*k*) Isolated with Gonococcus only................. 7 (4   per cent. of total Staph.)
                                                      (9   per cent. of mixed Staph.)

   (*l*) Isolated with 2 or more organisms............. 9 (5.1 per cent. of total Staph.)
                                                      (11.6 per cent. of mixed Staph.)

   (*m*) Isolated with acid-fast bacilli only............. 1 (0.5 per cent. of total Staph.)
                                                      (1.2 per cent. of mixed Staph.)

   (*n*) Isolated with diphtheroid.................... 1 (0.5 per cent. of total Staph.)
                                                      (1.2 per cent. of mixed Staph.)

   (*o*) Isolated with Gram-negative Diplococcus, not Gono-
         coccus................................... 2 (1.1 per cent. of total Staph.)
                                                      (2.5 per cent. of mixed Staph.)

TABLE 10—*Continued*

B. Streptococci:

(a) Isolated in pure culture................................ 16
(b) Isolated with undifferentiated colon group bacilli............ 10
(c) Isolated with bacilli of Bact. coli communior group........ 1
(d) Isolated with Staph. aureus............................ 1
(e) Isolated with Staph. albus............................ 3
(f) Isolated with undifferentiated Staph..................... 5
(g) Isolated with Pseudomonas pyocyanea.................... 4
(h) Isolated with acid-fast bacilli........................... 1
(i) Isolated with colon group bacillus and Proteus............. 1
(j) Isolated with colon group bacillus and Staph. undifferentiated. 1
(k) Isolated with colon group bacillus and Staph. albus......... 2
(l) Isolated with Staph. aureus and Proteus................... 1
(m)Isolated with bacillus of Bact. aërogenes group............. 1
(n) Isolated with Staph. aureus and Bact. coli communior group.. 1
(o) Isolated with colon group bacillus and Staph. and Pseudomonas
    pyocyanea and tetragenus............................ 1
(p) Isolated with colon group bacillus and Staph. and Pseudomonas
    pyocyanea.. 1

                          Total pure............... 16
                          Total mixed............. 34

                          Total Streptococcus........ 50

Streptococcus Summary:

Total... 50 (14 per cent. of total series)
                                                (22 per cent. of Gram-positive
                                                  cocci)
Pure.. 16 (32 per cent. of total Strept.)
Mixed... 34 (68 per cent. of total Strept.)
   (a) Mixed with undifferentiated colon group bacilli.... 10 (20   per cent. of total Strept.)
                                                  (29.4 per cent. mixed Strept.)
   (b) Mixed with bacilli of Bact. coli communior group.. 3 (6   per cent. of total Strept.)
                                                  (8.8 per cent. of mixed Strept.)
   (c) Mixed with bacillus of Bact. aërogenes group ..... 1 (2   per cent. of total Strept.)
                                                  (5.8 per cent. mixed Strept.)
       Total number isolated with Group I bacilli...... 14 (28   per cent. of total Strept.)
                                                  (41.1 per cent. mixed Strept.)
   (d) Isolated with Staph............................ 9 (18   per cent. of total Strept.)
                                                  (26.4 per cent. mixed Strept.)
   (e) Isolated with Pseudomonas pyocyanea............ 4 (8   per cent. of total Strept.)
                                                  (11.7 per cent. mixed Strept.)
   (f) Isolated with 2 or more organisms............... 6 (12   per cent. of total Strept.)
                                                  (17.6 per cent. mixed Strept.)

C. Staphylococcus tetragenus:

(a) Isolated in pure culture................................. 1
(b) Isolated in mixed culture............................... 1

Group II Summary (Staph., Strept. and Staph. tetragenus):

Total number cases.................................. 227 (65.7 per cent. of total series)
Total isolated in pure culture......................... 115 (50.6 per cent. of Group II)
Total isolated in mixed culture........................ 112 (49.3 per cent. of Group II)

Group III. Gram-negative Diplococci (Neisseria, S. A. B.).

TABLE 10—*Continued*

A. Gonococcus:
    (*a*) Isolated in pure culture.................... 7
    (*b*) Isolated with Staph. albus................ 5
    (*c*) Isolated with undifferentiated Staph......... 2
                 Total pure........... 7 (50 per cent. of Gc.)
                 Total mixed......... 7 (50 per cent. of Gc.)
                 Combined total.......14 (3.9 per cent. of Series)

B. Gram-negative diplococci not Gonococcus:
    (*a*) Isolated with Staph. albus................ 1
    (*b*) Isolated with undifferentiated Staph......... 1
                 Total............... 2 (0.5 per cent. of series)

Group IV. Proteus Group Bacilli:
    (*a*) Isolated in pure culture.................... 2
    (*b*) Isolated with Staph. albus................ 1
    (*c*) Isolated with undifferentiated Staph......... 1
    (*d*) Isolated with Staph. aureus and Strep....... 1
    (*e*) Isolated with Staph. aureus and diphtheroid.. 1
    (*f*) Isolated with colon group bacillus and Strep.. 1

                 Total pure........... 2 (28.5 per cent. of Group IV)
                 Total mixed......... 5 (71.4 per cent. of Group IV)

                 Combined total....... 7 (1.93 per cent. of series)

Group V. Pseudomonas pyocyanea:
    (*a*) Isolated in pure culture.................... 2
    (*b*) Isolated with Streptococci................. 4
    (*c*) Isolated with Staph. albus................ 2
    (*d*) Isolated with undifferentiated Staph......... 1
    (*e*) Isolated with undifferentiated Staph. and colon
          group bacillus.......................... 1
    (*f*) Isolated with colon group bacillus........... 2
    (*g*) Isolated with bacillus of Bact. coli communior
          group only............................. 1
    (*h*) Isolated with Actinomyces bovis............. 1
    (*i*) Isolated with colon group bacillus and Strept.
          and Staph. tetragenus.................... 1
    (*j*) Isolated with colon group bacillus and Strept.
          and Staph............................. 1

                 Total pure........... 2 (12.5 per cent.)
                 Total mixed.........14 (87.5 per cent.)

                 Combined total.......16 (4.4 per cent. of series)

Group VI. All Other Organisms.
  A. Actinomyces:
    A. bovis with Ps. pyocyanea....................... 1
    Actinomyces with tubercle bacilli................... 2

                 Total............... 3 (0.8 per cent. of series)
  B. Diphtheroid (related to Corynebacterium flavidum) in pure
    culture... 1
    Diphtheroid with Proteus and Staph. aureus............ 1

                 Total............... 2 (0.5 per cent. of series)
  C. Yeast in direct smear and pure culture (probably not
    pathogenic)..................................... 1 (0.2 per cent. of series)

TABLE 10—*Concluded*

SERIES SUMMARY

Group.	Total.	Percentage of series.	Pure.	Percentage of group.	Percentage of series.	Mixed.	Percentage of group.	Percentage of series.	Ratio of pure to mixed.
I. Gram-negative bacilli.......	192	53.9	128	66.6	35.9	64	33.3	17.9	2 : 1
II. Gram-positive cocci.........	227	63.7	115	50.6	32.3	112	49.3	31.4	1 : 1
Gram-negative cocci.... { III. A. Gonococci....	14	3.9	7	50	1.9	7	50	1.9	1 : 1
III. B. Not gonococci.	2	0.5	0	0	0	2	100	0.5	
IV. Proteus..................	7	1.9	2	28.5	0.56	5	71.4	1.4	0.33 : 1 (2 : 5)
V. Ps. Pyocyanea	16	4.4	2	12.5	0.5	14	87.5	3.9	1 : 7
All others { VI. A. Actinomyces....	3	0.8	0	0	0	3	100	0.8	
VI. B. Diphtheroid.....	2	0.5	1	50	0.28	1	50	0.28	1 : 1
VI. C. Yeast.........	1	0.28	1	100	0.28	0	0	0	

Pure.......256　71.9% of series.
Mixed......100　28.0% of series.
Ratio of Total Pure: Total Mixed—2.5 : 1.

While *bacilli of the colon group* usually occur in acid urine, this is merely because urine is usually acid, and these organisms do not alter its reaction, unless sugar be present, as in diabetes, when acid is produced. Indeed, Shohl[1] has shown that in sugar and protein-free urine the Bacillus coli even produces a slight amount of alkali—not enough to make the urine markedly alkaline.

Bacilli of the colon group may cause inflammatory reactions in any part of the urinary tract, and also septicemia. Abscesses may occur, with leukocytosis. The pus is yellow, and has a distinctive unpleasant odor. Superficial infections of mild but chronic nature are especially apt to occur, as for example in the renal pelvis. Abscesses and deep infections are likely to be less acute and severe than those caused by the pyogenic cocci[2] and colon group septicemia is of all septicemias the most benign, a large majority of the cases recovering spontaneously. In secondary infection of wounds of the urogenital tract, these organisms are usually present, owing to their ubiquity. They are occasionally seen in the urine in cases where it is impossible to find any definite lesion anywhere in the tract.

Of the Gram-negative bacilli which ferment carbohydrates with the production of acid but no gas, the *typhoid bacillus* is the most important. The urine shows an infection with the typhoid bacillus in from 20 to 40 per cent. of the cases of typhoid fever, but only occasionally are pus-cells present in considerable number. In sixty-eight autopsies in typhoid cases at the Johns Hopkins Hospital, only one presented an acute cystitis.

Chronic cystitis due to the typhoid bacillus is of great rarity. The first case was reported from this clinic[3] in May, 1898.

The patient had been admitted to the John Hopkins Hospital, service of Dr. Osler, with typhoid fever five years before, and the urine showed pus-cells in large amount. After recovering from typhoid fever he was discharged, but the urine still contained pus. In March, 1898 he was admitted to our service complaining of bladder trouble, and cultures showed a pure culture of the B. typhosus. Suprapubic aspiration was done to exclude urethral organisms and obtain an uncontaminated bladder culture.[3]

[1] Journal of Urology, 1920, iv, 371–378.

[2] Goldberg: Zeitschrift für Urologie, 1913, vii, 447–475.

[3] Young, H. H.: Johns Hopkins Hospital Medical Society, May, 1898; Johns Hopkins Hospital Reports, 1900, vii, 401–420 (Maryland Medical Journal, November, 1901).

Widal test with bacillus from urine and patient's blood—positive. Cystoscopic examination showed an ulcerative cystitis. In March, 1899, he acquired acute gonococcal urethritis. Aspirated urine still showed the typhoid bacillus in pure culture, and in January, 1900, following cystoscopy, the cystitis became much more acute, urination very frequent and painful; the urine was very cloudy, and cultures, obtained by suprapubic aspiration, showed now typhoid bacilli and also large numbers of gonococci, which were still present four months later.

In the same year Rovsing reported in his book[1] a case in which, eighteen months after an attack of typhoid fever, a severe chronic cystitis, due to the B. typhosus, was found.

In the following year Houston[2] reported a case of severe chronic cystitis of three years' duration also due to the B. typhosus. In this case the typhoid infection came from nursing a child with typhoid fever. The patient herself remained well, but soon afterward began to suffer with frequent urination. The blood gave the Widal reaction.

The kidney is occasionally the seat of suppuration due to the B. typhosus. In 1906 we were able to collect 6 cases of pyonephrosis and to these we added 2 cases of pus kidney, in which pure cultures of the B. typhosus were obtained.[3]

In our cases the typhoid fever had occurred eight and ten years before. In the center of a calculus removed from one kidney, a pure culture of B. typhosus was obtained.

Patients with urines infected with the typhoid bacillus may be "carriers" of the infection for months or years, and suffer little or no discomfort. Notorious cases, declared dangerous by public health officers, and cruelly quarantined for years are on record, (as in the case of "Typhoid Mary"). Now internal antiseptics bring hope of a cure of these unfortunates.

The significance of related forms, not definitely typhoid bacilli, which we have found in the urine is not known. A study of the cases shows that two had vesical calculi, one a renal calculus, one an infection of prostate and Cowper's glands, one renal pyuria and recurrent epididymitis, one double pyelitis with hematuria, one chronic cystitis with contracture following urethral stricture, and one the clinical picture of renal and genital tuberculosis. In this last case no tubercle bacilli were found, and the patient refused operation, so that no pathologic specimens were available.

The occurrence and pathologic significance of the *"paratyphoid" bacilli*, A (Bact. paratyphosum A, S. A. B.) and B (Bact. paratyphosum B, S. A. B.), in the urinary tract are like those of typhoid bacilli. Other members of this group are also found occasionally in the urine in various types of urinary infections.

Herrold[4] and Dudgeon[5] have shown that certain strains of the colon group are *hemolytic*. Herrold thinks the hemolytic strains more virulent, but the others more resistant.

GRAM-POSITIVE COCCI.—Most observers, with large series of cases studied place the group of *Gram-positive cocci* second to the colon group in point of frequence.[6] In our series (Table 10) they head the list. At all events, these two

[1] Infectiöse Krankheiten der Harnorgane, Berlin, 1898.

[2] British Medical Journal, 1899, i, 78–79.

[3] Young, H. H.: Johns Hopkins Hospital Reports, 1906, xiii, 455–478.

[4] Journal of Urology, 1922, vii, 473–479.

[5] Dudgeon et al.: Journal of Hygiene, 1922, xxi, 168–198.

[6] Mathé and Belt: Journal of Urology, 1922, viii, 281–299 (Lit.).

groups are by far the commonest invaders of the urogenital tract (excepting always the gonococcus).

Staphylococci occur much more frequently than streptococci. In the group of the staphylococci, efforts at classification everywhere have met with little success. There is no way in which we can divide the staphylococci which gives us the least useful information concerning source, pathogenicity, or treatment. The classic differentiation by means of pigment production into aureus, albus, etc., is of no practical value. Staphylococcus albus is just as apt to be virulent as Staphylococcus aureus.[1]

The original microbe discovered by Pasteur[2] in ammoniacal urine was a coccus ("Micrococcus ureæ"). This organism has never been identified with any known form, but apparently belonged to the staphylococcus group. Staphylococci are, however, frequently found in urine of normal acidity. Miquel[3] found sixty different organisms, cocci, bacilli, and sarcinæ, which fermented urea at different rates. A series of one hundred strains of staphylococci from various sources studied by us showed that only two decomposed urea at all strongly, and these not completely. Three others decomposed urea slightly. The majority of the remainder formed slight quantities of acid in the presence of urea. It is, therefore, obvious that most staphylococci will not produce an ammoniacal urine. It is possible that this ability to split urea is of importance in the bacteriology of the urinary tract, and such a test should be added to the routine of all urine cultures. We have already observed in our laboratory sixteen strains of staphylococcus obtained from the urinary tract, and only two of them decompose urea. The identity of the Micrococcus ureæ is still, therefore, undetermined.

Staphylococci may cause infections anywhere in the urogenital tract. Goldberg[4] notes that they are especially concerned in early and acute lesions. Baisch[5] found them in 85 per cent. of cases of fresh acute cystitis. They are often associated with other organisms. In the bladder they are often benign, but beneath the mucosa as in the kidney and seminal vesicle, abscess formation and destructive effect are more marked than with colon bacillus. When staphylococci are excreted by the kidney in experimental animals, the lesions found in the tubules are frequently very slight, in fact, some workers have not found any at all. In the pelvis, staphylococci may cause mild, chronic pyelitis just as do the colon group, but less frequently.

Staphylococcus septicemia may occur from urogenital lesions, and is much more fatal than colon group septicemia. According to Otten[6] 80 per cent. die, and Bertalsmann[7] gives 70 per cent. as the mortality rate.

Staphylococcus infections, except where superficial, cause leukocytosis and

---

[1] Winslow, Rothberg, and Parsons: Journal of Bacteriology, 1920, v, 145–167.

[2] Memoire sur les corpuscules organisés, qui existent dans l'atmosphere, Annales des Sciences Naturelles, partie zoölogique, 4e serie, xvi, 1861, 5–98; and Annales de Chimie et de Physique, 3e serie, lxiv, 1862, 5–110; Note sur l'alteration de l'urine, Comptes Rendus de l'Academie des Sciences, 1876, lxxxiii, 176–180; reprinted in Oeuvres de Pasteur, réunies par Vallery-Radot, Paris, 1922, ii, 247, and 459 et seq.

[3] Quoted by Flügge, Die Mikroörganismen, Leipzig, 1896, i, 211–213.

[4] Zeitschrift für Urologie, 1913, vii, 447–476.

[5] Beiträge zur Geburtshilfe und Gynäkologie, 1904, viii, 297–328.

[6] Deutsches Archiv für Klinische Medizin, 1907, xc, 461–500.

[7] Münchener Medizinische Wochenschrift, 1902, xlix (1), 521–525. (Quoted by Jochmann, Deutsches Archiv für Klinische Medizin, 1906, lxxxvii, 479–498.)

fever. The pus is yellow and odorless. Staphylococci may appear in exudates or in urine as flattened diplococci, when they will be mistaken for gonococci if the Gram stain is not used.

It must be remembered that the most common contamination of urine and prostatic cultures is a white staphylococcus. A few colonies should be viewed as a probable contamination, especially if no staphylococcus forms were found in the stained smears made at the time when the culture was taken.

Streptococci are found less frequently in the urogenital tract than staphylococci. In many cases they occur in mixed bladder infections where no special symptoms are noted. Rarely they are found in chronic pyelitis. As is well known, the virulence of various members of this group varies greatly, and it is difficult to determine whether the presence of streptococci in the urine denotes additional danger to the patient. Hemolytic varieties are considered most virulent, but the green-forming or Streptococcus viridans type, though less virulent, is generally fatal when found in the blood. Septicemia may occur, and is practically always fatal, quickly with the hemolytic variety, and more slowly with the viridans. The Streptococcus viridans septicemia is resistant to all known methods of treatment.

According to Rosenow and his co-workers, streptococci are capable of great specificity. Rosenow and Meisser[1] state that certain strains, obtained from human cases of pyelonephritis, will reproduce the disease in animals, and also that other strains from stone cases will produce renal calculi in animals with regularity. Meisser and Bumpus[2] have isolated a streptococcus which excites specifically a localized submucous cystitis, and this finding is confirmed by Hinman.[3] Some of these organisms were obtained from the urinary tract, others from foci at a distance, as dental abscesses. Further work of this kind should be of great importance to urology.

Streptococci may also be concerned in erysipelatous lesions about wounds of the urogenital tract or in urinary extravasations. Localization of streptococcus infection in the kidney may occur in other infections with these organisms, as tonsillitis, dental abscesses, sinus infections, carbuncles, infected hemorrhoids, impetigo, etc.

Pilot and Brams[4] found hemolytic streptococci in the preputial secretion in 9 per cent. of 100 healthy men.

The *Micrococcus tetragenus* (Staphylococcus tetragenus, S. A. B.) is occasionally found in the urine. It may appear with other organisms, or in pure culture. Its growth is usually superficial, and it apparently has low pathogenicity.

The *Pneumococcus* (Diplococcus pneumoniæ, S. A. B.) has been found in the urine or prostatic secretion in infections of the prostate, bladder, and kidneys, and in ulcerative lesions of the external genitalia. It occurs infrequently. Among 835 cases of upper urinary tract infections Mathé and Belt[5] found the pneumococcus only eight times. There is generally some association with respiratory infections in such cases.

The *Enterococcus* is a Gram-positive, encapsulated streptococcus, the differ-

[1] Journal of Laboratory and Clinical Medicine, 1922, vii, 702–712.
[2] Journal of Urology, 1921, vi, 285–298.
[3] Ibid., 1921, vi (discussion), 299–301.
[4] Journal of Infectious Diseases, 1923, xxxii, 172–174.
[5] Journal of Urology, 1922, viii, 281–297. .

entiation of which is not worked out as thoroughly as it should be. Heitz-Boyer reports several cases in which the Enterococcus appeared in the urine in cases of long-standing chronic upper tract infection. It has not been found in this country. Careful bacteriologic studies are necessary to differentiate the Gram-positive cocci. It is probable that when no note is made as to the presence of capsules, the Pneumococcus and Enterococcus may be overlooked. The Enterococcus occurs normally in the intestine, and French observers feel that it reaches the urinary tract through the blood in the same manner as that assumed for the Colon group.

GRAM-NEGATIVE COCCI.—The *Gram-negative cocci* are of especial interest because they include the gonococcus. This organism infects the urogenital tract more frequently than any other.   It is impossible to tell how frequently it occurs, but estimates have run from 40 to 95 per cent. of the entire male popula-

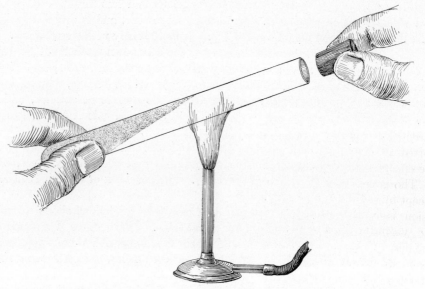

FIG. 50.—Culture method for gonococcus; heating tube with Bunsen flame to expel air (and reduce oxygen), rubber stopper then quickly inserted.   Swartz.

tion.   It is certain that it is extremely prevalent, and it occurs frequently in women as well, most of the pelvic inflammatory disease in this sex being ascribed to it.

Gonococcus (Neisseria gonorrheæ, S. A. B.) is highly parasitic, and easily killed by heat, cold, drying, sunlight, or germicidal substances. It may survive ten or eleven hours on damp towels.[1] It grows best when the oxygen tension is slightly reduced. It resembles closely other members of this group, but recent work[2] has shown that it may be cultivated without difficulty (Figs. 50, 51).   Its

[1] Engering: Zeitschrift für Hygiene und Infectiösen Krankheiten, 1923, c, 314–322.

[2] Swartz: Journal of Urology, 1920, iv, 325–345 (Lit.).   The medium used is a 1.5 per cent. peptone-beef-broth agar prepared in the ordinary way, and titrated with N/10 NaOH so that the reaction, after cooling and hardening, will be PH 7.4 (phenolsulphonephthalein is the best indicator).   Hydrocele, ascitic, or pleuritic fluid, collected aseptically and tested in the incubator to assure sterility, is added to the individual tubes of melted agar at 50° C. in the proportion of 1 c.c. fluid to 2 c.c. agar.   The tubes are cooled as slants, stoppered with rubber stoppers, and kept in the incubator.   When inoculation is to be made, the tubes should be warm at the time of inoculation, and not allowed to cool before reaching the incubator.   The oxygen tension is

identification by means of sugar reactions is comparatively simple.[1] Frequently this will be necessary, in medicolegal cases, in arthritis, in salpingitis, in chronic urogenital infections, etc., and is entirely within the powers of any well-equipped laboratory. A Gram-negative diplococcus of typical morphology, which will not grow on ordinary media, which grows only slightly upon enriched media unless the oxygen tension is reduced, which produces colonies of typical form, and which ferments glucose, but no other sugar, can be said definitely to be the gonococcus. Unless these simple criteria are fulfilled, the identification is not certain and all of them should be employed whenever cultures are made for gonococcus. Otherwise culture will give no more certainty than a Gram stain. All species of animals but the human have the most extraordinary and complete immunity against the gonococcus, so that experimental inoculations have never been successful except in men. Antigonococcus agglutinins in animals can, however, be increased by injections of the organism, and on this basis, vaccine therapy has been attempted in the human. While some apparently favorable results have been reported in gonorrheal arthritis, in general the effects are not striking.

The gonococcus is seldom transmitted except by sexual contact, when the primary lesion is in the urethra in males, and in the vagina, uterine cervix, or urethra in females. Children are sometimes infected when sleeping with adults. Extragenital infections occur in the rectum and conjunctiva—very rarely elsewhere. Discussion of non-sexual urethral infection is largely futile, since the facts can seldom be proved. Probabilities are always against it, because the gonococcus perishes so quickly outside the body.

The gonococcus causes an acute inflammatory reaction, with leukocytosis and often fever. In abscesses the pus sometimes has a peculiar brownish color and is odorless. In the chronic stage, scar formation is rather abundant. Spread may occur to any part of the urogenital tract.

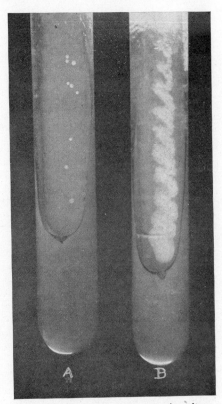

Fig. 51.—Gonococcus grown in culture. The medium is an ascitic fluid veal-broth agar. Tube A was stoppered with an ordinary cotton stopper, while in Tube B the oxygen tension was reduced and the reduced tension maintained by a rubber stopper. The resulting increase in the growth was very marked.

reduced by heating the part of the tube above the agar by passing it through the flame three or four times, then inserting the rubber stopper while the tube is still hot. As it cools in the incubator, the tension within drops. There should be a good growth of gonococcus in twenty-four to thirty-six hours.

[1] Swartz, Shohl, and Davis: Johns Hopkins Hospital Bulletin, 1920, xxxi, 449–452.

Marcel See has collected in his exhaustive monograph[1] all the information about the gonococcus up to 1896. He notes that Wertheim obtained stronger growths in cultures made over pyrogallic acid and potassium hydroxid (partial anaërobiasis). Finger and Gohn inoculated 7 persons who had just recovered from gonorrhea, with positive results in all, demonstrating that there is no immunity, or at least no effective urethral immunity. Heiman successfully inoculated a patient with a fever of over 40° C. Wertheim and Steinschneider failed to produce abscesses by subcutaneous inoculation. See was unable to find gonococci or pseudogonococci in any healthy urethra.

In 1893 Finger had stated:

With regard to the etiology of cystitis, it is a question whether it constitutes a direct blenorrhagic affection or is to be regarded as a mixed infection.

In 1900 we presented a series of cases which showed for the first time the ability of the gonococcus to produce chronic inflammations of· the upper urinary tract, viz., chronic cystitis, pyonephrosis, and also acute general peritonitis.[2]

Wertheim was the first (1895) to cultivate the gonococcus from cystitis. His patient, a girl aged nine years, was suffering from acute gonorrheal vulvovaginitis, acute cystitis, and arthritis of two joints. By means of the cystoscope he excised a small portion of the mucous membrane of the posterior wall of the bladder, and from this he obtained a pure culture of the gonococcus, as also from the urine. In microscopic sections of the tissue removed, a number of gonococci were seen in the epithelium, and in the submucosa "a great many venous capillaries were filled with gonococci, although the arteries did not contain any."

The second and last case in the literature in which the gonococcus has been cultivated from the bladder, was reported by Lindholm in 1896. A girl nineteen years of age had gonorrhea for one month when seen by Lindholm. She then presented acute urethritis and cystitis. A specimen of urine was obtained "with aseptic precautions," and in this gonococci were demonstrated and a pure culture obtained on cyst-fluid agar. Cystoscopic examination showed an inflammation of the entire vesical mucous membrane. The cystitis was rapidly cured by boric acid irrigations and nitrate of silver instillations.

I have had opportunity to obtain cultures by aspiration of the bladder in 5 cases of acute gonorrhea.

In all of them the posterior urethra was involved, and in three an acute cystitis was present, but in only one of these could a culture of the gonococcus be obtained, though in two other cases in which the cultures remained sterile, gonococci were obtained in abundance on coverslip, and decolorized by Gram. In the first case the urine contained a great deal of blood, while in the second and fourth cases no blood was present. The recent work of Colombini offers an explanation for this failure in obtaining cultures:

Colombini examined gonorrheal pus in 235 cases. He found it neutral twice, but in the other cases distinctly alkaline. He also showed that the gonococcus did not develop in urine, not because it was acid, but because it contains no albumin, and that albuminous urine furnishes a good culture-medium whether acid or alkaline.

In this same paper the subject of chronic gonococcus cystitis is discussed as follows:

The vast majority of cases of gonorrheal cystitis as seen clinically are of short duration, and in the few cases where the gonococcus has been found the observers have reported an early cessation of vesical inflammation.

[1] Le Gonococque: Thèse de Paris, No. 289, 1896, 1–359.
[2] Young: Johns Hopkins Hospital Reports, 1900, ix, 679–707 (Lit.).

Nowhere in the literature have I been able to find a suggestion that the gonococcus could produce a chronic cystitis and persist as the sole infecting organism.

The following case of very severe chronic cystitis of five years' duration in which the gonococcus was found alone in great number in the urine, and a pure culture obtained, seems to be the first recorded instance.

Surgery No. 6219. Chronic cystitis of five years' duration following gonorrhea. Double pyonephrosis. Atony of bladder. Retention of urine. Aspiration of bladder. Gonococcus pure in great number on coverslip and culture. Urine very foul and strongly alkaline.

A case of pyonephrosis (the first) due to the gonococcus (as proved by cultures) was also reported. Since then isolated cases of gonococcus infection of the kidney have been published. The following historical résumé was given:

Although Neisser announced his discovery of the gonococcus twenty years ago, it has only been during the last few years that evidence has been forthcoming to prove its peculiar and wide-spread powers of pyogenic infection. The chain of evidence is now practically complete, and is briefly as follows:

In 1879 Neisser demonstrated that this coccus was the cause of gonorrhea and ophthalmia neonatorum, but it was not till 1887 that it was successfully cultivated by Bumm. Since then it has been shown by pure cultures that the gonococcus may be the sole cause of various ascending and metastatic infections, viz.:

Arthritis, first demonstrated in pure culture by Lindemann, 1892.

Tenosynovitis, by Tollemer and Macaigne, 1893.

Perichondritis, by Finger, Ghon, and Schlagenhaufer, 1894.

Abscess, subcutaneous, by Lang and Paltauf, 1893.

Abscess, intramuscular, by Bujivid, 1895.

Salpingitis, by Wertheim, 1892.

Circumscribed pelvic peritonitis, by Wertheim, 1892.

Adenitis (glands of neck), by Pettit and Pichevin, 1896.

Pleurisy, by Mazza, 1894.

Endocarditis, by Thayer and Blumer, 1895.

Septicemia, by Thayer and Blumer, 1895.

Acute cystitis, by Wertheim, 1895.

Chronic cystitis, by Young, 1898.

Pyonephrosis, by Young, 1898.

Diffuse peritonitis, by Young, 1899.

Johnson and Hill[1] report a case of pyelitis due to the gonococcus, with bacteriologic proof, including the fermentation tests as given above. Hill has, after a study of the literature, found 54 so-called cases of gonorrheal pyelitis. These may be divided as follows:

TABLE 11

	Criteria.	Number of cases.
(a)	Smear only.....	20
(b)	No bacteriologic data available.....	11
(c)	Smear and "culture," no details of culture.....	10
(d)	Smear and culture, organism not growing on ordinary media.....	5
(e)	Clinical cases of gonorrhea, but cultures showed other organisms and no gonococcus	4
(f)	"Gonococcus present," no details of criteria.....	2
(g)	Smear and culture, organism conforming to all bacteriologic criteria, including fermentation test.....	1
(h)	Experimental human inoculation, cultures later negative.....	1

Only 6 of these cases, therefore (d and g), can be considered very reliable, and only 1 absolutely proved (g).

[1] Journal of Urology, 1924, xi, 177–187.

Gonococci may find their way into the blood, and cause arthritis, endocarditis, meningitis,[1] abscesses, or septicemia. Thayer[2] reports 198 cases of vegetative endocarditis studied at autopsy. Of these 22 (11.1 per cent.) were caused by the gonococcus. The septicemia is very serious, and often fatal. Of these complications, arthritis is the most common.

Other Gram-negative cocci are rare. It is possible, however, for the *Micrococcus catarrhalis* (Neisseria catarrhalis, S. A. B.) or related forms to be in the urethra, so that in case of doubt when any important issue is at stake, the gonococcus should always be identified culturally. Boyd[3] reports a case of acute purulent seminal vesiculitis with fever and leukocytosis, in which the Micrococcus catarrhalis was isolated from the vesicle contents, in association with staphylococcus and the colon bacillus. Pick[4] reports a case of epidemic cerebrospinal meningitis in which the *Meningococcus* (Neisseria intracellularis, S. A. B.) had caused a purulent seminal vesiculitis and ampullitis, the remainder of the urogenital tract being normal. The organism was thoroughly identified. Westenhoffer[5] found the Meningococcus in renal foci in two infants. In our series are 2 cases in which Gram-negative diplococci, not gonococcus, were recovered from the urine.

OTHER ORGANISMS.—A number of other organisms appearing less frequently in the urogenital tract may be mentioned briefly. The *Tubercle bacillus* (Mycobacterium tuberculosis, S. A. B.) is discussed in the section devoted to Tuberculosis.

Bacilli of the genus Proteus occur fairly frequently. They are usually in chronic cystitis, often that associated with stone, tumor, or obstruction, but may be found with other organisms in chronic pyelitis. The pathogenicity is not great. Both urea and protein are decomposed, so that urine in Proteus infections is ammoniacal and of fetid odor. These organisms may, therefore, be an important factor in causing a calculus to increase rapidly by phosphate deposits. Lenharz[6] reports a case of Proteus septicemia of renal origin.

The *Bacillus pyocyaneus* (Pseudomonas pyocyanea, S. A. B.) is a rather important invader of the urogenital tract. In our series it was present in 16 (4.4 per cent.) of 354 cases. Mathé and Belt[7] found it in only 16 (0.37 per cent.) of 4329 urine cultures. In 251 cases of infections of the upper urinary tract collected by them, 6 Pyocyaneus infections were found. It has also been isolated from infections of the testis and epididymis, and in septicemia. It does not as a rule give its characteristic color to the urine. It is not particularly apt to cause serious complications, but is very persistent and its resistance to most germicides is high. It also occurs in infected wounds.

The *Influenza bacillus* (Hemophilus influenzæ, S. A. B.) is sometimes found in the urine in cases otherwise infected by it. There may be evidence of renal infection.

In cases of *anthrax* with generalized lesions, the kidney may be involved,

[1] Prochaska, Deutsches Archiv für Klinische Medizin, 1905, lxxxiii, 184–196.

[2] Johns Hopkins Hospital Bulletin, 1922, xxxiii, 361–372 (Lit.), and later data presented before the Johns Hopkins Hospital Medical Society, 1923.

[3] Journal of Urology, 1923, x, 367–392.

[4] Berliner Klinische Wochenschrift, 1907, xliv, 994–998.

[5] Quoted by Salabert, Bulletin et Memoires de la Société Médicale des Hôpitaux de Paris, 1910, xxx, 3d series, 65–70.

[6] Virchow's Archiv, 1923, ccxlvi, 443–447.

[7] Journal of Urology, 1922, viii, 281–297.

the foci showing the same sort of gelatinous exudate as occurs elsewhere in the body. The bacilli (Bacillus anthracis, S. A. B.) may appear in the urine when there is no definite nephritis.

The *Bacillus melitensis* (Bact. melitensis, S. A. B.), the cause of Malta fever (Mediterranean or undulant fever), is found in abundance in the urine in cases of the disease. Occasionally a nephritis is caused. Orchitis occurs not infrequently, but the organism has not been cultivated from the testis.

The *Bacillus mallei* (Pfeifferella mallei, S. A. B.) (glanders) also occurs in the urine. The kidney may rarely be involved in cases of "internal glanders" but is spared in "cutaneous glanders" or the forms of the disease known as "farcy." The testis and tunica vaginalis may also be affected.

Plague bacilli (Pasteurella pestis, S. A. B.) may appear in the urine, especially in the septicemic form, but the kidney lesion is usually a toxic degeneration.[1]

In tetanus, yellow fever, and diphtheria the renal lesion is a toxic degeneration, especially severe in the case of yellow fever. *Tetanus bacilli* (Clostridium tetani, S. A. B.) are not found in the urogenital tract except as the result of local wounds. *Diphtheria bacilli* (Corynebacterium diphtheriæ, S. A. B.) also do not occur in the urine, but may cause local ulcerative processes on the external genitalia, especially in children. Diphtheria as a wound infection is of historical interest only.

Bacillus Thompsoni (Corynebacterium Thompsoni).—This organism has been found in our clinic by Thompson and Hill to be the cause of the specific sort of postoperative infection of wounds containing urinary fistulæ, which is characterized by ammoniacal urine, fetid odor, and gangrenous condition of the wound surfaces. It is a very small, almost coccoid organism which is Gram-positive. It grows readily and splits urea strongly, but dies out rapidly in an acid medium. It occurs often in conjunction with the Proteus, but may also occur alone. Infections of this organism are successfully treated by irrigations with dilute acetic acid.[2] Membrane formation occurs, but the organism does not produce an exotoxin.

Diphtheroid organisms of the most varied types are common in nature, and are sometimes found in the urinary tract. Most of them are non-pathogenic, but they may be concerned in genital ulcerations and possibly cystitis[3] often mixed with other organisms. The exact importance of their rôle in these cases is uncertain, but there is reason to believe that even if they occur only as secondary invaders, they may maintain the lesion after the primary causative organism has disappeared. (See the chapter on Ulcerative Lesions of the External Genitalia.)

Some members of this group, normally inhabitants of water, have high thermal resistance, and may be present in water otherwise sterile, especially that distributed through complicated systems of piping. If such water is used for irrigations of the urinary tract, these organisms may survive for some time in the urine and be recovered by culture. They are apparently non-pathogenic, and we have not seen any lesions due to them, or found any reported in the literature.

[1] Manson: Tropical Diseases, 5th ed., 1914.

[2] Hill and Shaw: Journal of Urology, 1925, xiii, 689–713.

[3] Townsend: Journal of the American Medical Association, 1913, lxi, 1605–1609; Rosenow: Journal of Infectious Diseases, 1909, vi, 296–303; Herbst and Gatewood: Journal of the American Medical Association, 1912, lviii, 188–191.

Various *mycotic organisms* occur in the urogenital tract and often cause lesions similar to those of tuberculosis. Among them may be mentioned, the Actinomycetes (Streptothrices) Leptothrices, etc. They are fully discussed in the chapter devoted to these infections.

Dysentery bacilli (Bact. dysenteriæ, paradysenteriæ, etc., S. A. B.) of the various types are found in the urine during the disease, sometimes accompanied by pus. A peculiar and fatal condition of symmetrical cortical necrosis of the kidneys[1] is seen in a few cases of dysentery, but the rôle of the bacillus in its pathogeny is not known.

An organism resembling the *Leishman-Donovan body* has been found in the lesions of granuloma inguinale (*q. v.*) both in this country and South America,[2] and is considered by Randall to be the cause of the disease.

The bacillus of *leprosy* (Mycobacterium lepræ, S. A. B.) may cause lesions of the external genitalia or testis, and more rarely of the other urogenital organs. The lesion is a proliferating granuloma, greatly resembling that of tuberculosis, with fibrosis, round-cell infiltration, giant-cells, and necrosis. The tendency to necrosis is perhaps somewhat less marked. The testicular lesion, unlike that of tuberculosis, begins in the testis itself.

Yeasts and *sarcinæ* may be found in the urine, but are probably not pathogenic. Grawitz found that moulds injected intravenously in animals are excreted in the urine, apparently without renal lesion. Thrush may involve the external genitalia, in which case the *Oïdium albicans* (Monilia albicans) is found in the lesions. Castellani[3] reports a case of urethritis due to this organism.

Amebæ may appear in the urine in lesions beginning in the intestine and perforating the urinary tract. It is possible that they may also reach the urinary tract by way of the lymphatics. McKenna reports a case in which amebæ were found in the vesicular and prostatic secretion of a patient who had suffered from amebic dysentery, and Warthin[4] one in which they were found in lesions in the testis and epididymis. Dobell[5] has covered the entire subject in his excellent monograph. Living and motile phagocytes may be mistaken for amebæ by the unwary.

The passage of gas from the urinary tract is known as *pneumaturia*.[6] According to Senator[7] such cases can be divided into three groups: (1) Where air is introduced from without; (2) where the gas enters the urinary tract through a fistula connecting with the intestine; and (3) where the gas is produced in the urinary tract by fermentation. The first group is of little importance, as the air is soon expelled. The second group is discussed elsewhere. The third group concerns us here. A further division can be made into cases with glycosuria, and those with sugar-free urines. In general, it may be said that this type of pneumaturia occurs usually

---

[1] Bamforth: Journal of Pathology and Bacteriology, 1923, xxvi, 40–45.

[2] Donovan: Indian Medical Gazette, 1905, xl, 414; Aragão and Vianna, Memorias do Instituto Oswaldo Cruz, 1913, v, 221–238; Randall, Small, and Belk: Journal of Urology, 1921, v, 539–548; Gage: Archives of Dermatology and Syphilology, 1923, viii, 303–325 (Lit.).

[3] Castellani and Chalmers: Manual of Tropical Medicine, 2d ed., 1913.

[4] Journal of Infectious Diseases, 1922, xxx, 559–568.

[5] The Amœbæ Living in Man, 1919, 125–129 (Lit.).

[6] Kelly and MacCallum: Journal of the American Medical Association, 1898, xxxi, 375–381.

[7] Internationale Beiträge zur Wissenschäftlichen Medizin, 1891, iii, 317–332.

in already infected urines, often with obstruction, stone, or neoplasm, and usually after instrumentation.

In cases with glycosuria, two types of fermentation have been observed. Senator[1] studied a case in which the organism present was a yeast, and the process was a true alcoholic fermentation, since the gas formed was carbon dioxid, and alcohol was found in the urine. Pere and others have described cases in which the Colon bacillus produced acid and gas from diabetic urine in the bladder just as it does from glucose bouillon in the incubator. Any other organism with this property might produce pneumaturia in a diabetic.

Fewer cases have occurred in which pneumaturia accompanied a sugar-free urine. Favre,[2] Schow,[3] and Heyse[4] report instances in which the organism is not definitely identified, but in the opinion of MacCallum[5] was probably the Bacillus lactis aëogenes in each case. Welch and Flexner found a bladder distended with gas at autopsy in a case with gas bacillus infection. In this case the gas was hydrogen. It is probable that anaërobic organisms are concerned in pneumaturia in other cases reported, but no cultural data have been found.

Oxygen, nitrogen, hydrogen, carbon dioxid, and methane have been found in these cases. The nature of the gas will depend on the organism, and also on whether sugar is present.

The gas-producing fermentation may be confined to the bladder, or, more rarely, involve the upper tract. When this is true, one side only is usually involved, since the gas formation is secondary to some other lesion. The gas may occur in a pyonephrosis, an infected retention cyst, or even be external to the kidney in a perinephric abscess (LeDentu[6]). A case has been reported in which the entire urinary tract was distended with gas.

After enterovesical fistulæ have been ruled out, careful aërobic and anaërobic studies should be made of all cases of pneumaturia to add to our knowledge of this interesting condition.

Anaërobic organisms in the urogenital tract deserve further study. DuMesnil de Rochemont[7] first called attention to them in 1896. Albarran[8] isolated a strictly anaërobic coccus from the fetid urine of a case of vesical neoplasm. Hartmann and Roger[9] report anerobic organisms in 5 cases of cystitis and Cottet[10] in 12 of perinephric and peri-urethral abscesses. In this country David[11] has isolated anaërobic organisms fourteen times in 10 cases. Among the organisms mentioned are the Diplococcus reniformis (Gram-negative), the Streptococcus parvulus, the Micrococcus fetidus, the Streptobacillus fusiformis, the Bacillus ramosus,

[1] Internationale Beiträge zur Wissenschaftlichen Medizin, 1891, iii, 317–322.

[2] Ziegler's Beiträge, 1888, iii, 159–188.

[3] Centralblatt für Bakteriologie und Parasitenkunde, 1892, xii, 745–749.

[4] Zeitschrift für Klinische Medizin, 1894, xxiv, 130–183.

[5] Kelly and MacCallum: Journal of the American Medical Association, 1898, xxxi, 375-381.

[6] Affections Chirurgicales des Reins, Paris, 1889, 484.

[7] Zur Pathogenie der Blasenentzündungen, 1896 (Berlin).

[8] Procés-verbaux, etc., de l'Association Française d'Urologie, 1898, iii, 6–76 (Albarran and Halle, Lit.); 83–97 (Albarran and Cottet). The first session (pp. 1–134) is entirely devoted to infection, and contains papers by Janet, Escat, Carlier, Desnos, Picqué, Loumeau, Genouville, and Hamonic.

[9] Presse mèdicale, 1902, x, 1107–1108.

[10] Thèse de Paris, 1899.

[11] Surgery, Gynecology, and Obstetrics, 1914, xviii, 432–437.

the Bacillus of malignant edema (Clostridium edematis, S. A. B.) and the Bacillus Welchii (Clostridium aërogenes capsulatus, S. A. B.). Most of the anaërobic organisms are proteolytic, producing decomposition products of offensive odor, and are, therefore, especially to be sought for in cases with putrid urine. The Bacillus Welchii has been reported from cases of cystitis with pneumaturia, and may cause generalized infections from lesions beginning in the urogenital tract. It may invade urinary extravasations. Little is known concerning the pathologic significance of anaërobic infections of the urogenital tract, but it is to be hoped that this lack will be remedied at an early date.

Bacteriologic studies of the urogenital tract are beset with difficulties arising principally from the danger of contamination during collection of the specimen. The preputial cavity in men, and the vagina in women, contain normally a great variety of organisms. Many urethræ, apparently normal, contain organisms. Rovsing[1] found, in healthy urethræ, practically all the forms occuring in urinary infection. Savor[2] studied 93 healthy women. In 31 the urethral cultures were sterile, while the colon bacillus was found in 14, the staphylococcus in 22, the streptococcus in 4, and "a diplococcus" in 9. In most cases where the prostatic or vesicular secretion is to be studied, the urethra is also infected. Kidney urine must be frequently obtained by catheterization across an infected bladder. We, in 1898,[3] reported a series in which bladder cultures were obtained by suprapubic puncture—a method entirely free from errors, but not suited to routine use. We further found that thorough irrigation of the urethra was an effective method of removing organisms from it. Player, Lee-Brown, and Mathé[4] report an ingenious method for obtaining vesicular and prostatic secretion without contamination from the urethra, and Klika[5] describes a complicated, but theoretically sound method for inserting a ureteral catheter without vesical contamination. Proper precautions to prevent contamination must always be taken; careless cultural work in the urogenital tract is simply time wasted.

In a great many cases when bacteria are few in number they will not be seen in stained smears, and can only be found by *culture*. It is also common for organisms to reappear after they have apparently been eliminated by vigorous treatment. For these reasons, cultural criteria alone are admissible to prove a cure of chronic lesions, such as pyelitis, and such cures should not be claimed unless supported by negative cultures on several occasions.

Urine cultures often show more than one organism, but it is usual for infections to be due at first to a single organism. Thus acute cystitis (Brown[6]) and epididymitis yield pure cultures in their early stages, and in early acute gonorrhea pure cultures of gonococcus are obtained in a great majority of cases.

The urine, as is well known, may be secreted either acid or alkaline. If infected, its *reaction* at the time of voiding will depend on whether or not the organisms concerned have altered the original reaction. Certain bacteria produce neither acid nor alkali in the urine, or else do so in such small quantities that the

---

[1] Die Blasenentzündungen, Berlin, 1910.
[2] Beiträge zur Geburtshülfe und Gynäkologie, 1899, ii, 103–147 (Lit.).
[3] Young: Maryland Medical Journal, 1898, xxxix, 630.
[4] Journal of Urology, 1923, x, 375–385.
[5] Zeitschrift für Urologie, 1923, xvii, 77–81.
[6] Journal of the American Medical Association, 1901, xxxvi, 1395–1397.

original reaction is not appreciably changed. In this class come the colon group and most of the Gram-negative cocci. Staphylococci may produce very small amounts of acid, while the bacillus coli has been shown to form fairly appreciable quantities of alkali. The colon bacillus never produces acid in urine unless it contains glucose. The urine is usually acid in colon infections solely because it is usually secreted acid.

Certain organisms make the urine strongly *alkaline* and *ammoniacal* because they decompose urea into ammonium carbonate. In this group are a very few of the staphylococci and the Bacillus proteus. There are no doubt others, but this point has not as yet been thoroughly determined. If a urea-splitting organism grows in the urine, a very large quantity of alkali is produced, so that any acid production by other forms is greatly surpassed, even in diabetic urines. This high alkalinity may serve to kill off certain forms formerly present, for example, the colon bacillus. If the urine is not ammoniacal, its normal limits of acidity and alkalinity are not wide enough to interfere seriously with the growth of any of the common organisms. Shohl and Janney[1] have studied the colon bacillus carefully in this regard, and find that it is impossible to alter the reaction of normal urine in either direction, by feeding or administering drugs, sufficiently to inhibit the growth of the colon bacillus in it. Some other explanation, therefore, must be found for the favorable action of alkalies or acids by mouth in certain cases of pyelitis.

In cases where the urine has a putrid, fetid, or otherwise offensive odor, it is due to the action of *proteolytic organisms* on albumin contained in the urine. This albumin may be present as the result of renal albuminuria, or of seropurulent exudations from the walls of the urinary tract.

Outline of Special Technic for Urologic Bacteriology.—Urology has bacteriologic problems all its own, which can only be solved by those who devote close attention to this work and understand the special circumstances under which it must be done. We desire to present the following practical outline, which is the result of daily experiences in the laboratory of our clinic for a number of years by Miss Justina H. Hill. It may confidently be followed as a reliable standard, and we recommend its adoption. Careless or incomplete bacteriologic work in urology is worse than none at all.

The lack of any similar work has forced us to prepare this outline for our own use. It is offered to those interested in the same problems with the hope that it will assist them in obtaining the bacteriologic information routinely needed in urology as accurately, quickly, and simply as possible. Because of the limited scope of routine urologic bacteriology, much subject matter has been eliminated from this outline which is necessarily included in more general manuals. On the other hand, special methods have been included which are omitted or not emphasized in works of broader scope. The material presented here is, therefore, essentially a condensation and selection of methods gathered from many different sources. Whenever possible, the procedures of the Society of American Bacteriologists have been followed. While bacteriologic methods, still far from perfect, are constantly changing and improving and although there is room for differences of opinion in these problems, the material given here seems to include the methods of choice at the present time.

[1] Journal of Urology, 1917, i, 211–229.

I. The Collection of Specimens for Culture.—1. *Urethral Cultures.*— These are best made by direct transfer of the material by means of a sterilized platinum loop from the urethra to the culture-medium. As these cultures are usually for the gonococcus, too much emphasis cannot be placed on the importance of having the medium used (see below) warm and moist and on the immediate return of the inoculated medium to the laboratory for incubation. If the culture is allowed to remain even a few minutes at room temperature, or exposed to light, negative results are valueless.

2. *Wound Cultures.*—The material for these may be obtained by means of sterile cotton swabs, which are kept for the purpose in sterile glass tubes in the wards and operating rooms. Immediate inoculation of the media from the wound with a platinum loop is still better. It is wise to use two swabs for each culture, one of which may be used for the inoculation of media, the other for smears, as otherwise, if the smears must be made after the cultures, there is often too little material left for a fair examination. It is important that there be no delay in sending these swabs to the laboratory, as they dry out rapidly and some of the organisms originally present may be lost.

3. *Urine Cultures.*—Before the patient voids the glans penis should be sterilized with an alcohol sponge and the anterior urethra then cleansed by injecting a mild antiseptic solution (1 : 1000 meroxyl, or 1 : 20,000 bichlorid of mercury). We use a rubber bulb syringe for this purpose. The first part of the urine is allowed to escape, thus further cleansing the urethra. The latter part of the voiding, but not the very last part, is caught in a culture tube. Urine should always be collected in sterile test- or centrifuge tubes. It is advisable to have these sterilized with paper caps in addition to the cotton plugs. These caps both protect the tubes before use and, if obviously untampered with, offer a greater degree of assurance that the tubes have not been opened and contaminated before use than is possible with the easily removed and replaced cotton plugs alone. Although, of course, it is possible to culture urines not collected in this way, the amount of time required to obtain pure cultures and the probability of error are greatly increased when specimens are collected in open glasses or carelessly sterilized containers. Great care must be used to avoid wetting the cotton stopper with urine at any time.

4. *Cultures of Prostatic Secretions.*—If these are for the gonococcus, the same precautions must be observed as have previously been stated, that is, there must be no chilling or exposure to light. The secretions should be obtained in sterile test or centrifuge tubes. When there is a sufficient quantity of secretion, it may be centrifugalized in a tube with as fine a tip as possible, but this can seldom be done. However, usually it is possible to fish from the secretion by means of a sterilized platinum loop the most purulent parts for smear and culture. When the secretion is clear, it is wise to culture all of it by transferring it by means of a sterile pipet to a solid medium, or similarly, by adding to it sterile broth.

Unless an examination for tubercle bacilli is to be made, the centrifuge tube is probably the best original container, for the specimen may be spun without transfer. The chief objection to the use of the centrifuge tube in this way is that the specimen is lost, if, as rarely happens, the tube is broken in the centrifuge. This danger may be obviated by transferring part of the specimen by means of a sterile pipet to a sterile tube before centrifugalization. However, if due care is taken, breakage occurs so seldom that the procedure is quite safe and it has the advantage of saving both time and handling. If test-tubes are used for the original containers, transfers must be made to centrifuge tubes by means of sterile pipets, never by pouring the urine from one tube to the other. If the specimen is especially clear, it is frequently worth while to reserve a portion of the uncentrifugalized urine for incubation, as the urine itself often furnishes an excellent medium for bacterial growth.

If an examination for tubercle bacilli is to be made, at least 2 centrifuge tubes should be used for each specimen, if the quantity of urine allows. In this way enough sediment is obtained for adequate smears, cultures, and guinea-pig inoculation.

The method of Jones[1] for finding tubercle bacilli should be tried in all urologic laboratories. The urine is centrifugalized at lowest speed for two or three minutes to remove the bulk of the pus. The cloudy supernatant is then decanted, one-half of it poured into a second centrifuge tube, to which is added one-quarter volume of 95 per cent. alcohol and one-quarter volume of distilled water. This mixture is then centrifugalized at highest speed until clear, forty-five minutes, the supernatant fluid discarded, and smears made from the sediment and stained.

Guinea-pig inoculations for tuberculosis are made with salt-solution emulsions of the urinary sediment. A lesion usually develops at the site of inoculation in from two to three weeks, and upon autopsy the organisms may be recovered from the retroperitoneal lymph-nodes. Inoculation should be made subcutaneously on one side of the lower abdomen, care being taken not to perforate the peritoneum, or, if this accidentally happens, not to puncture the intestine. This may be avoided by holding the pig with its head down and pointing the needle toward the inguinal glands. Very rarely well-developed tuberculosis is found upon autopsy without the appearance of a lesion at the site of inoculation, so that it is always necessary to check this. Pigs which fail to develop lesions are held two months before being killed and examined.

II. THE DIRECT SMEAR.—With the exception of cultures for the gonococcus, in which there must be no delay in getting them into the incubator, the examination of a direct smear of any specimen is always logically the first step. Choice of culture methods often depends on the findings in the smear, especially when more than one organism is seen. Also, the correlation of the findings of the smear with those of the culture is invaluable. Organisms may be found in the smear which are not viable on culture, especially after drug therapy. On the other hand, organisms may appear in the culture which were not seen in the smear. In urine cultures, for example, a scant growth of a Gram-positive coccus in forty-eight hours, which was not seen in the smear, may usually be interpreted as a contamination, unless repeated cultures disclose the same organism. However, there is undoubtedly a degree of infection in which the organisms are too few to be seen in the smear, but yet enough to give a few colonies on culture. This seems to be especially true in prostatic secretions, which by the usual methods often fail to show organisms in the smear, in spite of the presence of many white blood-cells, the nature of the infection being determined only by culture.

If smears are made at once after specimens are taken, a fair estimate may be

[1] A Method of Demonstrating Tubercle Bacilli in the Urine, Jour. Amer. Med. Assoc., lxxxiii, 1917, December 13, 1924.

made of the heaviness of the infection by determining the average number of bacteria per microscopic field. Such determinations are valueless if the specimens are allowed to stand at all. Unless the bladder has been emptied five minutes before the specimen is taken, a count of bladder urine is always valueless, because the bladder itself is an excellent bacterial incubator. But counts of fresh specimens are of use in following infections over long courses of treatment, although it must be remembered that a wide range of variation is to be expected.

In the preparation of smears for staining, the ideal is to obtain a smear in which the material is evenly distributed. In the case of specimens which show little or no macroscopic sediment, several loopfuls of material may be applied to one portion of the slide and the area so covered marked on the under side of the slide by a circle made with a glass pencil, in order to facilitate finding the area again. On the other hand, when the sediment is very heavy, one loopful must be spread out over a large area of the slide, in order to obtain a film thin enough for clear examination. In making slides for acid-fast staining as thick a smear should be made as is conducive to clear focussing. It is always wise to make two smears from every specimen, to allow for possible breakage of one of the slides, or in case there is some unusual finding which suggests special staining methods. In reporting findings from direct smears the presence of white blood-cells, red blood-cells, and epithelial cells should be noted, including their relative quantity, as well as the types and amount of bacteria present. Too much emphasis cannot be placed on the extreme morphologic variations of organisms seen in direct smears. The Colon Group bacilli may vary from organisms strongly resembling Leptothrices to diplococcoid forms. There are Gram-positive diplococci which, except for the Gram stain, could not be accurately distinguished from the gonococcus. That is, too much must not be concluded from the direct smear, which should be depended upon only to give an idea of the types of organisms to be found by culture.

III. STAINING METHODS.—By far the most useful stain for the urologic laboratory is that of Gram. It gives the most accurate picture, and saves time in the end by its clear differentiation of the various types of organisms usually found. Because there are many Gram-positive cocci which may closely resemble the gonococcus, it is the only scientific stain to use when this organism is in question. We feel very strongly that the use of methylene-blue or any other stain which does not differentiate these organisms cannot be too much condemned.

Although there are many Gram stains recommended, we prefer the following one-minute modification of Nicolle.

Stock solutions:

1. Saturated alcoholic solution of gentian or crystal violet.
2. Two and a half per cent. aqueous solution of phenol.
3. Gram's iodin solution, i. e.:

Iodin... 1 gm.
Potassium iodid..................................... 2 gm.
Distilled water.. 300 c.c.

4. Acetone 1 part and alcohol 3 parts.
5. Dilute carbolfuchsin, i. e., 1 of Ziehl-Neelsen to 20 of water.

Staining method:

A small graduate, with a bulb pipet fitted in the top by means of a cork is kept in a rack made for the purpose with drop bottles of Solutions 3, 4, and 5, in order of use. Every morning this graduate is carefully cleaned and in it is freshly prepared a mixture of 1 part of Solution 1 plus 9 parts of Solution 2, giving carbol gentian-violet. The staining method is as follows: After heat fixation of the smears, flood with the carbol gentian-violet solution for ten seconds, pour off, add Gram's iodin for ten seconds, pour off, decolorize with Solution 4 until the smear no longer streaks purple (usually one quick application suffices), wash quickly in tap-water and counterstain ten seconds or longer with Solution 5, wash in tap-water, dry, and examine under an oil-immersion lens.

By this method very clear-cut differentiation may be obtained. But, as is true of all Gram stains, to obtain the best results practice is necessary. It must also be remembered that organisms from old cultures stain irregularly and if the smear is uneven the best and clearest areas must be used for microscopic examination.

The Society of American Bacteriologists recommends two formulæ for the Gram stain[1] which others may prefer.

The only other stain essential for urologic work is the acid-fast stain. We use Ziehl-Neelsen's method, the methods which supposedly differentiate the tubercle bacillus from other acid-fast organisms being unsatisfactory. Ziehl-Neelsen's method is as follows:

Stock solutions:

1. Carbolfuchsin; saturated alcoholic solution of basic fuchsin, 10 c.c., 5 per cent. aqueous solution of phenol, 100 c.c.

2. Acid alcohol; 95 per cent. ethyl alcohol, containing 3 per cent. hydrochloric acid.

3. Löffler's methylene-blue; saturated alcoholic solution of methylene-blue, 30 c.c., 1 : 10,000 potassium hydroxid solution, 100 c.c. (Two drops of a 10 per cent. solution of KOH in 100 c.c. of water makes a 1 : 10,000 solution.)

Drop bottles of these reagents are kept in a rack in the order of use.

Staining Method:

After heat fixation of smears, stain five minutes with carbolfuchsin, heating gently, so that the stain steams, but taking care that it never dries off; wash in water; decolorize with acid alcohol until the best portions of the smear are a very delicate pink; wash in water; counterstain lightly with methylene-blue (usually merely pouring the counterstain on and off is enough), wash in water; dry, examine under oil-immersion lens.

For heating the smears we use the apparatus devised by C. F. Elvers.[2] (See Fig. 160.)

IV. CULTURES.—The clinical picture or examination of direct smears will indicate in which of the following groups a given specimen belongs and cultures can then be made according to such findings:

Group 1. Infection with Gram-negative bacilli.

---

[1] Manual of Methods for Pure Culture Study of Bacteria, Prepared by the Committee on Bacteriological Technic of the Society of American Bacteriologists, published by the Society of American Bacteriologists, Geneva, N. Y

[2] A New Apparatus for Heating Bacterial and Blood Smears, Johns Hopkins Hospital Bulletin, 1924, xxxv, 94.

Group 2. Infection with Gram-positive cocci:

    A. Streptococcus or Pneumococcus morphology.

    B. Staphylococcus or Micrococcus morphology.

Group 3. Infection with Gram-negative cocci.

Group 4. Mixed infection.

Group 5. No organisms seen in the direct smear.

Group 6. Infection with anaërobic organisms suspected.

Group 7. Infection with organisms other than those in the other groups.

Culture methods will be discussed under these group headings.

Group 1. Infection with Gram-negative Bacilli.—As by far the most common bacilli found in urologic infections are those of the Colon Group, the first medium to be inoculated should be one containing lactose. As it is possible that there may be more than one Gram-negative bacillus causing the infection, and in order to obtain separate colonies for fishing and subculture, the streaking of lactose agar plates offers the simplest and most satisfactory way of making a presumptive identification in the shortest time. Fresh lactose agar plates may be poured daily (for preparation of media, see Part V) or enough may be poured to last two or three days, the reserve supply being kept in the ice box. If a large number of bacilli have been seen in the smear, three plates should be used; if the number in the smear was small, two plates are enough. Using one loopful of sediment for all of the plates, they are given about eight streaks each, great care being taken not to open the Petri dishes any more than necessary at the time of inoculation. At the same time a tube of dextrose broth, either a fermentation tube or a large tube with a small one inverted in the bottom of it, should be inoculated, and a tube of sucrose broth or agar and a tube of plain broth without indicator. By these inoculations, it is usually possible after overnight incubation to obtain the following results:

1. To make a presumptive identification of the tribe and genus of the organism or organisms present, as follows:

(*a*) Acid and gas formed in dextrose and lactose, a presumptive identification of the genus Escherichia (Bact. coli group), or the genus Aërobacter (Bact. aërogenes group).

(*b*) Acid and gas formed from dextrose and sucrose, but not lactose, colonies usually showing characteristic spreading amæboid growth, presumptive genus Proteus.

(*c*) Acid and gas formed from dextrose, but not from lactose or sucrose, presumptive genus Salmonella (the paratyphoid group).

(*d*) Acid from dextrose, but no gas, lactose and sucrose may be fermented, but without gas, presumptive genus Eberthella (the typhoid and the dysentery group).

(*e*) No acid or gas formed, presumptive genus Alcaligines (Bact. alcaligines).

(*f*) Encapsulated, non-motile bacilli growing with the characteristic mucoid, viscid growth, presumptive genus Encapsulatus (Bact. pneumoniæ group).

(*g*) Motile organisms, producing chloroform-soluble blue pigment (see plain broth tube) presumptive genus Pseudomonas, species pyocyanea.

(*h*) Small bacilli, growing only in presence of blood or other serous fluids, Hemophilus of Ducrey.

It must be strongly emphasized that this identification is presumptive only and that it must be confirmed by further tests. Carbohydrate fermentation is sometimes delayed, as is chromogenesis. It is wise to incubate at least one of the plates for forty-eight hours to allow the growth of slow-growing organisms.

2. To fish one or more colonies from the lactose agar plates and so to obtain a culture suitable for subcultures.

3. By examination of one of the broth cultures by means of a hanging drop, to determine the motility of the organism, but if motility is not observed, a second broth culture should be made and examined not later than eighteen hours after inoculation.

When single colonies have been fished from the plates, care having been taken to select only entirely isolated colonies, subcultures may be made, varying with the presumptive identification of the organism.

(a) *Genus Escherichia* (Bact. coli group) or *genus Aërobacter* (Bact. aërogenes group).

1. The differentiation of these genera depends upon the production of acetyl-methyl-carbinol from dextrose by the genus Aërobacter, and the failure of the genus Escherichia to do this (Vosges-Proskauer test). To make this test, inoculate a tube of Vosges-Proskauer broth (see Part V) incubate five days at 37° C., then add 2 to 3 c.c. of 10 per cent. KOH and incubate one hour. A pink to red color indicates a positive test, that is, the presence of acetyl-methyl-carbinol, but if the red color does not appear within that time, the broth should be incubated overnight and then read.

2. Correlated with this is the Clark-Lubs test, made by inoculating the medium used for this purpose (see Part V), incubating five days at 37° C., then adding 4 to 5 drops of methyl-red indicator, the genus Escherichia, or Bact. coli group giving a red color, or positive test, an orange color indicating a negative test. The methyl-red indicator is prepared as follows:

Methyl-red powder	0.1 gm.
Neutral 95 per cent. ethyl alcohol	300 c.c.
Distilled water	500 c.c.

By these tests these two genera may be separated. We feel that for clinical purposes, generic identification is sufficient with organisms in these two genera, there being many species and an infinite number of varieties in each. The only manual of determinative bacteriology at present available which uses recent bacteriologic methods is that of Bergey[1] which was arranged by a committee of the Society of American Bacteriologists. It is to be hoped that a revised and enlarged edition of this book will soon be prepared. If specific identification is desired, Bergey's manual may be used, although the urologist will constantly encounter many organisms which do not correspond with any given in the manual. Bergey gives 22 species of the genus Escherichia (Colon Group) based on carbohydrate fermentations, especially sucrose, salicin, and dulcitol; motility, the reduction of nitrates, the action of the organisms on milk and the production of indol also being used. For the indol and nitrate tests, the reader is referred to the

[1] Manual of Determinative Bacteriology. A Key for the Identification of Organisms of the Class Schizomycetes, Arranged by a Committee of the Society of American Bacteriologists, David H. Bergey, Chairman; Francis C. Harrison, Robert S. Breed, Bernard W. Hammer, Frank M. Huntoon, Baltimore, Williams & Wilkins Company, 1923.

Manual of Methods for Pure Culture Study of Bacteria which is a necessary part of the equipment of any bacteriologic laboratory. Bergey has 6 species in his genus Aërobacter, classified according to the fermentation of sucrose, adonitol and dulcitol, motility and the production of indol also being important. The urologist will have difficulty in finding an organism which corresponds exactly to any species in either of these genera on account of the great variations in these organisms. The problem of bacteriologic classification and nomenclature is at present under active consideration. While preferring the more conservative usage which has the authority of the Society of American Bacteriologists, we have also included the more recent system found in Bergey's manual.

(b) *Genus Proteus.*—This genus is defined by Bergey as follows: "Highly pleomorphic rods. Filamentous and curved rods are common as involution forms. Gram-negative. Actively motile, possessing peritrichous flagella. Produce characteristic ameboid colonies on moist media and decompose proteins. Ferment dextrose and sucrose, but not lactose. Do not produce acetyl-methyl-carbinol. The type species is Proteus vulgaris Hauser."

Again we think that the specific identification of organisms in this genus is unnecessary for the clinician. However, it may be done on the basis of the fermentation of mannitol, sucrose, maltose, and salicin, by the liquefaction of gelatin and the production of indol, Bergey giving 6 species, one of which, inconsistently with the generic definition, is non-motile.

(c) *Genus Salmonella.*—This genus, which includes the paratyphoid bacilli, is not often found in urologic infections, but occurs frequently enough to make its identification important. Bergey defines the genus as follows:

"Motile forms occurring in the intestinal canal of animals, in various types of acute inflammatory conditions. Attack numerous carbohydrates with the formation of both acid and gas. In general do not form acetyl-methyl-carbinol. The type species is Salmonella schottmülleri."

There are 17 species given at present, the fermentation of mannitol, xylose, dulcitol, inositol, salicin, dextrin, raffinose, levulose, and maltose being important. The final test with these organisms is, however, the absorption of agglutinins. As these organisms are found so seldom in urologic work it is not usually worth while to keep the necessary immune sera for these tests on hand, but unless other serologic work is also being done, to have the culture tested in a general laboratory.

(d) *Genus Eberthella.*—This is important because it includes the typhoid and dysentery bacilli. The genus definition of Bergey is:

"Motile or non-motile rods, occurring in the intestinal canal of man, usually in different forms of enteric inflammation. Attack a number of carbohydrates with the formation of acid, but no gas. Do not form acetyl-methyl-carbinol. The type species is Eberthella typhi (Eberth-Gaffky), Castellani and Chalmers."

There are at present 25 species in this genus, differentiated by motility, indol production and the fermentation of lactose, inositol, levulose, maltose, dextrin, mannitol, sorbitol, salicin, dulcitol, sucrose, arabinose, rhamnose, and xylose. As in the preceding genus, the final test is agglutination.

(e) *Genus Alcaligines.*—This is defined by Bergey as:

"Motile or non-motile rods, generally occurring in the intestinal canal of normal animals. Do not form acetyl-methyl-carbinol. Do not ferment any of the carbohydrates. The type species is Alcaligines fecalis (Petruschky)." There are at present 9 species in this genus, differentiated by the liquefaction of gelatin, motility, the reduction of nitrates. Organisms of this genus are found infrequently in urinary infections, but they do occur.

(f) *Tribe Encapsulateæ, Genus Encapsulatus.*—The tribe is defined as follows: "Short rods, somewhat plump with rounded ends, mostly occurring singly. Encapsulated. Non-motile. Gram-negative. Ferment a number of carbohydrates with the formation of acid and gas. Encountered principally in the respiratory tract of man. Aërobic, growing well on ordinary culture-media." "The type species is Encapsulatus pneumoniæ (Friedlander)." There are at present 6 species, differentiated on the basis of the fermentation of dextrose, lactose and sucrose and the reduction of nitrates, although 1 species does not ferment any carbohydrates.

(g) *Genus Pseudomonas.*—The only species of this genus of interest to the urologist is Pseudomonas aëruginosa (Bacillus pyocyaneus), which may be identified best by the production of pyocyanin, a blue pigment soluble in chloroform.

(h) *Hemophilus Ducreyii.*—This minute bacillus is entirely different in its cultural requirements from the Gram-negative bacilli described above. It may be successfully cultured by the method of Teague and Deibert.[1] The essentials of this method are as follows:

"A rabbit is bled from the heart with a sterile 20-c.c. syringe and the blood is distributed in amounts slightly less than 1 c.c. in test-tubes about 100 mm. long and 10 mm. in diameter. The blood is allowed to clot at room temperature, is then heated for five minutes at 55° C., and is either used at once or is kept in the ice-box overnight and used on the following day. We found that instead of heating the clotted blood equally good results were obtained when the tubes were simply kept in the ice-box for from three to five days before they were used. Pieces of stiff iron wire, gage 18, about $5\frac{1}{2}$ inches long are bent upon themselves at one end for about $\frac{1}{8}$ inch. Ten or 12 of these wires are placed in a 6-inch test-tube and are heated in the dry sterilizer. The patient is told to remove the dressing, if he has one, and a bit of pus from the ulcer is picked up with the bent end of the sterile wire, the latter having been first rubbed gently over the base of the ulcer or under its undermined edge. The pus is then transferred to a tube of clotted blood and is quickly distributed in the serum by passing the wire several times around the clot. A second tube is inoculated in the same way with a fresh wire. After from twenty to twenty-four hours incubation at 37° C. the serum around the clot is thoroughly stirred with a platinum loop and then a smear is made and stained by Gram's method. Examination with the oil-immersion lens shows characteristic chains of small Gram-negative bacilli, sometimes apparently in pure culture, sometimes together with Gram-positive cocci or bacilli. If these characteristic chains are present, it is stated that the culture is positive for Ducrey bacilli." To obtain pure cultures, blood-agar plates may be inoculated from these primary cultures, but the nutrient agar used must be slightly alkaline, pH 7.2 or 7.3. The blood agar must not be dry nor too stiff.

Group 2. Infection with Gram-positive Cocci.—A. *Streptococcus of Pneumococcus Morphology.*—If organisms of this type are seen in the smear or are suspected, the best medium to use is plated blood agar, as in this way the action of the strep-

---

[1] The Value of the Cultural Method in the Diagnosis of Chancroid, Jour. Urology, iv, 543, December, 1920.

tococci on blood can be determined at once and separate colonies obtained for fishing. As it is wise to hold negative plates at least a week for incubation, thick plates should be poured, by increasing the amount of blood as well as agar used, or by first pouring a layer of plain agar and, after it has solidified, adding another layer of blood agar. For routine work this is enough. Suspected pneumococci may be fished, tested for bile solubility and typed, but they are found very rarely in urine. Streptococci, however, occur quite frequently.

B. *Staphylococcus of Micrococcus Morphology.*—Staphylococci are usually quite typical in their morphologic characteristics. When they are seen in smears, cultures should include Löffler's blood-serum or potato, as chromogenesis is apt to be more prompt on these media. Otherwise, they may be differentiated on the basis of the fermentation of lactose, sucrose, mannitol, and raffinose and by the liquefaction of gelatin.

There remains a large group of Gram-positive cocci found in urologic specimens which must for the present be classified as Micrococci. They may be differentiated by chromogenesis, gelatin liquefaction, action on milk, growth on potato, and the reduction of nitrates. From the point of view of the urologist, however, this is entirely unsatisfactory and it is hoped that the study of the Gram-positive cocci found in urinary infection can soon be undertaken, in order to increase our very meager and unsatisfactory knowledge of this large group of bacteria.

Group 3. The Gram-negative Cocci.—Neisseria gonorrheæ, or the gonococcus, is by far the most important species in this group to the urologist. Of the many culture methods suggested for this organism, we much prefer that of Swartz.[1] For the laboratory in which gonococcus cultures are made infrequently, it has the advantage over blood agar of keeping, for it may be made when convenient and kept in the incubator, ready for use at any time. The details of the preparation of this medium are given in Part V. It is essentially a veal-infusion-agar-hydrocele slant, the tubes being plugged with rubber stoppers. Only tubes which are uncracked and which show moisture at the bottom of the slant should be used for inoculation. They should be at body temperature when used and there must be no delay in putting them in the incubator. After inoculation the side of the tube opposite the slant is passed three or four times through the flame of a Bunsen burner, the stopper having been removed. The tube may be heated in this way even to the point of slightly coagulating the upper tip of the slant, without injuring the inoculum. By this heating, the air is driven out. The tube is then tightly plugged at once with the rubber stopper, so maintaining a state of reduced oxygen tension in the culture. Negative cultures should be held for incubation at least one week. If the presence of other organisms is suspected, veal infusion agar-hydrocele plates may be poured, inoculated by streaking, placed in a warmed desiccator, from which 10 to 25 per cent. of the air is then withdrawn by means of a water pump. The desiccator is then placed in the incubator and the plates examined at the end of twenty-four or forty-eight hours, or, if negative, held for further incubation. It is important to prevent the chilling of these plates after inoculation. If the growth on plates or slants is very scant at the end of twenty-four hours' incubation, it is wise to leave the cultures alone until the following day, by which time the growth will have become more luxuriant.

If a culture of a Gram-negative diplococcus is obtained by either of these

[1] A New Culture Method for the Gonococcus, Jour. Urology, iv, 325, August, 1920.

methods, a presumptive identification of gonococcus may be made. It is wise
to make a culture on plain agar at the time of the primary gonococcus culture,
as in this way, by the time growth has developed on the special medium, it will
be possible to know whether or not the diplococcus in question is also capable
of growing on plain agar. If it can, the organism is presumptively not a gonococcus. Subcultures of an organism presumptively a gonococcus must be made
to dextrose and maltose broths, as it has been shown by Elser and Huntoon[1]
that the gonococcus may be differentiated from the meningococcus by the fermentation of dextrose, but not maltose, the meningococcus fermenting both of
these carbohydrates. Only when this has been done can a final identification of
the organism as a gonococcus be made.

The other Gram-negative cocci, namely, Neisseriæ catarrhalis, sicca, perflava,
flava, and subflava, grow on simple media and may be differentiated by chromogenesis, and the fermentation of dextrose, maltose, levulose, saccharose, lactose,
and galactose.

Group 4. Mixed Infection.—The method of plating for the isolation of the
gonococcus has been given. If the direct smear shows a very large number of
Gram-positive organisms and a small number of Gram-negative ones, the former
may be inhibited by adding to the plates gentian-violet in a dilution of 1 : 100,000
or more. It must be remembered when this is done, however, that gentian-violet
also inhibits Gram-negative organisms somewhat, and for that reason a series
of dilutions should be used, for example, 1 : 100,000, 1 : 250,000, 1 : 500,000. If
Proteus is present, plates must be fished very early, before this organism has spread
over the entire surface. Blood-agar plates should be used if there is any reason
to believe that any of the organisms found will not grow on simple media. By
streaking a sufficient number of plates at least one is usually obtained which shows
colonies sufficiently isolated for fishing. Forty-eight hours of incubation is usually
better than twenty-four, because the colonies are larger and the presence of nearby
colonies can be more easily detected. After colonies have been fished, the identification of the organisms is carried out as previously indicated.

Group 5. No Organisms Seen in the Direct Smear.—With specimens of this
nature, two things should be done. First, a sufficient variety of media should be
used so that any of the organisms usually found would grow. Blood agar is excellent for such cultures, and also the gonococcus medium, in addition to the
simple ones. Second, it is wise to use as much of the specimen as possible, that is,
to be sure to incubate some of the uncentrifugalized urine, and to add broth by
means of a sterile pipet to the sediment remaining after culture.

In tuberculosis no organisms may appear in the smear. If this disease has not
been previously suspected, such a finding calls for careful search, in preparations
made with an acid-fast stain, for the tubercle bacillus.

Group 6. Anaërobic Cultures.—The simplest way of obtaining anaërobic conditions is to boil tubes of dextrose agar to drive out the air, cool rapidly to 42° C.
with cold water, inoculate, solidify as quickly as possible, and cover with sterile
vaselin, paraffin or albolin. Although this does not give complete anaërobiosis,
it is the method most suitable for the laboratory in which anaërobic cultures are
not made routinely. Otherwise the method of McIntosh and Fildes[1] as described
in the text-books may be used, or some of the older methods. It must be remem-

[1] Studies on Meningitis, Jour. Med. Res., xv, N. S., 373, June, 1909.

bered, however, that a pure culture of an anaërobe can probably be obtained only by use of the Barber[1] technic of culturing a single organism.

Group 7. Miscellaneous.—We believe that all of the bacterial organisms usually found in urologic infections have been discussed in the preceding groups. Occasionally, however, actinomycosis occurs. The genus Actinomyces Harz is defined by Bergey as follows:

"Organisms growing in form of a much-branched mycelium, which may break up into segments that function as conidia. Sometimes parasitic, with clubbed ends of radiating threads conspicuous in lesions in the animal body. Some species micro-aërophilic or anaërobic. Non-motile. The type species is Actinomyces bovis Harz."

The first point in connection with these organisms is that in direct smears the typical branching filaments may not be seen. Cultures should be both aërobic and anaërobic, and should include thick plates which are to be incubated at least two weeks, as the organisms often grow very slowly. The cultures show the characteristic branching forms. It is very important to run uninoculated controls when plates are held any length of time, to check possible contaminations.

Diphtheroids are occasionally found in the urine, usually with other organisms, but we have never seen one of proved pathogenicity, as they are usually found with other organisms. Their identification is seldom of interest to the urologist.

PART V. MEDIA.—For the preparation of simple media the methods of the Society of American Bacteriologists should be followed, as described in the Manual of Methods for Pure Culture Study of Bacteria.[2] We have used successfully in carbohydrate media double indicators, that is, a mixture of bromcresol-purple and cresol-red, 0.5 c.c. each of 1.6 per cent. alcoholic solutions of the two dyes to the liter of medium (Manual of Methods, B. 10). "When this combination is used, the media should be carefully adjusted to neutrality with bromthymol blue before adding any indicator. This mixture of indicators changes very slowly from purple to yellow through a long range (from about pH 8.0 to about pH 5.2), extending for a considerable distance each side of neutrality. By comparing with a blank tube of the neutral medium it is very easy to detect an increase either in acidity or in alkalinity." We have used agar slants containing the double indicator and the carbohydrate, rather than broth, as by making a stab as well as a surface inoculation the formation of gas is easily determined. Carbohydrate broths may be used if preferred.

Vosges-Proskauer Broth:

Difco peptone	10 gm.
Dextrose	10 gm.
Sodium chlorid	5 gm.
Distilled water to	1000 c.c.

Filter and tube about 10 c.c. per tube; sterilize ten minutes at 15 pounds in autoclave.

[1] A New Apparatus for the Isolation and Cultivation of Anaërobic Micro-organisms, Lancet, 1916, i, 768.

[2] Manual of Methods for Pure Culture Study of Bacteria, Prepared by the Committee on Bacteriological Technic of the Society of American Bacteriologists, published by the Society of American Bacteriologists, Geneva, N. Y.

Clark-Lubs Broth:

Difco peptone	5 gm.
Dextrose	5 gm.
Potassium acid phosphate	5 gm.
Distilled water to	1000 c.c.

Filter and tube about 10 c.c. per tube; sterilize ten minutes at 15 pounds in autoclave.

Gonococcus Medium (Swartz[1]).—"1. Agar medium. Five hundred grams of fresh lean meat—veal or beef—is finely minced and thoroughly mixed with 1000 c.c. of distilled water. This mixture is allowed to stand on ice for twenty-four hours. The liquor is then decanted and the remainder expressed through cloth, adding enough distilled water to make 1000 c.c. Boil until the albumin of the meat infusion coagulates. Correct to an acidity of pH 7.6 by the use of N/10 NaOH. In order to eliminate the effect of CO_2, which is acid to phenolsulphonephthalein, media should be titrated at as nearly 100° C. as possible, for then in subsequent sterilization the reaction will be less likely to be altered by driving off the CO_2 dissolved in the media. Boil again for a short time, filter, and make up to 1000 c.c. with distilled water. Add 10 grams peptone (Bacto-Difco), 5 grams NaCl (C. P.) and 15 grams agar, and boil until all is dissolved. If the media is to be used in hot climates or in the summer, 20 grams of agar should be used instead of 15 grams. This will give firm slants even after the addition of the hydrocele fluid. Let cool to 50° C. and then add the whites of three fresh eggs. Starting with a low flame, boil for ten minutes and again strain through cloth. Filter through a folded filter. This filtration is very slow, but can be hastened by placing flask and funnel in an autoclave at 10 pounds pressure. Place 5 to 6 c.c. of the medium in each tube, and plug with cotton stopper. The test-tubes best suited for this work measure about 150 mm. in length and about 16 mm. in diameter, and are made of heavy glass. Thin tubes are apt to crack when flamed and stoppered. These tubes are then autoclaved at 10 pounds pressure on three successive days. This sterilization changes the reaction from pH 7.6 to pH 7.4.

"The hydrocele, ascitic or pleuritic fluid, having been collected under the most rigid aseptic surgical technic, is tested to insure its freedom from any bacterial organisms. If sterile, it is kept in the refrigerator until needed.

"Freshness of the fluid is not an essential, as we have had just as good results with fluid kept in the refrigerator for six months, as with the fluid a few hours old.

"The tubes of agar are melted and placed on a water-bath at about 50° C. To this melted agar is then added hydrocele, ascitic or pleuritic fluid, in the proportions of 1 c.c. of fluid to 2 c.c. of agar. This proportion will permit the agar to harden into a firm slant and should produce about 0.5 c.c. of water of condensation in the angle of the slant when the agar is firm. Tubes are then slanted or Petri dishes poured and allowed to harden.

"The tubes are then stoppered so as to be air-tight, with sterile rubber stoppers, and kept in the incubator to insure their sterility and to have the media warm when wanted for use.

"2. Liquid medium. If fluid media is desired, it is made exactly as above,

---

[1] A New Culture Method for the Gonococcus, Jour. Urology, 1920, iv, 325.

except that the agar is omitted and after autoclaving, 1 c.c. of a 10 per cent. sterile solution of dextrose, maltose, or whatever sugar is desired, is added. The hydrocele, ascitic, or pleuritic fluid is added in the same proportions as above. More can be used if desired, but 2 to 3 c.c. per tube is sufficient to insure a good culture. These tubes are stoppered in the same manner as the agar slants, and kept in the incubator. This enables us to test the sterility of the medium as well as having it maintained at body temperature and ready for use at any time."

BIBLIOGRAPHY OF TECHNIC

In addition to the books cited in the footnotes in the text the laboratory should have at least one book for general reference. The following are especially recommended for this purpose:

Hiss, Zinsser, and Russell: A Text-book of Bacteriology, D. Appleton & Company, New York and London, 5th ed., 1924.

Stitt, E. R.: Practical Bacteriology, Blood Work and Animal Parasitology, P. Blakiston's Son & Co., Philadelphia, 7th ed., 1923.

Medical War Manual No. 6: Laboratory Methods of the United States Army, Lea & Febiger, Philadelphia and New York, 2d ed.

PATHOLOGY

Kidney.—It has been customary to divide the lesions occurring in infections of the kidney into three groups, namely, *pyelitis*, *pyelonephritis*, and *pyonephrosis*. These divisions are arbitrary, and they are to be considered as in no way separate diseases. In the past, it was suggested that lesions confined to the pelvis (pyelitis) or spreading from the pelvis (pyelonephritis) represented infections arriving by way of the ureter, while lesions confined to the parenchyma, or more intense there (acute nephritis, multiple abscesses, infected infarcts) represented the hematogenous infections. This distinction is no longer valid, since it has been proved that a hemogenic infection may set up a lesion essentially confined to the pelvis, and we now feel that the majority of kidney infections, where the ureter is normal, arrive by way of the blood. The application of names to the various kidney lesions, then, is purely on anatomic grounds, and they are descriptive of the condition found, but carry no inference as to the source of the infection.

A number of investigators have stated that bacteria may be excreted by the kidney without causing any lesion. Among them may be mentioned Lemierre and Abrami,[1] Patrick[2] (Bacillus typhosus), Rovsing,[3] Cuturi[4] (Bacillus coli), Biedl and Kraus[5] (staphylococcus) Mayer,[6] Heyn,[7] Kramer,[8] Buday,[9] Wyssokowitsch,[10]

[1] Journal d'Urologie, 1912, ii, 21–32.
[2] Journal of Pathology and Bacteriology, 1913, xviii, 365–378.
[3] Monatshefte der Harn und Sexualapparate, 1898, iii, 506–522.
[4] Annales des Maladies des Organes Génito-urinaires, 1911, xxix (i), 515–528.
[5] Archiv für experimentalischen Physiologie und Pathologie, 1896, xxxvii, 1–25.
[6] Virchow's Archiv, 1895, cxli, 414–434.
[7] Ibid., 1901, clxv, 42–79.
[8] Verhandlungen der Deutschen Pathologischen Gesellschaft, 1900, iii, 94–98.
[9] Virchow's Archiv, 1906, clxxxvi, 145–212.
[10] Zeitschrift für Hygiene, 1886, i, 3–46.

Rolly,[1] Cunningham[2] (Bacillus tuberculosis), Grawitz[3] (mold spores), and Honeij[4] (Bacillus lepræ). It has also been noted that finely divided inert matter may be excreted by the kidney, apparently without lesion.[5]   On the other hand, others have always found lesions in the kidney accompanying the bacteriuria, for example Wyssokowitsch[6] (with certain organisms), Pernice and Scagliose,[7] Sherrington,[8] Cotton,[9] Jahn,[10] Dyke,[11] Cabot and Crabtree,[12] and many others.   Dyke found with the staphylococcus very tiny lesions in the walls of the tubules, which might quickly heal and leave no trace if the examination of the kidney were long deferred. Cabot and Crabtree found that the lesions caused in the cortex by B. coli disappeared very quickly, leaving only a slight pyelitis.

During attacks of infectious disease, bacteria may be seen in the urine, often without pus, and a slight degree of pyelitis, caused by the colon bacillus or staphylococcus may persist for years with no direct evidence of kidney injury. If, however, we admit that lesions in the kidney always accompany the excretion of bacteria, a hematogenous infection would always be, or at least begin, as a disseminated nephritis, and become only later a pyelonephritis or pyelitis. The question is of considerable importance, but cannot be considered as settled. It is, however, evident that in any case we should make every effort to eliminate a kidney infection, wherever situated, and that if damage to the kidney has occurred, we are in a position to detect it in its early stages by means of functional tests.

It is obvious that in many cases where bacteria reach it through the bloodstream, the kidney either does not become affected, or else that the incipient lesions heal quickly and completely, so that no kidney disease can be detected, while in others, infections of varying degrees of severity are set up. One can only say that, here as elsewhere, the result is due to the balance between the virulence of organism, the number reaching the kidney, and the immune reactions of the body, both local and general. Any form of urinary obstruction, or the presence of stones or foreign bodies, predisposes to infection in the kidney.

When the infective agent arrives in overwhelming quantity, or the resistance of the kidney is greatly diminished for any reason, extensive and acute lesions are caused. This may be in the form of an *acute diffuse nephritis*. In certain cases of this disease, the etiology is unknown, micro-organisms cannot be demonstrated, and it appears to be mainly toxic in character. Usually, however, it is associated with some infectious disease, or with a localized portal of entry elsewhere in the body. These lesions determine the type of organism present, although in such conditions as scarlet fever, the organism, not being known, cannot be demonstrated.

[1] Münchener Medizinische Wochenschrift, 1909, lvi, 1873–1875.

[2] Annals of Surgery, 1912, lvi, 818–834; Transactions of the American Association of Genitourinary Surgeons, 1911, vi, 166–169.

[3] Virchow's Archiv, 1877, lxx, 546–598.

[4] Journal of Infectious Diseases, 1915, xvii, 376–387.

[5] Cohnheim: Vorlesungen über Allgemeinen Pathologie, 1882, ii, 188–295.

[6] Zeitschrift für Hygiene, 1886, i, 3–46.

[7] Deutsche Medizinische Wochenschrift, 1892, xviii, 761–765.

[8] Journal of Pathology and Bacteriology, 1893, i, 258–278.

[9] Quoted by Jahn (see note [10]).

[10] Centralblatt für Bakteriologie, 1910, Abteilung Originale, lv, 276–301.

[11] Journal of Pathology and Bacteriology, 1923, xxvi, 164–175.

[12] Surgery, Gynecology, and Obstetrics, 1916, xxiii, 495–537.

In the gross the kidney is swollen, dark, and congested. On section it is more friable than normal. The parenchyma is thickened. If suppuration has occurred, abscesses, large or tiny, may dot the cut surface, or a turbid, purulent fluid may exude from the whole surface. The pelvis is usually involved, the mucosa red, the pelvic urine turbid (Fig. 52). *Microscopically* (Figs. 53, 54), a cellular infiltration, mostly of polymorphonuclear leukocytes, is seen. These may be replaced by round-cells in certain cases, as scarlet fever and typhoid. The stroma is edematous. The tubular epithelium shows cloudy swelling and desquamation,

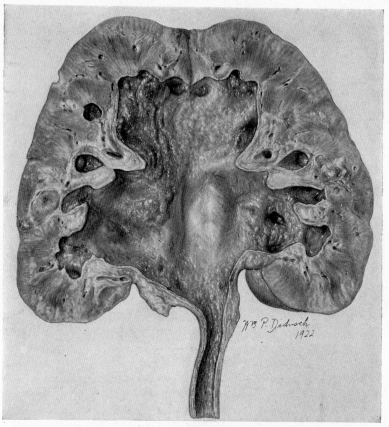

Fig. 52.—Autopsy specimen showing hydronephrosis, hydro-ureter, suppurative pyelonephritis, and intense pyelitis and ureteritis.

and in the tubules appear epithelial, pus and blood casts, and free blood. There may be hemorrhages in the stroma and glomerular capsules, and under the renal capsule.

In such a kidney, of course, the function is much diminished, and the urine contains blood, pus, casts, and micro-organisms (with exceptions as above). When bilateral, death may occur quickly, or the lesion may present any degree of lesser severity than the extreme condition just described. In such case, the progress may be by resolution, by suppuration, or by the assumption of chronicity. If the lesion resolves quickly, the kidney may be restored so that it appears quite normal, on examination or by functional test. The injured epithelium regenerates perfectly, although there is no evidence of the formation of new tubules.

This termination seldom demands treatment, but the others do. The existence of *suppuration* always indicates at least a certain degree of chronicity, and is usually associated with more or less fibrosis. The essential feature is the formation of abscesses, which may be large or small, single or innumerable. The exact point of origin is difficult to determine, but very early abscesses have been seen in the walls of the tubules and also in the glomeruli. At any rate, these abscesses

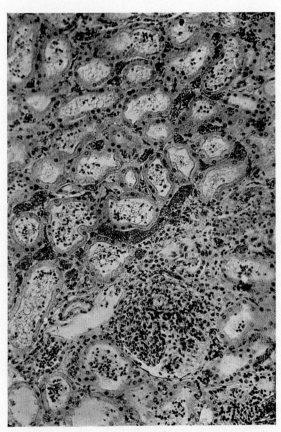

Fig. 53.—High-power picture of a section showing acute pyelonephritis. Note the dilatation of the tubules, the presence of an albuminous fluid within them, the thinning of the epithelium and the reduction of the number of nuclei within it, the vascular congestion, the swelling of the glomerular tuft, and the cellular infiltration.

destroy all of the kidney tissue where they exist, and in and around them may be seen masses of micro-organisms, sometimes in the blood-vessels. This picture gave rise to the idea that many such lesions were caused by the actual plugging of capillaries with masses of organisms transported from other parts of the body, with resultant anemic infarcts, which became infected. The name "infected infarcts of the kidney" was given, and the condition was usually described in connection with general pyæmia. In many of the cases, however, the picture was not typical of the regular pyramidal infarct of the kidney, and the term is now restricted to those cases of thrombophlebitis or endocarditis in which actual thrombotic emboli occur. The kidney condition usually constitutes a minor part of the picture in these cases, and is seldom, if ever, the occasion for local treatment.

If the patient survives, and the abscesses become more *chronic*, deposition of fibrous tissue in the peripheral portions ensues, and as a result, besides the damage caused by the abscess itself, otherwise intact tubules may be occluded. This may give rise to the formation of small or large cysts, or tubules may be seen to be much distended. The glomerular capsule does not distend, and while the glomeruli may be implicated in neighboring areas of fibrosis, they are often remarkable unchanged (Fig. 55). In general, the more widely disseminated the suppuration, the greater the damage. There may be only a few, or even a single abscess.

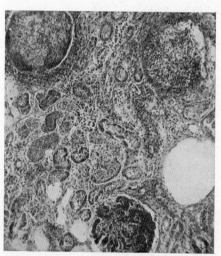

FIG. 54.—Section showing acute pyelonephritis. Note the edema and polymorphonuclear infiltration of the interstitial tissue. The three glomeruli show three different stages of the process. One is swollen, infiltrated, and has its capillaries filled with thrombi containing many organisms. The upper left glomerulus shows more advanced infiltration with beginning destruction of architecture, whereas in the upper right glomerulus the normal structure has entirely disappeared and it has become a small abscess. Collection D 27.

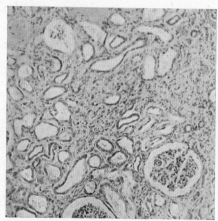

FIG. 55.—Chronic pyelonephritis. Section shows slight dilatation of the tubules, slight round-cell infiltration, slight fibrosis, some edema, two glomeruli, hypertrophic but with capsule unchanged, two others hyaline. B. U. I. Path. 4141.

Such an abscess may, in rare cases, become firmly encapsulated, and persist for a long period.

If the process is bilateral and extensive, as in the *surgical kidney* following operations on the lower urinary tract, the beginning of restoration will not save the patient's life. The entire renal tissue being the site of infiltration and abscess formation, renal insufficiency ensues and death follows from uremia (Fig. 56).

Fibrosis may occur without definite abscess formation, and is a feature of the *long-continued, milder types of kidney infection.* Its general characteristics are similar to those just described. It may sometimes be difficult to say whether a fibrotic process has been preceded, at some period, by suppuration, while in others, pictures simulating those of chronic interstitial nephritis, or the so-called arteriosclerotic kidney, may be produced. In general, the fibrosis produced in this manner is more patchy and irregular than that due to the other conditions, and may involve only a portion of the kidney. A final distinction is not possible, since we do not yet know just what the rôle of infection is in the ordinary chronic nephritis, or "Brights' disease."

In milder cases, the whole process may be continuous, in that new infectious material is constantly being brought, and new areas of inflammation set up.   In

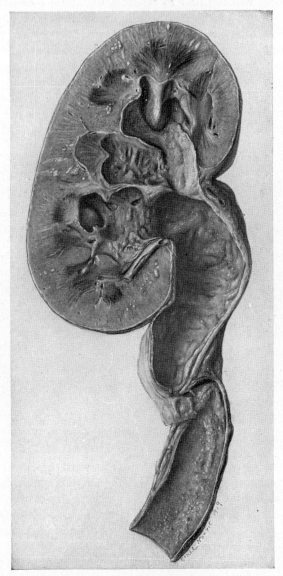

Fig. 56.—Autopsy specimen showing acute and chronic ureteritis, pyelitis, and pyelonephritis with multiple abscesses in the cortex.   Ureter and pelvis markedly dilated.   This is typical of the pathologic picture seen in cases of so-called surgical kidney following operative or other infection of the lower urinary tract in cases of obstruction.   Courtesy of Dr. M. C. Winternitz.

such a kidney one sees old scars alongside fresh abscesses, and in the course of time the scarring and destruction of the kidney become very great.

Acute infections of this sort are usually bilateral, but that they may be *unilateral* is now abundantly proved.   The unilateral lesion is, however, rare.   Sometimes the infection may be present in both sides, but much more pronounced on one. The reasons why a kidney infection should occur on one side only are not entirely clear, but the fact is of importance, since some such cases have been quickly cured by nephrectomy.

Singer,[1] in 1883, was the first to report a unilateral infection of the kidney. In his case, the affected kidney had been injured eighteen years before. Brewer[2] brought these cases to general attention, and performed experiments on animals. By injuring one kidney he was able to produce a localized infection after intravenous injection of various organisms in 8 of 16 animals. Of his 13 human cases, however, only 2 gave history of previous injury. Five had recently had some febrile disorder. All showed the usual signs of a general sepsis. While it is possible to produce a unilateral localization by injury to one kidney, we do not know the factors concerned in the localization in most of the cases reported. Microscopically, it

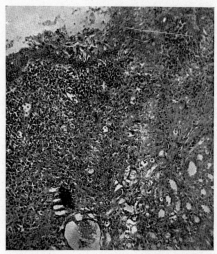
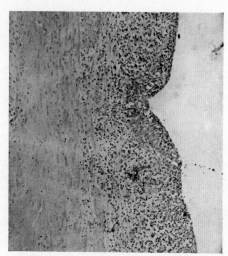

Fig. 57.—Section from the renal pelvis showing acute pyelitis. The epithelium is almost entirely destroyed. Subepithelial tissue shows edema and an intense cellular infiltration mostly polymorphonuclear. B. U. I. Path. 5106.

Fig. 58.—Section from the pelvis in a case of chronic pyelitis. Note the definite but superficial round-cell infiltration of the epithelium and subepithelial connective tissue. B. U. I. Path. 4818.

is clear that while typical wedge-shaped infarcts were present in some, in others there were simply multiple abscesses. It is, therefore, probable that infarction is not an essential feature of this form of infection. Unless the condition of the patient is grave from general sepsis, resolution is usually to be expected, and operation should not be performed without very definite indications, and absolute demonstration that the other kidney is healthy.

It has been stated above that in infections of the kidney the pelvis is usually involved, and when this is true, the condition is properly called *pyelonephritis*. The determination of the relative severity of the pelvic and parenchymatous lesions is too uncertain, in our opinion, to be of any great value; and in any case, it gives little or no indication of the prognosis or of the source of the infection. Infections of the parenchyma may, however, exist without pyelitis, and may even extend to the perirenal tissues without pyelitis or pyuria.[3] In these cases there are

[1] Quoted by Brewer (see note [2]).   [2] Surgery, Gynecology, and Obstetrics, 1906, ii, 485–497.

[3] Helmholz: Journal of Urology, 1922, viii, 301–306.

cortical abscesses, possessing a sufficient degree of chronicity to be sealed off, by fibrosis, from any connection with the pelvis through the tubules.

On the other hand, the pelvic inflammation may constitute practically the entire picture (Figs. 57, 58). The claim has been made that *pyelitis* without involvement of the kidney substance cannot occur. Rovsing[1] believes that all hematogenous infections of the kidney begin in the parenchyma. Cabot and Crabtree[2] support this view, and show that primary lesions of the tubules may heal quickly, so that in the later stages the inflammatory changes will be found in the pelvis only. It is, of course, true that the pelvic mucosa is so closely applied to the papilla that any inflammation not confined to the "parietal" portion of the pelvis must involve a little of the kidney proper. It is also probable that the kidney is affected to a certain extent in acute pyelitis, as this condition is some-times accompanied by albumin, casts, and diminished renal function. While an extension of a pelvic inflammation to the kidney parenchyma is always possible, and must be searched for in every case, it is frequently nothing more than a thin layer of cellular infiltration beneath the pelvic mucosa. That the infection may be ascending is indicated by the rare cases of pure gonorrheal pyelitis occurring in the course of gonorrheal urethritis.[3]

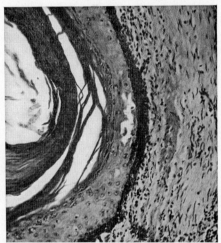

FIG. 59.—Section showing leukoplakia of the kidney pelvis. This specimen is from an ectopic kidney which was the seat of a severe pyonephrosis. Note the advanced degree of epidermization which is present. J. H. H. Autopsy 7345.

In *acute pyelitis* the mucosa may be slightly reddened and granular, or may show more severe changes with edema, formation of villi, diphtheritic membranes, or ulcers. The ulcers may be spontaneous, or occur in areas of contact with stones or foreign bodies. Ecchymoses are not infrequent, and may give rise to hemorrhage.

Microscopically, one sees essentially a cellular infiltration, polymorphonuclear in the *acute* cases, and mononuclear in the *chronic* cases (Figs. 57, 58). It involves a layer of varying thickness in the tip of the papilla in the "visceral" portions, and of the peripelvic fat, muscle, and connective tissue in the "parietal" portions of the pelvis. Small abscesses may occur in these areas. There are varying degrees of edema and vascular congestion in the mucosa, with rarely the formation of bullæ or even edematous polyps, as in the bladder. There may be extensive exfoliation of the epithelium, leading to ulcer formation. The small lymphatic nodules normally present may be increased in size.

The inflammation usually involves the entire pelvis, but may be confined to certain areas. This has been shown experimentally, especially in rabbits, and may explain why certain cases of pyelitis extend to the perirenal tissues, others to the cortex, etc., or cause the formation of adherent stones in the pel-

---

[1] International Congress of Medicine, London, 1913 (Section XIV, Urology, Part I), 137–149.

[2] Surgery, Gynecology, and Obstetrics, 1916, xxiii, 495–537.

[3] Johnson and Hill: Journal of Urology, 1924, xi, 177–188 (Lit.).

vis. In the chronic cases there may be a very thin layer of round-cell infiltration or the medulla and cortex may be involved to varying degrees, with round-cell infiltration and fibrosis.

Occasionally the pelvic epithelium may undergo a change to the squamous type, known as *leukoplakia* (Fig. 59). The significance of this has been the subject of much discussion.[1] (See the section on Infections of the Bladder.) It usually occurs in connection with chronic inflammation of long standing. It may give rise to squamous epithelioma. Cases have been reported where sheets of epithelium exfoliated from large patches of leukoplakia have caused ureteral obstruction and severe colic.

Patches of *malakoplakia* have also been found in the pelvis and ureter. (See Inflammations of the Bladder.)

An infection once established in the pelvis may involve *secondarily* the parenchyma. In this connection we know that materials deposited in the pelvis can ascend the tubules for some distance, and, in the presence of an obstruction, get into the venous circulation of the parenchyma.[2] The nature of the infecting organism is also of some importance, *e. g.*, colon is more apt to be the cause of mild chronic pyelitis, while the cocci, especially the streptococci, tend to set up more widely diffused inflammations. This rule is not without numerous exceptions. The pathologic picture is like that described for hematogenous infections, except that the generalized acute nephritis is not apt to occur.

Pyelitis, either acute or chronic, differs from the more severe infections in that it is about as often unilateral as bilateral. It may occur at any period of life.

The rôle of obstruction in the etiology of pyelitis has been the subject of a tremendous amount of discussion. There can be no doubt that it predisposes to infection, but to what degree can seldom be determined in an individual case. The reason why the pyelitis of pregnancy is more frequent on the right side has never been satisfactorily ascertained. The course of the right ureter over the iliac vessels may make it slightly more subject to pressure by the enlarged uterus, but just how is not entirely clear. Hunner feels that comparatively large caliber strictures of the ureter may determine pyelitis. Keith has shown that when the ureter is partially obstructed, infection is very prone to occur, even in dogs. We can say, therefore, that while obstruction cannot always be demonstrated, it is of prime importance when present, and demands treatment.

Obstruction complicates infection greatly, and adds to its seriousness. In addition, obstruction favors infection in cases where it is not yet present. This may be as a result of urinary stasis, or of lowering of the local resistance through back pressure, or in case of low obstructions, ascending infection may be favored. Infection obviously hematogenous frequently occurs in cases of obstruction, for example, in prostatic obstruction where the patient has never been catheterized, and where the urine has been clear and sterile up to the moment when pain and tenderness in the kidney region appear. When stone is present, its irritation must be added to the other factors favoring infection.

[1] Hinman and Gibson: Journal of Urology, 1921, vi, 1–50; Kretschmer: Surgery, Gynecology, and Obstetrics, 1920, xxxi, 325–339; Leçene: Journal d'Urologie, 1913, iii, 129–137; Cumming: Surgery, Gynecology, and Obstetrics, 1923, xxxvi, 189–195.

[2] Burns and Swartz: Journal of Urology, 1918, ii, 445–454; Hinman and Lee-Brown: Journal of the American Medical Association, 1924, lxxxii, 607–612.

If infection occurs in an *early obstruction* where no hydronephrotic change has yet taken place, the pathologic picture is much the same as has been described, except that the process tends to advance more rapidly and be more severe as a result of the obstruction. When hydronephrosis is present, changes similar to those described above add themselves to those caused by the hydronephrosis, intensifying and hastening the destructive process. In all cases the obstruction prevents the outflow of the products of inflammation, making more likely general symptoms, such as fever, leukocytosis, etc., supposed to be due to absorption of toxins.

In the case of an *infected hydronephrosis* the contents of the sac include pus-cells which may be in any proportion, varying from a slightly turbid, essentially urinous fluid, to thick pus. The latter condition accompanies the more advanced hydronephrosis, where the secreting tissue is extensively destroyed as the result of obstruction or of the infectious process itself, or else where anuria has resulted from complete obstruction. Thus it will be seen that if a partially obstructed kidney discharges thick pus into the bladder, it is an indication that the secretory elements are almost or quite destroyed.

When a distended kidney pelvis contains pus it is known as a *pyonephrosis,* but the term is not exact, since there is no definite

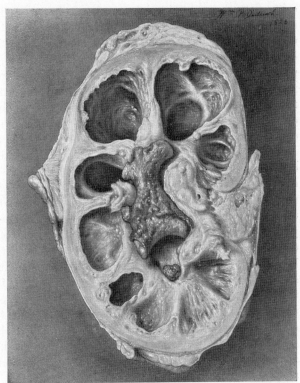

FIG. 60.—Specimen of pyonephrosis removed at operation. In this case the obstruction was due to a large renal calculus. The interior of the sac is extremely complicated and multilocular. Dull pain localized to back for eighteen months; no radiation. Worm-like stream of pus from left ureter. B. U. I. 10,678.

point of distinction between it and a slightly infected hydronephrosis. The interior of the pyonephrotic sac is irregular in shape, owing to the distention of the various calices, to communicating abscess cavities, or even to communications with the perirenal tissues, so that its proper drainage through the ureter or through an incision is often impossible (Fig. 60). Such cases lead often to intoxication or septicemia.

Infection in the kidney may itself lead to obstruction, or increase a pre-existent partial obstruction, by means of swelling of the mucosa, or scar formation, usually at the ureteropelvic junction. It is probable that this explains the slight dilatations of the pelvis often seen in chronic renal infections. Occasionally a return to normal is seen after the infection has cleared up.

In *infected nephrolithiasis* inflammation may produce enough scar tissue to occlude the pelvis at one or more points, giving rise to partial hydronephrosis. The effect of infection in the ureter will be considered later.

The end-result of a pyonephrosis may, in rare cases where there has been no interference, be a complete reduction of the kidney to scar tissue, within which the pus may become encapsulated and inspissated and the infectious process inactive. In such cases a secondary deposit of fat may be seen in the remains of the kidney tissue itself. The whole is bound to the surrounding tissues by adhesions, which may practically replace the perirenal fat.

Infection may extend to the *perirenal tissues* by various paths. In a few cases, little or no renal lesion may be made out, and in these cases, one deals with a hematogenous infection, arising here just as it does in an abscess or cellulitis elsewhere in the body. In some cases a hematoma following a blow or other trauma becomes infected. It appears that sometimes the portal of entry into the blood may be an infection of the lower urinary tract. Such an event is comparatively rare, however, and the process usually extends from the kidney. This extension may come from the pelvis, by way of the peripelvic fat and connective tissue, or from cortical abscesses, either by invasion of micro-organisms through the tissues or by rupture of an abscess, by rupture of an infected hydronephrosis, or by destruction of the true capsule by inflammation, pressure from a calculus, or growth of a neoplasm. In another class are the cases where the infection comes from some other organ than the kidney. They will be considered in a later paragraph. Infections arising from external trauma give a picture similar to that arising from the kidney if the kidney is involved in the trauma. A foreign body, usually a projectile of some sort, often complicates these cases.

Where the infection has come gradually by extension, the perirenal fat may become greatly scarred and distorted by fibrosis without the development of any abscess. Sometimes in these cases one sees firm, friable masses of typical infiltrated fat, containing great quantities of round or polymorphonuclear cells, without any frank pus. The bands of adhesions thus resulting may have important effects in obstructing the ureter or immobilizing the kidney. A change of this sort is the rule in all infectious conditions of the kidney which have existed for any length of time, and is appreciated at operation as the *"adhesions,"* often strong and numerous, which run across the perirenal fat. In extreme cases, the fat is entirely replaced by them, and the difficulties of surgery greatly multiplied.

When the process is more rapid, suppuration occurs, and a *perinephric abscess* forms. The site of this suppuration is oftenest posterior to the kidney, but it may spread readily through the loose perirenal fat, and for this reason the abscess may attain considerable size. It is at first contained by Gerota's capsule or the perirenal fascia, and later tends to burrow in certain directions. It may appear under the skin in the lumbar triangle just under the ribs, or follow down along the psoas muscle into the groin. It may perforate into the subdiaphragmatic space, or into the pleura, the peritoneum, the intestine, or even the renal pelvis itself. These perforations into other hollow organs may be followed by fistulæ.

A further complication which may ensue when the kidney cortex or the pelvis is ruptured or perforated is the *extravasation of urine*. This complication is rare, as the fibrosis already present usually prevents the spread of the urine. In this case the extension, although along the same lines, is more rapid, and the symptoms are more severe. Spontaneous or operative drainage may give rise to a long persisting urinary fistula, since in such cases some obstruction is usually present. Healing, with fibrosis, often follows drainage, but this will depend largely on the underlying condition in the kidney.

In some cases of perirenal inflammation or abscess the infection comes *from outside the kidney,* and these lesions may well be considered here. The kidney usually remains intact, protected by its true capsule. When this is true, study of the kidney by means of examination of the urine, pyelogram, and functional tests reveals no abnormality.

Rarely the kidney may be involved secondarily, oftenest perhaps in tuberculosis, and infected neoplasm. The possible sources of such infections are manifold, and among them may be mentioned appendical abscess (especially in cases of retrocecal appendix), spondylitis (especially tuberculous), empyema, abscess of the liver or gall-bladder, subdiaphragmatic abscess, perforating ulcer of the intestine (especially the duodenum), or of the stomach, pancreatic or splenic abscess, osteomyelitis of the ribs. Retroperitoneal infection or extravasation arising from the posterior urethra or the bladder may travel upward and finally reach the kidney region. After the perirenal tissue is once invaded the course is the same as in those infections arising from the kidney. It is possible for the source of the infection to escape detection, in which case the

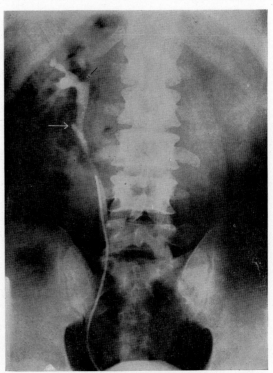

Fig. 61.—Ureteroduodenal fistula. Pyelogram demonstrating the fistula as a small knuckle or diverticulum seen projecting from the right ureter at the level of the upper border of the third lumbar vertebra.

perirenal inflammation will dominate the picture. If the kidney is invaded, the infection usually spreads through it from the point of entrance, since the preexistent lesion furnishes an abundant supply of infectious material. The pelvis, therefore, may be expected to be involved, and pyuria will be present. The process continues as described above, and may eventuate in complete destruction of the kidney. When the inflammation has started from a hollow viscus—usually the intestine—and involves the kidney, a fistulous connection may be set up. Several cases have been described of fistulæ between the duodenum and the right kidney, due presumably to retroperitoneal perforation of duodenal ulcer. An interesting case of this sort was reported[1] from this clinic by E. G. Davis (Figs. 61, 62). When this occurs, the intestinal contents set up a severe inflammation of the kidney, and may be detected in the urine. In the case mentioned, bile was found in the

[1] Davis, E. G.: Journal of the American Medical Association, 1918, lxx, 376–378.

fluid from the right ureter. The passage of urine into the intestine causes no trouble, since, as Hinman[1] has shown, the opposite kidney hypertrophies sufficiently to take care of the quantity of urine reabsorbed. In cases where both the kidney and another organ are involved, it may be impossible to state from the pathologic picture whether the infection originated in the kidney or outside it—in which event we must depend on the clinical history for the explanation.

The list of diseases in which infection of the kidney may occur includes every infectious disease. The infection may be caused by the organism producing the

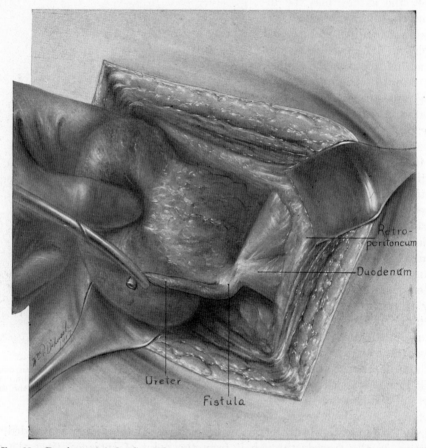

Fig. 62.—Duodenopelvic fistula. When traction was made upon the kidney a knuckle of duodenum was pulled into the wound, and the duodenum at this point was found to be intimately associated with the ureter just where the latter entered the mass of scar tissue constituting the pelvis and pedicle.

original disease, or by pyogenic bacteria as secondary invaders. In addition, there is toxic damage to the kidney in practically all febrile cases, as indicated by albuminuria, cylindruria, or hematuria. Pathologically, one sees cloudy swelling of the epithelium, sometimes a more extensive epithelial degeneration. Actual infection of the kidney has been observed in typhoid fever, yellow fever, cholera, dysentery, rheumatic fever, endocarditis of all types, septicemia, tonsillitis, osteomyelitis, furunculosis, localized abscesses, influenza, pneumonia, scarlet fever, meningitis, Malta fever, smallpox, glanders, anthrax, sprue, etc., sometimes

[1] Journal of Urology, 1923, ix, 289–314.

secondary and sometimes with the causative organism of the disease. Infections in tuberculosis, leprosy, and syphilis, and with the various mycotic organisms and protozoan parasites are considered under separate headings.

Ureter.—*Acute infection* of the ureter may occur by descent from the kidney, through reflux from the bladder, or by extension through the lymphatics. It is thus usually part of an infectious process involving other parts of the urinary tract. Localized metastatic infection may occur in the ureter. This is rarely seen except possibly in tuberculosis, and in cases such as that shown in Fig. 64.

Microscopically, the mucosa is the seat of cellular infiltration, either mononuclear or polymorphonuclear, edema, and vascular congestion. The epithelium may be desquamated. The picture generally is quite similar to that seen in inflammations of the pelvis or bladder.

Edema may be sufficient to obstruct the lumen markedly. We have seen a case in which a large acutely infected hydronephrosis was present without stone or other obvious obstruction. Owing to the serious condition of the patient, nothing was done except to open and drain the pelvis. The fistula closed spontaneously and the patient became entirely well. A pyelogram taken later showed the hydronephrosis decreased in size.

In the *chronic* forms of ureteritis the wall is invaded more deeply (Fig. 63) and with the deposition of fibrous tissue the lumen may be obstructed by contracture, and the elasticity and contractility of the ureter diminished. If the obstruction caused by such a stricture is sufficient, dilatation will take place above it. A localized inflammation may block or alter the peristaltic waves.

Inflammation spreading through the lymphatics may, according to Sweet and Stewart, Eisendrath, and others, cause the various acute or chronic changes

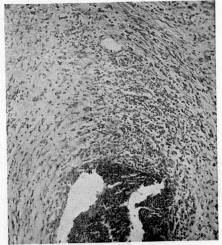

Fig. 63.—Chronic ureteritis. Note the hypertrophy of the mucosa and the fibrosis and edema of the ureteral wall. The kidney on the same side showed acute and chronic pyelonephritis with moderate distention of the pelvis. B. U. I. Path. 4818.

in the wall of the ureter with little or any involvement of the mucosa. They publish pictures showing the lymphatic spaces packed with leukocytes.

According to Hunner,[1] this intramural type of infiltration, with consequent *stricture*, is very common, especially in women. Exact pathologic data on the subject are difficult to obtain since the caliber of the ureter varies so much, and since muscular activity may affect the size of the ureter as seen in pyelograms. Catheters and bulbs placed in the ureters may excite changes in the peristaltic activity and even cause contraction rings, as shown by Wislocki and O'Conor. That it does occur is shown by the case pictured in Fig. 64. The inflammation was truly submucous, and the urine showed neither pus nor bacteria, as in submucous cystitis.

Inflammatory stricture at the ureteropelvic junction may occur as a result of renal inflammation when the remainder of the ureter is not markedly involved

[1] Cabot's Modern Urology, ii, 255–342 (Lit.).

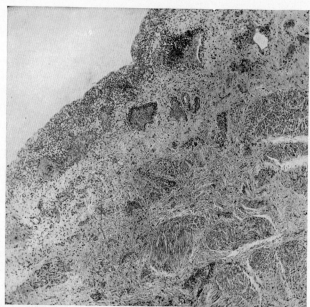

FIG. 64.—Submucous inflammation of the ureter. There is a round-cell infiltration of the submucosa and also a certain degree of fibrosis. In the muscular layer the round-cell infiltration is present, but less marked, while the fibrosis is more marked, separating the muscle bundles widely. The epithelium has been lost in preparation. In this case the ureteral wall was much thickened and there was definite dilatation above the lesion. Courtesy of Dr. Guy L. Hunner and Dr. Lawrence R. Wharton.

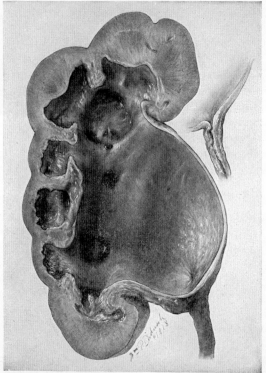

FIG. 65.—Inflammatory stricture at the ureteropelvic juncture with resultant hydronephrosis. Longitudinal section of specimen removed at operation. The wall of the ureter shows marked inflammatory thickening and the lumen is almost obliterated. The hydronephrotic sac has become infected and has become a pyonephrosis. B. U. I. 4822.

(Figs. 65, 66). Stone in the pelvis predisposes to this complication. It is distinguished from congenital narrowing at this point by the fibrotic thickening of the ureteral walls, and the lumen is usually irregular.[1]

Chronic *infections of the seminal vesicle and vas* may involve the ureter in scar tissue (Figs. 68, 69) at the point where the tip of the vesicle approaches the ureter. The wall of the ureter itself usually shows thickening, and the two organs may be bound together by a firm fibrous mass[2] (Figs. 68, 69).

The *intramural* portion of the ureter may be involved by an inflammatory process extending directly through the wall of the bladder, even when the meatus

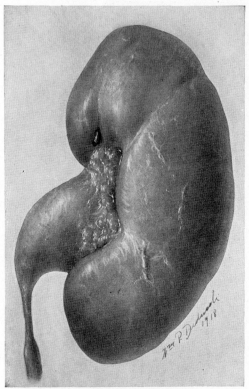

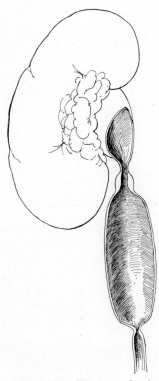

FIG. 66.—Medium-sized extrarenal hydronephrosis due to inflammatory stricture of the ureter just below the ureteropelvic junction. An aberrant artery shown entering the upper pole had nothing to do with the obstruction. B. U. I. 5281.

FIG. 67.—Diagram showing multiple strictures of the ureter with ureteral dilatation between the two strictures and hydronephrosis above. Patient of Dr. John T. Geraghty.

itself is removed from the affected area. This may lead to an extension upward along the lymphatics of the ureter, to fibrous tissue deposition, with stricture, or to ulceration with a new opening into the bladder (Fig. 70).

The ureter may be involved in infections extending from other organs, as the bones, muscles, intestine, peritoneum, female genital organs, etc. (Fig. 71). If there is ulceration in connection with a hollow viscus, as the appendix or intestine,

[1] Geraghty and Frontz: Journal of Urology, 1918, ii, 161–209. Figures 65–67 have been taken from this article.

[2] Young: Annales des Maladies des Organes Génito-urinaires, 1904, xxii, 1–20; Mark and Hoffmann: Journal of Urology, 1923, viii, 89–98.

a communicating fistula may be set up, as described for the renal pelvis. Otherwise, stricture may occur, and the infection may spread to the upper ureter and
kidney. We have seen a case (B. U. I. 10,140) in which such a sequence followed

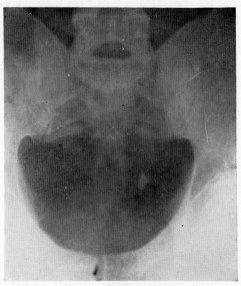

Fig. 68.—Shadow of concretion in left seminal vesicle. Adhesions about vesicle, constricted
ureter. This was thought to be a ureteral calculus, and the true condition was discovered at operation. B. U. I. x-Ray 3456.

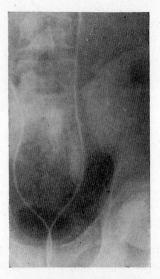

Fig. 69.—Ureterogram showing marked hydro-ureter. Same case as the preceding picture.
The obstruction was due to scar tissue resulting
from chronic seminal vesiculitis and surrounding
the ureter. B. U. I. x-Ray 3457.

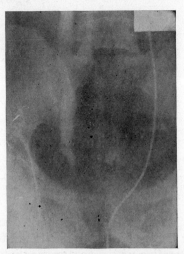

Fig. 70.—Ureterogram showing marked hydro-ureter due to inflammatory stricture at the
lower end of the ureter. There was also a hydronephrosis holding 90 c.c. Marked improvement
followed dilation of the stricture. B. U. I. x-Ray
2725.

a chronic adhesive peritonitis from an infected hernia operation many months
before. Autopsy showed the ureter involved in its lower third by a localized
peritoneal abscess, with stricture, hydro-ureter, and pyonephrosis.

Perforation of the ureter with involvement of the surrounding tissues is rare.

Areas of *leukoplakia* may occur in the ureter, being oftenest found when the tube is dilated and chronically infected.

Occasionally the ureter and pelvis may be studded with many little cysts, lined by a thin layer of epithelium, filled with clear fluid, and lying just beneath the surface. This condition is known as *ureteritis* (pyelitis) *cystica* (Figs. 72, 73). It is uncertain whether this is a result of inflammation, or a congenital anomaly.

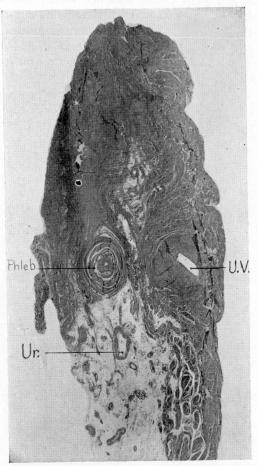

Fig. 71.—Autopsy case. Section showing chronic inflammation with fibrosis in the broad liga-ment in the region of the ureter. Slight dilatation of ureter above. The laminated structure is a phlebolith (Phleb.), to the right of this are the uterine vessels (*U.V.*), and below them the ureter (*Ur.*). Courtesy of Dr. Guy L. Hunner and Dr. Lawrence R. Wharton.

Bladder.—Inflammations of the bladder may be classified according to the depth to which they involve the wall, and also according to the severity of the lesion. Thus a superficial lesion may be severe, or a deep one indolent, chronic, and non-destructive.

Acute diffuse cystitis occurs very commonly in connection with other diseases of the bladder and with operations, either open or intravesical. Much more rarely it occurs in previously normal bladders, the usual sources being excretion of organisms through the kidney, acute gonorrhea, or catheterization. These three sources represent perfectly the three routes of infection—hematogenous, by extension, and by direct implantation. Any of these three routes may be concerned when cystitis occurs in the presence of other lesions, as for example, vesical calculus, vesical neoplsam, benign prostatic hypertrophy, or other forms of infravesical obstruction. The presence of stone, foreign body, tumor, ulceration, or residual urine predisposes to infection and maintains it when once established. Acute cystitis may be superposed on a chronic granulomatous process, as tuberculosis.

The normal bladder resists infection, due, no doubt, to its squamous epithe-

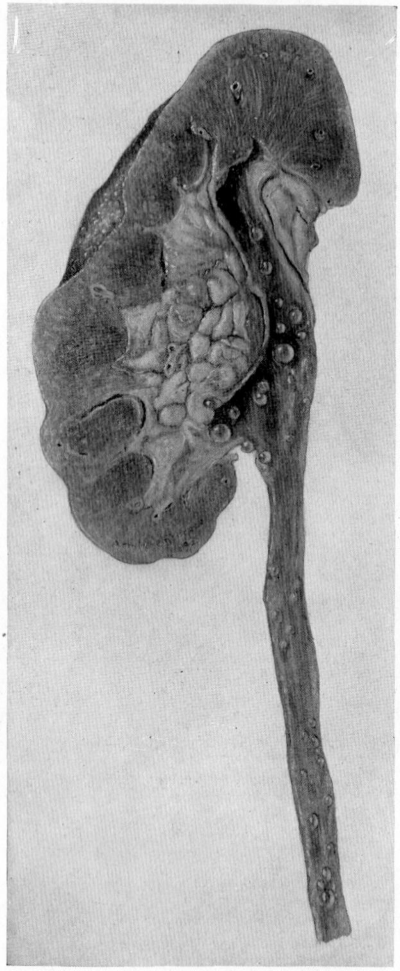

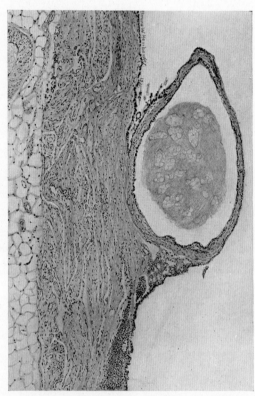

Fig. 72.—A rare specimen showing a very well-marked ureteritis cystica. This is exactly comparable to cystitis cystica, and is caused by the dilatation of small gland-like structures in the mucosa of the epithelium as shown in the following microscopic picture. The mucosa is inflamed and the kidney shows the changes of chronic pyelonephritis. By courtesy of Dr. M. C. Winternitz.

Fig. 73.—Microscopic drawing showing the structure of the cyst in the case of ureteritis cystica shown in the preceding figure. Note that the cyst is lined with epithelium and that while there is a definite round-cell infiltration of the ureteral wall, there is no edema and no resemblance to edematous polyps. By courtesy of Dr. M. C. Winternitz.

lium, few glands, and complete emptying at voiding. If uncomplicated infection occurs, it is usual for it to disappear spontaneously in a short time. It is easy to see how the above-mentioned lesions overcome these normal defenses. Of especial interest is *residual urine*. When the bladder empties normally, practically all the bacteria in the urine are expelled at each voiding, and usually, when cystitis

is present, more frequently than normal. Since we may assume that the number
of organisms present probably doubles every twenty or thirty minutes this is an
efficient check on their unlimited proliferation in the bladder. If, however, a
certain amount of residual urine remains, it acts as a culture medium and becomes
loaded to the limit with bacteria. It is a general rule, then, that we cannot expect
to eliminate infections of the bladder if residual urine (or diverticulum, which
acts in the same way) stone, foreign body, tumor, or ulcer be present. In the
same way, if the bladder is constantly being infected from the kidney, posterior
urethra (utricle), prostate, or seminal vesicles, these foci must be cleared up before
we can hope to influence the cystitis.

Acute cystitis as a complication of *gonorrheal urethritis* is not common, but
may occur. Wertheim[1] first demonstrated the organism, and we[2] obtained it by
suprapubic puncture in pure culture.

Acute cystitis occurs in young children and in women, especially during or
after childbirth. Heitz-Boyer[3] has shown
that in some, at least, of the cases in
women, the lesion can be referred to
bacteria, usually intestinal, which are
put out at intervals through the kidneys.
Pyelitis, however, is a frequent complication, and in this class of cases it is still
an unsolved problem whether the common path is through the kidneys or
through the urethra.

Acute cystitis, then, rarely, if ever,
occurs alone. It is practically always
associated with some other lesion or
pathologic condition, and a simple diagnosis of "cystitis" should seldom be made.
We may assume that in every case there
is an underlying cause which must be
removed before the cystitis can be cured.

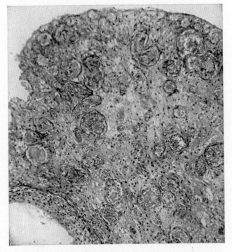

Fig. 74.—Acute cystitis with edema and
congestion showing part of a good-sized epithelium-lined cyst. Epithelium over surface is
desquamated. B. U. I. Path. 2134.

Microscopically, an early acute cystitis may show very little. The blood-
vessels are congested, accounting for the redness seen cystoscopically and some
degree of edema is present (Fig. 74). This edema may be very marked, and is
present especially in the loose submucosa. The epithelium may be raised up
into blebs, which appear translucent by cystoscope. This condition has been
called *bullous cystitis*, but has no special significance. The cellular infiltration
may be slight or marked, and contains a large proportion of polymorphonuclears.

Definite vesical pyuria may occur without any gross destruction of epithelium
(*catarrhal cystitis*). In other cases, when the lesion is severe, the epithelium is
sloughed off, and ulceration occurs. In very severe infections, the epithelium of
the whole bladder is largely destroyed, and the raw surface covered by a pyogenic

[1] Zeitschrift für Geburtshülfe und Gynäkologie, 1896, xxxv, 1–10.
[2] Young: Johns Hopkins Hospital Reports, 1900, ix, 679–707.
[3] Journal Medical Français, 1922, xi, 178–212.

membrane composed of fibrin, pus-cells, and organisms. This is called *diphtheritic cystitis*, but usually has nothing to do with the diphtheria bacillus.

The ulcerations of acute cystitis are usually shallow, and without indurated edges. As the lesion becomes less severe, they tend to heal rapidly. Involvement and perforation of the muscularis practically never occur. There may be edema and infiltration in the muscularis, diminishing the elasticity and motility of the bladder, and causing pain, but abscess formation and necrosis are very rare.

Bacteria may be found only in the most superficial layers of the epithelium, usually in association with slight lesions of the bladder wall, or they may penetrate deeply. In some cases, indeed, it seems as though the organisms were proliferating in the urine as a culture-medium, scarcely involving the bladder wall at all. Bacilluria and also cocciuria are not infrequently seen without any pus cells discernible even in centrifugalized specimens.

Any diffuse cystitis which persists becomes, of course, a chronic cystitis. While the changes of chronic inflammation appear, the acute process may continue. *Chronic cystitis* may be severe or mild, and in the latter case the amount of damage done to the bladder depends on the length of time the condition has persisted.

As stated above, cystitis is usually secondary to some other lesion, so that chronic diffuse cystitis usually indicates a persistent *renal, prostatic, posterior urethral,* or *diverticular* infection which keeps up the bladder inflammation, an *infravesical obstruction*, a *neoplasm* involving the bladder, or a *stone* or *foreign body*. Descending infection and infection by implantation have already been discussed. A chronic cystitis is often maintained by a chronic prostatic or vesicular infection. This may act by way of the urethra or by direct extension. That material from the prostate may reach the bladder is shown by the presence of pus and prostatic elements in the third glass of urine even when there is no cystitis. This back-flow probably occurs between urinations, when the entire bladder musculature is relaxed, and infection can occur in this way. The region of the prostate and vesical orifice is also supplied with very numerous, wide lymphatic spaces, anastomosing with those of the seminal vesicle and bladder. These no doubt play an important part in infections extending directly through into the base of the bladder.

The cystitis itself, if long continued, causes a deposition of fibrous tissue in the submucosa, and to a lesser extent in the muscularis of the bladder. The irritability of the bladder is heightened, and since the slightest stretching of the inflamed wall causes irritation, the muscle may remain in a state of almost continuous tonic contraction. If fibrous tissue is laid down under these conditions of diminished size, it prevents the normal stretching of the bladder, and consequently its capacity may be diminished even after the inflammation has disappeared. The fibrous tissue may, however, be gradually reabsorbed, and the bladder approach its normal size even after many months. Thus *"contracture of the bladder"* is a symptom, and not a disease *per se*. It may also be caused by localized cystitis, to be discussed later.

In the mucosa, chronic cystitis is characterized by cellular infiltration, by edema and congestion according to its severity, and by fibrosis according to its duration. Ulceration may occur as described above, and may be secondary to the trauma produced by stones or foreign bodies pressing on the epithelium. The bases of such chronic ulcers may become covered by granulation tissue, which, when it projects in irregular masses into the bladder, may resemble neoplasm. Not infrequently polyps occur (Fig. 75). Apparently they begin as edematous blebs, which later become filled with a growth of connective tissue and with cellular infiltration. The epithelium becomes somewhat thickened, and sends out rounded down-growths, which are usually solid, but may contain small lumina, and which are highly characteristic of these polypoid structures. Ordinarily the down-growths are not deeper than three or four times the thickness of the epithelium. If the lumina undergo cystic enlargement, *cystitis cystica* results, showing as small, transparent blebs (Fig. 76). The stroma is usually a loose edematous connective tissue, with plentiful blood-vessels. As the inflammation becomes less severe, the edema may lessen, and the base of the polyp contracts so that it becomes a thin pedicle. Such structures will

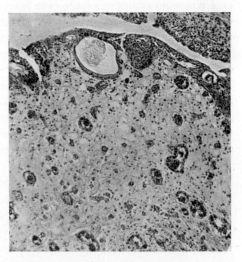

FIG. 75.—Chronic cystitis showing edema, congestion; polyp-like excrescence with some epithelial cysts (cystitis cystica). B. U. I. Path. 3643.

persist even after the causative inflammation has healed. The microscopic features mentioned distinguish them clearly from papillomata (*q. v.*).

Around the ureteral and urethral orifices, the fibrosis may have special effects, in the form of obstructions caused by contracture. The results of *contracture of the ureterovesical orifice* are the same as those of other lower ureteral obstructions.

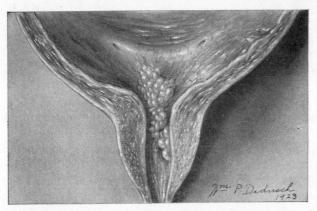

FIG. 76.—Multiple cysts or cystitis and urethritis cystica, occurring on the trigone and in the posterior urethra, in a case in which the symptoms were irritation and burning in the deep urethra and in which the urine was clear and microscopically negative and free from infection. These small cysts occupy the anterior part of the trigone, the median portion of the prostate, and the floor of the prostatic urethra to the verumontanum. B. U. I. 9676.

They are less apt to be bilateral than unilateral, but are fortunately quite rare. On the other hand, cicatricial *contracture of the vesicourethral orifice* is very common. This is not necessarily a sequel of diffuse chronic cystitis, but may also follow localized cystitis at the orifice and from its location, presupposes also involvement of the prostatic urethra and usually the prostate. It may result in a case where no symptoms have ever been present at any time except those of slight chronic urethritis and prostatitis, or if bladder symptoms have been present, they may have been no more than slight frequency and burning.

Gonorrhea, therefore, plays a prominent part in the etiology and the condition occurs often in young and middle-aged men below the age of prostatic hypertrophy. It may also follow chronic infections from other sources, such as catheter life, stone, or neoplasm, or result from trauma at operation or postoperative infections. Diverticulum is a frequent complication, probably, as pointed out by Hinman,[1] because the obstruction is of such gradual development. For the same reason symptoms begin insidiously. The effects on the kidneys, ureters, and bladder are

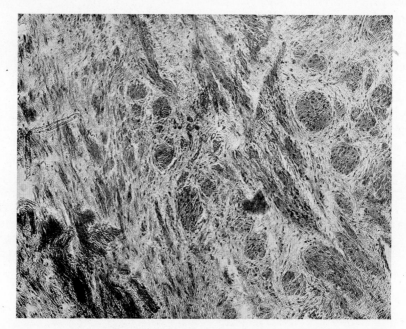

FIG. 77.—Sclerosis of internal sphincter.

those of an infravesical obstruction, described in the section on the Obstructive Uropathy.

The deposition of fibrous tissue about the orifice, in the sphincteric and trigonal muscles, interferes with its proper opening (Fig. 77). As the process advances, the orifice may become a very tiny aperture, with hard unyielding walls. Even before this the muscles may be so interfered with that residual urine occurs. The fibrous tissue may be present in greater amount on one aspect of the orifice, usually the posterior, when it is known as a median bar. In other cases, the contracture is nearly or quite circular, and is thought to result from cystitis rather than prostatitis alone.

The fibrosis of the orifice may be complicated in some cases, especially later in life, by hypertrophy of the prostatic glands at the orifice (Albarran's group).

[1] Journal of Urology, 1919, iii, 207–245.

The two processes can be seen side by side in the microscopic section. The contracture itself shows only a dense mass of fibrous tissue, enclosing here and there some bundles of smooth muscle, and usually with a round-cell infiltration. (See Benign Prostatic Hypertrophy; Chronic Urethritis.) If the prostatic hypertrophy is large, it, of course, overshadows the fibrosis, but the contracted orifice may require separate treatment after removal of the hypertrophied lobes.

Scar-tissue contractures following *operations* on the vesical orifice are the result of infection, often aided by imperfect operations, in which flaps or strands of mucosa are left in the orifice. In some cases where there is suprapubic drainage, the orifice may be completely closed by scar tissue. Epithelium grows over it, and a solid partition between bladder and prostatic urethra results.

Acute localized cystitis is rare, since an acute process tends to involve the entire bladder, and it is only mild, indolent infections which remain circumscribed.

Occasionally, especially in women, there may be a localized infection confined largely to the trigon and vesical orifice. Heitz-Boyer feels that this is due to organisms, insufficient in number or virulence to set up a severe infection, excreted by the kidney and poured out over the area between ureteral and vesical orifices. The usual picture is that of a rather superficial congestion and edema, characterized in the gross by reddening. There is some cellular infiltration, both round and polymorphonuclear, though the reaction may not be severe enough to cause pus-cells to appear in the urine, even when there is irritation and frequency. In more severe cases there may be some hemorrhage, and rarely shallow ulcerations. Study of the kidney urine may or may not disclose bacteriuria, but we know that renal bacteriuria may be intermittent.

If this condition persists, chronic changes supervene, consisting of polyps, small masses of granulations, sometimes covered by epithelium and with a raspberry appearance, and fibrosis. Similar changes occur in the upper urethra (*q. v.*).

Submucous or Interstitial Cystitis.—As we have seen, the majority of cases of bladder infection without urinary obstruction have their origin in infectious foci of the kidney or lower urinary tract. Everyone is familiar with the promptness with which the usual case of chronic cystitis clears up either spontaneously or as a result of local treatment following the eradication of the extravesical focus of infection. These are cases in which the pathologic process involves chiefly the mucous membrane, the changes in the deeper layer of bladder wall being comparatively slight or absent.

On the other hand, one occasionally finds cases in which bladder symptoms, sometimes of the greatest severity, resist all forms of treatment and no extravesical focus of infection can be found.

Nitze described these cases years ago, but their recognition in this country dates from 1913, when Hunner[1] reported a group of cases presenting symptoms of marked contracture of the bladder in which the urine was often perfectly clear and free of infection and the mucous membrane lesion insignificant or indefinite, the symptoms being out of all proportion to the cystoscopic findings. Further investigation of this condition showed that in many of these cases the mucosal

[1] Transactions of the Southern Surgical and Gynecological Association, 1914, xxvii; see also Frontz: Journal of Urology, 1921, v, 491–511; and Nitze: Lehrbuch der Kystoskopie, 1907.

lesion had practically disappeared, the predominant pathologic process being found in the deeper layers of the bladder wall.

The lesion in these cases is often small, consisting of a fibrosis replacing a portion of the loose areolar tissue of the submucosa. In those cases in which the process is circumscribed there is little or no increase in the thickness of the bladder wall at the point of involvement. In other cases in which the inflammatory process has extended through all the coats of the bladder, involving not only the submucosa but the muscularis as well, there may be great thickening at the site of the lesion. The mucous membrane covering these lesions may be intact, presenting only a slight reddening or edema. In other cases fissures or linear ulcerations are noted, these invariably being the result of previous overdistention of the bladder (Figs. 78, 79). It should be emphasized that the mucous membrane instead of lying upon the loose and mobile areolar submucosa of the normal bladder is attached to

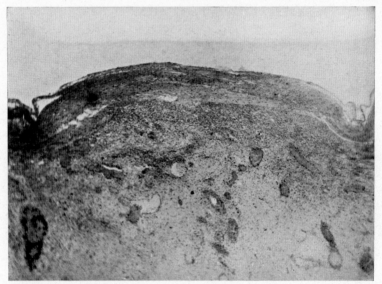

Fig. 78.—Photomicrograph showing a thin and intact layer of fibrosis lying upon a somewhat thickened submucosa. The bladder in this case was not subjected to overdistention preliminary to operation.

a dense and inelastic fibrosis, the unyielding nature of which results in tears when the bladder is subjected to overdistention. Our study of these cases has shown that the application of this observation provides an excellent means of accurately outlining the extent of the lesion, for when the bladder is overdistended the mucosa covering the dense scirrhous layer beneath is subjected to injuries which usually present themselves in the form of fissures. These linear mucosal lesions heal rapidly and at subsequent cystoscopy may be either absent or differently situated. This fact is responsible for the popular and misleading term "elusive ulcer" being applied to them.

Histologically except for the formation of the fibrous submucous layer, the microscopic picture differs in no respect from that seen in many cases of chronic cystitis. Round-cell infiltration in varying degrees of intensity is seen beneath the fibrous lamella which can sometimes be followed down between the muscle bundles as far as the serous coat. Usually there is marked vascular congestion and dilatation, and extravasation of blood is usually present, but the latter finding is thought often to be the result of trauma caused by distention.

The essential and consistent lesion in this disease is a dense submucous fibrosis—sometimes thin, sometimes thick. In the former cases the submucosa or a portion of it alone is involved; in the latter the process extends to varying depths in the muscularis.

Bacteria have not been found microscopically. In typical cases there are no pus-cells or bacteria in the bladder urine. Rosenow,[1] however, states that he has reproduced the lesion in animals by intravenous injection of streptococci obtained from a tooth abscess in a patient suffering from the disease, and Hinman[2] has accomplished the same result with a streptococcus grown from an excised human lesion. If the assumptions of these authors are correct, this condition provides the only common example of a direct hematogenous infection of the bladder wall.

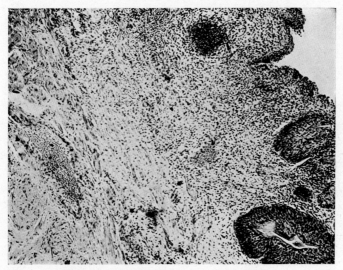

Fig. 79.—Chronic submucous inflammation.

In 1896 Fenwick[3] described a *solitary ulcer* of the bladder. This lesion consists of a very definite, rather punched out ulcer, with slightly elevated edges and an irregular base. The size is variable, as is also the depth. The muscularis may be included in the ulcerative process, but perforation is not reported. The usual site is in the base of the bladder, oftenest near the ureteral orifices. Fenwick states that the ulcer is always single, but Buerger[4] claims that the ulcers may be multiple. The remainder of the bladder may be normal, or the seat of a diffuse cystitis. In later stages, the ulcer becomes covered with an adherent membrane of exudate, which may be inspissated and rubbery, or heavily infiltrated with calcareous material.

The condition is distinguished by a long history, without, as a rule, antecedent

[1] Journal of Urology, 1921, vi, 285–298.
[2] Ibid., 1921, vi (discussion), 299–301.
[3] British Medical Journal, 1896, i, 1133–1135.
[4] Medical Record, 1913, lxxxiii, 656–661.

disease, negative kidney findings, painful urination, and most characteristic of all, prompt healing after thorough curettage. The cases are few, and no thorough pathologic study of a sufficient series has been reported. In the older cases, tuberculosis and other obscure causes are not satisfactorily ruled out. Where sections have been made, the picture was simply that of chronic inflammation. LeFur and others have suggested that the ulceration depends on a thrombosis or thromboangiitis of small blood-vessels, as has been proposed for gastric ulcer. No definite statement as to the etiology can be given. The diagnosis can only be made by exclusion, after the most thorough study of the entire urinary tract.

Leukoplakia of the bladder, ureters, and renal pelves has long been known, and was well described by Rokitansky in 1861. It is a condition in which the epithelium over irregular areas of varying size takes on the characteristics of squamous epithelium, and becomes covered with a cornified layer. This, according to Hinman and Gibson,[1] cannot be regarded as true metaplasia, but rather as a reaction to irritation. This is apparently a characteristic of all epithelium, since it is found in the cervix uteri, mouth, and elsewhere, while in normally cornified areas, the cornification is increased by irritation, as in corns and calluses. No glands, hairs, or other structures characteristic of skin are ever seen. The idea of Marchand that the process depended on a progressive epidermization through a fistula is not tenable.

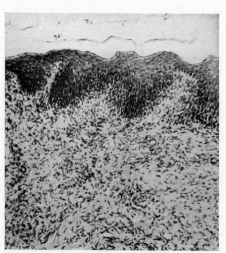

Fig. 80.—Section from the bladder showing leukoplakia. In this case there was a pyonephrosis on one side in an ectopic kidney. The leukoplakia was much more pronounced in this kidney than in the bladder. J. H. H. Autopsy 7345. (See Fig. 59.)

Leukoplakia is almost always associated with long-continued chronic infection, either tuberculous or non-specific. Very few uninfected cases are reported, but Leber reports a case, uninfected, in a child of four months.[2] The patches are surrounded by a zone of congestion and the thickened cornified layer gives a snowy white, unmistakable appearance. Flakes of this epidermis are thrown off constantly and are pathognomonic when found in the urine. Microscopically one sees the epithelium thickened, the outer layers flattened, and covered by a coherent layer of desquamated cells exactly like the epidermis. Beer[3] noted the presence of silicates, as in the skin. The lesion is slowly progressive, and we find no record of cure except by excision. Its principal importance is that it is apparently a necessary preliminary to epidermoid or squamous carcinoma (*q. v.*). We have recently seen a case (J. H. H. Aut. 7345) in which a pelvic ectopic kidney was the site of a severe pyonephrosis. The entire kidney pelvis and ureter were lined by a thick layer of keratinized epithelium (see Fig. 59) and the bladder epithelium was also keratinized, but to a lesser extent (Fig. 80). This is interest-

[1] Journal of Urology, 1921, vi, 1–50 (Lit.).

[2] Quoted by Kretschmer, Surgery, Gynecology, and Obstetrics, 1920, xxxi, 325–339.

[3] American Journal of the Medical Sciences, 1914, cxlvii, 244–246.

ing in view of the fact that the bladder inflammation was less severe than that in the kidney, and suggests that the degree of epidermization was dependent on the degree of inflammation. In another case very large rolled-up sheets of epidermis were voided. Ureter catheterization showed that these came from the left kidney.

Von Hansemann[1] described in 1903 a peculiar lesion which he called *malakoplakia*. There were small, round or oval, convex bodies rising above the surface, most numerous in the lower part of the bladder. In one case a few small ones were found in the ureter. All were slightly ulcerated on the surface, causing a characteristic umbilication. The color was of a yellowish hue, and there was a halo of congested vessels about each. Microscopically, the nodule was seen to have developed in the submucosa, pushing the epithelium out ahead of it, and having no connection therewith. The mass consisted of large cells, with good-sized vesicular nuclei, sometimes multiple, and containing rounded, colorless, highly refractile bodies of varying size in the cytoplasm. The largest ones were occasionally outside the cells. There was a delicate connective-tissue framework, and masses of short bacteria were found in the cells. A beautiful colored picture of the lesion is shown by McDonald and Sewell.[2]

Two cases described by Folsom[3] do not correspond to Von Hansemann's lesion. They were composed of cells like plasma cells, with phagocyted lymphocytes and red-blood cells. There were no cell inclusions and the color was not yellowish. They were apparently granulomatous. The nature of malakoplakia is entirely unknown. No symptoms are described. We have not seen a case of this interesting lesion.

Inflammation may extend to the exterior of the bladder (*perivesical inflammation*) by perforation of a malignant growth, or of an inflammatory ulcer (rare), by traumatic penetration of the bladder wall, as by an instrument, a missile, or a surgical wound, from neighboring organs, as the pelvic bones or intestines, or by injuries to the urethra or ureters in the neighborhood of the bladder. Infection of a retrovesical hydatid cyst or necrotic retrovesical neoplasm are rare instances. Wherever there is a direct communication with the cavity of the bladder, the infection is complicated by the extravasation of urine. If the development of the lesion is slow, as, for example, around some suprapubic fistulæ, the formation of scar tissue limits the spread of urine and prevents the phenomena of acute extravasation. Extravasation is discussed under Traumatism of the Bladder and Urethra. Owing to the usual presence of urine, with resultant necrosis, perivesical infections usually proceed quickly to abscess formation.

These infections are divided roughly into *prevesical* and *retrovesical* groups. Retrovesical abscesses may follow operations in the region of the seminal vesicles, prostate, and rectum, or extend from within the bladder, or seminal vesicles. If an operation tract exists, drainage will usually occur through it, though pus may be encysted and unable to drain in this way. If there is no tract, the spread tends to be upward, to the retroperitoneal space, and occasionally around the side of the bladder to the lower abdominal quadrant. Downward spread is prevented by Denonvillier's fascia and the lateral pelvic aponeuroses. In the upward direction such abscesses may even involve the kidney.

[1] Virchow's Archiv, 1903, clxxiii, 302–308.
[2] Journal of Pathology and Bacteriology, 1914, xviii, 1305 (Lit.).
[3] Journal of the American Medical Association, 1919, lxxiii, 1112–1114.

Retrovesical abscesses may open into the bladder or the rectum, although the latter is unusual. Communication with the rectum should be prevented, if possible, as the presence of intestinal contents complicates the infection, and, if communication with the bladder exists, at the time of opening into the rectum or later, rectovesical fistula may occur.

Prevesical abscess is especially caused from instrumental perforation of the urethra above the triangular ligament, the beak of the instrument passing up in front of the bladder. It may also follow infection of a suprapubic wound. The spread of these abscesses is usually first to the front, where they may point in the hypogastrium or groins. Later they dissect upward, and if mediăn, are contained laterally by the obliterated hypogastric arteries, but push between the peritoneum and posterior aspect of the recti muscles. They may appear at the umbilicus. As soon as they reach above the level of the vesical peritoneal reflection, they are separated from the abdominal cavity itself only by the thin peritoneum. This is of importance, as it may easily give rise to peritonitis. Such an event may be caused when in a case of infravesical obstruction an infected suprapubic fistula closes at the surface, so that the urine can be expelled with difficulty or not at all. In rarer cases, the infection may extend around the sides of the bladder. It does not, however, pass down beyond the upper margin of the pubis, Pouparts' ligament, or the triangular ligament unless the fasciæ at these points have been injured.

When a perivesical abscess has opened, spontaneously or by incision, urinary fistulæ result, always if the bladder is already penetrated, sometimes if it has not. As the infection clears up, these fistulæ will close, unless there is infravesical obstruction or unless the fistulæ themselves are indolent as in tuberculosis, neoplasm, or osteomyelitis of the pelvic bones.

Fibrosis follows perivesical inflammation as it does perirenal, but seldom causes serious interference with bladder function. Its principle importance is in the difficulties which it places in-the way of subsequent operations on the bladder. Contraction may pull the peritoneal reflection lower than normal, and the presence of dense scar tissue prevents its recognition and interferes with the pushing upward of the peritoneum.

Cases of very dense board-like chronic perivesical inflammation are seen.

Urethra.—Among infections of the urethra, that specifically due to the *gonococcus* is the most important. The gonococcus (Neisseria gonorrhœæ, S. A. B.) is a highly parasitic organism, affecting only the human species, and succumbing quickly outside the body to cold, heat, or drying.[1] This is why the infection is so seldom transmitted by any means but sexual contact. The gonococcus can cause infection in any part of the body when introduced under suitable conditions, and it is, therefore, only because sexual contact provides a ready means of transmission that gonorrhea is most frequent in the urethra.

Torrey[2] states that distinct strains of gonococci cannot be separated by immunologic tests. There is reason to believe that gonococcus vaccines induce some immunity, or increase a pre-existing immunity, in the human body. Immunity doubtless exists; it is striking that gonorrheal ophthalmia is such a rare complication of gonorrheal urethritis, although in many cases patients allow their hands

[1] Engering: Zeitschrift für Hygiene und Infectiösen Krankheiten, 1923, c, 314–322.

[2] Torrey and Buckell: Journal of Immunology, 1922, vii, 305–359.

and clothing to be constantly contaminated with gonorrheal pus. These factors in gonorrheal infection offer interesting possibilities for the future in therapy, and determine the progress and results of clinical gonorrhea.

The gonococcus is a pyogenic organism, and its first invasion incites a reaction of the most acute character (Figs. 81, 82). The noteworthy experiments of Finger[1] upon moribund patients provide almost our sole pathologic data on *acute gonorrheal urethritis*. His description follows:

The gonococci begin to proliferate on the surface of the epithelium which they are about to attack; they are not spread diffusely, but in small groups. At the end of thirty-eight hours, they have scarcely as yet penetrated into the epithelium, at the most they have slipped in among the superficial cells at the points presenting the feeblest resistance. If the epithelium is denuded at any point, exposing the connective tissue, the organisms penetrate there more rapidly. They invade the lumina of the crypts of Morgagni with extreme rapidity, and are

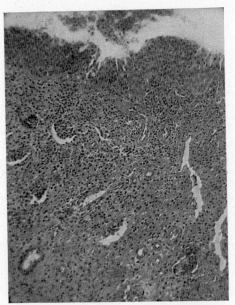

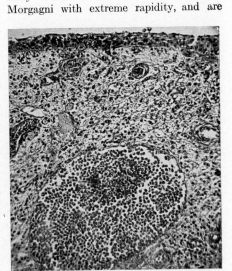

FIG. 81.—Section from the penile urethra of a case of acute gonorrheal urethritis. Note the extensive cellular infiltration consisting of both mononuclears and polymorphonuclears. Some leukocytes are also seen in the epithelium, and at the point where they are most numerous the epithelial cells are shrunken and clefts between them appear. Just outside this point is a mass of exudate in the lumen. J. H. H. Autopsy 6468.

FIG. 82.—Section from the penile urethra of a case of acute gonorrheal urethritis. The epithelium is intact. The subepithelial connective tissue shows some edema and an infiltration which is largely mononuclear. In the space in the lower half of the picture, possibly an enlarged lymphatic channel, is a dense collection of polymorphonuclears. J. H. H. Autopsy 6468.

found in them, lying free on the surface of the epithelium. From this moment, and, indeed, well before this, diapedesis has commenced, the leukocytes are everywhere numerous in the superior layers; a certain number have gained the surface, and one already finds intracellular gonococci.

At the end of three days the lesions have advanced remarkably. The entire surface of the mucosa is covered with a thick layer of pus-cells, which fill all the folds, crypts of Morgagni, and glands. The changes in the epithelium depend upon its nature: almost none at the level of the fossa navicularis, the stratified pavement of which has retained its solidity in spite of the leukocytes lying among its cells. The changes are accentuated in the cylindric epithelium which covers the rest of the affected portion. They are, however, not uniform. Although here and

[1] Finger, Gohn, and Schlagenhaufer: Archiv für Dermatologie und Syphilologie, 1894, xxviii, 3–24; 277–344. See also Motz: Annales des Maladies des Organes Génito-urinaires, 1903, xxi, 419–441.

there the epithelium has kept its cohesion in spite of the leukocytic infiltration, in other places it is dissociated even to the deepest layers. These places are not distributed in a haphazard way, but are constantly about the lacunæ, or have their point of maximum intensity at the reflection of the epithelium at the edge of a cul-de-sac. Furthermore, the epithelium of the lacunæ (crypts) undergoes identical changes, in an even more accentuated degree. It is the same with the ducts of the glands (of Littre), but the secreting portion of the acini shows only minimal alterations—a few leukocytes between the cells, which retain their original cohesion. The connective tissue shows dilated vessels packed with leukocytes, and an intense infiltration, becoming less marked toward the depths, but still visible in the trabeculæ of the corpus spongiosum. Like the epithelial changes, this infiltration is disposed in a perifollicular manner (*i. e.*, most intense about the crypts). Mast-cells are present in the subepithelial layers and near the vessels.

Gonococci are extremely numerous. The leukocytes which cover the surface are packed with them, those which fill the glands and lacunæ also contain them, although here more free cocci are to be found than on the surface. In the tissues, the distribution of the gonococci corresponds to that of the lesions. In the stratified pavement epithelium they penetrate practically not at all, and the leukocytes found between the cells contain none. In the cylindric epithelium they are relatively infrequent at the level of the interglandular folds, where they are intracellular, or insinuate themselves, pair by pair, between the cylindric cells, with little groups wherever larger spaces permit. They are, on the contrary, in enormous numbers in the perifollicular regions; the pus-cells which have invaded and broken up the epithelium are packed with them, and they push in in their usual manner in long lines between the deep cells, with here and there round colonies where space permits. They thus form a sort of network surrounding almost every cell. It is the same on the lateral walls of the crypts, but they penetrate less in the stratified epithelium at their extremities. It is also the same in the gland ducts, while gonococci are never found between the secreting cells of the acini proper. Finally, wherever the connective tissue is not covered and protected by a resistant epithelium, the gonococci push into its meshes and proliferate in the wider spaces, but here again they are much more abundant in the perilacunar foci. They may be intracellular, but are more often free in the tissue spaces.

The involvement of the urethral glands plays the important rôle in maintaining the infection in the face of treatment. Superficial ulcers often appear. A profuse purulent discharge is the rule, and leukocytosis indicates that a systemic reaction is occurring. Fever is not constant. Edema is generally insufficient to prevent free voiding, but infiltration of the corpus spongiosum may be of sufficient degree to destroy the elasticity of the urethra so that on erection the penis curves downward. This is known as chordee.

Cowper's glands may be involved, the infection being unilateral or bilateral. The process extends along the ducts, which being long and narrow, may easily be occluded. These glands are lined by tall cylindric epithelium which secretes mucus. The inflammation may be slight, with edema, moderate infiltration, and increased secretion of mucus, or it may be more intense, in which case the epithelium may desquamate, the secretion be reduced, and the lumina filled with pus. If the duct is occluded, the gland may become very tense from edema and infiltration, and may suppurate. Since it is located between the two layers of the triangular ligament, embedded in the external sphincter, the pus will tend to burrow, once the gland capsule is perforated, posteriorly into the ischiorectal fossa, where it may present at the skin surface. It is possible that in some cases the pus may follow the duct through the external layer of the triangular ligament into the anterior perineal triangle.

Since the infection comes directly from the outside, the lesion is at first confined to the pendulous and bulbous parts of the urethra, *i. e.*, the portion distal to the external sphincter. This portion is called, for clinical purposes, the "anterior" urethra, and we have, first, therefore, *acute anterior urethritis*.

The inflammation often spreads, in spite of all efforts, to the membranous and prostatic parts of the urethra—clinically the "posterior" urethra. *Acute posterior urethritis* occurs as a complication of acute anterior urethritis, and usually comes on eight to twenty days later. Our knowledge of how this occurs is deficient, since no autopsy material is available, and the disease cannot be reproduced in animals. It is, however, an ascending infection and may extend along the mucosa, or through the lymphatics, which pass in this direction, or by carriage of infectious material through the lumen. At all events, it occurs in about half the cases, in the absence of all instrumentation or retrograde injections past the external sphincter. Extension into this fresh field usually causes a recurrence of the acute inflammation and the posterior urethra becomes the seat of changes like those described for the anterior. Here, however, the gland system is much deeper than in the anterior urethra, and the urethral glands, the Albarran group, and the prostatic glands become involved in the inflammation. Acute generalized prostatitis is not the rule, occurring in only a small percentage of cases, but the inflammation, passing down along and around the ducts gains a foothold in this complicated organ, where it is apt to remain for very long periods, even though confined to the juxta-urethral portions.

In the anterior urethra resolution may occur, in a matter of two to six weeks, with complete disappearance of the lesion. The complexity of the gland system varies greatly in different individuals, and no doubt rapid healing is more likely with a simple than with a complicated system of glands. Ulceration also prevents healing. If healing does not occur, the condition passes into *chronic anterior urethritis*. The infiltration becomes more and more lymphocytic in character, and there is a deposition of fibrous tissue. The essential thing is that the process which was diffuse while acute now becomes localized. Edema of the mucosa and plugs of exudate occlude the urethral or Cowper's glands in early stages, and later this occlusion is continued by fibrosis. Thus foci of gonococci may be cut off from communication with the urethra, and sometimes give rise to peri-urethral abscesses. The discharge becomes mucoid or mucopurulent and usually reduced in amount. The little plugs of mucopus mentioned above may be washed out of the mouths of the glands, and are seen in the urine as the familiar "shreds." The amount of discharge depends on the extent of the lesion. The epithelium is often excoriated over the localized areas of inflammation, and these little ulcers may be heaped up with granulation tissue. Such masses of granulation tissue keep the infection alive, give rise to increased discharge, and may go on to polyp formation. In other places infiltration of the submucosa produces an inflammatory mass even where the epithelium is intact. In places where ulcers have occurred, or where an infected gland is cut off from the lumen, fibrous tissue formation is especially apt to take place. The deposition of fibrous tissue may be continuous if the chronic inflammation persists in the occluded ducts and peri-urethral tissue. If confined to one side of the urethra, such accumulations of scar tissue do not interfere with the passage of urine, but if they extend entirely around the urethra, its caliber will be diminished by contracture, giving rise to *stricture*. The stricture may be a simple ring, or the most complicated arrangement, really a conversion of the urethra into a highly irregular, fibrous, thick-walled tube. Stricture of the urethra may also occur as a result of urethritis in women. It is probably less uncommon than ordinarily believed.

Even where the flow of urine is not interfered with, patches of chronic inflammation, with fibrosis, infiltration, and occluded, infected glands, act as foci which may prolong a urethral infection indefinitely. They are sometimes known as "strictures of wide caliber," but scarcely merit the appellation of "stricture."

Chronic posterior urethritis is a very frequent sequel of acute posterior urethritis. As explained above, however, it is practically always associated with some degree of prostatitis, and it is difficult to separate the two clinically. The pathologic picture is similar to that described for the anterior urethra. In the membranous urethra the lesions are usually less pronounced, owing to the comparative absence of glands, while in the prostatic urethra the prostatic ducts and submucosal or suburethral glands take the place of Littre's glands. In addition chronic inflammation of the utriculus may occur, which in some cases goes on, through occlusion, to an empyema or pyo-utricle. The utricle may be infected when the prostate is comparatively normal.[1] If there is seminal vesiculitis (*q. v.*), the ejaculatory ducts may discharge infectious material into the prostatic urethra. Ulcers, granulations, and polyps occur here also.

In the posterior portion the membranous urethra remains comparatively free of strictures, owing to the paucity of glands to maintain infection. In the prostatic urethra the outcome depends on the conditions in the prostate. Early healing not infrequently occurs, but may be absent on account of the extremely convoluted gland system. Catarrhal inflammation of the ducts often persists. If so, infiltration and fibrosis occur in the stroma. The end-results in the prostate are discussed under that heading, but as that part of the prostate surrounding the urethra becomes more and more scarred and fibrous, the lumen of the urethra may be obstructed by its contracture, especially at the vesical orifice. This is part of a condition usually involving also the base of the bladder and the vesical orifice, and may be important from its obstructing effect. It is often known as "small fibrous prostate," but represents in a certain sense a stricture of the prostatic urethra. It is not as common as stricture of the anterior urethra, possibly because the caliber of the prostatic urethra is greater.

Ulcerations in the anterior or posterior urethra may become covered with granulation tissue masses which prevent healing. Irregularities of the mucosa may be due to *submucous infiltration* and proliferation of lymph-follicles. In long-standing cases *polyps* may arise, exactly as in the bladder, and oftener in the posterior urethra. Spots of *leukoplakia* are seen, but are rare. Obstruction of the ducts of the suburethral glands may give rise to *cysts*, which may be in the prostatic urethra or at the vesical orifice.

Cysts.—Obstructive retention cyst of the prostate was first stressed by Englisch,[2] who in 1873 reported 2 cases, both men, aged forty years, in which at autopsy a retention cyst was discovered in the median posterior portion of the prostate. After that, the subject received very little attention until 1900, when Abbe reported a case of acute retention of urine in a young man in whom on suprapubic cystotomy he discovered a cherry-sized cyst at the prostatic orifice "which acted as a ball valve." The cyst was transfixed, cut off, and the base sutured. Result excellent. Berkhart in 1902, and A. Cabot in 1906, reported similar cases, in which the cyst was also removed by suprapubic operation. In 1912

[1] Geraghty: Journal of the American Medical Association, 1911, lvi, 731–732.
[2] Wiener Medicinisches Jahrbuch, 1873, 1.

PLATE IV
URETHRAL DISEASES AS SHOWN BY URETHROSCOPE

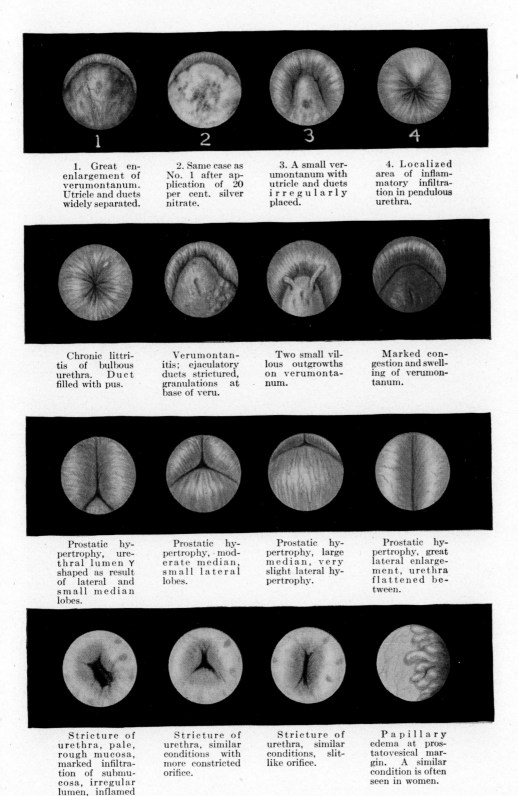

1. Great en-enlargement of verumontanum. Utricle and ducts widely separated.

2. Same case as No. 1 after application of 20 per cent. silver nitrate.

3. A small ver-umontanum with utricle and ducts irregularly placed.

4. Localized area of inflammatory infiltration in pendulous urethra.

Chronic littritis of bulbous urethra. Duct filled with pus.

Verumontanitis; ejaculatory ducts strictured, granulations at base of veru.

Two small villous outgrowths on verumontanum.

Marked congestion and swelling of verumontanum.

Prostatic hypertrophy, urethral lumen Y shaped as result of lateral and small median lobes.

Prostatic hypertrophy, moderate median, small lateral lobes.

Prostatic hypertrophy, large median, very slight lateral hypertrophy.

Prostatic hypertrophy, great lateral enlargement, urethra flattened between.

Stricture of urethra, pale, rough mucosa, marked infiltration of submucosa, irregular lumen, inflamed gland ducts.

Stricture of urethra, similar conditions with more constricted orifice.

Stricture of urethra, similar conditions, slit-like orifice.

Papillary edema at prostatovesical margin. A similar condition is often seen in women.

and 1913, we operated upon 3 patients, in 2 of whom the cyst was removed with the cystoscopic rongeur and in the third, removed intact suprapubically.[1] Recently Wesson[2] has collected all the cases from the literature, and added three of his own.

In most cases the obstructive retention cysts are located at the prostatic orifice and are due probably to closure of the prostatic ducts. The walls are thin, as seen with the cystoscope they are translucent and covered with very thin mucous membrane. They project more or less into the vesical cavity and may vary in size from that of a pea to an orange. In 25 cases collected, in which the size was stated, in 12 the cyst was the size of a cherry; in 3 the size of a walnut; in 2 the size of a small orange, and in the remainder of various sizes and shapes from that of a bean to the size of the thumb. The obstruction to urination produced varied greatly. In 2 cases it was very great (3500 and 3200 c.c.), in 1 case 1500 c.c. and in 2, 500 c.c. of residual urine was present. In the rest of the cases, the residual varied from nothing (2 cases) up to 400 c.c. Some of the cases were associated with vesical diverticulum and others evidences of obstruction. In some of the cases, death had resulted from renal destruction produced by back pressure. Prostatic hypertrophy was present in only 3 of the cases, and only 1 of these had hematuria, but bloody ejaculation was present in 1 case.

The ascent of the infection in the urinary tract usually stops at the internal sphincter, but may occasionally give rise to an acute cystitis, usually a trigonitis or a "basal" cystitis, with pure culture of gonococcus, or more rarely, a pyelitis. Less infrequently there is only a slight inflammation in the trigonal region and about the orifice, which causes frequency and burning, but is scarcely a real cystitis. This is known as trigonitis, cystitis colli, or collitis.

Extension to the peri-urethral tissues occurs through the blocking off of infected urethral or Cowper's glands by edema or fibrosis, by direct extension through the tissues or lymphatic spaces, or by traumatic rupture of the urethra. It may or may not be accompanied by extravasation of urine.

Extravasation of urine can occur only when there is an actual break in the mucosa, and is much increased if there is an obstruction (usually a stricture) in the urethra distal to the break.

The direction and extent of the invasion of the surrounding tissues by peri-urethral inflammation or abscess, or urinary extravasation, are determined by the pelvic, perineal, and penile fascias. While the main facts concerning these fascias are known, there is still discussion concerning minor points. This is due to the fact that all fascias are merely condensations of the fibrous connective tissue everywhere present, and may be dissected and split up in different ways by different workers.

The accompanying diagram (Fig. 83) represents the fascias as we understand them at present. The *triangular ligament* fills the space between the most anterior portions of the descending rami of the pubes. It is divided into two layers. The upper or internal layer is not particularly strong, being little more than the superior connective-tissue sheath of the external sphincter muscle. It fuses above with the prostatic and levator fascias laterally, and with the *fascia of Denonvilliers* posteriorly. The lower or external layer is much thicker and stronger. It is attached firmly to the lower borders of the pubic rami. It contains foramina for

---

[1] Reported in Keen's Surgery, 1913, vi, 670, and 1921, viii, 530.
[2] Journal of Urology, 1925, xiii (to be published).

the passage of the urethra and the ducts of Cowper's glands, and there is a hiatus at the apex of the pubic triangle for the nerves and vessels of the penis. The posterior border extends straight across from one pubic ramus to the other, and is sharp and well defined.

The *superficial perineal fascia* (Colles' fascia) is attached to the posterior border of the external layer of the triangular ligament, and to the rami of the pubes. It runs around the dorsal aspect of the superficial transverse perineal muscles, then down, and forward under the skin of the perineum and scrotum, forming the outermost fibrous sac of the testicle. This conformation encloses the anterior

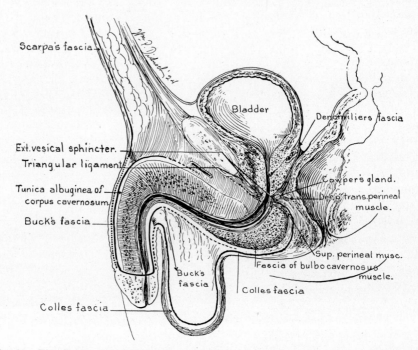

FIG. 83.—This diagram represents the present state of our knowledge of the fascias of the perineum. Note that the deep layer of the triangular ligament is much less well defined than the superficial layer, that it fuses with the superficial layer near the symphysis, and that posteriorly it is apparently continuous with Denonvilliers' fascia. The recto-urethralis muscle fuses with the external sphincter. Buck's fascia is shown in dotted lines in its perineal portion since we are not certain of its exact relations at this point. Colles' fascia is shown in dotted lines in the penis since we are not certain whether it runs down on the penis or not. Adhesions between Colles' fascia and Buck's fascia at the root of the penis are shown. It is these which prevent infiltration of the penis until after the anterior perineal triangle, scrotum, and lower abdomen are infiltrated.

perineal triangle everywhere except anteriorly about the root of the penis, and extravasations cannot escape anywhere else unless they penetrate Colles' fascia or the triangular ligament. Extension down the penis is opposed by a close application of Colles' fascia to the deeper fascias of the penis proper at its root, so that the only remaining path is upward to the abdomen. As Colles' fascia comes up from the perineum, it is continuous with the *superficial abdominal fascia* (Scarpa's fascia), so the areolar space beneath Scarpa's fascia communicates with the anterior perineal triangle through the region just in front of the symphysis.

In addition to Colles' fascia, each erectile body of the penis is provided with a fibrous investment of its own, known as the *tunica albuginea*. Each of these tunics is separate except that in the pendulous portion the two adjacent faces of the corpora cavernosa are fused, forming a median septum (septum pectiniforme). Surrounding the entire penis is *Buck's fascia*, which, according to Buck's original description, sends a partition between the corpus spongiosum and the corpora cavernosa, so that it makes two compartments in the penis, a small one ventrally containing the corpus spongiosum, and a large one dorsally containing the two corpora cavernosa. These relations are borne out by injection experiments made to simulate extravasations.

At the end of the penis, the corpora cavernosa end at the proximal surface of the glans, while the more superficial investments (Buck's) are inserted all the way around at the corona glandis. The tunica propria of the glans is in close relations and practically continuous with the tunica of the corpus spongiosum.

The above-mentioned features may be taken as proved and reliable, but other points are more uncertain. The relations of Buck's fascia and Colles' fascia, both in the perineum and in the penis, are disputed. In Buck's original description[1] he describes the continuation of Buck's fascia in the perineum as identical with Colles' fascia. On the other hand, Wesson[2] pictures Buck's fascia as continuing upwards internal to Colles' fascia, more closely applied to the corpora, dividing to surround each, external to the bulbocavernosus and ischiocavernosus muscles, and finally passing up in front of the transversus perinei to fuse with the external layer of the triangular ligament.

Similarly, it is often taught that Colles' fascia fuses with Buck's fascia about the root of the penis, and does not extend down over the penis. Wesson, however, believes, as the result of injecting fluid in the perineum which, after the pressure became quite high, passed down the penis outside Buck's fascia and inside a more superficial fascia, that Colles' fascia, although rather adherent to Buck's fascia at the root of the penis, passes down separate from Buck's fascia and envelops the entire penis except the glans.

In spite of these divergences of opinion, however, the main clinical facts are obvious enough. If an extravasation takes place in the penis, the penile fascias, especially Buck's, confine it and produce a circumscribed swelling. The above described septum usually protects the corpora cavernosa from involvement, and even if the dorsal compartment of Buck's fascia is invaded, there is still the tunica propria of the corpora cavernosa to be penetrated.

In the perineum, the tunics surrounding the bulb, and the connective tissue trabeculæ of the anterior perineal triangle, serve to circumscribe at first an abscess or extravasation, but it may eventually fill the entire triangle. Colles' fascia then interposes an effective barrier, preventing spread posteriorly, to the ischiorectal fossæ, and laterally, to the thighs. As a result, the tumefaction invades first the scrotum, then passes up beneath Scarpa's fascia on the abdomen, and usually last of all extends down the penis to the coronary sulcus.

Buck's and Colles' fascias, and the triangular ligament may, however, be penetrated by inflammatory processes or neoplastic growths, so that the above mentioned rules have some exceptions. We have seen a case (B. U. I. 9972) in which a cord of induration reached back from the midportion of the bulb to the superficial region of the right ischiorectal fossa, evidently passing directly through

[1] Transactions of the American Medical Association, 1848, i, 367–372.
[2] Journal of the American Medical Association, 1923, lxxxi, 2024–2029.

Colles' fascia. When extravasations are complicated by necrosis, the fascias may be destroyed, and the further involvement follow unexpected paths.

Since the membranous urethra is short and usually devoid of glands, peri-urethral inflammation and abscesses above the triangular ligament commonly take the form of prostatitis and prostatic abscess (*q. v.*). Suffice it to say that these abscesses are usually led backward by the triangular ligament to its rectal edge, and thus to the ischiorectal fossa, where they usually appear when they come to the surface. They may break into the rectum.

If a *peri-urethral abscess* originates in a submucous inflammation, or the inflammation of a gland cut off from the urethra by fibrosis, it will contain no urine. If extensive and severe, secondary opening into the urethra may occur. In this case, the severity of the *extravasation* depends on whether stricture is present below the point of origin. If so, the pressure of urine at the time of voiding, necessary to force it past the stricture, will now force it into the tissues. Urinary extravasations are guided and limited by the fasciæ as described above. When very extensive, extravasations from the penile or bulbous urethra, escaping between the upper portion of Colles' fascia and the pubis in the region of the suspensory ligament, may infiltrate the wall of the lower abdomen external to the muscles, up even as far as the axillæ. If the communication with the urethra is small, there may be only enough urine extravasated to make the inflammation more severe and rapid.

If there is no stricture, or if a stricture is present above the point of origin, very little urine will escape from the urethra. Even a small quantity, however, causes necrosis and, therefore, hastens abscess formation. Peri-urethral inflammations without urinary connection may be merely an induration, with edema, cellular infiltration, and in the later stages fibrosis. Abscess formation, however, is the rule. When such an abscess opens to the outside, spontaneously or by incision, it may heal without ever discharging urine, or the urethral wall may subsequently be penetrated by the inflammation, when a urinary fistula will ensue.

When connection with the urethra is present, the presence of urine makes the process more rapid, and suppuration usually occurs. If the connection is proximal to a stricture, the extravasation may be rapid and extensive and quickly pass beyond the bounds of the original inflammation. Wide-spread necrosis occurs, and the condition is a very serious one (see Wounds of the Urethra). When such an abscess is opened, a *urinary fistula* follows at once. In the penis, the tissues involved are thin, and the distance short, which make the fistula less apt to heal spontaneously. In the perineum, the more abundant connective and muscular tissue surrounding the longer fistula make healing the rule, if urethral obstructions are removed.

If the inflammation has become wide-spread before incision or rupture, these fistulæ may be numerous and complicated. Chronicity leads to fibrosis, so that their walls become thick, inelastic, and unyielding. In extreme cases, multiple sinuses and urinary fistulæ, surrounded by indurated masses of scar tissue, penetrate penis, scrotum, and perineum in every direction, exuding urine and pus. Such conditions are especially noted in the colored race, in which fibrous reaction to inflammation is more abundant than in the white race. Healing cannot be expected except after extensive removal of the tissues involved, and restoration of the urethral lumen.

Acute inflammations of the urethra due to organisms other than the gonococcus are rare except when infection is introduced instrumentally or at operation, but undoubtedly they do occur as a result of coitus with women having severe non-specific infections of the vagina and uterus. We have seen a case of acute anterior and posterior urethritis, with the Staphylococcus aureus in pure culture, and due to coitus with a wife who had a cancer of the uterus and a severe leukorrhea. Numerous cases of urethritis have been reported in which the gonococcus was never found and in which the colon bacillus or other organisms appeared in the discharge. Cases of urethritis due to descending infections of the urinary tract coming from foci in tonsils, teeth, and elsewhere are rare, but do occur. Urethral discharge is said sometimes to occur spontaneously in cases of multiple arthritis.

Chemical inflammation of the urethra may result from too strong injections or irrigations for prophylactic or thera-peutic purposes. While these are sterile at the beginning, secondary infection may ensue, or they may heal quickly without infection. When very strong chemicals are used by mistake, there may be exten-sive necrosis of the epithelium, with peri-urethritis, stricture formation, etc.

Definite statements about such cases are difficult to make. One can never depend upon histories of no exposure, and in some cases with definite exposure gonococci are never found in the dis-charge. We must, however, feel that non-gonorrheal infection is at least possi-ble, and draw no inferences not based on actual demonstration of the organism. This will usually be possible if careful study is made by smear and culture.

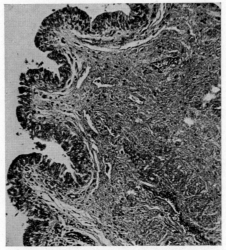

Fig. 84.—Section from the urethra of a case which came to autopsy after having had a retention catheter in the urethra for more than two weeks. Note the remarkably slight degree of inflammation which is present. B. U. I. Path. 4891.

The urethra is remarkably resistant to descending infections, but may be involved in the posterior portion in some cases of chronic renal bacteriuria. Local-ized infection may follow instrumental injury. Urethral calculi are usually asso-ciated with infection.

The most frequent cause of non-gonorrheal urethritis is *catheterization*. It frequently follows repeated catheterization, and always accompanies a retained catheter. Figure 84 shows, however, how little reaction may be produced by a catheter á démeure. Here traumatism is important in the origin and maintenance of the lesion.

Secondary infection of gonorrheal infections is more apt to occur the longer they persist, although rare in the early stages. The peristence of gonococci in the lower urinary tract is a matter of some dispute. It is claimed by some[1] that they are extremely resistant, and may be discovered in almost any case of chronic

[1] Nogues and Durupt: Journal d'Urologie, 1923, xv, 133–136; Janet, ibid., 205; Player, Lee-Brown, and Mathé: Journal of Urology, 1923, x, 377–385; Young, Geraghty, and Stevens: Johns Hopkins Hospital Reports, 1906, xiii, 271–384.

urethritis or seminal vesiculitis if cultures are made by the proper technic. Others claim that the gonococcus regularly dies out in a year or so, if there be no reinfection, that the chronic changes in urethra and prostate are caused by secondary invaders, and that the organisms recovered in late states are Micrococcus catarrhalis or other pseudogonococci. This point should receive further study. At all events, much of the damage in chronic urethritis and its complications must be laid to the secondary invaders.

Catheter urethritis may give rise to prostatitis, peri-urethral inflammation and abscess just as does gonorrhea. Epididymitis is as common as in gonorrhea, and is more apt to go on to suppuration. Stricture is apparently uncommon, unless trauma, mechanical or chemical, be present. In general, complications are less frequent, and complete healing more likely to occur. The explanation is, doubtless, that the gonococcus, in its initial attack, finds no immunity to combat, and, therefore, becomes more deeply intrenched behind areas of fibrosis and in-

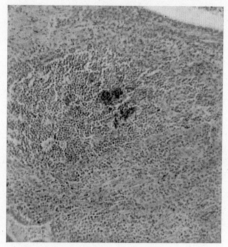 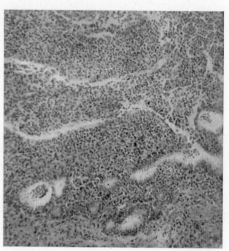

FIG. 85.—Acute prostatis showing polymorphonuclear infiltration of stroma and beginning abscess formation. B. U. I. Path. 4136.

FIG. 86.—Another area in the same prostate showing a more chronic change; round-cell infiltration of stroma, polymorphonuclear exudate in acini. B. U. I. Path. 4136.

filtration resulting from the primary damage. Colon bacilli, staphylococci, etc., meet a pre-existent immunity which restricts their activity from the beginning.

Prostate.—*Prostatitis* occurs as a complication of gonorrheal or other urethritis, and on occasion secondarily to upper tract infections with infected urine. Some have claimed that bacteria may be rubbed through from the rectum by too vigorous massage, but this is not proved. The only cases of undoubted hematogenous prostatitis are those found in conditions of general pyemia.

Prostatitis, with colon bacillus or other organisms in the secretion, does occasionally occur without demonstrable infection anywhere else in the urinary tract. Whether such cases represent hematogenous infections is usually impossible to say.

Acute prostatitis is much less often seen or recognized than the chronic form and usually results from an active process in the prostatic urethra. The prostate shows edema, congestion, and great infiltration of the interstitial tissue with polymorphonuclear leukocytes (Fig. 85). The swelling is often sufficient to compress the urethra and make voiding difficult or impossible. The process may subside, giving place to ordinary chronic changes, or not infrequently suppuration may occur, causing *abscess of the prostate*. The abscess may involve only a single group of tubules, or a large part of the prostate (Figs. 85, 87). One sometimes sees the urethra suspended across the cavity of an abscess which has completely surrounded it. The inflammatory reaction blocks the tubules, cutting off communication with the urethra—otherwise abscess would probably not occur. The abscess then must rupture anew into the urethra if the pus is to escape that way; and frequently does so. If in the median portion of the prostate, rupture may occur through the trigonal region into the bladder. Denonvilliers' fascia offers a strong

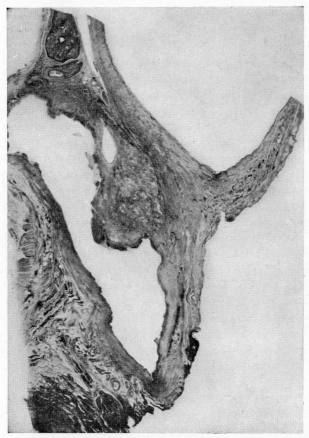

Fig. 87.—Low-power magnification of a sagittal section, taken slightly to one side of the midline, and showing the bladder, prostate, and seminal vesicle. The large open space in the prostatic region is an abscess cavity. The abscess was a sequel of impermeable stricture of the urethra. From Dr. Henry Wade.

barrier posteriorly, and retains the abscess within the prostate for a long time. Occasionally, however, it is penetrated, and then the process spreads to the periprostatic tissues; *periprostatic abscess*. Below it is contained by the triangular ligament, but posteriorly it presses toward the rectum. The recto-urethralis muscle and central tendon constitute a firm barrier in the midline, and, therefore, the pus usually goes to the side, down past the posterior margin of the triangular ligament, and into the ischiorectal fossa, where it appears in one, or sometimes almost simultaneously in both. Rupture may then occur to the surface in the ischiorectal fossa, or into the rectum. Rarely the prostatic abscess ruptures directly into the rectum. A prostatic abscess usually does not burrow toward the prevesical space, unless there is a false passage.

If a prostatic abscess is opened by an extra-urethral route, urinary fistula does not always occur, probably because the abscess has originated in the prostate at some distance from the urethra. Healing usually occurs in a very effective way, without stricture, fistula, or recurrence. Being a complication of acute urethritis, prostatic abscess is not often seen in the presence of stricture, so that urinary extravasation is a rarity.

The pathology is practically the same in gonorrheal and non-gonorrheal cases. The colon bacillus is usually present, and makes itself known by its characteristic odor, while if the gonococcus is in pure culture, the pus is odorless and often of a dark brown color.

Chronic prostatitis is an exceedingly common condition, indeed, it is almost as common as gonorrheal urethritis.

It is probable that posterior urethritis can never occur without at least some involvement of the prostate. In gonorrhea, this is oftenest not in the form of acute generalized prostatitis, but localized in the portions surrounding the urethra. Chronic infection of the prostate, usually slight, may occur as a result of catheterization and other instrumentation. This explains the chronic infection usually found in hypertrophied prostates. Infection may spread directly to the prostate, or through the prostatic urethra, from cystitis, either generalized, or localized in the form of trigonitis. Infection may be introduced by false passages made through the prostate by instruments. Descending infections from the seminal vesicles occur in tuberculosis, and perhaps in other cases where the vesicles are infected from the blood. This sequence has not been proved except in tuberculosis. Direct hemogenic infection of the prostate is possible, but has not been proved definitely. It has been postulated in cases where prostatitis is found, without history of antecedent urinary infection, in cases with metastatic infection elsewhere, as in the joints, from teeth, tonsils, or other foci.

The *bacteriology* of the prostate has scarcely received the attention it deserves. It is not uncommon to find no organisms in the stained smears of purulent prostatic secretion, and the statement has been made that "sterile inflammations" are not uncommon. It is our experience that organisms can be cultured from most, if not all, of these cases, indicating that they escape observation in the smear by reason of their small numbers.

The results of cultures in 100 cases studied by J. H. Hill at the Brady Institute are given in the following table:

TABLE 12

SUMMARY OF DIRECT SMEARS AND CULTURES OF PROSTATIC SECRETION AND URINE OF 100 CASES

Number and percentage.

Group 1.—No organisms in smears from prostatic secretion or urine; cultures from both sterile...... 30

Group 2.—No organisms in smears from prostatic secretion or urine, but cultures from one or both positive...... 30

Group 3.—Organisms found in smears from prostatic secretion or urine, or both, and cultures positive...... 40

100

Subdivision of Group 2:

	Number.	Group percentage.	Total percentage.
(1) Cases showing growth in both prostatic secretion and urine:			
(a) Staph. albus..	15	50	15
(6 of these scant or only after forty-eight hours incubation.)			
(b) Colon group bacilli.................................	3	10	3
(c) Staph. aureus..	1	3.3	1
(d) Streptococcus..	1	3.3	1
(e) Undifferentiated micrococcus.......................	1	3.3	1
Totals......................	21	70	21
(2) Cases showing growth in urine, but none in prostatic secretion:			
(a) Staph. albus..	7	23.3	7
(5 of these showed growth only after forty-eight hours.)			
(b) Gram-positive spore-forming bacillus, only after forty-eight hours..	1	3.3	1
	8	26.6	8
(3) Cases showing growth in prostatic secretion but not in urine, 6 colonies of Staph. albus..............................	1	3.3	1
Group 2 totals.................	30	100	30

Note on Group 2.—In this group fall the organisms which do not appear in large enough numbers to be seen in the direct smears, that is, light infections or contaminations. It is of interest to note the large percentage of Staph. albus cultures, 76.6 per cent. of the group, and the fact that of these 23 Staph. albus cultures, 12 appeared only after forty-eight hours or were scant.

Subdivision of Group 3:

	Number.	Group percentage.	Total percentage.
(1) Direct smear and culture of urine positive but prostatic secretion negative:			
Staph. albus..	3	7.5	3
(2) Direct smears and cultures of both prostatic secretion and urine positive:			
(a) Colon group bacilli................................	9	22.5	9
(b) Staph. albus......................................	9	22.5	9
(c) Streptococcus.....................................	3	7.5	3
(d) Gonococcus..	1	2.5	1
(e) Staph. aureus.....................................	1	2.5	1
(f) Ps. pyocyanea.....................................	1	2.5	1
(g) Undifferentiated Gram-positive coccus..............	1	2.5	1
(3) Direct smears of urine only positive, but cultures from both urine and prostatic secretion positive:			
(a) Colon group bacilli................................	5	12.5	5
(b) Staph. albus......................................	3	7.5	3
(c) B. mucosus capsulatus.............................	1	2.5	1
(d) Staph. albus and Streptococcus....................	1	2.5	1
(4) Prostatic secretion showing no organisms in smear, but 1 colony of Staph. albus in seventy-two hours; urine showing Gram-negative bacillus in smear and colon group bacillus in culture.	1	2.5	1
(5) Prostatic secretion showing Gram-negative bacillus in smear; urine showing Gram-negative bacillus, Gram-positive coccus in smear; cultures from both prostatic secretion and urine showing colon group bacillus, Staph. aureus, and Staph. albus........	1	2.5	1
Group 3 totals.................	40	100	40

Note on Group 3.—In no case was there growth in the prostatic secretion with the urine sterile. On the other hand, in 11 cases there was growth in the prostatic secretion of organisms observed in direct smear in the urine only. In only 1 case was a different organism obtained from the prostatic secretion than from the urine and the nature of this growth would indicate a probable contamination.

Several significant facts appear from this table. Organisms were seen in the smears in only 40 per cent., while the cultures were positive in 70 per cent. It frequently happens that the prostatic secretion is sterile in cases with infected urine, but in only 1 case with sterile urine has growth been obtained from the prostate. In this case there were only six colonies of Staphylococcus albus, which may easily have been a contamination.

In addition, there was only 1 case which showed in the prostatic secretion any organism different from those found in the urine—a single colony of Staphylococcus albus, probably a contamination. We may conclude, then, that an infected urine does not necessarily infect the prostate, but that with an infected prostate, the urine is always infected, and with the same organisms.

Staphylococcus albus and colon group bacilli were the most frequent invaders, with Staphylococcus albus slightly in the lead. Streptococcus was present in but 5 cases, pyocyaneus in 1, and gonococcus in 1. This corresponds with the results obtained by Young, Geraghty and Stevens, Mathé, Player, and Lee-Brown, and other observers. We cannot agree with those who find gonococcus present in a large proportion of these cases; or with those who believe that a prostatitis can occur without organisms.

When infection occurs from the urethra, as is the rule, it enters the prostate by way of the ducts. At the time material is usually available for *microscopic* study, one sees the ducts surrounded by zones of round-cell infiltration, continuous with that in the submucosa of the urethra (Fig. 86). This in some cases is only near the openings into the urethra, but later may spread along the ducts to the remote portions of the prostate. At first the glandular portions are unaffected, but late in the process become involved, and are also surrounded by halos of infiltration. Desquamation of the epithelium may be increased. In the acinar spaces one sees numbers of desquamated cells undergoing fatty degeneration, and often mixed with them a certain number of polymorphonuclear leukocytes, although the infiltration in the stroma may be entirely mononuclear. As the process becomes older, areas of plasma-cell infiltration occur, and eosinophil leukocytes become numerous—a characteristic finding. Fibrous tissue is laid down, and by its shrinkage causes marked distortion of the entire architecture. Certain groups of glands appear to be compressed in the fibrotic mass; they are reduced in size or flattened out, irregularly placed, with the epithelial cells small, deep staining, and having pyknotic nuclei. In other groups, dilatation of acini, and the presence of increased quantities of desquamated cells indicate that the scarring has caused duct obstruction. The ducts may be compressed and irregular. Their epithelium may undergo a progressive change, so that it becomes many layers thick, and presents bizarre pictures which may be mistaken for carcinoma by the uninitiated. Rarely, the acinar epithelium also becomes thickened, sometimes taking on an almost squamous appearance. Young, Geraghty, and Stevens[1] describe a few cases studied microscopically in which there was slight chronic prostatitis with normal prostatic urethra.

The irregular induration and shrinkage are manifested externally by increased consistence of the gland, and loss of the normal smoothness and regularity. The fibrosis, however, is seldom as dense as in tuberculosis, nor is the nodularity so marked; indeed, in some cases, good-sized areas may show a smooth induration of

[1] Johns Hopkins Hospital Reports, 1906, xiii, 271–384.

moderate degree. As in the kidney, inflammation of the prostate causes changes in the surrounding tissue, and bands of fibrous tissue make their appearance, most marked, on rectal examination, at the upper and outer angles of the gland, and in the lateral sulci between the prostate and the inferior pubic rami. On dissection, one finds that they also involve the posterior surface, and may bind the rectum to the prostate, obliterating the "éspace décollable rétroprostatique" of Proust. Where the inflammation is slight, and central, the surface of the prostate may feel normal.

Contracture occurs when fibrosis is present throughout the entire gland, and its total size may be markedly diminished. At the same time, its contraction compresses the prostatic urethra, and causes urinary obstruction which produces the same symptoms and changes in the urinary tract, as benign prostatic hypertrophy, or other infravesical obstructions of moderately slow development. (See Obstructive Uropathy.) The average age for this condition is some years less

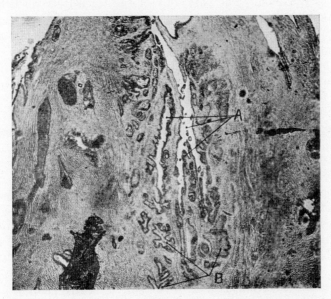

Fig. 88.—Photomicrograph showing the structure of the utricle, indicated by *A*, longitudinal section, and by *B*, cross-section. After Rytina.

than that for benign hypertrophy. Where found at operation, it is spoken of as "small, fibrous prostate," but may well be considered as a form of urethral stricture. The obstruction, however, is usually at the vesical orifice. Here chronic prostatitis and urethritis combine with general or local inflammations of the bladder to produce fibrous *"contracture of the vesical orifice"* (Fig. 77). (See Chronic Cystitis.)

The formation of *calculi* in the prostate is usually associated with chronic prostatitis. (See Urinary Lithiasis.)

The *verumontanum* and its associated structures are involved in posterior urethritis. The mucous membrane covering the surface partakes of whatever changes occur in the urethra. The prostatic *utricle* is also very apt to become inflamed. Being the remnant of the fused Müllerian ducts of the embryo, it varies considerably in length and complexity. The ordinary limits, for length, are from 5 mm. to 2 cm., but rarely, a duct several inches long may persist, even reaching to the vicinity of the epididymis. The structure of the normal utricle is that of a central lumen (Fig. 88), surrounded on all sides by a complicated system of short, racemose tubules, lined by epithelium morphologically similar to that of a prostate. The general architecture is reminiscent of that of the seminal vesicle.[1] In these convoluted passageways infection lodges and becomes chronic in the same manner as in the prostate. The utricle, therefore, may become a nidus of infection serving to keep up a chronic posterior urethritis.[2]

The *ejaculatory ducts* become infected from the urethra in the same manner as the prostatic ducts. Young, Geraghty, and Stevens show that they may remain uninfected in the presence of chronic posterior urethritis. Their length and smooth surface, however, usually prevent a rapid spread upwards. Acute infections doubtless occur, but have no special symptom picture. In chronic infections, fibrosis about the duct occurs as elsewhere, and may lead to definite *stricture* formation, or occlusion. The pathology of the ejaculatory ducts has not been thoroughly studied, but it appears that complete occlusion does not usually occur except from destructive lesions beginning outside the ducts. On the other hand, fibrotic changes in the posterior lobe of the prostate may stiffen the walls of the duct, and possibly by scar-tissue contraction enlarge its lumen, so that, in rare cases, urinary reflux through the duct may occur, the urine appearing in perineal or inguinal fistulæ leading to the seminal vesicle or vas deferens.

The verumontanum itself is supplied with many blood-vessels, lymphatics, and nerve endings. During sexual excitement it becomes greatly congested, and this condition may become practically permanent in certain cases of sexual neurosis, especially those associated with premature ejaculation. It is doubtful whether this is the cause or the result of the sexual abnormality. In other cases, sometimes associated with impotence, the veru is small, smooth, and pale. As a result of inflammation or long-continued treatment with caustics, the veru may be converted into a mass of scar tissue, which scarcely rises above the level of the urethral surface. There may be stricture of the ejaculatory ducts at their mouths. No constant relation between this condition and sexual symptoms has been definitely established.

Occasionally the verumontanum is the seat of severe pain. Examination of excised specimens discloses no special lesion to account for it, and the excision itself often fails to relieve the pain. In so far as this condition is not purely psychogenic, it must be accounted a true neuralgia.

Seminal Vesicle.—The pathology of infections of the seminal vesicles has not received the thorough attention it deserves. Most text-books ignore the subject, or speak of it in very general terms. Dillon and Blaisdell[3] have recently supplied the only systematic study which exists, and it is to be hoped that more such work will soon place our knowledge on a sound basis.

Infection of the seminal vesicles from the blood-stream is possible, but it usually occurs secondarily, from the urethra or epididymis. Other paths of infection are by direct extension from the prostate, bladder, ureter, or rarely, the peritoneum. Lymphatics, no doubt, play a rôle in this process. Infection from

[1] Rytina: Journal of Urology, 1917, i, 231–261.
[2] Geraghty: Journal of the American Medical Association, 1911, lvi, 731–732.
[3] Journal of Urology, 1923, x, 353–366.

the rectum has been suggested, but not proved. Oppenheim and Löw[1] believe that infectious material may be carried upward in the vas deferens to the vesicle or epididymis by reverse peristalsis and have actually observed this phenomenon in rabbits after stimulating the hypogastric nerves or region of the verumontanum. Extension along the mucosa of the ejaculatory duct or its accompanying lymphatics also occurs.

From the epididymis, the process may spread along the vas to the vesicle in the same manner. There is also good reason to believe that infectious material may pass down the lumen of the vas to the vesicle, eventually setting up inflammation there, where it stagnates, even though the vas is not involved. Simmonds[2] found pus containing tubercle bacilli in essentially normal vesicles when there was tuberculosis of the epididymis. Boyd[3] has found vesicles, not indurated, but distended with pus, in cases of acute epididymitis.

The common form of *seminal vesiculitis* depends on infection of the posterior urethra, and, therefore, accompanies and follows this disease. The frequence of its occurrence as a complication of posterior urethritis is still uncertain, since the means of diagnosis are not exact, and investigation of the vesicles is often deferred until late stages. The figures given by various workers are divergent: Petersen,[4] 4 per cent. of all cases of gonorrhea; Chute and O'Neil,[5] 11.1 per cent. of 540 cases of "various sorts of genito-urinary disease"; Mayer,[6] 45 per cent. of all cases of gonorrhea, 60 per cent. of all cases of posterior gonorrheal urethritis. Lewin and Böhm[7] studied 1000 cases of gonorrhea; 371 had anterior urethritis, in 629 the posterior urethra was involved. Of the 629 posterior cases, there were 218 cases (35 per cent.) of seminal vesiculitis (right 32, left 47, bilateral 139). In 38 cases, the vesicles were involved alone (6 per cent.) and in 180, seminal vesicles and prostate together (29 per cent.). The prostate alone showed changes in 385 (61 per cent.) while in only 16 of the 629 cases was the rectal examination negative. Of the cases of seminal vesiculitis, 76 had epididymitis, distributed as shown in the following schema:

TABLE 13

		Seminal Vesiculitis.			
		Right.	Left.	Bilateral.	No note.
Epididymitis.........	Right......	14	1	18	
	Left........	3	8	19	
	Bilateral....	0	0	19	
	No note....	..	..	..	4

142 of the 218 vesiculitis cases had no epididymitis.

It will be seen that as attention has turned toward the seminal vesicles, more and more involvements have been found. There is no doubt that this is a frequent and important disease.

[1] Virchow's Archiv, 1905, clxxxii, 39–64.

[2] Aschoff's Pathologische Anatomie, 1909, ii, 549, et seq.

[3] Journal of Urology, 1923, x, 387–392.   [4] Quoted by Lewin and Böhm (see note [7]).

[5] Boston Medical and Surgical Journal, 1901, cxliv, 577–580.

[6] Zentralblatt für die Krankheiten der Harn und Geschlechtsorgane, 1903, xiv, 5–12.

[7] Zeitschrift für Urologie, 1909, iii, 43–64.

The lumen of the normal seminal vesicles is convoluted, and almost filled with a multitude of thin trabeculæ or villi which project into the lumen and anastomose with one another (Figs. 89, 90). This produces a sponge-like structure of almost inconceivable complexity. Surrounding it is a wall of smooth muscle of moderate thickness. This muscle contracts on stimulation of the hypogastric nerve. When ejaculation occurs, it forces the vesicular contents out through the ejaculatory duct. The convolutions of the main lumen vary in different individuals; in a very few the tube is simple and straight, in others in addition to convolutions of the main lumen, there are many small subsidiary side-lumina. It is supposed that the vesicular epithelium has a secretion and examination of the expressed contents shows that it is a thick tenacious mucus. Experiments have failed to show that it has any activating influence on the spermatozoa.[1] The structure of the ampulla is exactly the same as that of the vesicle, and from a

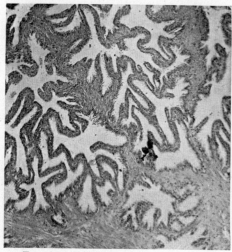 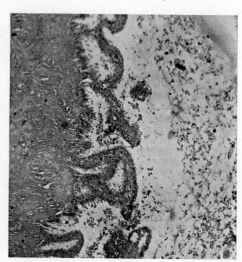

Fig. 89.—Normal seminal vesicle, empty. Showing thin, complicated trabeculæ. B. U. I. Path. 4963.

Fig. 90.—Normal seminal vesicle, dilated. Section from another portion of the same specimen. The lumen is dilated with secretion and the apparent complexity of the trabeculæ surrounding it is very much reduced. B. U. I. Path. 4963.

pathologic point of view, it should be considered part of the same organ. Infections involving the one usually involve the other.

Unfortunately, we have no thorough pathologic study of the effects of infection on the ejaculatory duct, and our conclusions must be drawn from clinical observations. We know that strictures of these ducts occur, for they can be demonstrated on probing. We also know that temporary complete obstruction, probably the result of edema, can occur, since it may be impossible to empty a vesicle manually on one occasion, while a few days later the contents can be expressed without difficulty. The vesicle, like other hollow organs, shows the effects of obstruction. Kaufmann[2] states that cystic dilatation follows partial obstruction of the ejaculatory duct, while atrophy results from complete atresia. These statements must be accepted with the same reservations as similar ones made

[1] George Walker: Johns Hopkins Hospital Reports, 1911, xvi, 223–255.

[2] Lehrbuch der Speziellen Pathologischen Anatomie, 8th ed., Berlin and Leipzig, 1922, 1186–1188.

for the kidney, which have been shown to be inaccurate. Animal experiments and observations on eunuchs show that the seminal vesicles and ampullæ atrophy after castration.

Acute seminal vesiculitis, according to Simmonds,[1] may show edema and congestion of the mucosa, without involvement of the deeper structures. The contents is thin, losing its mucoid character, but containing blood, polymorphonuclear leukocytes, and flakes of pus. With severe inflammations desquamation of the epithelium may occur—in short, the typical picture of acute catarrhal inflammation of any mucous surface.

Simmonds also states that the vesicular contents may be purulent in acute inflammations of the epididymis, without obvious involvement of the vesicle itself, the pus having come down the vas.

In *chronic infections*, the infecting agents penetrate beneath the epithelium, and round-cell infiltration and fibrosis ensue in the submucosa and muscularis. As a result, the trabeculæ are thickened (Fig. 91), and herein lies the characteristic feature of chronic vesiculitis (Dillon and Blaisdell[2]). Free outflow from the labyrinthine spaces in interfered with by this swelling, and later this is further hindered by actual coalescence of the thickened tips of the trabeculæ. In this manner enclosed spaces containing infectious material are created, the number of which may be very great. The process advances more rapidly nearest the lumen, where the tips of the trabeculæ become great club-shaped masses of fibrous tissue, which eventually coalesce and even occlude the entire lumen. At the periphery,

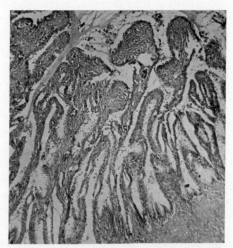

Fig. 91.—Section from seminal vesicle showing early inflammatory change. The tips of the lumen are moderately thickened and club shaped with slight round-cell infiltration. This is the first pathologic indication of inflammatory changes in the vesicle proper. B. U. I. Path. 4963.

a halo of epithelium-lined spaces may persist for a long time. Coincident with these changes, the muscular wall is usually involved, and becomes greatly thickened by infiltration and fibrosis.

The above-described changes may involve only a portion of the vesicle-ampulla, neighboring areas remaining practically normal, or may include the entire organ. Drainage through the ejaculatory duct is impossible, owing to the wide spread occlusion, and to this obstruction is later added loss of contractility of the muscular coat, from infiltration and fibrosis. In the late stages, the architecture of the vesicle cannot be made out, and the swollen organ is beset with innumerable foci of infection resulting from the isolated labyrinthine spaces. Eventually the epithelium lining these spaces may be destroyed by the infection, when the entire organ becomes a mass of inflammatory tissue.

Associated with the various stages of this process may be the results of obstruction, in the form of dilated, cystic spaces, lined by thinned-out epithelium. These cysts may become converted into abscesses.

[1] Aschoff: Pathologische Anatomie, 1909, ii, 549 et seq.   [2] Journal of Urology, 1923, x, 353–365.

In some cases the muscular wall is involved early, and the changes in it are more pronounced than in the epithelial structures. In these cases, the architecture of the vesicle, while persisting, is much distorted, and compression atrophy may occur.

Extension to the perivesicular tissues is common. It is probable that lymphatic channels play a part in this distribution. The inflammation is usually contained posteriorly by Denonvilliers' fascia (retroprostatic fascia). The fat and fibrous tissue become edematous and infiltrated with polymorphonuclear or round-cells. This may occur on the bladder side, and Fuller[1] describes cases in which the edema and congestion involve the bladder wall sufficiently so that the outline of the vesicles can be traced on the base of the bladder by means of the cystoscope.

Abscesses may develop in the vesicle or ampulla, or in the perivesicular tissues. Drainage through the ejaculatory duct is usually impossible, on account of the above described occlusions. Vesicular abscesses may extend into the perivesicular tissues. Denonvilliers' fascia directs perivesicular abscesses upward and backward toward the tip of the vesicles, where they may involve the ureter, or, coming in contact with the peritoneum of the rectovesical pouch, may cause pelvic or general peritonitis. Rarely, the intestine may be involved and perforated, giving rise to fistulæ to the bladder or rectum. If Denonvilliers' fascia is penetrated, the abscess may present in the ischiorectal fossa, or perforate into the rectum, or it may travel upward behind the peritoneum. Abscesses located on the vesical aspect of the vesicles may rupture into the bladder. Occasionally severe destructive lesions may give rise to rectovesical or other intestinovesical fistula.

Normally, the *ejaculatory duct*, probably by muscular contraction, always prevents reflux of urine through it, but if its walls are stiffened by inflammatory infiltration, or its lumen widened by cicatricial contraction, such reflux may occur. Where the urine is infected, it may help to maintain the vesicular infection. In a few of our cases vesiculectomy has been followed by perineal fistula which discharged only minute quantities of urine at the time of each voiding. In another case (B. U. I. 10,104), after simple epididymectomy, the reflux extended up the vas and urine escaped through a fistula in the groin. In the latter case the urine certainly came through the ejaculatory duct from the urethra. In the former the urine probably escaped through the divided ducts and not through a urethral fistula.

The pathology of vesicular infections is such that we can easily conceive of them serving as *foci of infection* giving rise to general manifestations such as chronic arthritis, endocarditis, etc. More careful study, however, including consideration of the general symptoms in specific cases, is necessary to enable us to know which types of vesicular lesions may be responsible for these generalized infections, and to plan the treatment intelligently.

Marchildon[2] describes 2 cases of typhoid fever, in one of which the seminal vesicles were the seat of an abscess containing typhoid bacilli. In the other case, there were many small abscesses in the prostate, also containing the specific organism. Such conditions may well account for typhoid bacilluria following the disease in some cases where no renal lesion can be demonstrated.

Vas Deferens.—In infections of the seminal vesicle, or epididymis, or both,

---

[1] Annals of Surgery, 1905, xli, 902–913; Medical Record, 1909, lxxvi, 717–724.

[2] American Journal of the Medical Sciences, 1910, cxl, 74–80.

the vas deferens may be involved, or may remain unaffected. We suppose that in the first case, the infection has extended along the mucosa or lymphatics of the vas, and in the second, infectious material may have been carried through the vas, without causing infection of its walls. If the vas is involved, the ordinary acute changes occur, and later fibrosis of its walls ensues, causing thickening and occasionally occlusion. In some cases the mucosal changes are in the foreground, while in others those of the wall are more pronounced, suggesting lymphatic involvement. Kaufmann states that a moderate degree of cystic dilatation may occur above an atresia. Extension to the surrounding tissues is rare. Not infrequently an epididymal infection will extend a short distance along the vas. Urinary reflux through the vas is unusual, but may occur as described above. The careful study of Brams[1] shows that injection of irritant substances, such as collargol, into the vas may lead to atresia.

Epididymis.—The epididymis, being so much more accessible than the seminal vesicle, has received more careful study. Since it is sometimes infected very quickly after instrumentation, it has been thought that antiperistalsis might carry infectious materials upward to the epididymis. Absolutely conclusive experimental proof for this sequence has not been secured; we can only say that it seems quite reasonable. Epididymitis may occur by infection from the blood-stream. It is sometimes seen in typhoid, tonsillitis, septicemia, etc., or may come on suddenly in patients, apparently healthy, but in whom, presumably, there is some hidden focus of infection. In the great majority of cases, however, epididymitis is secondary to infection of the posterior urethra, and the infection is supposed to travel through the lymphatics of the vas, by contiguity along its mucosa, or by reverse peristalsis.

The subject of the mode of infection of the epididymis is discussed further in the section on Urogenital Tuberculosis, Chapter IV.

Epididymitis sometimes follows a blow or other injury to the scrotum, and may present all the signs and symptoms of serious acute infection, without the presence of urethritis or prostato-vesiculitis. Whether these cases represent hematogenous infection or arise from very latent infections of the lower tract is impossible to say.

Epididymitis is frequent in gonorrhea, and also occurs in any kind of infection of the posterior urethra. Lewin and Böhm[2] found epididymitis in 12.4 per cent. of 1000 cases of gonorrhea. Simultaneous bilateral involvement occurs in 10 per cent. or less of the cases, but secondary invasion of the opposite side is more frequent. Practically every organism found in the urogenital tract has been isolated from inflamed epididymes. As Kretschmer and Alexander[3] point out, the pathologic picture is identical in all types of infection, excepting the chronic granulomata (tuberculosis, syphilis, mycoses, etc.), and there is nothing characteristic about gonorrheal epididymitis except the presence of the gonococcus (which is usually in pure culture).

The epididymis is divided into the head, or *globus major*, the *body*, and the tail, or *globus minor*. The vas deferens enters the globus minor. The organ is composed of a single highly convoluted tube.

That the infection comes along the vas, either by the lumen or by the lymphatics, is indicated by the fact that the initial lesion is commonly in the globus minor. The onset of epididymitis is usually acute, regardless of the organism

[1] Journal of Urology, 1923, x, 383–404. [2] Zeitschrift für Urologie, 1909, iii, 43–64.
[3] Journal of Urology, 1923, x, 335–352.

concerned (again excepting the granulomata), but may involve only a part, or the whole of the organ.[1] In the *acute* state, the epididymis is swollen, red, and tender. The surrounding tissues are involved in varying degree, being the seat of edema and congestion. If the subcutaneous layer is involved, the skin loses its normal mobility, and is red and tense. Since the visceral layer of the tunica vaginalis covers the epididymis, it is usually involved here, and may be covered with a fibrinous exudate. In other cases the entire cavity of the tunica vaginalis is affected, with fibrinous exudate and a moderate degree of hydrocele (*acute inflammatory hydrocele*). In 33 cases of acute gonorrheal epididymitis seen at operation, Hagner[2] found an acute inflammatory hydrocele in 31, and a plastic fibrinous exudate of the cavity of the tunica vaginalis in the other 2. The fluid is turbid, and contains flakes of pus and usually red blood-cells. The serous lining of the cavity is reddened and its surface dulled and roughened.

The process may spread quickly through the epididymis, or more seldom, remains confined to one portion.

Microscopically, one sees edema and polymorphonuclear infiltration of the stroma. Often the leukocytes appear in thick masses, which may be in the stroma or in the walls of the tubules. The submucosa is involved in the changes and the ciliated epithelium often desquamates, so that it may be impossible to tell whether an inflammatory focus or small abscess has originated within the tubule, or in its wall. Where the epithelium is preserved, the lumen is often enlarged, and filled with a polymorphonuclear exudate. Spermatozoa are usually absent from the areas of most marked inflammation.

When such an area is incised, purulent fluid will exude even if there is no frank abscess.

The outcome of the process is by resolution, with restitution practically to normal, by suppuration, or by the assumption of chronicity. The exudate may be reabsorbed, and the continuity of the duct preserved. Benzla reports that one-half of a group of patients who had bilateral gonorrheal epididymitis subsequently begot children.

Suppuration is common. Multiple small abscesses are seen, or coalescence takes place into a larger abscess which gives typical fluctuation. Such an abscess may perforate through the skin in an adherent area, or may first spread to the scrotal tissues. It is rare for an abscess to involve the cavity of the tunica vaginalis, as the layers usually adhere together in the neighborhood of the abscess. If one part of the epididymis suppurates, the remainder, while involved, will be the seat only of edema and congestion. Like changes may occur in the lower end of the vas, and in the tissues of the spermatic cord.

If suppuration occurs, the damage is practically always sufficient to destroy the duct at one or more points, and the process of repair completes the occlusion. Spermatozoa are therefore no longer able to leave the testis. The infection itself usually clears up after evacuation of an abscess.

The process may become *chronic* without suppuration, or, more rarely, will continue in chronic form even after evacuation of an abscess, particularly if the evacuation is incomplete. The edema and congestion diminish, the infiltration

[1] Cunningham and Cook: Journal of Urology, 1922, vii, 139–152. Kretschmer and Alexander: Journal of Urology, 1923, x, 335–352.

[2] Medical Record, 1909, lxxvi, 944–946.

becomes round-cell in character, and fibrosis begins.   Plasma-cells and eosinophils may be present, sometimes in large numbers.   The duct may be obliterated at points where its epithelium has been destroyed, or may be compressed and distorted in masses of fibrous tissue.   The fibromuscular walls of the duct become much thickened.   The stroma becomes markedly thickened, and in the gross the organ is irregular or even nodular.   Lymphoid follicles become hyperplastic. The epithelium occasionally shows an extraordinary overgrowth, becoming 5 to 25 cells thick, and almost or quite filling the lumen.   The blood-vessels are often increased in number, and show intimal hyperplasia.

The surrounding tissue is involved, and bands of fibrous tissue may run between the epididymis and the scrotal tissues and adjacent skin.   The serosa of the tunica vaginalis becomes adherent, usually in the measure in which the fibrinous inflammation has occurred in the acute stage.   In some cases the parietal layer is bound to the epididymis, in others the epididymis is bound to the testis, the digital fossa being obliterated in whole or part.   Occasionally the entire cavity is obliterated by adhesions, though sometimes small serous-lined cavities or cysts may be left in the meshes of the dense adhesions which bind testis and epididymis to the scrotal tissues.

Chronic *sinuses* may occur, especially after improperly drained abscesses, but are very rare, and may usually be considered pathognomonic of tuberculosis.

In chronic cases the hyperemia may eventually lead to a great increase in number of the small arteries and veins in the tissues about the epididymis and cord.   These vessels persist after the capillary engorgement has disappeared, and are important on account of the hemorrhage which may occur from them at operation.   They are larger than capillaries, and being the results of inflammation, are often thick walled, and do not collapse.   For this reason bleeding may be persistent, and unless enormous numbers of hemostatic ties are made, postoperative hematoma is to be feared.   There is never any difficulty about recognizing these cases.

Epididymitis may occur in *cryptorchid testicles*, and sometimes gives rise to cellulitis or abscesses in the surrounding tissues.   In abdominal testes or in cases where the tunica vaginalis retains its open communication with the peritoneal cavity (congenital or sliding hernia) epididymitis may give rise to local or general peritonitis.   The statement is made that an abnormal position of the testicle increases the liability to epididymitis.

The chronic process may continue for months or years, or may cease after a shorter time.   Although often persistent, infection does not seem quite as tenacious here as in the prostate or seminal vesicles.   After it has ceased, the depositions of fibrous tissue are slowly absorbed, but some induration and distortion may be permanent, and apparently if the duct is once occluded, its function is never restored spontaneously.

The effect of *occlusion of the duct*, or of the vas deferens, on the testis has been much studied.   Gross changes in the testis do not usually occur.   Tournade,[1] working with rats, found a constant atrophy of the spermatogenic apparatus, the interstitial cells being unaffected.   In man this may occur, as indicated by absence of spermatozoa from fluid squeezed out of the testis, but usually the testis seems substantially unaffected, and spermatozoa have been found in it as much as

[1] Thèse de Lyon, 1903.

nine years (Simmonds) and fifteen years (Chevassu) after occlusion of the duct. When portions of the efferent apparatus are congenitally absent, the testis may appear normal. Dimitresso found spermatozoa in an epididymis, in a case of congenital absence of the vas deferens. If the occlusion of the vas occurs before puberty, the picture is usually different. It is the rule for the tubular epithelium to atrophy, and the testicle becomes smaller. The interstitial cells too may be sometimes but not always included in the degenerative process.

Careful studies of the epididymis by Regaud and Tournade[1] and Cruveilhier and Savariaud[2] show that the tubules proximal to the obstruction may be somewhat dilated, and are filled with thick masses of spermatozoa, often arranged radially about a central point (Figs. 92–94). These masses sometimes become so compact that they may be turned out of the epididymis like little pearls or white calculi (Delbet and Chevassu[3]). (Similar structures may be found oc-

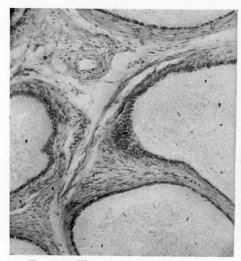

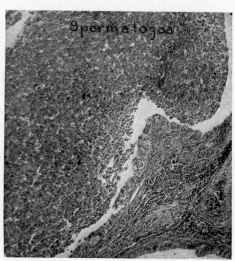

Fig. 92.—The epididymis above an inflammatory occlusion of the duct showing a marked dilatation of the lumen containing many spermatozoa. B. U. I. Path. 4917.

Fig. 93.—A more advanced stage of the same process showing slight round-cell infiltration of the stroma, epithelial hyperplasia, and dense masses of spermatozoa filling the dilated duct. B. U. I. Path. 3390.

casionally in the seminal vesicles, the "samensteine" of the German authors.) Around these masses the epithelial cells of the duct persist, and seem to take on phagocytic activity, so that the spermatozoa are resorbed. Multinuclear masses, resembling foreign body giant-cells, and containing within their cytoplasm spermatozoa, are described. This process may explain how the spermatozoa constantly being formed by the testis are disposed of in cases of obstruction.

Testis.—In the past it was not customary to distinguish clinically between infections of the testis and epididymis, inflammations of the scrotal contents being indiscriminately called "orchitis." In Europe, especially in France, the later tendency has been to treat the two together, as "orchi-epididymitis," while

[1] Quoted by Sebileau and Descomps, in Nouveau Traité de Chirurgie, LeDentu and Delbet, 1916, xxxii (Maladies des Organes Genitaux de l'Homme).

[2] Ibid.

[3] Ibid.

in this country a more complete separation has been made. We feel that the latter course is desirable, for the following reasons: (1) The mechanism and occurrence of infections of the epididymis and testis are almost entirely different, and it is remarkable how frequently one organ remains intact in the presence of infection of the other; (2) by careful palpation the distinction can be made clinically, and; (3) if it is found that the epididymis alone is involved in cases requiring surgical treatment, the testis can be saved by performing an epididymectomy. The term "orchitis" should, therefore, not be used unless involvement of the testis itself can be demonstrated.

Inflammations of the testis proper arise, in the great majority of cases, as blood-borne infections. It is also possible for infection to spread from the epididymis to the testis by means of the tubuli recti, the lymphatics, or by direct extension; from the tunica vaginalis by direct extension (glanders); and occasionally through the general lymphatic system (filariasis). In certain cases of blood-stream infection there is reason to believe that the process begins as an infected thrombosis of the pampiniform plexus, which eventually involves the testicle. In such cases the epididymis and testis are usually affected equally, and gangrene may occur.

In general, any infectious process in the body may become localized in the testis, as in the kidney. For this reason the list of diseases here given which can involve the testis may not be complete, but it includes all the more important ones.

Further, in any infectious disease, the testis may be infected with the causative organism of the disease, it may undergo secondary infection with ordinary pyogenic organisms, or it may be damaged by toxins without actual infection. In

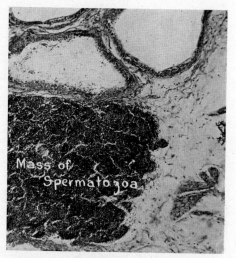

FIG. 94.—Epididymis showing dilatation of the duct, some edema of the stroma, and a curious mass of extravasated spermatozoa lying in the stroma. B. U. I. Path. 4723.

diseases where the infectious agent is unknown it may be difficult to say whether the testicular lesion is toxic or infective. Where secondary infection occurs, it may well be that the organ is first damaged by toxins, allowing the other organisms to invade it easily, either by way of the vas deferens and epididymis or the bloodstream.

Jäckh[1] found tubercle bacilli in the tubules of apparently normal testes in cases of generalized tuberculosis. From this observation has been built up a theory of the testicular excretion of bacteria, as in the kidney, and this theory has been used to explain the frequent hematogenous infections of the testis. It must be said that the theory rests on no further experimental evidence than the finding mentioned above. Biedl and Kraus[2] found organisms and particulate matter in urine and bile after intravenous injection, but never in the secretions of the pan-

[1] Virchow's Archiv, 1895, cxlii, 101–133.
[2] Zeitschrift für Hygiene, 1897, xxvi, 353–376.

creas, salivary gland, or trachea (mucous glands). No analogies can justifiably be drawn from these experiments in regard to the testis. We feel, however, that insistence on an excretory function of the testis has little point.

Regardless of the source of the infection, the microscopic appearance of *acute pyogenic orchitis* is the same. Location of the lesion near the hilus may indicate origin from the epididymis, while blood-stream infections may occur in any part of the testis, or as multiple disseminated foci. The entire organ may be converted into a single abscess before rupture or incision.

In the gross, the testis is swollen, tense, and if the lesion is localized, there are nodules to be made out on the surface, or, by palpation, in the depths. The

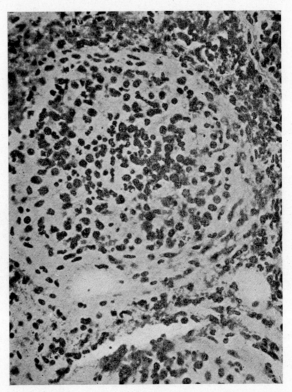

Fig. 95.—Acute pyogenic inflammation of the testis: A seminiferous tubule as shown in cross-section. The germinal epithelium is much altered and the lumen is occupied by a number of polymorphonuclear leukocytes. Others are also seen in the surrounding tissues.

blood-vessels are congested. The organ may swell, in spite of the thick tunica albuginea, to two or three times its normal size.

The internal pressure apparently varies, as in some cases incision of the capsule is followed by herniation of tubular tissue, in others there is none. Abscesses may rupture externally, in which case herniation or *fungus* formation may occur, especially if the abscess is large and acute. This process often goes on with gradual extrusion of testicular tissue until the entire testis is destroyed.

Microscopically one sees edema and polymorphonuclear infiltration (Fig. 95). The spermatogenic epithelium undergoes degeneration. The tubules contain leukocytes, and it is usually impossible to say whether the process is essentially intratubular, subepithelial, or interstitial. Most authorities believe that the spread is by way of the stroma. Necrosis involving all elements precedes *abscess* formation. If a portion of the testis is not involved, the tubules there remain unaffected, and capable of spermatogenesis. Abscess formation in the pyogenic infections is common. On the other hand, the testis does not become the seat of a chronic, indolent inflammation as does the epididymis. Chronic fibrotic changes occur only in the wall of an abscess, or as the result of specific, non-pyogenic infections (mumps, syphilis) or toxic degenerations.

Abscesses may perforate the capsule into the cavity of the tunica vaginalis, the scrotal tissues, or to the outside. Spontaneous rupture is preceded by subcutaneous involvement and fixation of the skin. *Sinuses* may persist, especially while necrotic testicular tissue is being discharged. The epididymis, if intact, may be secondarily involved by contiguity. The arteries of the testis radiate from the hilus, and if a principal one is occluded, gangrene of a part of the testis may occur.

The *tunica vaginalis* is usually involved in acute processes, and may be reddened, while the cavity contains a fibrinous exudate, and a small or moderate quantity of turbid hydrocele fluid.

In pyogenic orchitis, there have been found Bacillus coli, Bacillus mucosus capsulatus, streptococcus, staphylococcus, Bacillus typhæ, Bacillus pyocyaneus (Pseudomonas pyocyanea), and other organisms. Gonococcal infection of the testis is rare, extends from the inflamed epididymis, and usually involves only part of the testis.

Among *specific types of orchitis*, a few may be mentioned.

Orchitis occurs in about 20 per cent. of cases of *mumps*, though in some epidemics the incidence is much greater. The infection may be entirely confined to the testes, the parotid glands escaping. Wolbach, in an article by Smith,[1] states that the process is an acute inflammation, involving some groups of tubules, which are distended and whose epithelium is destroyed, while adjoining areas of the testis are normal. The exudate consists of polymorphonuclear and endothelial leukocytes. The tubules show hyaline degeneration. The stroma is edematous, with some hemorrhages. In some normal tubules, the lumen is filled with polymorphonuclear leukocytes, while other tubules are involved over only a part of their circumference, suggesting that the process is essentially in the stroma, with secondary invasion and destruction of the tubules. The tunica albuginea is edematous, and the blood-vessels show endothelial proliferation. The interstitial cells may be involved, so that in bilateral cases eunuchism may result. This is, fortunately, rare. The epididymis may be swollen and congested, and there may be a small inflammatory hydrocele.

Severe damage is caused by the inflammation so that regeneration often does not occur, but there is fibrous tissue deposition and the testis shrinks. This atrophy ensues in about 30 per cent. of the cases (Laveran and Catran). If the involvement has been slight, restitution to normal occurs. Cultures made from these testes show no growth.

According to Chiari, Berand, and Esmonet, orchitis occurs in from 60 to 85 per cent. of all cases of *smallpox* coming to autopsy. Sebileau and Descomps[2]

---

[1] Boston Medical and Surgical Journal, 1912, clxvii, 323–325.

[2] Nouveau Traité de Chirugie (Le Dentu and Delbet), 1916, xxxii (Maladies des Organes Genitaux de l'Homme).

state that this disease involves the testis more frequently than any other. It has escaped attention because it is slight and benign. Macroscopically, the testis may appear quite normal, even on section, or it may be slightly swollen and congested. Councilman[1] gives the best description of the microscopic picture:

> Lesions most difficult of interpretation are those of the testicle. There is absence of spermatogenesis in the cases in which convalescence is established. Normal spermatozoa are absent in the lumina of the tubules, and there is degeneration of the spermatogenetic cells. This affects both cytoplasm and nuclei and the degenerating nucleus assumes forms which present some similarity to certain of the intracellular parasites in the epithelial cells of the skin. This degeneration is not peculiar to smallpox, but may be found in typhoid fever. These lesions are absent in the undeveloped testes of children.
>
> In addition to diffuse degenerative lesions there are found, in adult and child's testes, focal lesions, as characteristic of the disease as the skin lesions. Lesions begin as an infiltration of the intertubular tissue with both ordinary lymphoid cells and large mononuclear basophilic cells. The tubules in the foci are unaltered. From such lesions as these, which are best compared with small interstitial foci in the kidneys, the process extends. The area enlarges, the cellular infiltration extends and finally there is complete necrosis in the center, with fibrin and hemorrhage in the surrounding interstitial tissue. The necrotic tubules often contain numbers of phagocytic cells. The blood-vessels in the foci are obliterated in some cases by thrombi, but chiefly by the pressure of the cells. Acute endarteritis with accumulations of mononuclear cells is often found.
>
> The lesions vary in number, some testicles showing large numbers of them, while in others they are found only after prolonged search. The smallest lesions and those best adapted for study are in the undeveloped testes of children. They show a general relation to the duration of the disease, the most advanced cases occurring late in the course.
>
> Notwithstanding its apparently specific nature no parasites were found in the testicular lesions of man.

Esmonet adds that the exudate may contain eosinophils and plasma-cells. The epididymis is usually quite normal. There may be slight hydrocele. Suppuration is possible, but seldom ensues; the usual termination is by restitution to normal, though a few cases of late atrophy are mentioned.

A true orchitis occurs in about 0.25 per cent. of cases of *typhoid fever*, usually during convalescence. The epididymis is often involved, the lesion is acute, and suppuration is not uncommon (about 20 per cent., Beardsley[2]). Inflammatory hydrocele occurs. The typhoid bacillus is found in the testis. In a few cases the picture begins with thrombo-angiitis of the veins of the spermatic cord, and spreads to the testis.[3] Pathologically, the lesion is like that described for pyogenic orchitis.

Involvement of the testis may occur in any form of *septicemia*, though it is not common. It also occurs in the various conditions in which we assume that organisms are carried about in the blood, though there is no actual blood-stream infection. In this class are *tonsillitis, furunculosis, osteomyelitis, endocarditis, localized abscesses*, etc. Barney[4] has described cases of apparently *idiopathic* infections of the testis, in which an acute orchitis appears without other symptoms and the primary focus or portal of entry is never discovered.

In experimental and diagnostic infections of animals with *glanders*, inflammation of the testis is early, constant, and pathognomonic. The process has been

---

[1] Osler and McCrea's Modern Medicine, 2d ed., 1914, i, 791–792.
[2] Journal of the American Medical Association, 1908, l, 1014–1016.
[3] Kinnicutt: Medical Record, lix, 801–803.
[4] Surgery, Gynecology, and Obstetrics, 1914, xviii, 307–313.

studied by Straus[1] and Duval.[2]   In human glanders, also, involvement of the testis is not uncommon.   The path of infection is rather characteristic, since the tunica vaginalis is first affected, apparently from the blood-stream.   The involvement of the testis and epididymis is secondary.   In animals, the inflammation is confined to the serous surface in 90 per cent. of the cases, the testis remaining free.   The lesions are acute or chronic.   Acute forms show marked necrosis with karyorrhexis, polymorphonuclear and mononuclear infiltration, and some fixed tissue reaction.   Older lesions are surrounded by fibrosis, the infiltration is round-celled, and giant-cells are present, the whole resembling somewhat tuberculosis.   In general, glanders, while a granulomatous lesion, is more destructive and less chronic than tuberculosis.[3]

A few cases of orchitis complicating *influenza* have been reported.   Wolbach[4] describes an apparently toxic lesion, with epithelial degeneration and fibrosis. In autopsies of cases dying of streptococcus and of pneumococcus pneumonias, Mills[5] found regularly a lesion consisting of aspermatogenesis, epithelial degeneration, giant-cell formation, and slight fibrosis.   In similar cases, which recovered, no lasting damage was observed and the orchitis was usually negligible clinically.

Malta fever (undulant or Mediterranean fever) is not infrequently accompanied by an orchitis which is usually mild.[6]   It is stated that the organism has been grown, and in other cases where cultures were unsuccessful, the fluid removed agglutinated the Bacillus melitensis.

An orchitis may occur in certain cases of *leprosy*.   This lesion is primary in the testis itself, but otherwise resembles tuberculosis, being a proliferative granuloma, which may undergo necrosis.   Fibrosis, round-cells, epithelioid cells and giant-cells are present.   The bacilli are present in much greater numbers than in tuberculosis.

Inflammations of the testicle and epididymis occur in the course of epidemic cerebrospinal meningitis, malaria, scarlet fever, rheumatic fever, vaccina, typhus, and other infectious diseases, but their exact relation to the causative organisms of these diseases has not been determined.

SYMPTOMS AND DIAGNOSIS

Kidney, Symptoms.—The symptoms of renal infections vary with the nature of the lesion.   In *acute fulminant infections* there are fever, chills, prostration, and pain in the kidney region.   The onset is often sudden.   Hematuria is frequently noticed, but frank pyuria may be absent.   Pain, however, is sometimes absent, in which case there may be tenderness over the kidney region.   In short, the picture is that of an acute general infection, with only pain to suggest its location in the kidney, unless the patient has seen blood in the urine.   If both kidneys are heavily

[1] Archives de la Medicine Experimentelle et de l'Anatomie Pathologique, 1889, i (1 serie), 460–462.

[2] Ibid., 1896, viii, 361–370.

[3] MacCallum: Text-book of Pathology, 2d ed., 1920, 587–589.

[4] Johns Hopkins Hospital Bulletin, 1919, xxx, 104–109.

[5] Journal of Experimental Medicine, 1919, xxx, 505–529.

[6] Poinsiller: De l'orchite maltaise, Thèse de Montpellier, July, 1910.   Eyre, Kolle and Wassermann's Bacteriology, 1912, iv, 438.   Bassett-Smith: British Medical Journal, 1904, ii, 324.   Castellani and Chalmers: Nelson's Loose Leaf Medicine, 1920, ii, 209–211.   Yount and Looney: Arizona Medical Journal, April, 1913, No. 4.

involved, renal function is impaired, and the symptoms of uremia begin to appear quickly. These patients are very ill, and the diagnosis usually rests on the results of examination, rather than on any special symptom complex.

Acute renal infections occurring *de novo* or in the course of other urogenital conditions, or after operations on the urinary tract, may have a sudden onset, or may be insidious, probably because masked by other conditions present. Chill is often the first symptom, and fever is practically always present, usually of a remittent type. Pain is inconstant; it may be severe, or the kidneys may be painless, even when pressed upon. A mild delirium may occur, especially in old persons, and this may pass insensibly into uremic coma. This transition is more rapid if the kidneys are already damaged before the acute infection begins. In certain mild cases, there may be no more than slight fever and lumbar pain, the general condition remaining unaffected. We are, therefore, often unable to tell whether there is a real disseminated nephritis, or simply a pyelitis, possibly ascending.

Renal colic is infrequent, and indicates the passage of masses of pus or blood-clots. Ureteritis may increase these obstructive symptoms if present.

In general, the symptoms are only roughly parallel with the extent of the involvement. In debilitated individuals lack of reaction may mislead as to the severity of the infection.

In the more *chronic forms* there is the same variation in the severity of the symptoms, but no definite dividing line can be drawn between "pyelitis" and "pyelonephritis" on the basis of the symptomatology. The treatment and prognosis depend, however, on the severity and extent of the lesion, so that one must form the most accurate idea possible of the pathologic picture.

The principal symptoms are fever, with chills and sweating, local pain, pyuria, polyuria, tumor, and the features of general intoxication. In addition, there may be symptoms due to irritation or actual infection of the lower urinary tract, as frequency, burning, dysuria, urgency, difficulty or tenesmus. Hematuria is rare in these chronic forms except when the picture is complicated by stone, or in case of acute trigonitis or posterior urethritis.

Fever is constant in the severer cases, and frequent even in mild cases. High remittent fever, with chills and sweats usually indicates a suppurative process, often with dammed-up pus, and a general intoxication. A sudden fall in such fever may be accompanied by the discharge of a quantity of pus in the urine. In mild cases the fever is often of a low hectic type, with slight evening rises, so that tuberculosis or endocarditis may be suspected. Finally, there are some cases, apparently of superficial infection, without fever, or with afebrile periods.

Pyuria is constant, though the pus may be insufficient in quantity to be noticed by the patient. Deposits of phosphates or urates may be mistaken by the laity for pus. As stated above, pyuria may be intermittent, indicating a suppurative focus which discharges at intervals. Coherent masses of pus indicate an abscess or pyonephrosis, though little reliance should be placed on this point. Pus diffused in the urine may settle into masses at the base of the bladder if there is no great frequency. Rarely worm-like casts of the ureter may be passed, but they do not usually have sufficient coherence. Pyuria may cease suddenly, indicating a blocking off of the infected area. This event is sometimes followed by fever, pain, or development of a mass.

Polyuria is an indication of renal damage, and is often associated with partial or intermittent obstruction. The urine is usually light colored and of low specific gravity. This polyuria may give rise to a frequency independent of any involvement of the bladder, and one should always inquire as to the quantity passed at each voiding. Drinking large quantities of water will cause an artificial polyuria.

Tumor is seldom large enough to attract the patient's attention unless pyonephrosis or perinephric abscess is present. The tumor of pyonephrosis may vary in size or disappear from time to time. The disappearance may be accompanied by a discharge of pus in the urine.

The *general condition* of the patient is of great importance. In the severe cases, the suppurative process causes loss of weight, weakness, anemia, and jaundice, or a pasty appearance of the skin. The jaundice is hemolytic, and bile pigments may appear in the urine. Attacks of furunculosis may occur. The picture is not infrequently such as to suggest malignant disease. In milder cases, these symptoms are all lessened. Frequently intermittent attacks occur, when with fever and pyuria, the patient will experience malaise, weakness, and some loss of weight, becoming practically normal again between attacks. In still other cases the general health is apparently unaffected. In late cases with severe destruction, uremic symptoms may supervene. Often they are confused with those due to the intoxication from the infection. In some cases coma may come on rapidly, without antecedent symptoms, as in anuria.

The bladder symptoms require no special notice. Sometimes they are the only ones which annoy the patient, so that careful examination is necessary to disclose the kidney lesion.

Extension to the perinephric tissues, if acute, is marked by an increase in the local and general symptoms, but chronic infection of the fatty capsule, resulting in much fibrosis, may exist with no symptoms. Abscess formation is frequent in the more acute cases. Symptoms of intoxication are more constant, for there is no way for the pus to escape. The pain is usually quite severe. It may be referred downward, or to the hip-joint, and involvement of the psoas muscle may cause flexion of the hip and pain on movement. The spine may be held stiffly. Pyuria may be present or absent, depending on whether the perirenal focus communicates with the kidney pelvis. The abscess may break, and sinuses appear in various places, enumerated in the section on pathology. In very chronic and indolent cases, there may be no symptoms but the appearance of a small sinus in the loin. In some of these cases connection with the kidney is never suspected.

Ureteritis is practically always associated with infections of the kidney, and has no distinctive symptoms of its own. When it becomes chronic, stricture formation may occur, when the symptoms are those due to the effects of obstruction on the kidney, which are treated under Obstructive Uropathy.

Kidney, Diagnosis.—The diagnosis of infections of the kidney includes not only (1) the determination of the presence of an infection, but also (2) the identity of the infecting organisms, (3) the source of the infection, (4) the severity and extent of the lesion, (5) the amount of damage done to the secreting renal parenchyma, and (6) whether any obstruction is present. If obstruction is present, its nature must be discovered.

Physical examination gives important information. Fever, emaciation, anemia, tenderness, and masses are sought for. Tenderness may be accompanied by definite muscle spasm, which includes the abdominal wall over the kidney and ureter, or in some cases only the spinal muscles on the affected side. Spasm of the psoas may be made out by extending the hip-joint manually. In perirenal inflammation, there will often be puffiness and redness of the skin in the loin, or one may see an abscess pointing to the surface. The mass of a pyonephrosis is usually fairly definitely outlined, while in perinephric inflammation it will be more of a diffuse fulness, which may also be appreciable to inspection. Percussion, especially with distended colon, may sometimes help in distinguishing from gall-bladder disease.

Examination of the urine is next in order. Doubt often remains after the physical examination, and in the presence of upper abdominal symptoms pus and organisms in the urine are strong evidence, although not absolute proof, that the kidneys are at fault. The urine may be normal, however, in perinephric abscess, or in closed unilateral pyonephrosis. One should take the specific gravity and the reaction of the urine. *Low specific gravity* indicates renal damage, and a strongly *alkaline ammoniacal urine* indicates an infection with urea-splitting organisms. Phenolphthalein is the best indicator. *Albumin* is of minor value, since well-marked quantities may arise from pus and blood, and we are never sure, in the presence of an infection, just how much of the albumin has really passed through the kidney. *Microscopic examination* shows the amount of pus roughly, and also whether red-blood cells are present. In case of doubt the benzidin test for blood may be applied. The presence of pus is of prime importance as it distinguishes bacterial renal infections from acute Bright's disease and most of the toxic nephritides. A *stained smear* of the sediment from a centrifuged specimen is studied carefully. Bacteria are proof positive that an infection exists somewhere in the urinary tract. If cocci are found, a Gram stain should be made, and the acid-fast stain for tubercle bacilli should never be omitted. Facilities should be available to make careful *cultures*, after first disinfecting the meatus and irrigating the urethra (see section on Bacteriology) and catching the latter part of the urine in a sterile tube. It is well to take the first culture before any instruments are used, if possible.

The decision to carry out *cystoscopy* and *ureter catheterization* immediately or to wait, depends on the condition of the patient. Perinephric abscess may demand immediate treatment. Wherever a nephrectomy is contemplated, or even regarded as a possibility, study of the divided urines must be carried out at all costs, and if the condition of the patient offers no contraindication, we should take these measures in any event to make our diagnosis exact.

They are preceded by a total *phenolsulphonephthalein test, blood-urea* determination, and a plain *x-ray*. If the total phthalein is diminished, there is probably a bilateral destructive lesion or obstruction. The blood urea tells us if accumulation of waste products in the blood has already begun. The *x*-ray discloses stones, if they are present, and should show also the size, shape, and position of the kidneys.

The intravesical examination has two objects: (1) To tell us whether the infection is really in the upper urinary tract, and (2) to determine the relative functional ability of the kidneys. In addition we can see if the bladder is involved, whether there is any obstruction, calculus, or tumor present there, and find out if the infection is confined to one kidney or is bilateral. The first-named object is important, as occasionally a pyuria arising in the prostate or elsewhere in the lower urinary tract may coexist with upper abdominal symptoms due to a lesion not in the urinary tract. The second also, as it avoids operating on a patient with an atrophic or destroyed kidney on the other side.

The *ureteral orifices* (Plate XVIII) are studied for signs of inflammation, and the stream of urine from each closely observed. Abnormalities in the *rate* of ureteral peristalsis are noted. If no urine appears to come from an orifice, obstruction is suggested. In this work it is better to have the bladder filled with sterile water than with salt or other solutions, as the higher specific gravity of the urine produces refractive phenomena which make it visible as it flows into the water-filled bladder. This occurs with clear urine, and must be distinguished carefully from the cloud produced by an admixture of pus or blood. When the urine is clear the pseudocloud is very vague and details of the bladder wall are seen through it, but somewhat distorted. This appearance ceases instantly when the orifice closes and the flow stops. A real cloud of *blood* or *pus* (Plate XVIII) actually conceals the bladder-wall picture momentarily, and, most important of all, persists for a mo-

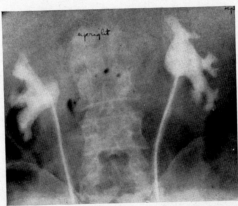

Fig. 96.—Bilateral pyelogram in a case of chronic pyelitis. While the extrarenal portions of the pelves are large, the minor calices are normal, and no obstruction was ever demonstrated. The patient's symptoms persisted even after long treatment, and the urine did not become sterile. B. U. I. *x*-Ray 2643.

ment after the flow stops, and before the particles of the cloud disperse into the bladder contents. When the quantities of pus or blood are greater, there can be no doubt, and they appear as flakes or clots. If a worm-like stream of pus which retains its shape for a time in the bladder is discharged from the ureter, one can be sure that very little urine is coming from that side, and, therefore, that there is pyonephrosis present. In intense or long-standing cases of renal infection *edema* or *ulcers* may appear around the ureteral orifice.

After the *ureter catheters* are inserted, specimens from the two sides are carefully examined, and it is well to take cultures. A very few widely scattered organisms may escape detection by the microscope. Blood and epithelial cells are now of minor importance, since these elements will appear from the trauma of the catheters. The concentration of the urine is studied with the *hydrometer* and by the *hypobromite* test, using the Doremus tube. Markedly lower concentration on one side indicates a damaged kidney.

A *divided phthalein test* gives the respective functional states of the two kid-

neys. (For technic see the section on Obstructive Lesions of the Urogenital Tract.)
The *transvesical* leakage, if any, must be determined, and the sum of the functions
of the two sides should check with the previous total phthalein before definite
conclusions are drawn from this test.

In acute cases a *pyelogram* is usually best omitted, but in chronic cases will
often give valuable information. It may decide whether a suspicious shadow is
really a ureteral or renal calculus (this can also be told by an x-ray taken during
ureter catheterization with a shadowgraph catheter), will disclose any dilatation
due to a slight or obscure obstruction (Figs. 96, 97) and also any ptosis or other
malposition of the kidney which may
be helping to maintain the infection.
It will also help greatly to rule out
neoplasm, tuberculosis, or other lesions
of the kidney often associated with
secondary infection. In the ureter,
zones of constriction are not to be interpreted as strictures unless dilatation
exists above, since they may be due to
muscular contraction and lateral movements of the ureter during the radio-

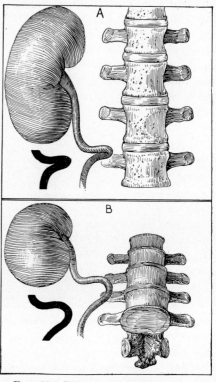

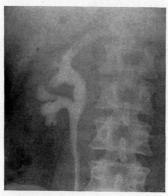

FIG. 97.—Pyelogram showing a mild degree
of hydronephrosis, with slight blunting of the
calices. This patient had a very chronic pyelitis
in the kidney shown. The pelvis is also a beautiful example of bifid pelvis. Note shadow of kidney
outline. B. U. I. x-Ray 2085.

FIG. 98.—Diagram showing how an easy
curve in the ureter may be shown on the x-ray
plate as a kink if taken from certain angles. A
is the ordinary view; in B the ureter and kidney
are viewed obliquely from below.

graphic exposure. Similarly, apparent kinks may be due to easy curves viewed
from certain angles, as illustrated in the diagrams (Fig. 98). Infectious lesions
in the ureter itself may occasionally appear as irregular areas, with ragged outline. A stereoscopic pyelo-ureterogram is of great assistance in correctly interpreting ureteral pictures.

A thorough study of this sort enables us, first, to decide whether obstruction
of any kind is involved, and whether such other lesions as tuberculosis, neoplasm,
or calculus are present. Even in cases where a pyonephrosis or perinephric abscess
has demanded immediate surgical incision, the study should be carried out after
the patient has recovered from his acute illness, in order to plan the subsequent
treatment intelligently.

If the upper abdominal symptoms are due to a lesion outside the urinary tract, the urologic examination will be necessary to exclude the kidney. Suppurative processes near the urinary tract are sometimes associated with hematuria, as appendicitis. In addition a secondary renal infection occurs, in rare instances, in such conditions as appendicitis and cholecystitis, etc. These cases often provide very difficult diagnostic problems, and mistakes are easy. Attacks of pain due to appendicitis, partial intestinal obstruction, biliary colic, gastric ulcer, or neoplasm, etc., may give rise to confusion and call for urologic examination.

If renal infection is present, we divide the cases into those *with* and those *without obstruction*. Obstruction of any kind, of course, requires its surgical removal. Cases without obstruction can be divided into those with additional lesions, as stone, neoplasm, or tuberculosis, and those without. Such lesions must be treated surgically whenever possible. In all these cases, and in those without obstruction or additional lesion, the treatment of the renal infection itself is decided according to the findings, on the general principle that a kidney showing little or no functional impairment is treated conservatively; the greater the renal destruction, the more radical measures can be employed.

Where symptoms are largely or entirely those arising in the lower urinary tract, a renal lesion must be sought with great care. The discharge of organisms through the kidney is often intermittent, so that repeated examination may be necessary. Sometimes the bacteria are present in very small numbers, so that they may be missed if cultures are not made. Cultures and smears are always required, as certain cases of colon group infection of the kidneys are practically without pus. Reliance on the naked-eye appearance of pus is no longer allowable; it must always be confirmed microscopically.

Diagnostic measures must now include thorough overhauling in search of the portal of entry for renal infections. The teeth, tonsils, paranasal sinuses, gall-bladder, intestine, rectum, and genital organs are those most commonly implicated. Heitz-Boyer[1] feels that, in women especially, renal infections are often associated with deficient intestinal motility involving the cecum and ascending colon, stasis in the descending colon being of less importance. Bismuth x-ray studies of the intestine are necessary to determine this point.

Bladder, Symptoms.—*Frequency* and *burning* are the classic symptoms of cystitis. Owing to the great annoyance they give the patient, they are most often the principal source of his complaint. In connection with *pyuria*, they do indeed make the diagnosis of cystitis almost certain; however, the physician should not be misled, like the patient, by the predominance of the bladder symptoms, but should seek out the underlying cause of the bladder infection.

The urinary *frequency* of cystitis is caused by (1) increased irritability of the bladder from inflammation, or (2) actual decrease in the size and elasticity of the bladder from fibrosis and infiltration. The highly irritable and painful bladder of acute cystitis may have a normal capacity under anesthesia, while the contracted, inelastic bladder of chronic cystitis may be incapable of holding more than a few cubic centimeters under any circumstances; symptomatically they are alike, because in either the presence of a small quantity of urine causes an urgent and often painful desire to void. The frequency is usually most marked in the day time, as movements of the patient increase the irritability. The severity

[1] Journal Médical Français, 1922, xi, 178–212.

of the symptom is best indicated by the quantity passed at each voiding, as the intervals, and number of voidings, will depend largely on the amount of fluid ingested.

Painful sensations in the bladder are increased by contractions of the bladder muscle. It frequently happens that no pain is perceptible when the bladder is relaxed, but it is felt when contraction occurs before or during urination. This condition is spoken of as *dysuria*. When pain is felt at all times, it is invariably increased at the time of voiding, though it may be somewhat relieved for a period immediately afterward, when the bladder is both empty and relaxed. Since the sensory nerves of the bladder are parasympathetic, the pain is usually not well localized, but usually referred, and oftenest to the tip of the penis or along the course of the urethra. The patient is frequently unaware, for this reason, that the source of his pain is in the bladder. Less frequently, the pain is referred elsewhere in the distribution of the sacral nerves, as the scrotum, perineum, rectum, or even the upper inner surface of the thighs. When the pain is more pronounced and constant, it is appreciated over the suprapubic region or groins, indicating that some sensory fibers may go by way of the hypogastrics. The quality of the pain is generally described as "burning," "stinging," or "scalding," especially during urination; the constant pain may be of an aching character.

The inflammation of the bladder wall not only causes painful sensations, but makes the muscle hyperirritable, so that it contracts oftener and more strongly than normal. This gives rise to the feeling of an urgent necessity to void at once, and often the patient cannot retain the urine more than a few moments. When this *"urgency"* of urination becomes severe and frequent, the patient seeks relief by an almost constant emptying of his bladder, and when this becomes habitual, he may believe that he suffers from a true incontinence. Such patients often have recourse to rubber urinals. When inflammation is very pronounced, the muscular contractions may cause the most exquisite pain, and may persist after the bladder is empty, even for considerable periods, perhaps squeezing out from time to time a few drops of mingled pus, blood, and urine, and accompanied by the feeling that the bladder is not empty. This is known as *tenesmus* or *strangury*, and is oftenest associated with acute cystitis, or with extensive ulcerated cystitis of a more chronic nature. Strangury is often marked in the acute cystitis colli of gonorrhea.

Vesical irritation which is not specifically associated with infection may be caused by irritation resulting from the excretion of certain chemical substances (turpentine, urotropin, cantharides, etc.). There are frequency of urination, sensations of burning or actual pain, urgency, tenesmus or strangury, pyuria, hematuria, and occasionally dribbling or partial incontinence. In chronic cases cicatricial obstructions may cause difficulty of urination.

Pyuria of a varying degree is constant in cystitis. The amount of pus may be small in mild superficial cystitis, increases with the severity of the infection and is perhaps greatest in the cystitis associated with diverticula and cellules in obstruction. Ordinarily the pus is uniformly mixed with the urine, but when large quantities occur, it may settle in the bladder and be more plentiful in the last portion of the urine.

Hematuria occurs in severe acute cystitis and in ulcerative forms or those with granulation tissue formation. The blood is usually small or moderate in quantity, and well mixed with the urine, but there is nothing specific about the appearance of it to distinguish from the hematuria of stone, neoplasm, tuberculosis, or other diseases. The blood may appear at the end of urination only, and is then presumably due to the mechanical disturbance of the muscular contraction.

Cystitis most commonly has its origin from catheter infection, and is generally accompanied by no change in the patient's symptoms. The "classical" burning and irritation are often absent, and the urine may be clear to the naked eye, although markedly infected. Later pus may be manifest and with it vesical discomfort.

On the other hand, bladder infection may be ushered in by chill and high fever, shortly after instrumentation.

Patients under treatment—particularly if catheterized for residual urine—should have immediate urinalysis for bacteria on each visit. Only by diligence in antiseptic prophylaxis and treatment may serious infections be avoided.

Patients with residual urine, accompanying prostatic obstruction in men or the postpartum period in women, may go months or years without having infected urine, if they are not catheterized. Conversely, in many cases infection occurs early, without any instrument having been inserted.

In cases with a long history of cystitis, *difficulty of urination* may gradually develop, due to a scar-tissue contracture of the vesical orifice. This in turn may give rise to dilatation of the bladder, trabeculation, diverticula, and functional or anatomic damage to the kidneys, the symptoms of which are given in the chapter on Obstructive Uropathy. It is characteristic of this condition that its development is extremely gradual. It usually brings the patient to the physician earlier in life, however, than benign prostatic hypertrophy, Hinman[1] giving the average age for this condition as fifty-five, as compared with seventy for prostatic hypertrophy. The causative cystitis may have been so mild and chronic that its symptoms were ignored by the patient, but careful questioning will usually elicit the story of frequency, burning or pyuria, perhaps transient or slight, but over a long period.

If inflamed surfaces become covered with *calcareous incrustations*, bits of gravel may be passed. Very fulminant acute cystitis occasionally causes extensive loss of epithelium, so that large pieces of it, even the entire lining of the bladder may be passed in the form of thin, rolled-up, usually ragged membranes.[2]

Leukoplakia is associated with chronic cystitis, but has a very characteristic symptom of its own, namely, the passage of flakes or sheets of desquamated epithelium, with a pearly white appearance.

The *solitary*, or *Fenwick ulcer*, has no characteristic symptoms, but gives those of a chronic cystitis.

Submucous (or "interstitial") *cystitis* causes frequency and pain, which may gradually increase over many years with, eventually, urgency and tenesmus. The symptoms are often very pronounced when only a portion of the bladder is involved. If secondary infection has not occurred, the urine may be perfectly normal, and this is the most characteristic feature. In advanced cases, the symptoms may be of extreme severity, with intense pain and voiding every few minutes,

[1] Journal of Urology, 1919, iii, 207–245.

[2] Dawson: Johns Hopkins Hospital Bulletin, 1898, ix, 155–159.

leading to complete incapacitation of the patient. In earlier cases there may be no more than a slight frequency and burning. Hematuria may occur, and while usually transient, due to a splitting of the lesion, may be terminal and more persistent.

Radium Ulcer.—When radium has been used in the treatment of vesical neoplasms, an ulcer is frequently left at the site of the tumor, especially where the dose of radium has been large. These ulcers are like radium ulcers on the surface of the body in their chronicity and painfulness. This is supposedly due to a destructive effect on the neighboring blood-vessels, making the formation of normal granulation tissue impossible. There is also marked inflammation about the ulcer, producing symptoms sometimes as severe as those caused by the original lesion, and sometimes more so. They consist of frequency, dysuria, and occasionally the most distressing tenesmus. There may be slight hematuria.

Cystitis may occur at any *age*. However, the forms associated with gonorrhea are most frequent in the third decade, while those accompanying stone, neoplasm and prostatic hypertrophy have the same age incidence as these diseases, in later life. Submucous cystitis is a disease of middle life. In Frontz's[1] studies of 26 cases from our clinic the ages were as follows: ten to twenty, 1; twenty to thirty, 4; thirty to forty, 6; forty to fifty, 7; fifty to sixty, 8.

In cystitis in general there is no distinction as to *sex*, except that cystitis as a complication of obstruction is practically confined to males, infravesical obstruction being a rarity in females. It is remarkable, therefore, that cystitis is so common in females. Cystitis coming on with no evident cause is more common in females than in males, although modern methods are elucidating more and more of these cases, which may result from renal bacilluria, pelvic inflammatory disease, etc., and may be prolonged by the residual urine following pregnancy, by urethral granulations, polyps, etc.

Uncomplicated cystitis causes remarkably few general symptoms. Fever is usually an indication that the infection involves more than the bladder. The state of nutrition is not affected by the cystitis, but often a persistent chronic cystitis, with pain and frequency, will by its nervous and physical strain, wear the patient down. The result will be not only anorexia, anemia, and emaciation, but psychic depression as well.

Perivesical inflammation usually occurs in cases where previous events give a suggestion of what has happened; for example, forceful or unsuccessful instrumentation, or operations upon the bladder. The symptoms are fever, with chills and sweating and pain. There may also be visible swelling, especially in prevesical abscess, and reddening of the skin. If extravasation accompanies the inflammation, tumefaction is more extensive, and prostration and toxemia soon supervene. Retrovesical abscess may give rise to painful, and, if of large size, difficult defecation. Extension to the peritoneum gives typical symptoms of peritonitis, pain, distention, muscle spasm, and prostration. The pain of perivesical inflammation depends on the location; if posterior, it is located in the rectum and perineum, and if anterior, in the lower abdomen.

Bladder, Diagnosis.—*Acute cystitis* in young individuals, especially as a complication of urethritis, usually offers no difficulties of diagnosis. If there is no obstruction, and no extension to the renal pelves, the early resolution usually

[1] Journal of Urology, 1921, v, 491–511.

makes the diagnosis sure, and makes further effort unnecessary. The *urine* is, of course, studied in all cases. The *three-glass test* should not be omitted. In the presence of a cystitis, all three glasses are always cloudy, but the same may be true in certain cases of prostatitis. The urine examination, therefore, must be considered in conjunction with the clinical symptoms. In the *stained smear* pus and organisms are sought for, and the nature of the organisms determined by *culture*. If no organisms are found, but pus is present, tuberculosis or stone is suspected. The culture will usually show a pure growth of one organism. The urea-splitting bacteria are infrequent in acute cystitis. One must keep in mind the infrequent cases of chemical cystitis, where organisms are absent, and where the history is that of the injection of irritant substances, or the ingestion (or inhalation) of turpentine, urotropin, cantharides, etc.

The real diagnostic and therapeutic problems appear when *chronic cystitis* supervenes. The questions which are to be answered concern, (1) the nature of the cystitis; (2) the infecting organism or organisms; (3) the source of the infection; (4) the presence of complicating or additional lesions, as calculus, neoplasm, obstruction, etc., and (5) the involvement of other parts of the urogenital tract, especially the kidneys, prostate, and seminal vesicles.

Examination of the Urine.—This should be done immediately after the patient has voided in 3 glasses. This method can also be used in women, if the vagina is cleaned beforehand by a douche. For the reaction, phenolphthalein is the best indicator. If the urine is alkaline enough to produce the deepest red color of this dye, it is pH 8 or over, a point which is seldom if ever reached without urea-splitting organisms. If the color is a light pink, the urine is mildly alkaline; if colorless, it is neutral or acid. If further information is wanted, a drop of phenolsulphonephthalein is added. This will give a pink color unless the urine is more acid than pH 6.5, when it will be yellow. If a true alkaline cystitis is present, the ammoniacal odor of the urine will be unmistakable. One should rule out glycosuria by the Fehling or Benedict reaction.

The second glass of urine is chosen as the best index of the bladder urine. A drop of urine, uncentrifugalized, and a drop of the centrifugalized sediment, are next examined. The first gives an idea of the amount of pus or other elements present. Bacilli can usually be seen with the simple high power. The second enables us to examine these elements more closely. The high-power lens should be used. One notes the character of the pus-cells, of the epithelial cells, and the relative numbers of the two. It is impossible to identify epithelial cells from different parts of the urinary tract, and diagnoses based on the supposed differences are fallacious. In addition, one looks for shreds, red blood-cells, crystals, bacteria, casts, flakes of leukoplakic epithelium, tumor fragments, etc. Triple phosphate crystals indicate an alkaline urine, while neutral or slightly acid urine, when cooled, may show a deposit of urates, which will redissolve on further acidification. In the fresh urine one rarely sees many crystals. Much confusion is thus avoided. The number of organisms can be roughly estimated, and their motility noted. In urine that has stood, bacteria are of little significance, except Bacillus tuberculosis which is sometimes brought out by incubation.

The *stained smear* of centrifugalized sediment confirms the impressions previously gained concerning the cells present. The morphology of the bacteria is noted, and their numbers roughly estimated. When few, this may be expressed by the average number seen in an oil-immersion field, when more numerous, by +, ++, +++, or ++++. In addition, there should be a Gram stain and an acid-fast stain. When no pus is present it may be difficult, when the bacteria are scarce, to obtain a sediment which will stick to the bottom of the tube when it is emptied to make a loop smear. A fine capillary glass tube may be used to pick up the slight sediment. Egg-albumen may also be used to make it stick to the slide.

Cultures are made by the previously described technic.

In the three-glass test, clear urine in the second and third glasses rules out cystitis. Pus in the third glass may occasionally come from the prostate, but usually pus evenly distributed through the second and third glasses indicates an infection above the vesical orifice.

If pus and organisms have been found and symptoms of cystitis are present, we must determine whether the prostate and kidneys are involved. The prostate is investigated by the methods described in the succeeding section. If no pus or organisms are found, we suspect at once (in the presence of frequent and painful urination) submucous cystitis. If pus is present without organisms, tuberculosis or stone is suggested. If there is blood, one thinks of neoplasm, calculus, or tuberculosis, but it is essential to make sure that the blood is not coming from the kidneys.

For these reasons, and others, *cystoscopy* is necessary; and should certainly never be omitted in cases of chronic cystitis.

The patient is requested to void before the instrument is inserted, so that the *residual urine*, if any, can be determined. The bladder is then filled, and its *capacity* noted, as well as the *vesical tonus* and the ease, or difficulty, with which it can be *washed clean*. A careful systematic study of prostatic orifice, trigone, ureteral orifices, posterior, lateral and anterior walls is then made, prostatic hypertrophy, calculus, neoplasm, trabeculation, diverticulum, or other *complicating bladder lesion* being thus eliminated. The *vesical mucosa* is now carefully examined everywhere. In slight infections there is often only a congestion of the blood-vessels noted. If there is a diffuse reddening (Plate VI, *e*), a superficial lesion is indicated, and this appearance may be confined to the trigonal region. Irregularities of the *ureteral orifices*, or localized areas of inflammation about them, suggest renal involvement (Plate V, *a*). The urine flowing from them is observed for turbidity due to pus or blood. In more severe lesions, the mucosa may show edema, in advanced grades of which the epithelium is raised up in blebs, the so-called *bullous cystitis*. When localized, this appearance may be taken for neoplasm (Plate VI, *e*). Bullous cystitis often exists in the neighborhood of tumors, and in many cases only experience can make the distinction. The bullæ usually transmit light, giving a peculiar opalescent appearance. In trabeculated bladders, the inflammatory changes may be more marked on the summits of the ridges.

Blood clots and shreds of mucopus are often seen in the bladder, and may conceal localized lesions. They should be washed out during cystoscopy by the irrigating stream, or displaced by a ureteral bougie if suspicion exists, since in searching for ulcerations, etc., one must be sure to inspect the entire bladder. Ulcerations appear as areas usually reddened, with slightly elevated and inflamed border (Plate VII). Shreds of exudate often cling to the base of the ulcer, and sometimes there is a crust or membrane, which may vary in color from almost

PLATE V

URETERAL ABNORMALITIES: ULCERS, TRABECULATION

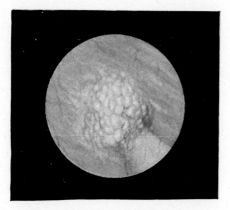

A. Bullous edema of mucous membrane in region of right ureter, obscuring orifice.

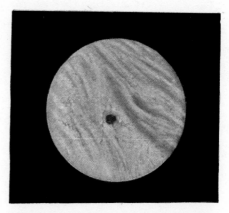

B. "Golf-hole" ureter frequently seen in tuberculosis of ureter and kidney.

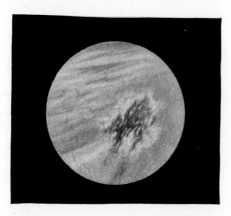

C. Tuberculous ulceration surrounding left ureteral orifice.

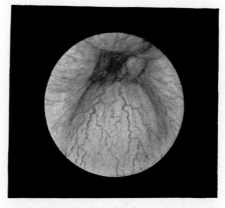

D. Enterovesical fistula; carcinoma of ileum adherent to and involving bladder wall. B. U. I. 8398.

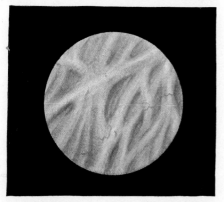

E. Trabeculation of bladder in case of prostatic hypertrophy. Note the heavy trabeculations.

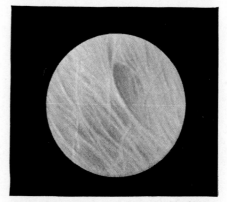

F. Trabeculation of bladder in case of tabes. Note the very fine character of trabeculations.

black to a shiny white, indicating calcareous deposits. Occasionally, when shallow and without much halo of inflammation, ulcers may be almost invisible.

In infections of long standing, the mucosa may be much thickened, and abnormalities in the form of masses of *granulation tissue, papilliform structures, polyps* (Plate VI, *f*), etc., appear. Some of these simulate neoplasms closely, so closely in fact that occasionally only microscopic examination can make the distinction. The papilliform structures are rare, but are seen to spring from many points, usually about an ulcer, branch little if any, and are not arranged in a single tree-like growth as are papillomata. Polyps may be large or small, single or multiple. Some are sessile, and resemble large blebs of bullous cystitis. Others are pedunculated, and may be plump or slender. They are frequently translucent, and blood-vessels can be seen through the thin, normal-looking epithelium. They are most common about the vesical orifice. Polyps are easily distinguished from papillomata because they are not branched. The exact nature of the so-called *cystitis cystica* is not altogether clear. It is probable that this name has been applied, by some to bullous cystitis, and by some to conditions with sessile polyps. Cystitis cystica properly speaking is a condition characterized by epithelium-lined cysts beneath the surface. Its appearance may resemble that of bullous cystitis, but the inflammation may be absent. The appearance of this lesion in the ureter is shown in Fig. 72.

The cystoscopic appearance in *submucous cystitis* may be entirely negative. If this is the case, one distends the bladder forcibly, under anesthesia if necessary (rare) to "bring out" the lesion. More often there will be visible irregular areas of localized reddening, and edema, with perhaps some ecchymotic spots (Plate XIV, *d*). There may be very shallow ulcers, scarcely more than excoriations. Even when lesions are thus visible, distention should be employed, as it usually shows them to be much more extensive than suspected. After the distention, it will be found that the thickened inelastic submucosa has split at certain places over the involved areas. These splits are shallow, and moderate hemorrhage takes place from them. A day or two later it will often be found that the splits have become small irregular, or linear ulcerations. Such ulcers, however, heal fairly rapidly, and one may be surprised by their disappearance, all symptoms persisting as before. If secondary infection has occurred, the other changes of bacterial cystitis may be superposed. The distention method, however, may be relied upon to disclose these lesions in practically all cases where they are present.

Areas of *leukoplakia* are quite unmistakable, having a smooth, pearly white surface. The rounded, elevated, yellowish nodules of *malakoplakia* are also, according to those who have seen them, unmistakable. Fenwick's *solitary ulcer* is chronic looking, with thickened borders and adherent membrane of exudate. It cannot be diagnosed by its cystoscopic appearance, but only by the exclusion of other conditions, such as tuberculosis, and by its amenability to treatment. It seems that the designation of "solitary" ulcer is hardly correct, as multiple ulcers having exactly similar characteristics may occur. Geraghty[1] believes that the disease is not specific, but merely a result of chronic inflammatory changes in the bladder; according to this view, chronic ulcerations sometimes seen on intravesical lobes of hypertrophied prostates would belong in the same class.

The diagnosis of cicatricial *contracture of the vesical orifice* is most important,

[1] Personal communication.

since this condition not only favors the continuance of a bladder infection, and renders treatment useless, but also subjects the patient to the danger of obstructive renal damage. For the cystoscopic diagnosis, the reader is referred to the section on Diagnosis under Benign Prostatic Hypertrophy, where all obstructive lesions at the vesical orifice are treated together, for the sake of convenience.

Complicating lesions may alter the appearance of cystitis. Trabeculation has already been mentioned. If multiple cellules with small orifices are present, they may be converted by inflammation practically into small abscesses. In such cases the cystitis is absolutely intractable; the visible mucus membrane is intensely congested and edematous, and it is very difficult to wash the bladder clean enough to get a clear view. The edema often conceals the orifices of the cellules, and the issue of pus from them may not be seen with the cystoscope. Occasionally the situation is not entirely clear until operation, when upon pressure, the pus will be seen flowing from the cellules. Small stones are often present in these cellules as well, and are very helpful in diagnosis since, while invisible at cystoscopy, they appear in the *x*-ray.

Diverticula in like manner form niduses of infection which maintain bladder inflammations. The presence of a diverticulum may often be suspected merely from the large quantity of purulent débris recovered on irrigating the bladder. The orifice is usually visible, though sometimes it may be concealed by edema and masses of pus. When it is possible to insert the cystoscope in the diverticulum, the degree and nature of the inflammation of its walls can be studied directly. Otherwise one must estimate it by the amount of pus recovered.

Intense cystitis on the surface of hypertrophied median *prostatic lobes* projecting into the bladder, with congestion, edema, bullæ, ulcers, hemorrhage, etc., may simulate neoplasm. The location and shape of the mass help in the diagnosis, and the practised eye learns to distinguish the inflammatory lesions, characterized especially by the smoothness and translucency of edema, from the more irregular and opaque-looking structures associated with neoplasm. The diagnosis is confirmed, however, by noting the changes which occur after catheter drainage and antiseptic irrigations have ameliorated the cystitis.

Cystitis is frequent in association with *bladder neoplasm*, and inflammatory changes always occur after treatment of any kind directed at the tumor. Here experience alone can be depended upon to identify the papillary structures or indurated areas of the tumor, often in the midst of an intense inflammatory reaction. The cystitis due to bacteria or following fulguration has the characters already described, and can be expected to subside in the course of time; that due to radium however is different. *Radium burns* heal very slowly, ulcerations sometimes persisting three to four months. Due to this chronicity, the edges may become indurated, and the base appears grayish and indolent. Surrounding the ulcer is a halo of congestion and edema. Correct diagnosis is often difficult, but one depends upon the observations made at the time of destruction of the tumor as to whether it was completely removed, and watches carefully during the period of healing of the radium ulcer for signs of renewed neoplastic growth.

Vesical *calculi* in most cases intensify cystitis. If the cystitis is alkaline, phosphatic deposits occur on the stone, and its growth becomes more rapid. It is doubtful if the pressure of stones causes ulceration, unless the bladder is completely filled by masses of calculi or a large single stone. Ulceration is frequent, however, and if the cystitis is alkaline, these ulcers will show phosphatic incrustations in addition to the calculi proper. This process often causes large quantities of sand or gravel to be present.

The x-ray is of no assistance in the diagnosis of cystitis proper, but very valuable with the complicating lesions. The plain x-ray discloses calculi in bladder, cellules, or diverticula, and the cystogram shows trabeculation, cellules, diverticula, the relaxed sphincter of a paralyzed bladder, and ureteral reflux or dilatation. In the case of large neoplasms or intravesical lobes, they may be revealed in cystograms taken with opaque media or air.

In the course of the routine examination of all patients, the examiner will learn the condition of the prostate and seminal vesicles on rectal palpation, and will have studied the prostatic and vesicular secretions. If marked infection is present here, and if there are no symptoms from the kidney regions and the phthalein excretion is normal, one may treat the prostatic and vesical infections in the hope that the amelioration of the former will bring about the cure of the latter. If complicating lesions of the bladder (obstruction, stone, neoplasm) are present, and if there is no sign of acute renal infection, one proceeds at once to the treatment of these lesions, in the expectation that the cystitis will improve after they have been removed. In any case, however, where the cystitis proves rebellious for any length of time, or where renal symptoms appear, one should proceed to study the kidneys by means of *ureteral catheterization*. That is, in any chronic cystitis which resists treatment we must assure ourselves that there is no focus of infection in the kidney, for if there is, treatment of the bladder alone is useless. One sometimes sees patients who have received bladder irrigations for years without improvement, in whom examination of the kidneys quickly shows the source of the trouble in a chronic pyelonephritis, calculus, etc. The renal studies are carried out by the technic described under Renal Infections, Renal Calculi, etc. The passage of ureteral catheters through the infected urine of cystitis to healthy kidneys is practically without danger, but one should not neglect to inject through the catheters a few cubic centimeters of some effective germicide (meroxyl, mercurochrome, etc.) as they are being withdrawn.

To recapitulate, cystitis is practically always *secondary*, with the possible exception of submucous cystitis, and the important thing, therefore, is to discover the *source of the infection*. This will be usually found in the kidneys, prostate, or vesicles, or there will be some complicating lesion in the bladder itself (obstruction, calculus, neoplasm). If these factors are ignored, local treatment of the cystitis is inevitably doomed to failure.

Occasionally after the cure of a chronic cystitis, the bladder will be *contracted* from the residual fibrosis, giving a frequency entirely without pain or discomfort. This should never be mistaken for a cystitis.

The diagnosis of *perivesical inflammation* depends on the history and the general and local examination of the patient. The cystoscope may show compression or contracture of the adjacent bladder wall.

The general signs of infection are present; *fever*, often with chills and sweats, and *leukocytosis*. There is not the prostration of acute perinephric inflammation, unless the process is far advanced or accompanied by extravasation. *Pain* is constant, and there will be *tenderness* in the corresponding localities. For the *prevesical region*, the abdomen is carefully palpated, and distention and free fluid

carefully noted, since, in traumatic cases, we are often not sure whether the peritoneum is involved. If there is such involvement, the usual signs of acute peritonitis will quickly dominate the picture. In the lower abdomen, tenderness is
outlined, *masses* felt for, and surface redness or swelling noted. There may be
muscular rigidity, but in the absence of peritonitis this is localized. Characteristically, the fulness is noted in the midline, or extending outward and upward
in one or both groins parallel with Poupart's ligament. Rarely signs of inflammation are seen at the umbilicus. *Fluctuation* may not be elicited, even when pus
is present, owing to the thick abdominal wall.

For the *retrovesical region*, examination must be per rectum. A large suppuration pushing upward retroperitoneally may be felt on abdominal palpation, but
smaller lesions will not be found unless the rectal examination is made. One
searches for tenderness, induration, and fluctuations, extending the finger upward
as far as possible. When the abscess is here, there is usually also painful and difficult defecation. The position of the lesion is determined by noting its relation
to the seminal vesicles and prostate. Bimanual palpatation, with one hand on the
abdomen, may be of assistance with lesions high up.

In certain cases the lesion cannot be located by palpation, especially when
low down in front, behind the pubis, or in the groins. In these cases the diagnosis
must rest on the history, the fever, the leukocyte count, and the symptoms of
intoxication. If the fever becomes hectic, suppuration is to be inferred. Occasionally the diagnosis is confirmed only on exploratory incision. If extravasation
is present, the course is more rapid and the tumefaction more pronounced. See
the section on Traumatism of the Bladder.

Urethra, Prostate, and Seminal Vesicles; Symptoms.—URETHRA.—The common symptoms of acute urethritis, regardless of the cause, are urethral *discharge*
and *burning* on urination. Less frequently there are *painful and persistent erections* and there may be slight *fever*, with chills.

In *gonorrheal urethritis* the incubation period, during which no symptoms are
noticed, may be from two to twelve days, five days being about the average. A
slight tickling or burning is first felt, then redness and congestion about the meatus.
At first discharge may be obtained only by compressing the urethra; soon, however, it becomes abundant enough to issue from the meatus spontaneously. It
is purulent, and usually quite thick. There may be no other symptoms, but usually
the passage of urine is painful. There is no frequency of urination at first, or
later, unless the inflammation extends to the vesical orifice or bladder.

Erections may be painful, and in some cases very persistent. If the penile
urethra is deeply involved and indurated it may, by its rigidity, cause the penis to
curve downward on erection. This condition of "chordee" is always very painful. It is occasionally complicated by trauma, with edema, hematoma, etc., the
result of the barbarous custom, among ignorant people, of "breaking the
chordee."

If *extension to the posterior urethra occurs*, there may be an increase in the discharge, frequency, and pain in the perineum. Inflammation in the region of the
prostate and sphincters causes pain to be especially marked at the end of urination. Other possible complications are *peri-urethral infection, seminal vesiculitis,
cystitis*, and *epididymitis*, described elsewhere. The surface of the glans and interior
of the prepuce may become infected, often with erosions and purulent discharge

(*balanoposthitis*). The inguinal glands may be enlarged and tender, and may suppurate (*bubo*).

Intense congestion of the prostatic urethra may give rise to *hematuria*, which is usually slight or moderate, and terminal. In rare cases there is hemorrhage from an acutely inflamed anterior urethra, which is characterized by its occurrence independent of voiding. When the patient does void, the blood is washed out of the urethra at the first gush, the remainder of the urine being free from it. In other cases the blood is only sufficient to give a slight reddish tinge to the pus.

The symptoms described above may be of any degree of severity. In certain cases, the discharge is slight and thin, and there are no other symptoms. In other cases the discharge, pain, and inflammation are intense, and the patient is acutely ill, with general malaise and definite fever. In general, however, fever of more than 1 or 1½ degrees indicates a complication. The *duration* of the acute symptoms is variable. They may disappear, rarely, in a few days, even without treatment; the average duration is from ten days to three weeks, and occasionally they persist for several weeks. In this latter group of cases reinfection, alcoholic indulgence, undue physical exertion, or even coitus, are often to be blamed, and complications are likely.

Acute urethritis may end by complete restoration to normal, but in a large percentage of cases becomes *chronic*. The chronic changes may be confined to the anterior portion, or may involve the whole urethra. The symptoms of acute inflammation disappear, but the discharge, instead of ceasing, becomes thinner, less purulent, and less profuse. In *chronic anterior urethritis*, there is no dysuria, but often there are sensations of tickling in the urethra, aching in the perineum, or an indefinite feeling of "weakness" in the genitalia and perineum. The discharge is often so slight that it is seen only in the morning (the "morning drop"). This is because it collects during the night, and in the daytime is washed away by urination before there is enough present to fill the urethra. It was once so common in the French army that it was called "la goutte militaire."

Chronic posterior urethritis is always associated with a greater or smaller degree of chronic prostatis, and the subject is discussed more fully under the latter heading. The principal symptom is again a chronic discharge or "morning drop," but this may be accompanied by pain, referred to the perineum, testis, or penis, and frequent and burning urination.

In the later stages of chronic urethritis frequency, difficulty, and dribbling, with diminishing size of stream indicate *stricture* formation, and may lead to complete retention. The urinary abnormalities with stricture are different from those of obstruction at the vesical orifice, and have already been discussed in the section on Obstructive Uropathy. A very characteristic symptom is the small stream, which may split and fork more than the normal stream. Dribbling at the end of urination comes from the gradual emptying of the distended, dilated urethra above the stricture. In late stages the urine comes only in drops. Sudden complete retention is not nearly so frequent as in prostatic hypertrophy, and usually occurs after unsuccessful attempts at instrumentation. Obstructive damage to the kidneys, with uremic symptoms, may occur, but is very rare, since in stricture the bladder, if it can empty at all, usually empties completely. Chronic urethritis is not very rare in women, and is often associated with trigonitis, the symptoms being frequent and painful urination.

In *prostatic cysts* the symptoms present in a series of 33 cases were frequency and difficulty of urination in 21 cases, complete retention of urine in 7 cases. Pain, indefinite in character, was present in some of the cases, not stated in others. The symptoms were not described in 2 cases, and in 4 cases no symptoms were produced by the cyst. The diagnosis was made by the cystoscope in 17 cases, by autopsy in 9, by suprapubic operation in 5, by endoscope in 1, and by rectal examination in 1.

PROSTATE.—Prostatitis can best be considered at this point, as it is so closely associated with posterior urethritis.

Acute prostatitis occurs generally as a sequel to acute gonorrheal urethritis, but it may also follow catheter or other non-specific urethritis. The symptoms are pain, fever, often with signs of general febrile intoxication, and painful and difficult urination. A pre-existent urethral discharge may be increased, or if the prostatic ducts are occluded, as in *abscess* formation, the discharge may be markedly decreased. The pain is usually severe, and is usually located in the perineum and rectum. Referred pain is uncommon. The pain is markedly increased on defecation. The fever may be high, and accompanied with chills and sweats. Not infrequently the patient is quite prostrated, with anorexia, vomiting, or mental confusion. There is marked *dysuria*, and a pre-existent dysuria is always increased. As the prostate becomes more congested and swollen, *urination* is *difficult*, and *complete retention* is by no means uncommon. Since this obstruction is at the vesical orifice, it means residual urine, and acute functional damage to kidneys may occur, with uremic symptoms. Indeed, the vomiting and mental confusion mentioned above may well be uremic, though no doubt in some cases, a generalized urinary infection with pyelitis or pyelonephritis may exist. One is unable to determine this, except by palpation of the kidneys, as no instrumentation is permissible in the acute stage. If abscess formation occurs, there is no distinctive change in the symptoms, but the history of a sudden discharge of a quantity of pus, with immediate relief of symptoms, indicates that an abscess has ruptured into the urethra or bladder. Suppuration may also be accompanied by a change of the fever to a hectic type.

Chronic prostatitis is an exceedingly common disease. It is often entirely without symptoms, and may be discovered accidentally, and it is usually associated with vesiculitis. The prostate may be the source of a persistent *urethral discharge*. It may take on any character, and may be indistinguishable from the morning drop of chronic urethritis. It is oftenest watery and turbid, when it is known as a "gleety" discharge, but may be purulent. "Prostatorrhea" and "spermatorrhea" were formerly supposed to be associated with prostatitis, but the accuracy of this supposition is doubtful. The majority of cases of prostatitis, even the most severe, do not show these symptoms, but cases having them often show signs of prostatic infection.

Many cases of chronic prostatitis are not associated with urethral discharge or even gluing of the meatus. The urine may, however, contain *shreds* in all 3 glasses. Where the inflammation does not involve the prostatic urethra, but is confined to the prostatic ducts, shreds (of the "comma" variety) are often seen in the last urine voided, having been squeezed out of the ducts during the final spasmodic contractions of micturition.

Pain and *abnormal sensations* of various sorts are often associated with prostatitis. Pain may be subdivided as follows: (*a*) Dysuria, at the beginning, during, or at the end of urination; (*b*) local pain—prostatic, deep urethra, vesical neck, penis, perineum, rectum; (*c*) referred pain—to various regions of the body according to the dicta of Head.

The table of Young, Stevens, and Geraghty[1] may well be reproduced here. In 358 cases of prostatitis, they found the following referred pains:

TABLE 14

PAIN IN CHRONIC PROSTATITIS

		Cases.
In the back (low lumbar)		64
Over kidney region { right side, 5 / left side, 1 / both, 2 }		8
Simulating renal colic, 10 cases { right side / left side / not stated }		6 / 2 / 2
Suprapubic		22
In neck of bladder		4
In penis or urethra		14
In groin (one or both)		18
In testicles (one or both)		18
Over sacrum		5
In buttocks		2
In hips (one or both)		10
In thighs		12
In the knee (one or both)		4
In the legs (one or both)		4
Simulating sciatica		5
In perineum		35
In rectum		13

Sensory symptoms may be such that they do not reach the dignity of real pain, when they are described as sensations of fulness, gnawing, constriction, burning, or coldness. They may have the same sort of distribution as the pain.

All of the pains referred to may be constant or intermittent. Sometimes asymptomatic periods of several weeks may be interspersed in the course of a chronic prostatitis.

As noted in the table, *pain in the lower back* is the most frequent and most characteristic referred pain in chronic prostatitis (Figs. 99–101). It is often considered by the laity a sign of "kidney trouble." It is a very distinctive feature of this pain that it is at its worst when the patient arises in the morning, and wears off in the course of the day, while arthritic pains usually become worse as activity increases.

The prevalence of referred pain from the prostate is not surprising, since its innervation is entirely sympathetic and parasympathetic. Head[2] has shown that fibers ending in the prostate arise all the way from the tenth dorsal to the third sacral segments, so that it is possible for prostatic pain to be referred to any point innervated by any of the corresponding spinal nerves. This would include the entire body below the diaphragm.

[1] Johns Hopkins Hospital Reports, 1906, xiii, 271–384.

[2] Studies in Neurology, London, 1920. See also Sherrington, Integrative Action of the Nervous System, New York, 1906.

A possible exception must be made in the case of pains simulating renal colic, which may possibly be related to actual obstruction of the ureter following seminal vesiculitis. The local pain may be slight, or severe and persistent.

In chronic prostato-vesiculitis there are often no *urinary symptoms*. Frequency, dysuria, and urgency, if present, are usually associated with inflammatory changes involving the vesical orifice and trigone. Frequency, difficulty, and dribbling suggest cicatricial contracture of the vesical orifice or prostatic urethra. In the latter case, complete retention may eventually occur, and there may be the symptoms of obstructive damage to the bladder and kidneys. The former

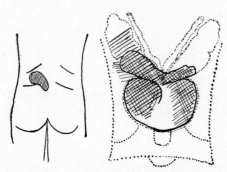

FIG. 99.—Rectal findings and location of pain in the left side of the back. The induration of the prostate and seminal vesicles is much more marked on the left side. History of chronic gonorrhea for seven years. Symptoms were chronic urethral discharge, pain in the back, and occasional pain in the right inguinal region. Prostatic secretion contained pus. B. U. I. 935.

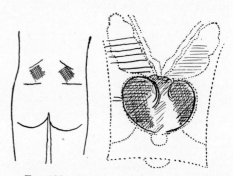

FIG. 100.—Location of pain in the back due to prostatitis. There was a history of chronic gonorrhea. The prostate is seen to be markedly indurated, but not enlarged. Secretion contained a large amount of pus. B. U. I. 1185.

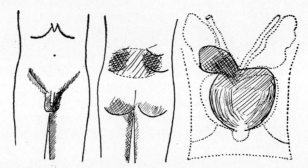

FIG. 101.—Rectal finding and distribution of pain due to prostatitis. History of chronic gonorrhea for three years. Symptoms are morning drop, loss of sexual power, and pain in the back, buttocks, inner side of thighs, groins, and scrotum, as indicated in diagram. No discharge. Prostatic secretion composed mostly of pus. B. U. I. 935.

symptoms, which are irritative in character, may be slight or severe, but, as a rule, only slight discomfort, such as burning on urination, is present. Pain on urination is variable, and has no distinguishing feature on which to rely.

In view of the fact that the prostate is essentially a sexual gland, it is remarkable that *sexual symptoms* are not more common and severe than they are.

In considering abnormalities of the sexual function, one must take into account the great importance of psychologic factors. It is undoubtedly true that in many cases of the most extensive chronic prostatitis, with large amounts of pus in the prostate, desire, erection, and ejaculation are entirely unaffected, or even, for a time, increased. In those cases with sexual deficiencies, neurotic tendencies are often noted. Further still, many individuals with entirely normal genitalia suffer from the greatest variety of sexual symptoms, which can only have a psychic basis. Persons of introspective nature may become impotent, the trouble dating definitely from a single instance of failure, due usually to (1) premature ejaculation following exceptional sexual excitement, (2) failure of erection following too prolonged excitement, or (3) failure of erection or ejaculation, or both, following alcoholic intoxication, fatigue, worry, or preoccupation. In many cases this type of impotence is cured at once by a few words of sensible advice from an authoritative source coupled with tonic treatment. Where the mental state is less stable, more subtle influences may have far-reaching results. Among them may be mentioned worry over early masturbation, or over fancied physical deficiencies, and feelings of sexual inferiority, due often to association with a very zealous partner. Lastly, the existence, even at some past time, of a diseased condition, such as urethritis or varicocele, often leads to impotence from worry.   Unwise advice, lay or medical, exaggerates this condition. Nothing is more disturbing to the average patient than the fear of the loss of sexual power.

On the other hand, definite pathologic conditions in the prostate and vesicles undoubtedly do cause sexual symptoms. In any acute case, or in cases associated with severe pain or other troubles, sexual activity ceases—and the patient may forget all about it. In other cases, pain is increased by coitus, or occurs only on coitus. Inflammation sometimes increases genital irritability, so that nocturnal emissions are more frequent, ejaculation more premature than normal, or erection more frequent and persistent than normal (Fig. 102). Such erections are sometimes painful.

The physician should attempt to obtain from the patient's history an idea of the significance of his sexual symptoms, and as to what elements in them have basis in local inflammation, and what are purely psychogenic.

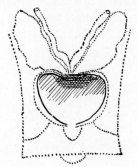

The *subsequent course* depends largely on the source of the symptoms. As the prostatitis improves, symptoms with a real pathologic basis will improve. We know that quite extensive changes of a fibrotic nature, even with occlusion of the ejaculatory ducts, do not preclude normal sexual function. The course of the psychogenic symptoms depends on the malignancy of the psychic disorder. It may be that advice, encouragement, and sympathy will effect an early cure; it may be

Fig.   102.—Involvement, confined largely to the upper median portion of the prostate. History of gonorrhea three years before.   The symptoms were excessive nocturnal emissions, no pain. B. U. I. 9777.

that only the most expert psychiatric treatment will bring about an improvement, or it may be that a severe psychosis is present, and that there is no means whatsoever of arresting its progress.

SEMINAL VESICLES.—Since *seminal vesiculitis* so frequently accompanies prostatitis, and since seminal vesiculitis practically never occurs without prostatitis, it is not possible to differentiate accurately the symptoms peculiar to diseases of either. Urethral discharge and local and referred pains may occur with vesiculitis much as described for prostatitis. Hematospermia, pyospermia, painful emissions or coitus, suggest disease of the ejaculatory ducts, ampullæ, or seminal vesicles, as do recurrent attacks of epididymitis. Renal colic may rarely result from inclusion of the ureter in scar tissue about the tip of the vesicle, but we have seen several cases of typical "renal colic" which were simply referred pains from the prostate. In 1 case blood from a congested verumontanum made the picture more suggestive of renal calculus.

Infections of the urethra, prostate, and seminal vesicles may *spread to the surrounding tissues*. Indurated and painful *nodules* occur along the course of the urethra. There may be *urethral rupture*, sometimes, but not always, with formation of urinary *fistulæ*. If the inflammation involves the corpora of the penis, as it seldom does, painful and continuous complete or partial erection may occur. Suppuration is frequent in *peri-urethral inflammation*. It may involve penis, scrotum, or perineum. The direction of spread of the various kinds of *abscesses* is given in the section on Pathology. A sudden flow of pus from the urethra may indicate intra-urethral rupture of an abscess. Fever and leukocytosis occur. Pain is usually severe, but may be so slight that attention is not directed to the site of the abscess. We have noted this in the case of a patient with a retention catheter, and it should be kept in mind, as it may involve serious delay in discovering the source of the fever and toxemia. *Peri-urethral abscess* is practically never accompanied by extravasation unless there is a stricture distal to it. In this case the symptoms of stricture, already described, will precede the pain and tumefaction of the peri-urethral inflammation.

Periprostatic inflammation, giving symptoms, seldom occurs except when a prostatic abscess ruptures through the capsule. The previous symptoms of inflammation are intensified, though a urinary retention may be relieved. Pain and swelling may be noted in the ischiorectal fossa. Rectal symptoms are increased with painful and difficult defecation. If the extension has been upward—a rare occurrence—symptoms of peritoneal irritation will be noted. A sudden discharge of pus per ano indicates rupture into the rectum.

Extension to the perivesicular tissues is more common in vesicular infections, but has no distinguishing symptoms. If *abscess* formation occurs, or if a vesicular abscess ruptures posteriorly, the symptoms will be like those of retroprostatic abscess. On the bladder side frequency and dysuria may result from an extension of the inflammation to the wall of the base of the bladder. Very common are the adhesions which bind the prostate or vesicles to surrounding structures and which lead to a great variety of local or referred nervous symptoms—sciatica, lumbago, pain in hip, or sacrum, or sacro-iliac joint, or in the buttocks, etc.

Infections of the urethra, prostate, and bladder may give rise, as portals of entry, to various *metastatic infections*, some with symptoms suggesting the source. Acute arthritis, with great pain, redness, and swelling, involving various joints in succession, especially the knee, sternoclavicular, and mandibular joints, occurring in the course of a gonorrheal urethritis, is probably a gonorrheal arthritis. Gonorrheal septicemia and endocarditis occur, and are not really so very rare. The symptoms are not specific for this organism, but the history will usually give the clue. Chronic arthritis of various sorts, as well as other obscure disorders, are ascribed to chronic prostatic and vesicular infections, often without convincing proof. However, in view of this possibility, and in the absence of other discoverable portals of entry, we often feel obliged to apply the therapeutic test.

In the pelvis itself, urogenital infections may be complicated by *thrombophle-*

bitis of the prostatic and vesical venous plexuses. *Embolism* may occur, or the process may spread, especially to the saphenous and femoral veins, with the characteristic pain and swelling in the affected leg.

Urethra, Prostate, and Seminal Vesicles; Diagnosis.—The proper diagnosis of infections of the urethra, prostate, and seminal vesicles depends on local examinations which, to be complete, must be carried out conscientiously, and according to a regular systematic sequence.

In acute cases some of the maneuvers employed in chronic cases must be omitted. Instrumentation and all but the gentlest palpation are contraindicated.

In *acute urethritis*, if non-specific, the cause will usually be apparent from the history—retention catheter, irritant injection, traumatism, etc. Microscopic examination of the urethral discharge and of the urine, voided in 3 glasses, will usually reveal the causative bacterium or the absence of the gonococcus.

The *discharge* is first examined, before urination, and treatment should be deferred until all possible microscopic data have been secured. A number of smears of the discharge are made—at least three. These should be studied after *staining* by Gram's method. The routine use of a simple stain, as methylene-blue, for this purpose is to be condemned, as Gram-positive cocci not infrequently simulate gonococci morphologically. Where any doubt exists, a *culture* should be made by the method of Swartz, which is simple and practical. This is especially important, as it has been conclusively shown that Gram-negative diplococci which are not gonococci do occur in the urethra, prostate, and vesicles.

After the discharge has been studied and any *visible lesions of the external genitalia* noted, the patient voids, dividing the urine equally in *three conical glasses*. The first glass contains any discharge or shreds which may have been washed out of the urethra. The second glass is free of urethral pus and shreds, and, if the bladder urine contains no pus or shreds, the second glass is clear. The last urine voided into a third glass also passes through a clean swept urethra, but in the final spasmodic act of micturition, pus and shreds may be squeezed out of the ducts of the prostate and appear in the third glass. If, however, the production of pus in the posterior urethra has been considerable it will generally have passed back into the bladder, thus clouding the urine, which when voided will be cloudy in all three glasses (Fig. 103). The same is true with cystitis and pyelitis, all three glasses of urine being cloudy. Cloudiness may be due to phosphates or carbonates in the urine; they will disappear on acidifying with dilute acetic acid. It is always wise to confirm the purulent nature of a cloud by *microscopic examination*. If no discharge has been obtained, even on compressing the urethra, owing to its small quantity, it may be washed out in the first glass, and may be studied by centrifugalizing the urine. The glass test may be used in women, where only two glasses are necessary, owing to the absence of the prostate. The vagina must be cleansed by a douche before the urine is voided.

The *external genitalia* are carefully *palpated* for nodules of peri-urethral inflammation, buboes, epididymitis, etc.

Rectal examination may be carried out even in apparently simple acute gonorrhea, but should be gentle. The prostate of acute prostatitis is enlarged, and may be tense and exquisitely tender, but is usually smooth. If an abscess of some size is present, fluctuation can usually be elicited. Any abscess between the prostate and rectum, originating in either organ, may be mistaken for prostatic abscess. In such cases, the outline of the prostate cannot be made out.

Acute vesiculitis is characterized by a distended, tender vesicle. In acute gonorrhea massage should be avoided, but later purulent secretion can be expressed and will usually appear at the urethral meatus. In other cases the duct is occluded. If perivesiculitis is present, the tumefaction is more extensive, and the contours of the vesicle are obscured. The prostate can be outlined below the vesicles if not involved. For abscess we have to depend on fluctuation.

It is, of course, important to distinguish cases of *gonorrheal urethritis*. Gonorrhea may be present where the lesion began as a chemical or traumatic urethritis. The two conditions most apt to give rise to serious mistakes are syphilis and tuber-

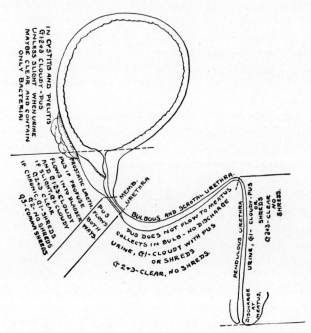

Fig. 103.—The "water-sheds of the urethra." Diagram intended to show the direction which pus will follow along the urethra. In pendulous urethra secretions gravitate toward meatus. Pus produced in bulbous urethra may not pass over suspensory ligament. Pus produced in prostatic urethra is prevented from passing downward by external sphincter, and, if considerable, flows into bladder. The three-glass test for these various regions is indicated.

culosis. Certain cases of tuberculosis have a purulent urethral discharge as the first symptom, and are sometimes treated for a long time as gonorrhea. Only vigilance can detect them. Undue frequency, dysuria, and hematuria, or renal pain, and failure to follow the normal evolution of gonorrhea, should arouse suspicion. Intra-urethral chancres give rise to urethral discharge, which is usually thin and milky, and contains the Treponema pallidum. The chancre can be felt along the course of the urethra as an indurated and painless nodule. Intra-urethral chancre may come on in the course of a gonorrhea, when it is not difficult to overlook them. Small chancres in the midst of a gonorrheal balanoposthitis may also easily escape observation.

Patients with *chronic infections* may come under observation with the condition already established, it may develop from an acute condition while under treatment, or it may be detected by the thorough examination always carried out before discharging acute urethritis as cured. The examinations to be described may, therefore, be taken as a model for the procedure to be used to determine whether a cure of acute urethritis has taken place.

The *urethral discharge* and *urine* are studied as described for acute urethritis. Urine from the third glass should, however, be centrifugalized and the sediment studied *microscopically* to determine the presence of urinary infection. *Cultures* from the urine are also made if indicated. *Shreds* are "fished," spread on slides, and examined for pus and organisms.

After *inspection* and *palpation* of the *external genitalia* and *perineum*, one proceeds to the *rectal examination*. The rectal examination should not be made before the urine is voided, as the urinary picture is obscured by prostatic secretion pressed into the urethra or bladder, while the prostatic secretion is contaminated with urethral discharge. It is made just after voiding, when the urethra has been washed clean by the urine.

The examiner must be thoroughly familiar with the normal anatomy of the prostatic region. The patient bends forward and rests the elbows on the knees.

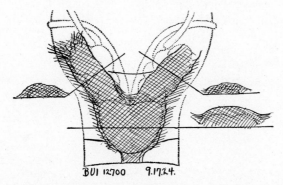

BUI 12700   9.17.24.

Fig. 104.—Rectal finding in an extreme case of chronic prostatitis and seminal vesiculitis. History of chronic gonorrhea for eleven years. Chronic arthritis for nine months.   Note how cross-section of the vesicle may be indicated as well as of the prostate.   The induration is extensive, but has nowhere extreme hardness and irregularity characteristic of carcinoma or tuberculosis.   Treated by intravenous medication, with marked improvement.

It is best first to insert the left index-finger directly in the midline as far as possible, noting various landmarks which will be useful in keeping oriented later on. The distance of the upper and lower borders of the prostate from the anus (giving the length of the prostate) can be noted, and put on the chart (Fig. 104). A chart similar to the one pictured should be used for recording the results of all rectal examinations. The outlines of the various organs are drawn in, and the varying degrees of induration indicated by shading as shown. The finger is then passed around the prostate on either side, noting its size and contour, and whether adhesions are present. On reaching the apex, the membranous urethra is investigated in the same way. Then proceeding to the seminal vesicles, one notes enlargement, induration, nodularity, compressibility, and adhesions, as far up as one can reach. It should be remembered that the vesicles slope backward as well as outward and upward from the prostate, so that they are palpated with the tip of the finger rather than the ball. The notch between the vesicles is palpated for adhesions and induration, and at the same time induration or tenderness of the base of the bladder can be noted. One attempts to distinguish the ampullæ of the vasa deferentia, but they are often covered by the vesicles or obscured by coalescence with them. Indurated glands in the vicinity of the vesicles are searched for. Returning to the prostate, firm pressure is exerted, beginning at the outer upper margin, and rolling the finger toward the midline rather than stroking it. This serves to express the prostatic contents, and also allows the consistence of the organ to be determined. One notes the depth and contour of the median furrow, and the location and extent of any areas of induration present. The secretion is collected on a slide as it appears at the urethral meatus. It may be necessary to strip the vesicles and prostate vigorously and to force the secretion from the prostatic into the bulbous urethra by massaging the urethra from the perineum downwards. One may attempt to separate the prostatic and vesicular secretions

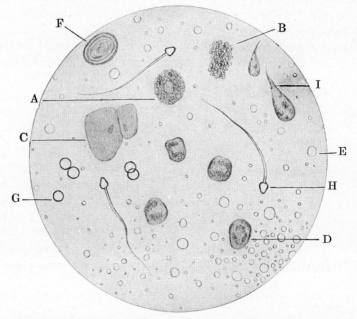

FIG. 105.—Prostatic secretion with normal and pathologic cells from a case of mild chronic prostatitis: A, Prostatic epithelial cell (compound granular cell); B, same, in which nucleus has disappeared; C, flat epithelial cells; D, pus-cell; E, lecithin bodies; F, corpus amylaceum; G, red blood-cell; H, spermatozoön; I, mucus.

by exerting no pressure on the vesicles until after the prostate has been emptied and the secretion collected. The urethra may then be irrigated and the vesicular secretion pressed out in the same way, but it is usually better to reserve this for the next visit. The results of this maneuver are not very satisfactory.

The normal *prostatic secretion* is fluid and milky. The quantity obtained varies. The reaction is very slightly alkaline. Microscopically, it contains a few epithelial cells, lecithin bodies (Fig. 105), which are round, refractile structures, varying in size, but all much smaller than any of the cells, and "compound granular cells," which are usually without nucleus and contain a mass of round refractile granules or droplets. Sometimes the cytoplasm has entirely disappeared, and one sees only the mass of granules. These cells are prostatic epithelial cells, which after desquamation, normally undergo a fatty degeneration, very reminiscent of the process in the mammary gland in the formation of milk. The fat or myelin droplets coalesce as the cell grows older, so that they become quite large. They stain with Sudan III or Scharlach R., but disappear entirely in preparations dried, fixed, and stained, since they are dissolved by the fixative, or melted by heat. They have, therefore, no pathologic significance. Prostatic secretion is usually mixed with some seminal vesicle contents, so that spermatozoa are to be expected and should show motility. Small corpora amylacea are infrequently seen.

The *contents of the vesicles* and *ampullæ* is characterized by being mucoid and tenacious; it does not mix at once with the prostatic secretion, and gelatinous masses of it may be seen in the fluid obtained by massage. Within these masses are normally groups of spermatozoa which show little or no motility until they are free from the mucoid material. There are no characteristic cellular elements. In normal secretion the lecithin bodies preponderate greatly; granule cells are few, spermatozoa vary according to the source of the fluid.

The examination is made of *fresh, unstained* material, using a cover-glass and the high dry lens. *Stained specimens* are useful only for bacteria, and must, therefore, be taken with precautions against urethral or urinary contamination. Naked eye examinations are inaccurate and should not be depended on. Not infrequently in the secretion expressed at the first examination only normal cells are seen, whereas in the second and third "strippings" many leucocytes are found. This fact shows the importance of not remaining content with a single test, especially if areas of induration are present or if the prostate is suspected of harboring a chronic infection.

The *pathologic elements* to be sought are pus-cells, red blood-cells, and bacteria. (See Fig. 105.)   In cases of sterility, absence (azoöspermia) or non-motility of spermatozoa is to be noted. The question of the presence of pus-cells in normal prostatic fluid has been much discussed. There is little doubt that polymorphonuclears will appear in the secretion of uninfected prostates after one or two vigorous massages, and possibly also after great sexual excitement. In routine work, therefore, the presence of a small number of pus-cells, ordinarily expressed as 8 to 10 per high-power field, is considered of little significance. On the other hand, it is possible that where the infiltration is largely interstitial, the pus-cells will not appear in the secretion. In general, however, there will be little doubt, and the presence of numerous polymorphonuclear leukocytes is of diagnostic importance. Sometimes in a secretion otherwise practically normal, definite clumps of pus-cells will be found on searching. These indicate definitely an inflammation. A drop of 1 per cent. acetic acid may be added at the edge of the cover-slip to bring out the nuclei.

Pus from the vesicles can often be identified by finding it entangled in the mucoid masses. In other cases the inflammation dissolves and dilutes the mucoid material, so that the distinction cannot be made.

Red blood-cells not infrequently result from massage, so that their significance is small, unless present in quantity, or in semen which has been ejaculated.

Bacteria are not found nearly as often as one would expect, at any rate in stained smears. Large amounts of pus may be present without demonstrable organisms. The statements made concerning the results of cultures are conflicting. Nogues and DuRupt[1] found Gram-negative diplococci, which they identified as gonococci,

[1] Journal d'Urologie, 1923, xv, 133–136.

in 80 per cent. of cases of chronic prostatitis following gonorrhea. White and Gradwohl[1] confirm these findings. The figures are astonishing; Nogues and Du-Rupt admit that the organism they find, while like gonococcus in all other respects, grows much more luxuriantly, and survives at room temperature. They call it an altered, avirulent gonococcus. Also from clinical observation the wives of patients with this organism do not contract gonorrhea. Player, Lee-Brown, and Mathé,[2] on the other hand, found the expressed fluid sterile in 57 of 118 cases, while in the rest only 2 harbored Gram-negative diplococci, and these were identified as Micrococcus catarrhalis. The remainder were principally "B. coli" and hemolytic streptococcus. The cultures were made with great care to avoid contamination.

In our laboratory we have recovered gonococcus from prostatic fluid but rarely. Surely the statement that it occurs in 80 per cent. of chronic prostatitis must be taken with great reserve.

The fact that bacteria are frequently undemonstrable in prostatic fluid in cases of chronic prostatitis led older observers to assume that there was an abac-

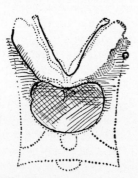

FIG. 106.—Marked prostatitis with very extensive adhesions about the prostate and seminal vesicles. Phlebolith on right side. History of recurrent gonorrhea. Symptoms were constant pain in the back, but no discharge. B. U. I. 952.

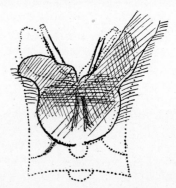

FIG. 107.—Very extensive involvement with enlargement and induration of the prostate, more marked in the upper part, and of both vesicles with marked adhesions. The ampullæ are also definitely thickened. Denies gonorrhea. Recurrent febrile attacks. Severe pain in right lumbar region, less marked between attacks. Slight dysuria and frequency. B. U. I. 1238.

terial inflammation. This now seems illogical, and we believe that bacteria are always present in true prostatitis, but may be few in number and concealed in the stroma or in occluded ducts. Gonococci may persist in the prostate for considerable time, but the consensus of opinion is that they die out in three years or less, if no reinfection occurs. Secondary invaders are frequent, and often survive after the gonococcus can no longer be found.

Where suspicion exists, an acid-fast stain should be made. Search should be careful, as tubercle bacilli when present are usually in small numbers.

The results of the examination of the expressed fluid are taken in conjunction with the *findings on palpation*. Prostatitis is appreciated as *areas of induration*, and as *adhesions* between the prostate, seminal vesicles, and surrounding tissues (levator ani muscles, rectum, etc.). The induration is often most marked along the

[1] Journal of Urology, 1921, vi, 303–319.
[2] Ibid., 1923, x, 377–385.

lateral borders of the gland, and the adhesions most frequent at the upper outer angles of the gland. Enlarged Cowper's glands are sometimes palpable just above the triangular ligament. A few typical diagrams are shown, cases of tuberculosis and carcinoma being shown for comparison (Figs. 106–112). The prostate may be somewhat *nodular*, but the extreme degrees of nodularity and induration suggest tuberculosis or carcinoma. It is infrequent indeed to find a prostate in which some slight abnormalities cannot be noted after the age of twenty-five or thirty, consequently we believe that one should be conservative in diagnosis; usually where the prostate is causing any serious trouble, the pathologic findings will be distinct and unmistakable.

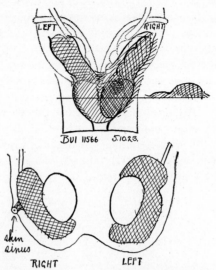

In some cases the normal *seminal vesicles* are not palpable, but many perfectly normal vesicles are easily felt, especially when distended. If a vesicle feels tense and full, but cannot be emptied on massage, obstruction of the duct is indicated. Inflammation is shown by *induration, enlargement, irregularity, adhesions,* and *tenderness* (Figs. 110–112). Here again definite findings should be required.

FIG. 108.—Rectal and scrotal findings in a case of bilateral genital tuberculosis. Entire tract is involved, but the findings are much more marked in the right seminal vesicle and right half of the prostate. Patient had had pulmonary tuberculosis for two and one-half years. Testicular swelling for three months. Radical removal of epididymes, vasa, seminal vesicles, and part of the prostate was done. One year later patient was much improved, with no urinary symptoms.

While many cases of arthritis have benefited by operations on the vesicles, an even larger number has failed to do so, often because the diagnosis of vesiculitis was based on conviction more than on definite findings.

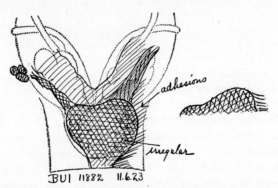

FIG. 109.—Involvement of the entire prostate, which is enlarged, indurated, and nodular in carcinoma of the prostate. The seminal vesicles are enlarged and corded, but do not show stony induration of actual involvement. Indurated lymph-nodes are felt at the tip of the left seminal vesicle. Membranous urethra markedly thickened. No urinary symptoms. Pain in the back for two years. x-Ray showed bony metastases. No operation.

Unless the above described examinations have been entirely negative, the condition of the *interior of the urethra* is now investigated by means of the "*bougie à boule,"* selecting a good-sized instrument, about No. 18 or 20 French. The bulb is introduced to the bladder, and then withdrawn slowly by a series of short, rhythmical pulls. Irregularities and areas of induration impart through the bulb a sense of resistance as it passes over them, very distinct from the smoothness of the normal mucosa. The external sphincter gives some resistance, not to be mistaken for a stricture. If a stricture of any severity exists, the bougie of course cannot be inserted past it. This gives an idea of its location, while smaller instruments, tried in succession, give an idea of its caliber. When areas of induration are located, they can be palpated between the fingers and the bulb of the bougie.

A quiescent infection can sometimes be stirred up, and organisms, gonococci or other, obtained for smear or culture. This procedure is useful in confirming cure, or determining the organism concerned in a chronic infection. The methods employed are: (1) Passage of sounds, (2) moderately irritating injections or irrigations, (3) drinking of beer or other alcoholic drinks, and (4) coitus. In general,

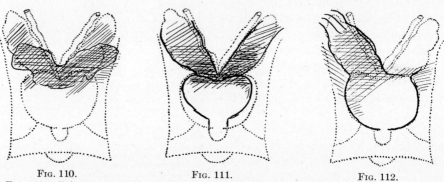

Fig. 110.   Fig. 111.   Fig. 112.

Fig. 110.—Enlargement and induration of the lower part of both seminal vesicles and the upper part of prostate. History of chronic gonorrhea for ten years. The symptoms were morning drop, weakened sexual power, and occasional prostatorrhea. Marked adhesions are also present around inflamed areas in this case. B. U. I. 822.

Fig. 111.—Induration in the upper part of the prostate and the lower part of both seminal vesicles. History of chronic gonorrhea for fifteen years. Symptoms were slight pain in back, slight urethral discharge, prostatorrhea, and faulty erections. B. U. I. 1138.

Fig. 112.—Moderate induration of the left lobe of the prostate and enlargement and induration of the left seminal vesicle. History of gonorrhea thirty-eight and eighteen years before. Symptoms were chills, fever, dysuria, and uncomfortable sensations in the perineum. Urethral stricture was also present. B. U. I. 1178.

these methods are not to be recommended; usually the instrumentation of treatment will suffice without any special measures.

Urethroscopy is not done as a routine; it is reserved where the other examinations do not clear up the diagnosis. The instrument, of whatever type, is usually inserted to the bladder, and the examination begun at the vesical orifice. One notes congestion, edema, ulcer, granulations, polyps, leukoplakia, cysts, etc. In chronic inflammations, localized infiltrations, interpreted by some as hyperplastic lymphoid follicles, may sometimes give a characteristic nodular appearance to the posterior urethra with intact mucosa. The size and shape of the verumontanum is observed. With probes one locates the utricle and ejaculatory ducts, and strictures can then be detected in the lowermost 3 cm. of the ducts by resistance to the probe, and "hang" on its withdrawal. Opaque media can be injected in the vesicles, and x-ray pictures made (Fig. 113). The utriculus masculinus is investigated in the same way. Its depth is noted, pus coming from it is observed, and smears can be made.

In the remainder of the urethra the procedure is similar. Often the infiltrated and indurated areas are well seen. The mouths of infected glands of Littré and urethral sinuses are rarely seen when normal on account of their small size, but when infected are often clearly visible. Urethroscopy is particulary valuable in women with chronic urinary symptoms, since chronic urethritis, with granulations, polyps, etc., is so often associated with trigonitis and bacilluria. (See Plate IV.)

The *complement-fixation test* for gonorrhea is of no value for acute urethritis, and it fails in a certain number of cases of chronic urethritis and prostatitis. A negative test is, therefore, inconclusive. Positive tests are oftenest obtained in deeper invasions of the disease, as pyelitis, arthritis, endocarditis, and septicemia. Caution is necessary, as syphilis may cause a positive reaction. Consequently, unless the Wassermann is negative, a positive complement-fixation test is inconclusive.

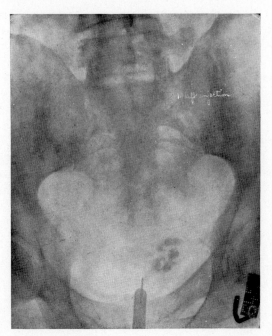

Fig. 113.—Vesiculogram. Note urethroscopic tube; injecting needle in left ejaculatory duct; left vesicle and vas injected with thorium nitrate, 15 per cent.

In most of the cases where absence of other evidence makes the complement-fixation test most desirable, it is difficult or impossible to confirm positively, at any later time, the results of the test. We believe, therefore, that while this test may furnish corroborative evidence in cases of chronic vesiculitis, prostatitis, pyelitis, arthritis, salpingitis, etc., it should not be depended upon alone.

If the above series of examinations is carefully made, one will usually know just where the infective process is located in the lower urogenital tract. Rebellious infections which resist ordinary treatment do so because they are intrenched in some place where they are not reached. The places especially culpable in this regard are (1) glands of Littré (urethral glands), para-urethral sinuses, and lacuna magna, if present; (2) Cowper's glands; (3) utricle; (4) prostate, and (5) seminal vesicles. In addition, productive changes, such as granulations, polyps, and indurated ulcers, may provide the resistant focus of infection. If any such focus is present, it must be located, otherwise treatment is aimless and usually ineffective.

At the same time, the *upper tract* is not to be forgotten; the prostate may be secondarily involved if the kidney is producing an infected urine—so also more rarely the urethra, though it is much more resistant. Renal infection or cystitis may be secondary to chronic prostatitis or vesiculitis—whether by extension, ascending infection, or through the blood-stream we usually cannot tell. Obstruction, as from contracture of the vesical orifice, aids ascending infection. Pain in the loin or persistently purulent bladder urine should indicate study of the kidneys by ureteral catheterization. In case of doubt, this examination should not be long deferred, as it is advantageous to neither patient nor doctor to treat a renal infection by prostatic massage.

Chronic prostatitis is the rule in *benign prostatic hypertrophy* after instruments have been used. It is of no significance unless severe, when fibrotic changes may make operation difficult. Acute infections and abscesses are fortunately rare, but must always be ruled out by a careful rectal examination when unexplained fever and toxemia occur in the preoperative period.

Boyd[1] has called attention to acute infections of the seminal vesicles after prostatectomy, with or without epididymitis. Rectal palpation shows a distended, tender vesicle, and pressure will force out a quantity of purulent material into the wound, urethra, or bladder, according to the conditions present at the moment.

The presence of *sexual symptoms* complicates the diagnosis, and often, in addition, produces difficult problems in the personal relations with the patients. We feel that new conceptions of these syndromes are urgently needed, and that the relations existing between sexual symptoms and local urogenital disease should be reviewed in the light of recent psychiatric advances.

We may first analyze roughly the various sexual symptoms from the point of view of the mechanism by which they are produced. The symptoms are as follows:

Painful erection.

Painful ejaculation.

Hematospermia.

Incomplete erection.

Absence of erection.

Premature ejaculation.

Excessive nocturnal emissions.

Delayed ejaculation.

Absence of ejaculation.

Flaccidity and coldness of genitalia.

Deficient or absent sexual desire.

Of this list, painful erection, painful ejaculation, and hematospermia, are the most apt to be the result of definite local pathologic conditions. Deficiencies in sexual desire, when not the result of senility, endocrine disorders, poor general health, or loss of testicular substance, are practically always of psychic origin. The others occupy an intermediate position, and may equally well be due to local disease or psychic abnormalities. Absence of erection and ejaculation following section of nerves, usually the pudics, at operation or by traumatism, will usually

[1] Journal of Urology, 1923, x, 387–392.

be apparent from the history. Similar conditions occur in spinal cord lesions which only rarely will give rise to any confusion.

Other cases may be roughly divided, for convenience of description, into *three groups*, with the understanding that the boundaries between these groups are not very definite. They are: (1) Cases with definite local pathologic findings, in which the sexual symptoms do not seem out of proportion to the severity of the disease present; (2) cases with definite local pathologic findings, in which the sexual symptoms seem out of proportion to the severity of the disease present, and in which a "nervous disposition" or "neurotic tendency" is noticeable; and (3) cases without definite local pathologic findings, in which nevertheless the sexual symptoms are pronounced: the typical and familiar "sexual neurasthenic." In the first group, we may expect to see the sexual symptoms disappear concomitantly with the local disease, in the second group they may, or may not do so, while in the third group no effects can be expected from local treatment unless accompanied by encouragement, advice, or other forms of psychotherapy.

The examinations described above will disclose the amount of local disease present. We no longer believe that slight, scarcely demonstrable lesions, merely because they are in the genital organs, have any semimysterious powers of bringing about the severest mental and physical disorders. It may be taken as a guiding principle that when local disease is causing serious trouble, it will usually be immediately demonstrable. Definite induration, irregularity, and adhesions of the prostate and seminal vesicles, pus in the expressed secretion, urethral discharge, ulcers, granulations, or polyps in the posterior urethra, purulent utriculitis, contracture of the vesical orifice, basal cystitis, all indicate real disease of the lower urogenital tract. As such, local treatment is demanded, provided there be no contraindication. If nothing can be found but a congested verumontanum, with no sign of actual infection, it will usually be true that this is the result, not the cause, of the disordered sexual function.

On the mental side, the experienced urologist is usually able to recognize instinctively the "neurotic" individual. The following list of diagnostic features will help in doubtful cases.

A. *From the History.*—(1) The duration of the sexual symptoms; (2) ideas of sexual inferiority, such as bashfulness, convictions that the genitalia are too small, too cold, etc.; (3) worry over the results of early or recent masturbation, or venereal disease; (4) sexual history, including rate of intercourse and previous occasions of premature ejaculation, excessive nocturnal emissions, or impotence; (5) state of mental anxiety about condition, including especially growing irritability, and palpitation and shortness of breath.

B. *From the Examination and Observation of the Patient.*—(1) Frank expressions of great worry and depression; (2) state of disability, even invalidism, with excessive desire to see the doctor at frequent intervals and to be constantly reassured (which makes these patients a pest to the doctor); (3) repeated spontaneous inquiry by the patient as to the ultimate effect of his condition on his sexual power; (4) the response of the patient to common-sense advice and answers to his questions: the normal person will quickly take courage and cease to worry, the abnormal one is impervious to reason; (5) finally, taking these observations and the physical findings together, a *disproportion* between the sexual symptoms, mental depression, etc., and the amount of local disease actually present.

The prognosis depends more on the extent of this *disproportion* than anything else. Definite local disease, with mild sexual symptoms of short duration, may be expected to do well. Marked sexual symptoms of long duration have a bad prognosis. If the depression and lack of response to advice approach the point of being real delusions, the case is a psychiatric one, and distressing consequences may follow neglect of the mental features. There may be suicide, or even homicide, sometimes with the doctor as the victim.

Vas Deferens, Symptoms.—Infection of the vas deferens (vasitis) is usually associated with disease of the epididymis, seminal vesicle, or both, and has no important symptoms peculiar to it. If inflammation spreads to the tissues of the spermatic cord, pain and swelling along its course are produced (funiculitis).

Vas Deferens, Diagnosis.—The vas may be palpated from the inguinal ring to the epididymis, and also by rectum at its opposite end, where it enlarges into the ampulla. In tuberculous vasitis it may be sometimes palpated in the inguinal canal and even above it by deep abdominal pressure. The ampulla is usually involved with the seminal vesicle, and is, therefore, better considered with that organ. Inflammation of the vas in the region of the spermatic cord is indicated by enlargement, induration, and tenderness. Tuberculosis is differentiated by the beaded character of the induration which is often present, or great enlargement. One also draws inferences as to the character of the inflammation in the vas by the findings in the vesicle and epididymis. When induration, edema, and tenderness are present in the tissues of the cord—funiculitis—one examines carefully to try to isolate the vas and determine its condition. Funiculitis, beginning as thrombophlebitis of the pampiniform plexus, is usually preceded by some infectious disease or other febrile condition, and the vas at first is uninvolved. Suppuration is indicated by areas of fluctuation.

Epididymis, Symptoms.—The symptoms of *acute epididymitis* are generally the same whatever the causative organism is. The onset is usually fairly rapid. *Pain* and *tenderness* appear first, then a *swelling* is noticed in the scrotum. This swelling may be slight, or may increase to great size. The skin becomes reddened, and often tense and shiny. Tenderness is exquisite. There are usually some *fever* and *leukocytosis*, and not infrequently prostration, due in part at least to the pain. Where gonorrheal urethritis is present, the discharge may disappear during the acute stage of an epididymitis. This phenomenon has been ascribed to the fever, as it has also been noted in other febrile conditions, as typhoid and malaria.

The *course* of acute epididymitis is usually fairly short, from six to twelve days, by which time resolution or, more rarely, suppuration may be expected. A subacute stage may occur, however, in which the epididymis remains swollen, hot, and tender for weeks or months.

Chronic epididymitis may be marked by recurrent acute attacks, the intervals between which are practically symptomless. In other cases pain, without much swelling, is the important feature, and in still others a painless swelling gives trouble. Finally, there may be sterility, when the tubules of the epididymes or the vas have become obliterated by inflammation. Hunner and Wharton[1] investigated the husbands in 279 cases of childless marriage, and found 56 (20 per cent.) sterile.

[1] Southern Medical Journal, 1924, xvii, 269–277.

Funiculitis as a complication is marked by pain and swelling in the cord and over the external inguinal ring. The pain may radiate upward and outward.

Epididymis, Diagnosis.—*Acute epididymitis* is generally sufficiently evident, and the principal diagnostic problems are to determine the source of the infection, and to rule out tuberculosis, syphilis, tumor of the testis, and acute orchitis.

If gonococcal pus can be demonstrated from the urethra, it is usually safe to assume that the epididymitis is *gonorrheal*. It is wise always to examine the urethra carefully in all cases of acute epididymitis, as gonococci are sometimes present when not expected. A history of recent gonorrhea, or chronic urethral discharge, points toward gonorrheal epididymitis, but the absence of these points from the history is inconclusive, as they may be concealed by the patient. A rectal examination, revealing a chronic prostatitis or seminal vesiculitis, may explain the etiology. A *culture* of gonococcus obtained by puncturing the epididymis is proof positive, but is not often necessary.

In *non-gonorrheal epididymitis*, the source will usually be apparent from the history, as the usual causes of this condition are urethral instrumentation, catheterization (especially a retention catheter), surgical procedures or traumatism about the prostatic urethra, and sometimes upper tract infection.

If epididymitis occurs in the course of an *infectious disease*, without previous urethritis, it is often due to the organism of the disease. Absolute proof can be had only by puncturing the epididymis and culturing the organism.

Hematogenous epididymitis occurring suddenly and alone can be diagnosed only by excluding local sources, as urethritis, and culture is the only way of determining the organism concerned.

Traumatic epididymitis follows injury and may present all the symptoms and signs of a serious acute infection, without any evidence of urethritis or prostatovesiculitis.

In acute epididymitis the skin is *hot, red*, and often *tense*, with obliteration of the normal rugæ. There is usually a slight *acute hydrocele* present, which may obscure the testis. The epididymis is felt as an *indurated, enlarged*, very *tender* mass. The outlines are generally partially obscured by *edema* in the surrounding tissue. The *globus minor* is usually the part in which induration first appears in cases where the infection comes from the urethra, but, as a rule, the inflammation spreads rapidly to the remainder of the epididymis. Gonorrheal epididymitis rarely leads to abscess formation, and usually resolves spontaneously.

Suppuration is indicated by fluctuation, though it may be impossible to detect the pus when present in multiple small foci. *Extension to scrotal tissues* or spermatic cord is shown by edema, induration, and tenderness. Such areas, especially in the cord, must be palpated carefully for fluctuation, as deep-set abscesses may occur and spread to considerable distances if not detected.

Acute tuberculous epididymitis may simulate pyogenic infection exactly. History of tuberculosis elsewhere may give a clue, but sometimes it is only the course of the infection which makes the distinction. If induration persists, and becomes firmer, and especially if sinuses appear, tuberculosis is to be suspected. Rectal examination of the prostate and vesicles, and careful study of the urine and prostatic secretion for tubercle bacilli are indicated.

Syphilis will seldom cause confusion, but a gumma may become secondarily infected, with onset of pain and swelling. The induration of the gumma, usually in the testis, the Wassermann test, the history, etc., will make the diagnosis. The epididymis is generally free from trouble and palpable on the posterior surface of the testicle.

Acute orchitis is comparatively rare, except those cases associated with mumps. Occasionally the testis will become secondarily involved from the epididymis. The diagnosis can only be made by careful, thorough palpation, distinguishing the epididymis from the testis, and outlining the size, contour, and consistence of each. In some cases this may be greatly facilitated by removing an excess of fluid from the sac of the tunica vaginalis. There is no longer any excuse for designating any intrascrotal inflammation as merely "orchitis" or "epididymo-orchitis" —the distinction can be made, and should be, for the prognosis, course, and treatment of epididymitis and orchitis are quite different. Acute epididymitis, both gonococcal and that due to other organisms, is rarely accompanied by pronounced orchitis.

Chronic Epididymitis.—Here one is required to distinguish between a chronic, persistent inflammation, and the scarring resulting from pre-existent but now

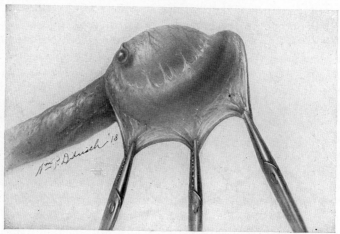

Fig. 114.—Painful testicle due to adhesions, as seen at operation, between epididymis and testis. Adhesions resected, tunica vaginalis everted. B. U. I. 6822.

healed infection. It is also necessary to exclude tuberculosis, syphilis, mycotic infections, and neoplasm.

A history of *recurrent acute attacks* suggests that the infection is still present and active. In elucidating this question it is necessary to examine also the urethra, prostate and seminal vesicles. An active vesicular infection may be present, or, according to Kaufmann, the vesicle may be distended with pus, supposedly from the epididymis, without any marked infection of its own substance. Boyd has seen striking improvement in epididymitis after expressing a quantity of purulent material from the seminal vesicles. In the epididymis itself, redness, heat, tenderness, fluctuation, edema, all suggest an active inflammation. Induration, increase in size, and irregularity, however, may indicate inflammation, or only the scarring resulting from a previous infection.

Painful epididymes are often associated with adhesions in the cavity of the tunica vaginalis (Fig. 114), so that obliteration of the digital fossa should be felt for in these cases. Careful palpation will often disclose a single tender point. Another cause of pain or tenderness on pressure is adhesions resulting in a cyst between the epididymis and the testis.

If the complaint is *sterility*, one should first make sure that sterility is actually present. The patient's wife should also be examined by a competent gynecologist, the examination to include preferably inflation of the fallopian tubes. The epididymes of the patient are carefully studied, although areas of induration do not necessarily mean obstruction. If motile spermatozoa are found in the expressed secretion, sterility on the part of the male is practically ruled out. If not, it is not conclusive, and a positive opinion should not be given until after 2 or 3 condom specimens have been examined. Lack of motility of the spermatozoa is of no significance unless the specimen is examined while fresh and still warm. One should distinguish between absence of spermatozoa and non-motility of spermatozoa, both included in *azoöspermia*. Absence indicates usually obstruction of both epididymal ducts, while lack of motility indicates that they are open, but that something along the genital tract, usually an infection, destroys the motility of the spermatozoa. There are recorded a few cases of congenital azoöspermia of unknown origin.

The distinction between chronic pyogenic epididymitis and *tuberculosis* is sometimes difficult. The history is valuable, though one must remember that an epididymitis coming on after gonorrhea may prove later to be tuberculous. In the same way, tuberculosis may cause a discharge simulating gonorrhea. The induration occurring in the two diseases may be similar, though the tuberculous epididymis is apt to be less acute, harder, and more irregular. Examination of the prostate and vesicles may disclose typical tuberculous induration, and tubercle bacilli are to be sought for in the urine and prostatic secretion (after cleansing to eliminate smegma bacilli). A ruptured abscess in the epididymis gives rise to a sinus, but that from a pyogenic process usually closes promptly, while an indolent sinus points toward tuberculosis. Any epididymis large, hard, and chronic enough to suggest tuberculosis may well be removed, when microscopic examination will give the diagnosis.

Mycotic disease simulates tuberculosis, and the same diagnostic considerations apply.

Gumma and syphilitic *fibrosis* of the testis are usually easily excluded by a careful local examination, since in these conditions the enlargement and induration are in the testis, not the epididymis (compare Chapter V). Syphilis rarely invades the epididymis, and when it does so, other lesions will usually be well marked.

Neoplasms of the testis are distinguished in the same way. Fibroma of the lower end of the spermatic cord may give rise to confusion, and in such cases the diagnosis may not be clear until operation. This condition is rare. Small cysts embedded in the epididymis may simulate nodules of induration, but these cysts are quite round and smooth, and usually movable enough to be easily diagnosed. They usually occur at the upper end of the epididymis.

If the testicle is *undescended*, the diagnosis is more difficult. It is said that in monocryptorchids the retained organ is more apt to become the seat of a gonorrheal epididymitis than the scrotal one. Epididymitis may be very serious if the testicle is intra-abdominal, or if the vaginal process remains patent (congenital hernia), as it may set up an acute peritonitis. Occasionally serious mistakes are made in these cases through failure to notice the absence of a testicle from the scrotum.

Testis, Symptoms.—The principal symptoms of *orchitis* are *pain* and *swelling*. There are local *redness, heat,* and *edema,* and in acute cases, *fever*. In mumps, a febrile condition is already present, so that only local symptoms call attention to the orchitis. In later stages *atrophy* of the testis may attract the patient's attention, but only if both testes are entirely destroyed by inflammation or subsequent atrophy do the symptoms of eunuchism appear. (See Chap. IX.)

The *onset* of acute orchitis is usually rather sudden, and the course short or only moderately long. The end-result is resolution or suppuration. Atrophy may follow resolution. The testicle is a parenchymatous organ, and pyogenic infections do not usually become chronic in it unless the infection is constantly renewed from the blood. In such cases the course may be silent, and the first symptom noted a fibrous atrophy.

Testis, Diagnosis.—Examination of the scrotal contents discloses the testis *enlarged, firm,* and *smooth*. It is only in later stages, with marked fibrous change, that *irregularities* are palpable through the tunica albuginea. *Fluctuation* is not easily made out, but appears when large abscesses are present. It must not be confused with hydrocele. Involvement of the subcutaneous tissues and cord, with redness, edema, and tenderness, is not uncommon, but changes in the epididymis are in the background, since it is seldom simultaneously involved. If an abscess has ruptured, masses of testicular tubules will frequently be seen in the opening.

If no symptoms of an infectious disease are present, they should be looked for at once, as orchitis is sometimes the first manifestation, especially of *mumps*. If any localized infection is present elsewhere in the body, a possible connection is to be considered. The teeth and sinuses may also be examined.

If an infectious disease is present, one may assume that the orchitis has resulted from it, though it may be impossible to prove this unless specimens of pus or tissue are obtained by puncture or operation.

True orchitis and *epididymitis* are often confused, and indeed until comparatively recent years the distinction between them was not made clinically. In both the scrotum is enlarged, reddened, hot, painful, and exquisitely tender. On palpation, however, one can feel, in epididymitis, the swollen, usually irregular epididymis, with the vas running directly into it. The testis may be palpated separately, or it may be entirely obscured by the enlarged epididymis, the edema of the scrotal tissues, or the inflammatory hydrocele, which is practically always present in acute cases.

Urethritis, or sign of some inflammation in the lower urinary tract, is usually present, but may be undiscoverable. In true orchitis, however, the enlargement is due to the testis itself and it is seldom irregular. The disease is independent of urethritis or lower urinary tract infections. Since, as we have seen, the epididymis is scarcely ever involved in true orchitis, it can be palpated alongside the enlarged testis, and is found not to be enlarged (Figs. 187, 188). This is the most important point in the differential diagnosis.

As to the occurrence of acute orchitis as a complication of epididymitis, it is usually impossible to be sure of it clinically, but Hagner,[1] who has had a large

---

[1] Medical Record, 1906, lxx, 565–568, and 1909, lxxvi, 944–946; Annals of Surgery, 1908, xlviii, 876–882.

experience with epididymotomies in cases of gonorrheal epididymitis, states that he has never seen the testis involved. He does an open operation, incising the tunica vaginalis, which gives opportunity to inspect the testis closely.

Torsion of the cord may cause a condition in the testis resembling orchitis. In some cases such a testicle becomes secondarily infected. The onset of torsion is very sudden, more sudden indeed than that of acute orchitis. The tenderness is extreme. Where edema does not prevent palpation, the epididymis will be found involved equally with the testis, unlike orchitis. Torsion must be suspected in all cases where scrotal pain and swelling occur without any pre-existent or concomitant lesions whatever, such as are often associated with orchitis. The diagnosis is difficult, however, and may have to be deferred until operation.

Strangulated hernia should give less trouble. The history, the sausage-like outline of the tumor, running to the inguinal ring, and most important of all, the discovery of the testicle at one side of the tumor, will make the diagnosis. Differentiation is more difficult if the testis is undescended.

Toxic necrosis occurs in certain infectious diseases, and resembles orchitis very closely. It may become infected. In any case, the differential diagnosis is difficult, and really of minor importance, since the treatment is the same as for orchitis.

Tuberculosis usually begins in the epididymis, and will, therefore, even when acute, seldom be confused with acute orchitis. If the testis is secondarily involved, it may become enlarged, or suppurate, but the chronic history distinguishes from pyogenic infections.

Acute orchitis in an *undescended testicle* may give quite a different picture. If well up in the inguinal canal, palpation may be impossible, and exploratory operation may be necessary. Symptoms of peritonitis may ensue if the infection extends through to the peritoneum.

Chronic pyogenic orchitis, as stated above, is practically non-existent. Chronic infections of the testis are practically always syphilitic or tuberculous. The diagnostic features of these are given elsewhere. Rarer conditions, as glanders, leprosy, mycoses, etc., occur in the course of infections of these kinds elsewhere in the body, and will be recognized as such.

TREATMENT

GENERAL CONSIDERATIONS

Antiseptics.—Since the discovery of bacteria, efforts have been continually in progress to treat infections of all parts of the body by destroying the causative organisms with germicidal substances. The two important problems have always been, and still are (1) to bring the germicidal substances in contact with all the bacteria, and (2) to obtain germicides which will kill bacteria and at the same time harm the body tissues as little as possible.

Germicidal substances have been applied *locally*, and given internally, either by *mouth*, by *inunction*, or by *intravenous injection*.

Mercury and silver were used for urethral injections in the pre-antiseptic period. Indeed, with the exception of astringents, represented by zinc chlorid, zinc acetate, zinc sulphate, lead acetate, and copper sulphate, they finally came to be about the only drugs used. We must assume that in those empirical days, these two substances survived through a long process of trial and error. Charles

Musitanus, who lived from 1635 to 1714 (quoted by Astruc,[1] who disapproved of the method), used the following prescription as an abortive treatment, guaranteed to cure gonorrhea in three days: "Plantain water, 8 ounces, in which dissolve some sweet mercury (mercuri sublimati dulcis) reduced to a very fine powder; inject 1 ounce in the urethra three times a day." Later Carmichael in England and Debeney in France[2] were the protagonists of silver nitrate injections in the early stages of "blenorrhagia," using strong solutions of from 15 grains to 1 dram in 1 ounce of distilled water. Most urologists, however, recoiled from the effects of this treatment, and utilized the silver injections only in the chronic stage, for their "tonic and alterative" effects (Wallace[3]), although muriate of mercury, $\frac{1}{2}$ grain to the ounce, was sometimes substituted.

After the discovery of the gonococcus, efforts were at once made to apply the newly appreciated principles of antisepsis to the treatment of urethritis. Of these the most noteworthy was that of Halsted, who used large quantities of weak solutions of bichlorid of mercury with the idea of supplementing the antiseptic action of the drugs by a mechanical washing away of pus and organisms. Later, Janet introduced in France the use of permanganate of potassium in a similar way. Following the lead of Lister, carbolic acid was also used.

Nitrate of silver was still considered a valuable drug, but its strongly irritant qualities caused efforts to be made to obtain a milder silver compound. Halsted[4] showed that metallic silver had a powerful germicidal or inhibitive action and explained the raison d'être of Marion Sims' epoch-making surgical results. Halsted's work led to Credé's[5] experiments resulting in the production of a colloidal silver compound, collargol, and later argonin, protargol, argyrol, and many other similar substances were made, in which the silver is maintained in colloidal suspension through the presence of a "protective" albumin. Credé imagined wide usefulness for collargol, and foreshadowed the "therapia sterilizans magna." His idea was to introduce silver into the body by inunctions.

Salol and other drugs were thought of as urinary antiseptics, but were not effective. In 1894 Nicolaier[6] introduced hexamethylenamin under the name of urotropin, which liberated formaldehyd in the urine. Burnam,[7] Smith,[8] Hinman,[9] and Shohl and Deming,[10] at this clinic, have elucidated its manner of action, showing that the formaldehyd is freed only in acid urine, and that the urine must be concentrated and markedly acid in order to contain enough formaldehyd to be at all effective. In spite of enthusiastic early reports, experiences with urotropin have not been very favorable. Tests show that in a majority of cases

---

[1] A Treatise of Venereal Diseases (English translation), London, 1754.

[2] Vidal: Traité des Maladies Vénériennes, Paris, 1853.

[3] Treatise on the Venereal Disease, London, 1838.

[4] Johns Hopkins Hospital Bulletin, 1894, v, 33; American Journal of the Medical Sciences, 1895, N. S., cx, 13–17; John Hopkins Hospital Bulletin, 1903, xiv, 210 (footnote); Journal of the American Medical Association, 1913, lx, 1119–1126.

[5] Archiv für Klinische Chirurgie, 1897, lv, 861–871.

[6] Centralblatt für die Medizinischen Wissenschaften, 1894, quoted by Nicolaier, Zeitschrift für Klinischen Medizin, 1899, xxxviii, 350–416.

[7] Archives of Internal Medicine, 1912, x, 324–334.

[8] Boston Medical and Surgical Journal, 1913, clxviii, 713–716.

[9] Journal of the American Medical Association, 1915, lxv, 1769–1775.

[10] Journal of Urology, 1920, iv, 419–437.

even the minimum effective concentration of formaldehyd in the urine is never reached. This drug, however, stands out as the first example of a proved internal urinary antiseptic, and, it is to be hoped, the forerunner of a long line of more effective ones.

During the great war interest in antiseptics was revived by the work of Carrel and Dakin[1] with hypochlorite combinations. Browning[2] and his co-workers in England discovered that some of Ehrlich's aniline dyes were strongly bactericidal, and obtained good results with brilliant green, acriflavin (trypaflavin), and proflavin in infected wounds.

It was noted that Pseudomonas pyocyanea (Bacillus pyocyaneus) was sensitive to acids, and that acetic acid applications gave good results in these infections.

Certain patients with gonorrhea who were also being treated for syphilis by Janet and Levy-Bing[3] showed a cessation of discharge after novarsenobenzol, which led them to use it in a case of gonorrheal arthritis successfully. Gross[4] tried the drug in cases of pyelitis, with favorable results.

Beginning in 1916 we began a systematic clinical and laboratory study in an effort to produce more effective antiseptics. Later on we shall describe how Dr. E. C. White, chemist of the Brady Urological Institute, undertook, at our suggestion, to make combinations of phenolsulphonephthalein which would be antiseptic, and when eliminated through the kidneys would act as urinary germicides. The investigation was extended to take up a multitude of other dyes and combinations made from them. A series of clinical papers dealing with these experiments by White, Davis, Swartz, and others were published.[5] As a result of this work some 265 combinations, many of which were new, were studied in the laboratories, and from these the most promising were also studied in the clinic. Of these, Number 220, to which we gave the name of mercurochrome, was described by Young, White, and Swartz[6] in 1919, who presented a series of clinical reports which indicated that mercurochrome possessed considerable value as a local germicide in urology. Mercurochrome not only proved to be remarkably non-toxic and non-irritating, but it did not coagulate serum or blood, or precipitate urine, and had remarkable penetration. Its germicidal strength was also excellent. In urine it was found to kill B. coli in one minute in strength of 1 : 800 to 1 : 1000. Staphylococcus aureus was killed in five minutes in 1 : 5000. In hydrocele fluid B. coli and Staphylococcus aureus were both killed in one hour in strength 1 : 1000. Tests of the action of mercurochrome on the gonococcus in our laboratories showed that five-minute exposures killed the organism in a dilution of 1 : 4000; failed in dilution of 1 : 6000. A twenty-minute exposure killed in 1 : 16,000, failing in 1 : 32,000. Twenty-minute tests on B. coli by the same technic showed

[1] Carrel and Dehelly: The Treatment of Infected Wounds, New York, 1917.

[2] Browning, Gulbransen, and Kennaway: British Medical Journal, 1917, i, 73–78; Browning, Gulbransen, and Thornton: British Medical Journal, 1917, ii, 70–75.

[3] Gazette des Hôpitaux, 1913, lxxxvi, 326, 327.

[4] Wiener Klinische Wochenschrift, 1917, xxx, 1381–1384.

[5] Davis, E. G., and White, E. C.: Journal of Urology, 1918, ii, 107–127. Young, White, and Swartz: Journal of the American Medical Association, 1919, lxxiii, 1483–1491; Journal of Urology, 1921, v, 353–388; Journal of the American Medical Association, 1921, lxxvii, 93–98. Swartz and Davis: Journal of the American Medical Association, 1921, lxxvi, 844–846.

[6] Journal of the American Medical Association, 1919, lxxiii, 1483–1491.

complete killing in 1 : 400 and failure in 1 : 800.   In the original article and in subsequent papers, Young, White, and Swartz[1] presented an extensive series of clinical
cases in which it was shown that mercurochrome could be used with safety
in wounds and mucous membranes in strength of 1 per cent., and that not infrequently remarkably quick sterilization of infections could thus be produced.   It
was also shown that it was not safe to leave mercurochrome or other strong
mercurial in deep wound cavities where it might be absorbed and produce stomatitis.

As a result of our further study of germicides, Young, White, Hill, and Davis[2]
presented "253," to which they gave the name meroxyl, as an efficient local germicide.   Meroxyl differs from mercurochrome in that it is colorless, does not stain,
has not the same penetration, and is slightly more toxic and irritating than mercurochrome.   However, it has the advantage of being much more germicidal and,
therefore, of value for irrigations of the urethra and bladder and the local treatment
of wounds where a disagreeable stain is to be avoided.   Meroxyl was found to kill
B. coli in 50 per cent. serum in one minute in a strength of 1 : 6000, and in salt
solution in 1 : 8000, in one hour a strength of 1 : 20,000 sufficed in 50 per cent.
serum, and a strength of 1 : 600,000, even, succeeded in killing the B. coli in normal
salt solution in one hour.   B. pneumoniæ was killed in one hour in salt solution
in strength of 1 : 1,000,000, thus showing the drug to have very powerful germicidal
action.

Mercurochrome and meroxyl have accordingly been used in a great variety
of urologic cases in this clinic, the details of treatment and results of which will
be given for the various diseases.

INTRAVENOUS USE OF ANTISEPTICS.—*Therapia Sterilisans Magna.*—In 1913
Ehrlich, in a brilliant address before the last International Medical Congress in
London, summed up his work on chemotherapy.   In this address, after detailing
the successive stages by which he arrived at his great discovery, and the possibility of a therapia sterilisans magna in the treatment of syphilis by the use
of salvarsan, Ehrlich finished his address with the following prediction for the
future:

I believe definite and sure foundations have been laid for the scientific principles of chemo-
therapeutics.   In diseases due to protozoa and spirilla, extraordinarily favorable results have
already been gained.   There are many favorable indications that in a series of other diseases and
above all, the infectious diseases, that the prospects of success are brightening.   I shall put
forward the view that within the next five years we shall have advances of the highest importance to record.   Considering the enormous number of chemical combinations which must be
taken into consideration with the struggle against disease, it will always be a caprice of chance
or fortune or of intuition that decides which investigator gets into his hands the substances
which turn out to be the best for fighting diseases.   In spirillar diseases the principle of therapia
sterilisans magna has proved most successful.   This form of therapeutics remains unassailed,
but in the case of the hardier bacteria—such as the Bacillus typhosus—the possibility of sterilization is not beyond hope.   The chance of finding a real cure and so winning the big prize will
naturally increase with the number of those who occupy themselves with the problem.

Ehrlich's great address thrilled all of us who heard it.   At the Brady Urological
Institute in 1917 we began a systematic search for better germicides and antisep-

---

[1] Journal of the American Medical Association, 1921, lxxvii, 93–98.
[2] Surgery, Gynecology, and Obstetrics, April, 1923, 508–521.

tics. For several years we had been impressed with the wonderful selective action of the kidney upon phenolsulphonephthalein and it occurred to us that with this dye, which could be injected intravenously with such impunity, we might, following the footsteps of Ehrlich, make some combination which would be eliminated as a germicide through the kidney and sterilize the urinary tract.

It was first necessary to find a chemist expert in dyes, and in our search we found one who had already done experimental work with phenolsulphonephthalein, Dr. E. C. White, who consented to join our staff and soon began a systematic effort to make combinations with phenolsulphonephthalein in the effort to produce our much wanted intravenous urinary germicide. This work led to the study of many other dyes and some 265 different combinations, many of which were new, were made in our laboratories and successively studied by members of the staff.

We have not space to refer to all the papers which have resulted from these laboratory and clinical studies. In our search for germicides the following desiderata were sought for: stability, germicidal strength, absence of toxicity and irritation, absence of tendency to coagulate blood or precipitate urine, absence of irritation to tissues and particularly to veins, elimination in urine in bactericidal strength, penetration as a dye and lasting efficiency.

Mercurochrome.—We soon chose drug No. 220, to which we gave the name mercurochrome, as best answering these requirements. We set about to give it thorough clinical trial against various forms of infection and infectious disease. It was soon shown that it could be used with impunity in wounds and on mucous membrane in a strength of 1 per cent., at which strength it was rapidly germicidal to both the bacilli and cocci of ordinary infections. It was found to be eliminated in the urine in germicidal strength when administered intravenously, and, when given by mouth, to reduce greatly the bacteria in the stools and to be eliminated in the bile in sterilizing quantity. Injected into the blood it was found to produce no irritation of the veins and practically no injury to the kidney or other viscera in a strength of 10 mg. per kilogram in animals, and 5 to 8 mg.-kg. in human beings. When so treated, the blood was shown to be bacteriostatic and sometimes germicidal. In a strength of 1 : 1000 it will kill the colon bacillus and the staphylococcus in one minute.

Following our two publications of its clinical advantages as a local and urinary germicide, numerous papers appeared relative to its value in many forms of infections, the consensus of which was that a new germicide of low toxicity, marked penetration and great clinical value had been found.

The question of general infections had always been before us. In 1899 we published a case of general septicemia cured by intravenous injections of large quantities of sodium chlorid solution.[1]

J. H. Hume, of our clinic, had also published interesting cases of septicemia apparently cured by intravenous injections of large quantities of mild solutions of nitrate of silver.

Credé, as before mentioned, following Halsted's demonstration of the bactericidal value of metallic silver, produced collargol, a silver compound, which was used intravenously in a few cases of septicemia, but no further progress has been made with it for many years.

Trypaflavin and colloidal silver have also produced a few isolated cures. Stann-

[1] Young: Maryland Medical Journal, xlii, November 19, 1899.

oxyl, sulphate of copper, and eusol have also been reported to cure occasional cases of general infection.

Piper,[1] confirming our demonstration that mercurochrome could be safely used in animals in 1 per cent. solution up to 5 or 10 mg. per kilogram, injected women about to die of puerperal septicemia, with doses of 5 mg. per kilogram without evidence of injury. He then used the drug in 5 puerperal septicemias, 3 of whom died, but the 2 others got well after a prolonged convalescence. Concerning these results Piper stated:

> These cases are not definitely conclusive that in mercurochrome we have found a specific cure for blood-stream infections, but we feel that we may perhaps, after more extensive observations, find a way to increase the dosage so that our subsequent results will be better.

In the meantime, working along the same lines, we injected mercurochrome intravenously in a man with general septicemia due to colon bacillus. Blood cultures showed 120 colonies per cubic centimeter and the patient was unconscious and practically moribund. He was given 34 c.c. of a 1 per cent. solution (5 mg. per kilogram) by Dr. Colston; in a few hours he was conscious, in twelve hours the blood was sterile, and on the following day he was practically well. The urine became sterile and he has remained cured—the first positive demonstration of a therapia sterilisans magna with mercurochrome.

The second case was that of a woman with bilateral pyelonephritis due to Bacillus lactis aërogenes. Within twenty-four hours the urine was sterile and the patient cured.

A young man with extensive retroperitoneal abscess due to the colon bacillus, with a large indurated mass in the left side and temperature of 104° F., received 27 c.c. of a 1 per cent. solution intravenously. Within twelve hours the temperature was normal and the mass had begun to disappear, and in two days it was completely gone and the urine sterile.

In a series of papers[2] we reported these and other cases, among which was that of a man with staphylococcus septicemia and extensive subcutaneous abscess of chest and back following a cutting injury on the shoulder from a circular saw. The patient was delirious, temperature 104° F., chest, back, shoulder, and arm extensively infected, and blood-culture showed quantities of staphylococci. Three intravenous injections of 10 c.c., 1 per cent. solution mercurochrome, administered by Dr. Grantham were followed by a rapid disappearance of the infection and cure of the septicemia.

General and local streptococcus infections were also shown to be curable by this treatment. This was especially shown in a case of scarlet fever, complicated by erysipelas, streptococcic sore throat, abscess of tonsils and glands of neck, and septicemia.[3] Blood-culture showed 38 colonies of Streptococcus hemolyticus per cubic centimeter. The patient could not swallow, the temperature was 105° F., and he was drowsy and delirious. Erysipelas extended over the face and head. When this case was considered practically hopeless, the patient was given 15 c.c.

[1] American Journal of Obstetrics and Gynecology, 1922, iv, 532.

[2] Young: New York Medical Society, Buffalo, October 4, 1923; Transactions Southern Surgical Association, December 11, 1923; Johns Hopkins Hospital Bulletin, 1924, xxxv, 14–16. Young and Hill: Journal American Medical Association, 1924, lxxxii, 669–675.

[3] Young and Birkhaug: Journal American Medical Association, 1924, lxxxiii, 492–494.

1 per cent. solution (equal to 7.5 mg. per kilogram). The transformation was indeed remarkable. Within a few hours he was conscious and drinking water; within twelve hours the blood was found to be sterile. The infection of the throat, tonsils, glands of the neck, and the erysipelas disappeared completely within two or three days. The urine which was infected and contained streptococci in large numbers became sterile and the patient was discharged well in about a week.

As a result of these publications much interest was aroused and we began to receive numerous reports from physicians all over this country and from some foreign countries. These men did not hesitate to use mercurochrome intravenously, not only in the types of general, local, and urinary infections which we had reported, but in various other conditions and infectious diseases.

In a paper which we prepared for an address in Cleveland it was possible to collect 255 cases, which included puerperal, postoperative and other septicemias, erysipelas, many genito-urinary infections, cases of gonorrhea and its complications—arthritis, epididymitis, myalgia, etc.—arthritis and other rheumatic conditions of non-gonorrheal character, 14 cases of pneumonia, 2 cases of typhoid fever, 2 of meningitis, 2 of epidemic encephalitis. While many of the case reports were too brief for scientific use, they were sufficiently convincing to add further proof to the statements which we had already made that in mercurochrome we had found a drug which could be introduced intravenously without injury to the patient and often with remarkable cures of general, local, and urinary infections. In a brief publication of this study we[1] stated:

In analyzing these 255 cases, we found many septicemias in which the case was practically hopeless and a fatal outcome almost certain until intravenous therapy with mercurochrome was begun. In many cases it frankly failed, this being particularly true in Streptococcus viridans endocarditis and B. coli pyelonephritis. In 15 staphylococcus cases, 10 of which were general septicemia, it failed in only 1 case complicated with osteomyelitis. Making every allowance, I believe I can safely say that mercurochrome has already saved many lives and assisted the body defenses in throwing off grave local and general infections. It does not supplant surgery, but does, in many instances, turn the tide for the patient.

In a later more detailed study of all cases, where fairly complete notes were at hand, we[2] stated:

The records here cited are definite in showing that in such diseases of the skin as erysipelas, furunculosis, cellulitis, and in infections of soft parts, including abscess, really astoundingly rapid clearing up of the infectious process often follows intravenous injections of mercurochrome—220 soluble. In arthritis the disappearance of pain, swelling, and limitation of motion has in some cases been extremely striking and rapid. We have recorded 24 really amazing recoveries in septicemias, and in pneumonia, particularly in children, a number of really remarkable results have been cited. Freeman and Hoppe seem justified in the claim of having reduced the mortality from pneumonia in children from 39 to 8 per cent. in a series of 46 cases. In the treatment of gonorrhea and its complications there have been many failures due, we believe, to insufficient treatment, but some very striking results—particularly in arthritis—have been secured.

Technic.—We have recommended the injections of 1 per cent. solution made up with freshly distilled water from the granular form of mercurochrome-220 soluble. Warm water may be used in making the solution, but it should not be boiled, as disintegration may occur. In the

[1] Young: Surgery, Gynecology, and Obstetrics, January, 1925, 97–104.

[2] Young, Hill, and Scott: The Treatment of Infections and Infectious Diseases with Mercurochrome-220 Soluble. Analysis of 210 Cases that Furnish Many Definite Examples of a Therapia Sterilisans Magna, Archives of Surgery, 1925, x, 813–924.

adult the injection is usually made into the arm vein. In children, and patients with very small veins, the external jugular or the veins of the thigh may be employed, and in infants the peritoneal cavity may be used. We have never seen evidence of irritation of vein or thrombosis in any of our cases. In the majority of cases a dosage of 5 mg. per kilogram of body weight has been employed (23 c.c. of a 1 per cent. solution per 100 pounds of body weight). In a few instances this dosage has been exceeded, 7 and even 8 mg./kg. in succession having been employed without untoward result, and with some remarkable recoveries. In some instances the dose has been much smaller and we believe many of the negative results herein recorded are directly due to the small dosage used and consequent insufficient treatment employed.

Reactions.—In rare instances even doses of 5 mg./kg. or over have been followed by little reaction. In most cases there is a pronounced reaction consisting of nausea, vomiting, and frequent stools, and occasionally some shock. In febrile cases there may be a rise of from 1 to 5 degrees within three or four hours after the injection, often accompanied by a chill. In one case a temperature rise to 107.5° F. was recorded, but the patient recovered from a severe septicemia. An initial rise in temperature is almost always followed by an early drop, not infrequently to normal. There have been only 2 deaths that we can discover which were possibly traceable to the drug—one a case of multiple osteomyelitis and septicemia, and the other pemphigus—both diagnosed as probably fatal cases before injection. After much experimentation on animals and very careful study of a large series of cases we are convinced that little or no damage is done to the kidneys and that the drug may be used with safety even in patients with albumin, casts, and urinary infection, and with little risk. By giving small doses of mercurochrome (2 to 3 mg./kg.) little reaction is usually encountered, and multiple treatments may be used without producing stomatitis. In rare instances, stomatitis may occur early from small dosage. It is interesting to note that even with large doses the reaction is progressively less with the second or third injection.

The whole subject of reaction can, therefore, be viewed with little concern. In order to give adequate dosage in desperate or very severe cases, it is necessary to inject at least 4 or 5 mg./kg., and in so doing one may expect some marked reactions, but although these produce great discomfort, they are transitory in character and apparently lead to no permanent damage. The severity of the reaction (especially febrile) may play an important part in the elimination of the infection.

In a later study we[1] felt justified in stating:

Sufficient laboratory and clinical work, however, is at hand to prove conclusively that with both mercurochrome and gentian-violet the long sought for Therapia Sterilisans Magna of Ehrlich is possible in certain bacterial infections—both general and local—and the prediction which Ehrlich made in 1913 is now true. I have every confidence that I am speaking with moderation when I say that I believe in the very near future we shall see the proof of one of the greatest conquests of disease in the history of medicine.

The following tabulations and summaries show the results obtained with intravenous mercurochrome in the treatment of septicemia, pneumonia, genitourinary infection, arthritis, and skin infection.

Analysis of cases of *septicemia* reported. Of these 57 cases of septicemia, it will be seen that under "cure probably due to M-220" we have listed those cases, 28 in number, in which the physicians in attendance have thought that the cure was almost solely due to and immediately coincident upon the use of intravenous injections of mercurochrome. Under "great improvement after M-220" are listed 8 cases in which the patient improved immediately after the intravenous injection and eventually got well. In these cases the attending physicians thought the drug was an important factor in the cure. In the column "improvement, but

---

[1] Young: Federation of American Societies for Experimental Biology, Washington, December 31, 1924.

TABLE 15

FIFTY-SEVEN CASES OF SEPTICEMIA TREATED WITH INTRAVENOUS MERCUROCHROME

Group.	Classification by origin.	Total number.	Cure probably due to M-220	Great improvement after M-220	Improvement, but later complications.	Action M-220 doubtful.	Failed.
A	Urinary.	2	1	..	..	..	1
B	Traumatic or postoperative.	12	5	4	1	..	2
C	Throat infection.	6	5	..	..	..	1
D	Ear or lateral sinuses.	2	1	..	..	..	1
E	Osteomyelitis or abscess.	6	2	1	..	..	3
F	Puerperal.	20	11	3	1	1	4
G	Endocarditis.	7	2	..	..	..	5
H	Focus not found.	2	1	..	..	..	1
Totals.............		57	28	8	2	1	18

TABLE 16

TWENTY-FOUR CASES OF SEPTICEMIA SAID TO HAVE BEEN CURED BY INTRAVENOUS MERCUROCHROME

Archives Case No.	Age.	Septicemia and, in addition, the following:	Blood culture.	M-220, I. V. Number.	M-220, I. V. Dose mg./kg.
1	40	Pyelonephritis.	B. coli.	1	5
3	30	Traumatic; cellulitis.	Staph.	3	1.7, 1.7, 1.7
4	2	Tonsillitis.	Strep.	5	4.3, 4.4, 6
5	46	Postoperative.	Staph. albus.	2	5.5
6	58	Traumatic; cystitis.	Staph.	2	5 (?), 5 (?)
7	?	Osteomyelitis.	Strep. vir., staph.	1	5
8	Adul	Cellulitis.	Staph. aur.	3	3, 2, 1
15	4	Scarlet fever, tonsillitis, adenitis.	Strep. hemol.	1	7.5
16	6	Pharyngitis.	Strep. hemol.	2	8, 8
18	38	Pharyngitis.	Pneumococ. IV	2	5, 7.5
19	..	Tonsillitis; phlebitis.	Diploc.	1	5 (approx.)
21	7	Mastoiditis.	Strep.	1	5
23	3	Osteomyelitis.	Staph. (?).	2	6 (?)
24	40	Furunculosis. Abscess of groin.	Staph. aur.	4	4 (?), 3, 2, 4
29	16	Pelvic abscess. Furunculosis.	Staph. gonococcus.	1	5
30	25	Puerperal.	Staph.	6	3, 3, 5, 5, 5, 5
31	24	Puerperal.	Strep. and pneum.	2	5, 5
32	32	Puerperal; pneumonia.	Strep. and pneum.	1	5
33	20	Puerperal.	Strep. (?).	6	3, 4, 3, ?, ?, ?
34	18	Puerperal.	Strep. (?).	1	5 (?) approx.
35	23	Puerperal.	Strep. (?).	2	4.6, 4.6
36	22	Puerperal.	Strep. (?).	1	5
49	22	Endocarditis; arthritis.	Strep. hemol.	3	5
56	9	No focus found.	Strep. hemol.	1	5

TABLE 17

Twenty-two Cases of Pneumonia Treated with Intravenous Mercurochrome

Case No.	Age.	Diagnosis.	Condition stated.	Mercurochrome, I. V.		Doctor's comments.
				Number of injections.	Dose.	
58	?	Pn. dental abscess. Mul. arthritis.	"Condition desperate."	1	5 mg./kg.	"Saved her life."
59	..	Pn. after influenza.	"Almost moribund."	1	5 (approx.)	"A marvelous success."
60	2½	Bronchopneumonia.	"Patient in stupor."	2	5, 3 mg./kg.	"Rapid recovery."
61	5½	Bronchopneumonia. Otitis media.	"Desperate condition."	1	5 mg./kg.	"A spectacular recovery."
62	6½	Bronchopneumonia after measles.	"Fair condition."	1	5 mg./kg.	"Rapid recovery."
63	11 m.	Bronchopneumonia. Otitis media. Measles.	"Fair condition. Temp. 104° F."	2	6 mg./kg.	"Rapid fall in temperature."
64	1	Lobar pn. Stomatitis.	"Almost comatose."	2	4.6 mg./kg. 6 mg./kg.	"Rapid resolution."
65	9 m.	Bronchopneumonia following measles.	"Marked cyanosis."	1	5 mg./kg.	"Recovery uneventful."
66	5	Bronchopneumonia. Otitis media. Stomatitis.	"Grew gradually weaker."	3	5, 5, 5 mg./kg.	"Died."
67	6	Lobar pneumonia.	"Temp. 105.5° G."	1	5 mg./kg.	"Remarkable change. Well."
68	3	Lobar pneumonia.	"Temp. 104.4° F."	1	5 mg./kg.	"Recovery rapid."
69	8	Lobar pneumonia.	"Very ill."	2	5 mg./kg. 4.6 mg./kg.	"Lungs promptly cleared."
70	5	Bronchopneumonia.	"Moribund."	1	1.5 mg./kg.	"Died one hour later."
71	8	Lobar pneumonia.	"Rt. lower lobe."	2	5 mg./kg. 4.6 mg./kg.	"Marked benefit. Well."
72	8 m.	Bronchopneumonia following measles.	"Both lungs involved."	1	4.6 mg./kg.	"Spectacular recovery."
73	3	Lobar pneumonia.	"Desperate condition."	1	5 mg./kg.	"Rapid recovery."
74	10 m.	Lobar pneumonia.	"Temp. 105.2° F. Both lungs involved."	2	5 mg./kg. 5 mg./kg.	"Total duration sixty-four hours. Well."
75	inf.	Bronchopneumonia.	"Both lungs involved."	2	5 mg./kg. 5 mg./kg.	"Lungs clearing rapidly."
76	?	Lung abscess or pneumonia.	"Temp. 103.5° F."	1	21 c.c., 1 per cent.	"Cleared at once."
77	21	Lobar pneumonia.	"Both lungs involved. Temp. 105.2° F. Delirious."	2	10 c.c., 2 per cent.	"Salivation. Pneumonia cleared. Empyema. Recovery."
78	2½	Lobar pneumonia and appendicitis.	"Condition critical."	2	18 c.c., ½ per cent.	"Definite improvement."
79	4	Pneumonia. Empyema. Otitis media.	"Condition very poor."	1	2 mg./kg.	"Apparent improvement, but death later, being unable to withstand the continued infection."

later complications" have been included 2 cases in which the blood became sterile and the patient's condition much better, but local abscesses, which required ultimate drainage, occurred, the patients finally recovering. In the next column, "action M-220 doubtful," is 1 case in which the action of the drug was thought to be doubtful, the surgeon being unable to attribute the final recovery of the patient to the use of the drug, and in the last column there are 18 cases in which the drug failed.

There are thus recorded 39 recoveries (69 per cent.) in patients suffering with general septicemia, most of whom had more or less pronounced local infectious processes, and 18 deaths (31 per cent.).

TABLE 18

THIRTY-TWO CASES OF GENITO-URINARY INFECTIONS TREATED WITH INTRAVENOUS MERCURO-CHROME

Case No.	Age.	Diagnosis.		M-220.		Result.
				No.	Dose.	
80	17	Retroperitoneal abscess.	Urine infected B. coli.	1	5 mg./kg.	Abscess resolved, urine sterilized.
81	22	Perinephric abscess.	Staph.	2	5 mg./kg.	Abscess resolved, urine not sterilized.
82	..	Perinephric abscess	....	1	3.5 mg./kg.	"Cured" in two days.
83	..	Perinephric abscess.	....	2	3.1, 2.3 mg./kg.	Much improved.
84	..	Bilateral chronic pyelitis.	B. aerogenes.	1	5 mg./kg.	Urine sterilized.
85	63	Acute pyelonephritis.	Condition too desperate for operation.	1	5 mg./kg.	Marked improvement.
86	45	Pyelonephritis.	Staph.	2	3 mg./kg.	Urine sterilized.
87	45	Pyelonephritis.	Staph.	3	4, 5, 5 mg./kg.	Urine sterilized.
38	4	Pyelitis.	B. coli. sepsis.	5	8, 2.5, 2.5, 2.5, 2.5 mg./kg.	Life saved; urine not sterilized.
89	..	Pyelitis.	....	1	5 mg./kg.	"Cured."
90	54	Pyelonephritis.	....	2	....	"Cured."
91	65	Pyelitis, cystitis, furunculosis, arthritis.	....	1	3 mg./kg.	Urine sterilized, marked improvement.
92	55	Pyelocystitis.	....	2	....	Urine sterilized, marked improvement.
93	40	Pyelonephritis.	Bilateral Staph. and B. coli.	1	4.2 mg./kg.	Urine sterilized.
94	23	Pyelitis. Cystitis.	Strept. Staph. and B. coli.	1	2.2 mg./kg.	Urine sterilized.
95	34	Pyelonephritis.	B. coli.	1	30 c.c.	"Cured."
96	19	Pyelitis, cystitis.	B. coli.	3	3.8, 3.8, 1.5	Clinical cure.
97	35	Pyonephrosis, cystitis.	B. coli.	2	24 c.c., 24 c.c.	"Cured."
98	34	Pyelitis.	....	1	3.1 mg./kg.	Much improved.
99	31	Pyonephrosis.	In stupor.	1	4.5 mg./kg.	Much improved.
100	45	Pyelitis.	B. coli.	2	4.7 mg./kg.	Much improved.
101	..	Pyelitis.	Staph. aureus.	2	20 c.c., 15 c.c.	No result.
102	..	Pyelitis.	B. coli.	1	5 mg./kg.	Infection persisted.
103	..	Pyelitis.	B. coli, ureteral stricture.	1	5 mg./kg.	Infection persisted.
104	..	Pyelitis.	....	2	30 and 30 c.c.	Infection persisted.
105	..	Pyelitis, prostatitis, ureteral stricture.	B. coli.	2	25 and 25 c.c.	Infection persisted.
106	..	Pyelitis.	....	2	....	Infection persisted.
223	11	Pyelitis.	Atypical B. coli.	6	5, 5, 5, 5, 5, 5 mg./kg.	Urine sterilized.
107	60	Chronic cystitis.	Staph. and B. coli.	1	3 mg./kg.	Urine sterilized.
108	26	Cystitis and prostatitis.	B. coli.	7	3, 3, 3, 3, 3, 5, 5 mg./kg.	Urine sterilized.
109	..	Acute cystitis.	....	3	20, 30, and 30 c.c.	All symptoms subsided.
110	39	Cystitis.	Staph.	2	30 and 30 c.c.	Little effect.

In analyzing the failures we find that 3 cases were practically moribund when treated. Five cases were of endocarditis due to a streptococcus, 2 recognized as viridans, notoriously resistant to all therapy. The 3 others may also have been Streptococcus viridans. In 2 cases, however, with streptococcus endocarditis the patient did recover, and 2 Streptococcus viridans endocarditis also recovered.

In 7 cases which ended fatally, 3 received only one injection each, 2 received two injections of small dosage, and 2 received three of moderate size. In none of these 8 cases did the patient receive two injections of 5 mg./kg. It seems fair to state, therefore, that either the treatment was inaugurated too late or was not as vigorous as was given in successful cases cited in the table.

It seems evident, therefore, that in septicemias doses of 5 mg./kg. should be used and repeated as often as necessary or as possible.

Analysis of *pneumonia* cases reported. Total, 22 cases, 3 deaths (1 moribund before injection). Nineteen recovered, of whom 5 were in desperate condition, 1 "almost moribund" and 1 "almost comatose." Of the recovered cases, 10 received only one injection, generally of 5 mg./kg., and 9 cases received two injections of 5 mg./kg. (approximately). In only 1 case was the reaction severe and apparently in no case did nephritis follow. Of the three failures, No. 70 was said to be moribund, No. 79, complicated with empyema and otitis media, showed marked improvement after one injection of 2 mg./kg., but died one week later, and No. 66 died after three full doses of 5 mg./kg.

It seems fair to deduce that with large and if necessary multiple doses (5 mg./kg. each) a large percentage of recoveries may be expected in certain pneumonias, particularly in children. The number of adult cases is still too small to warrant positive assertions. In children the results appear to be really brilliant.

Analysis of cases of *genito-urinary infection* reported. A. Perinephritis: In the 4 cases of perinephric abscess the results were apparently uniformly good and in our 2 cases very striking, especially in Case 80, in which a large inflammatory mass disappeared quickly. The total number of cases, however, is still too small for definite conclusions. In Nos. 80 and 81 the dosage was 5 mg./kg., in No. 82, 3.5 mg./kg., and in No. 83, 1 and 2.5 mg./kg.

B. Pyelonephritis, 24 cases: In 8 cases the urine was sterilized and the patient relieved of all signs and symptoms. In 2 of these cases with urine cultures: staphylococcus pure, Case 86 received 3 and 3 mg./kg. and Case 87, 5, 5, and 4 mg./kg. In 2 cases of staphylococcus and other organisms, Case 23 with B. coli received 4.2 mg./kg. and Case 94, B. coli and streptococcus, received only 2.2 mg./kg.

Three cases with B. coli in pure culture: Case 95 received 5 mg./kg.; Case 96, 3.8, 3.8, and 1.5 mg./kg., and Case 223, six injections of 5 mg./kg. each.

Number 84, due to B. lactis aërogenes, was sterilized by one dose of 5 mg./kg.

In apparently none of the 8 "cured" cases cited above was any other treatment used. In 3 cases cultures and doses are not given, but the patient is said to have been "cured." Improved greatly, 7 cases: In No. 88 the child was desperately ill, the dosage was 8 mg./kg. and four injections of 2.5 mg./kg.; "the patient's life was saved," but the urine still contained B. coli. In No. 85, a man very ill with left pyonephrosis and urine culture, B. coli, streptococcus and staphylococcus after M-220, i. v., 5 mg./kg., B. coli disappeared, and after gentian violet, i. v., 5 mg./kg. staphylococcus disappeared, streptococcus alone remaining in the urine. Fever and toxemia and all kidney symptoms disappeared and his life was unquestionably "saved."

In Cases 87, 97, 98, 99, 100 great improvement was noted, disappearance of fever and pain, but the record does not show that the urine was sterilized and the patient "cured." Bacillus coli present in 3, streptococcus and staphylococcus in 1, cultures not noted 2.

In all of the 18 cases (cured or greatly improved) there was no doubt in the mind of the reporter that M-220, i. v., had been of great benefit. The dosage employed was generally high and multiple—only 4 times below 4 mg./kg. Two or 3 cases of 4 or 5 mg./kg. were often employed.

Failures, 6 cases: In all of these cases fairly good doses were used, but only 1 received as much as three of 4 mg./kg. Bacillus coli were present in 3, staphylococcus in 2. In 2 cultures not recorded.

Summarizing: In B. coli pyelonephritis, 7 were sterilized, and 3 were not. In 6, organism not stated, B. coli was more probably present, 3 "cured," 3 not sterilized. In 5 cases with staphylococcus present all were sterilized. The B. coli cases are thus shown to be variable in results; this corresponds to the great variation in resistance shown by Miss Hill in an exhaustive study of 150 strains of B. coli.

Among the "improved" cases are some which were finally sterilized by pelvic lavage. It seems probable that bacteria growing in the urine or the urethra may not be reached by intravenous drugs in some cases and may require antiseptic lavage of the urinary reservoirs to sterilize them.

With eradication of the primary focus of infection, pelvic lavage, and intravenous mercurochrome we believe the great majority of pyelonephritis cases can be sterilized. Combined treatment is, therefore, indicated.

Analysis of *gonorrheal urethritis* cases reported. Twenty-six cases: 12 "cured." In the reports of these 12 cases it is positively stated that the discharge disappeared completely and in most cases that the urine was clear and gonococci absent. In all the reports the physician considered that the disease was eradicated. In only a few cases were provocative injections and cultures from the prostatic secretions obtained. Nevertheless, a clinical cure was apparently achieved in these 12, or 46 per cent., of the cases. In 4 acute cases (gonococci noted) the dosage employed was, in Case 112, four doses (5, 3.7, 3.7, 5 mg./kg.); in Case 113, five doses (2.4 mg./kg.); in Case 115, five doses (from 10 to 25 c.c. of 1 per cent. solution); in Case 122, one injection 10 c.c. and four of 15 c.c. All were sterilized. In 8 cases, chronic in duration, gonococci were noted in 5 and not in 3. Only Case 123 was said to have been "cured" by one injection, 31 c.c. 1 per cent. Two received two injections of 5 mg./kg. and 2 of 4 mg./kg. (112, 120). Case 121 received three injections (1 per cent., 10, 23, 15 c.c.). Two received four injections (Case 118, 2.5 mg./kg. each, and Case 116, 10 to 20 c.c., 1 per cent.). Case 115 had five injections varying from 10 to 25 c.c., 1 per cent. Case 117, 6 of 10 to 14 c.c., 1 per cent. None of these 12 cases received any local treatment. In most of these 12 cases the injections were given intravenously at intervals of forty-eight hours, and in all but 3 several treatments (three to six) were given. In many cases the goncocci disappeared after the first or second injection, but additional treatments were given. While it is evident that multiple small doses (2 or 3 mg./kg.) may be effective, larger doses are to be preferred. In 5 cases (124, 5, 6, 7, and 137) the reporter states positively that they were cured, but to be conservative we have classed them as greatly improved, because other treatment was sometimes employed. Large doses (4 to 5 mg./kg.) and several injections were generally used. In 9 cases (34 per cent.) we have classed the results as failures. Four of these cases (132 to 135) were reported by Lavandera, who gave much smaller doses than have usually

TABLE 19

TWENTY-SIX CASES OF GONORRHEAL URETHRITIS TREATED BY INTRAVENOUS MERCUROCHROME

Case No.	Age	Diagnosis.		M-220.		Results.
				No.	Dosage.	
112	23	Acute gonorrhea, old chronic gonorrhea.	Gonococci present.	4	5, 3.7, 3.7, and 5 mg./kg.	Urethra sterilized.
113	32	Acute gonorrhea.	Gonococci and Staph.	5	2 to 4 mg./kg.	Infection cleared completely.
114	..	Acute gonorrhea.	Gonococci present.	6	10 to 25 c.c.	Discharged as cured.
115	25	Chronic gonorrhea.	Gonococci present.	6	10 to 25 c.c.	Discharged as cured.
116	22	Gc. prostatic abscess.	Gonococci present.	4	10 to 25 c.c.	Discharged as cured.
117	36	Chronic gonorrhea, prostatitis.	Gonococci present.	6	10 to 14 c.c.	Cultures sterile.
118	..	Chronic gonorrhea, prostatitis.	Gonococci present.	4	2.5 mg./kg.	Apparently cured.
119	..	Chronic gonorrhea, primary syphilis.	Gonococci present.	3	5, 5, and 4 mg./kg.	Complete healing.
120	..	Chronic gonorrhea.	Gonococci present.	2	2 and 4 mg./kg.	Discharge terminated.
121	26	Gonorrheal epididymitis.	....	3	10, 23, and 15 c.c.	Secretions became normal.
122	45	Acute gonorrhea, epididymitis, adentitis.	....	5	1 of 10 and 4 of 15 c.c.	Apparently cured.
123	..	Chronic gonorrhea.	....	2	31 c.c.	Discharge disappeared.
124	..	Chronic gonorrhea.	Gonococci present.	5	4 to 5 mg./kg.	Discharge and gonococci disappeared.
125	..	Chronic gonorrhea, prostatitis, vesiculitis, epididymitis.	....	..	....	Marked improvement.
126	4	Gonorrheal infection, preputial abscess.	....	2	4 mg./kg.	Complete recovery.
127	36	Acute urethritis and endocervicitis.	Gonococci present.	3	6, 8, and 10 c.c.	Marked improvement.
128	..	Acute urethritis.	Gonococci present.	5	3 mg./kg.	Not benefitted.
129	..	Chronic gonorrhea, prostatitis.	No gonococci.	5	4 of 2.3 mg./kg.; 1 of 46 mg./kg.	Result doubtful.
130	..	Chronic gonorrhea.	Gonococci present.	3	2.5 mg./kg.	Not benefitted.
131	.	Chronic gonorrhea.	Gonococci present.	4	....	"Cured."
132	34	Chronic gonorrhea, arthritis of toe.	....	4	10, 14, 15, 18 c.c.	Apparently cured; relapse.
133	..	Acute urethritis, epididymitis.	Gonococci present.	4	10, 11, 15, 15 c.c.	Infection persisted.
134	19	Gonorrhea, epididymitis.	....	3	10, 11, and 15 c.c.	Unimproved.
135	22	Chronic gonorrhea, prostatitis.	Urethral smear negative.	3	10, 15, and 15 c.c.	Unrelieved.
136	..	Chronic gonorrhea.	Gonococci present.	4	2 to 4 mg./kg.	Great improvement.
137	..	Chronic gonorrhea.	Gonococci and Staph.	4	4 mg./kg.	Organisms and discharge ceased.

been necessary (10 to 15 c.c., 1 per cent., possibly only 1.5 to 2 mg./kg.). Three were chronic cases without gonococci, 1 acute, with epididymitis. Four other cases were chronic, but with gonococci present. The dosage was small. One acute case of four days' duration received 3 mg./kg. five times at our clinic and gonococci were still present in the discharge.

Résumé: It is apparently proved that gonococcus urethritis may sometimes be rapidly sterilized and all symptoms of disease may disappear after several intravenous injections of M-220; but that doses of 4 and 5 mg./kg. should be employed to secure results. With smaller doses reactions may be avoided, but the patient may not be cured. In many cases the treatment failed.

It seems probable that gonococci may be eradicated from the tissues and yet live and multiply in the urethra. On this account antiseptic injections should also be employed. In dealing with this dread malady every valuable weapon of offence should be used.

TABLE 20

FIVE CASES OF GONORRHEAL ARTHRITIS TREATED BY INTRAVENOUS MERCUROCHROME

Case No.	Urethral discharge.	Urine.	Prostatic secretion.	Joints involved.	Temperature.	No. of injections.	Dosage, c.c. or mg./kg.	Results.
139	Negative.	Staph.	Staph.	Both knee-joints.	No note.	2	5 mg./kg.	Urine and prostatic secretion sterilized. Arthritis disappeared; function good.
143	Gonococcus.	Cloudy and contains shreds.	No note.	Right wrist very swollen and painful.	No note.	6	15, 15, 15, 20, 20, 10 c.c.	Urine became clear. Wrist freely movable and normal in size. No pain.
144	Gonococcus.	Cloudy.	No note.	Right sterno-clavicular and right shoulder.	No note.	5	10 c.c.	Arthritis and urethritis disappeared completely.
145	Gonococcus.	Cloudy.	No note.	Right sterno-clavicular and right shoulder.	100° F.	3	10, 10, 12 c.c.	Urethral discharge ceased and arthritis cured.
146	Gonococcus.	Cloudy.	No note.	Arthritis right elbow and knee.	No note.	6	10, 12, 12, 12, 14, 14 c.c.	Ultimate cure. Urethral discharge ceased.

Analysis of cases of *gonorrheal arthritis* reported. Among the 12 cases of gonorrheal arthritis recorded, in 5 the results are apparently cures—complete disappearance of the arthritis and initial infection. Gonococci were found in 4 and staphylococci in 1.

The dosage in Case 139 consisted of two injections of 5 mg./kg. and the urethra, prostatic secretion, and urine were completely sterilized and the two badly involved joints became absolutely normal in twenty-seven days. In the other cases from three to six injections of similar dosage were employed, 10 to 20 c.c. at intervals of two or three days. The results in these 4 cases (143, 144, 145, 146) were excellent. In every case the joint became practically normal and urethral discharge and infection disappeared completely.

Four cases (138, 140, 141, 142) may be classed as greatly improved (not shown in table). Gonococci were present in all in the urethral smear. In Case 138, with arthritis in the sternoclavicular, shoulder, knee, and tarsal joints, there was almost complete disappearance of the arthritis. The urethral discharge disappeared and the urine became sterile after two doses of 5 mg./kg. In Case 141 only one dose, 5 mg./kg., was given, and there was said to be great improvement in the knee-joint involved, but no note is recorded as to the infection. Case 142 received seven small doses (1.4 mg./kg.) and was greatly improved. In Case 140, which received seven small doses of 10 c.c., there was great improvement of extensive arthritis of the knee, the urethral discharge continuing and gonococci being present.

Dr. N. S. McLeod has studied an additional 12 cases of gonorrheal arthritis in the dispensary of the Johns Hopkins Hospital. Six of the cases were acute, 3 of them showing gonococci, 3 being sterile. All 6 obtained rapid improvement of the arthritis as a result of the intravenous treatment and all got completely well both of the arthritis and also of the urethral infection and discharge. Urethral irrigations were given in the 3 cases showing organisms. Treatment varied from five injections of 2 mg./kg. to some receiving repeated injections of 3, 4, and 5 mg./kg., to a maximum in 1 case of eighteen injections of 2 mg./kg., two days apart, one injection of 4 mg./kg. and three injections of 5 mg./kg.

Six cases of chronic multiple arthritis were treated. One case was not improved. All of the others showed definite improvement, 1 case being absolutely cured both of the arthritis and of a coccus infection of the prostate.

TABLE 21

FIVE CASES OF NON-GONORRHEAL ARTHRITIS

Case	Age.	Diagnosis.	M-220 I. V.		Results.
			No.	Dose mg./kg.	
149	32	Multiple acute arthritis, both knees, shoulders, heels and right elbow, four months' duration.	?	1, 5, 3 times a week.	Arthritis gone by end of month.
150	38	Chronic arthritis. Prostatitis (streptococcus).	2 6	4 mg./kg, 3 mg./kg.	Arthritis greatly improved. Prost. secretion sterilized.
151	23	Polyarthritis after tonsillitis. Diagnosis, acute inflammatory rheumatism.	3	3, 4, 5 mg./kg.	Recovery.
152	?	Multiple arthritis, one week's duration.	5	12 to 15 c.c. daily.	Recovery. "Result remarkable."
153	?	Inflammatory rheumatism following tonsillitis.	3	3, 3, 4, 1.4 mg./kg.	Recovery.

Analysis of cases of *non-gonorrheal arthritis* reported. These cases show that excellent results may be obtained in the treatment of non-gonorrheal arthritis, both chronic and acute.

Dr. N. S. McLeod has treated 4 cases in the dispensary of the Johns Hopkins Hospital. Two were of urinary origin. One patient, who was brought in on a stretcher and unable to walk, was completely cured. He received six injections of 3 mg./kg. every other day, four injections of 4 mg./kg. every second day and three injections of 5 mg./kg. every other day, the treatment totalling 49 mg./kg. No albumin or casts appeared in the urine and no stomatitis developed. The other urinary case had lumbar arthritis which was greatly improved, the accompanying bilateral B. coli pyelitis not being sterilized. Of the 2 cases of non-urinary focal infection, 1 showed marked improvement and 1 slight improvement.

Analysis of cases of *erysipelas* reported. Eight cases; 8 cures. In these cases we have some of the most striking results with intravenous mercurochrome. The erysipelas varied in duration, type, and extent. In some cases it was merely facial, in others very extensive, and in one involved the neck, body, and arms. Several of these cases were desperately sick, the organism streptococcus, and the temperature high. The disappearance of the erysipelatous lesions was in almost all cases, indeed, extraordinary. The dosage in almost every case was high (about

TABLE 22
EIGHT CASES OF ERYSIPELAS

Case No.	Age.	Diagnosis.		M-220.		Results.
				No. of injections.	Dosage.	
15	4	Erysipelas of face, scarlet fever, strept. hemol. septicemia.	....	1	7.5 mg./kg.	Rapid recovery.
154	..	Erysipelas of face extensive, back, neck, and arms.	Two weeks' duration, moribund.	4	25 to 30 c.c.	Marked improvement, recovery.
155	44	Erysipelas of face, neck, and chest.	....	1	5 mg./kg.	Apparently cured in less than twenty-four hours.
156	24	Erysipelas of face.	Previous attacks.	1	0.3 gm.	Gone overnight.
157	19	Erysipelas and cellulitis of leg; sepsis.	....	1	30 c.c., 1 per cent.	Rapid recovery.
158	54	Erysipelas and osteomyelitis of leg.	Condition critical.	1	5 mg./kg.	Marked improvement, recovery after 1 injection 5 mg./kg. G. V.
159	65	Erysipelas of leg.	Previous attack.	1	5 mg./kg.	Rapid recovery.
5	26	Erysipelas in wound.	....	1	30 c.c., 1 per cent.	Rapid recovery.

5 mg./kg.) and in 1, 7.5. As a result, in 6 cases only one injection was necessary to effect a complete cure with startling rapidity. One case received four, and 1 two injections. Not a single case of failure in the treatment of erysipelas has reached us, and we feel that we can confidently state that the results obtained in our case No. 15 (which was the first published record showing the effect of mercurochrome in erysipelas) have been equalled in the 7 other cases here recorded.

TABLE 23
SIX CASES OF FURUNCULOSIS

Case No.	Age.	Diagnosis.	M-220 I. V.		Results.
			Number.	Dose.	
160	64	Interstitial nephritis and carbuncles of forearm.	1	5 mg./kg.	Furunculosis cured.
161	55	Furunculosis of thigh and lower leg of eight weeks' duration.	2	4 mg./kg.	Lesions healed.
162	16	4 or 5 boils on each arm.	1 of	10 c.c.	Finally cured.
163	29	Large carbuncle of lower lip.	1	4.6 mg./kg.	Recovery.
24	?	Multiple furunculosis with septicemia.	2 of 1 of 1 of	20 c.c. 15 c.c. 10 c.c.	Dr. Sanmartin considers that the drug saved his life.
29	16	Furunculosis with puerperal sepsis and pelvic abscess.	1 of	30 c.c.	Rapid recovery.

The following case is a good example of the effects of mercurochrome intravenously in severe skin infections: Case 163. Carbuncle. M-220 i. v., 1 per cent., 4.6 mg./kg. Recovery. A. B., aged twenty-nine, weight 145 pounds, admitted April 1, 1924 with large carbuncle involving entire lower lip which was 3 cm. thick and everted. Temperature 100.4° F. Was given intravenous mercurochrome 1 per cent., 30 c.c. (4.6 mg./kg.). Little reaction. This injection was repeated the following day. No operation. The infection subsided rapidly and he was discharged on the 13th with practically normal lip. I believe that M-220 was of distinct benefit.[1]

Analysis of cases of *furunculosis* reported. The 6 cases above stated are the

[1] F. S. Hopkins: Boston Medical and Surgical Journal, 1924, cxci, 732–736.

first to be recorded showing the really remarkable effect of intravenous injections of mercurochrome in furunculosis. Cases 160 and 161, which were treated at this clinic, are excellent examples of the rapidity with which extensive staphylococcic boils may disappear. The case of carbuncle was equally striking, as were Cases 24, 29, and 162 of generalized furunculosis. In one of our cases (160) the entire group of boils disappeared after one injection of 5 mg./kg. In Case 161 two injections of 4 mg./kg. were equally efficient. In the other cases from 3 to 5 mg./kg. were used, one to three doses being employed.

TABLE 24

SEVENTEEN CASES OF CELLULITIS AND ABSCESSES

| Case No. | Age. | Diagnosis. | M-220 I. V. | | Results. |
			No. of injections.	Dose.	
164	19	Extensive cellulitis and sloughing of leg, streptococcus wound infection.	3	10 c.c.	Recovery.
165	?	Cellulitis of face after trauma, gandular involvement.	1	10 c.c.	Marked improvement, second injection not necessary. Marked reaction.
166	52	Multiple abscesses and cellulitis following fracture of first lumbar vertebra, lower sacrum, and coccyx. Streptococcus infection.	1	50 c.c.	No reaction; lesions healed.
167	?	Large pharyngeal abscess unimproved by drainage.	1	23 c.c.	Recovery.
168	17	Streptococcus hemolyticus, multiple local infection. Illness two months with high temperature.	3	10, 12, 19 c.c.	Prompt recovery.
169	43	Gangrene of thigh following extensive trauma. Probably gas gangrene.	2	20, 15 c.c.	Infection cleared up.
170	64	Cellulitis of hand, tenosynovitis of finger. Incision, amputation.	2	30 c.c.	Recovery after amputation.
171	..	Infected hand, enormous cellulitis of forearm. Persistant brawny induration after incision.	1	30 c.c.	Striking improvement; recovery after drainage of abscess.
172	..	Extensive lacerations of right thigh and leg, infection.	3	2.7 mg./kg.	Swelling subsided, wound sterilized.
173	31	Subpectoral abscess, streptococcus hemolyticus; delirious.	1	30 c.c.	Delirium cleared in two hours. Recovery (incision and antistreptococcus serum also given).
174	..	Infected nephrectomy wound.	2	1.4 mg./kg.	Condition cleared; salivation.
175	..	Cellulitis of leg after injury.	1	3.8 mg./kg.	Rapid recovery.
176	..	Infected finger, adenitis.	1	10 c.c.	Rapid recovery.
177	37	Diabetic gangrene of toe.	1	30 c.c.	Marked improvement.
178	62	Infected herniotomy wound.	1	30 c.c.	Doubtful.
179	34	Extensive injuries, fractured skull, laceration of brain, traumatic amputation of arm.	2	30 c.c.	Lived twelve days without infection.
180	71	Streptococcus cellulitis of leg, acute.	2	30 c.c.	No reaction, no benefit.

Analysis of cases of *cellulitis and abscesses* reported. Seventeen cases. In these 17 cases we have grouped together a great variety of superficial and deep infections of skin, subcutaneous tissue, and soft parts. The pathologic processes have been very varied. The streptococcus was isolated from 5 cases, the staphylococcus from 2, and in the others no record is at hand. The clinical description, however, justifies the diagnosis in practically every case. In the first 11 cases here recorded (164 to 176) the rapid disappearance of the lesion and the recovery of the patient is sufficiently definite to class them as cured. In several of these abscess were present, in others only a brawny induration, or deep cellulitis of the skin, in one an extensive gangrene of the thigh, Case 169.

Dosage employed in these 11 cases: In 6 only one dose was used, varying from only 10 c.c., 1 per cent., to 6 mg./kg. In the other 4 cases two or three injections, varying from 1½ to 3 mg./kg. were used. In 4 cases the patients recovered and the local infection seemed to be greatly improved as a result of the intravenous injections. Five mg./kg. was used in each of these cases. In one case (No. 178) the effect of the injection was doubtful and in 2 cases (Nos. 179 and 180) the patients died.

Summarizing, we can safely say that 15 of the 17 cases of cutaneous and sub-cutaneous infections and abscess have been markedly improved by the use of M-220, the effect of which in most cases was, indeed, very striking and rapid.

Although the powerful direct germicidal action of mercurochrome has been proved, when the drug is used intravenously the problem of its mode of action at once becomes extremely complex. We have shown that the germicidal action of mercurochrome is reduced in the presence of serum, and it is therefore improbable that the destruction of bacteria in a remote focus of infection, such as a carbuncle, is due entirely to the direct killing power of the drug, which reaches such a focus only after great dilution in the blood-stream. Such direct action may occur when conditions allow the drug to reach the organisms in killing concentrations, and there must be also in many cases marked inhibitive action, by which the bacteria may be so weakened that the body defences can complete the process of destruction. It also seems probable, however, that fully as important as any direct action of drug upon organism is an indirect stimulation of the body defences. It remains to be determined whether such a modification is due to changes in the blood or in enzyme activity, in alteration of antibody titer, or in some effect the nature of which has not yet been conceived. There is a striking parallelism in the reaction following the intravenous injection of mercurochrome and of foreign protein. The obvious complexity of these problems makes their solution extremely difficult, but it is hoped that researches now in progress and a correlation of previously deter-mined facts about drug action will in time yield further knowledge along these lines of fundamental importance.

Gentian-violet.—The remarkable germicidal action of this drug for Gram-positive staphylococci was demonstrated by Churchman[1] in our clinic in 1912. Since then Churchman has presented numerous other interesting papers which have shown that this drug possesses great value in local infections. In a recent paper Churchman[2] wrote:

Tri-phenyl-methane dyes may be injected into the circulation of rabbits in pretty large doses without harm to the animals, and the blood of the injected animal possesses the selective bacteriostatic property of the dye itself. But only for a short time. At the end of one and three-fourths hours it has entirely disappeared. This power which the blood possesses cannot be interpreted as an activation of the serum, but is due solely to the presence in the blood of the unchanged dye. When the dye is changed, as it is in a relatively short time, the power disappears. It seems probable, since all dyes are rather unstable, that a similar change takes place in other dyes. I have never been able to kill organisms circulating in the blood by intra-vascular injection of gentian-violet. There is some evidence in the literature that it may at some time prove possible to produce a sterilisans magna in this way; but certainly at the present time there is nothing to suggest that it is now possible to do for bacteria what quinin does for malaria.

In our experimental and clinical work on antiseptics we have been greatly impressed with the value of gentian-violet in the local treatment of staphylococcus

[1] The Selective Bactericidal Action of Gentian Violet, Journal of Experimental Medicine, 1912, xvi, 221–248.

[2] The Selective Bacteriostatic Action of Gentian Violet and Other Dyes, Journal of Urology, 1924, xi, 1–18.

infections. We therefore decided to investigate the feasibility of employing it as an intravenous germicide. Accordingly, animal experiments were undertaken.

We have studied the toxicity of gentian-violet by intravenous administration of the drug to normal rabbits. An injection of 20 mg. per kilogram killed in five hours. However, single doses of 5 mg. per kilogram (3 rabbits), 7.5 mg. (2 rabbits), and 10 mg. (4 rabbits) have been well tolerated in every case. Repeated injections, given three times a week, have shown that of 3 rabbits given 5 mg. per kilogram, 2 died after the seventh injection, 1 tolerating seven injections well. Two rabbits died after four doses of 7.5 mg. per kilogram. Of 4 rabbits given 10 mg. per kilogram, 1 died after the fifth dose, 1 after the fourth, and 2 after the second, an average of about three doses. Further experiments with repeated injections of smaller doses are now in progress in connection with pathologic studies. The series here reported, however, indicates that single doses of 5, 7.5, and 10 mg. per kilogram have so far been without toxic effects on rabbits, while repeated doses of these amounts have been sufficiently toxic to indicate that when series of injections are contemplated, smaller doses should be used or, possibly, the intervals between injections lengthened.

The fact that urine may become bactericidal for staphylococci after the intravenous injection of gentian-violet is shown by the following experiment:

The animal was catheterized with aseptic precautions, five minutes before injection, and one, three and five hours after injection. Two c.c. of each specimen so obtained was placed in a sterile test-tube and inoculated with one standard loopful of the test organisms. One minute after inoculation 0.1 c.c. of this urine-organism mixture was removed, diluted, and plated to determine the number of bacteria present. Similar tests were made by dilution and plating one, two, and twenty-four hours after inoculation. In this way it was possible to estimate the increase or decrease in the number of bacteria, and so to determine the antiseptic or germicidal action of the urine. The marked increase in the number of bacteria in the urine taken before drug administration indicates that the urine was not normally antiseptic. The findings are expressed in terms of number of bacteria per cubic centimeter in Table 25.

TABLE 25

ANTISEPTIC ACTION OF URINE AFTER ONE INTRAVENOUS DOSE OF GENTIAN-VIOLET, 10 MG. PER KILOGRAM[1]

	Staphylococcus aureus per cubic centimeter.				
	One minute after inoculation.	One hour after inoculation.	Two hours after inoculation.	Twenty-four hours after inoculation.	Uninoculated control.
Urine obtained by catheterization one hour after injection.	3,300,000	1,160,000	430,000	0	0
Urine obtained by catheterization three hours after injection.	1,040,000	630,000	410,000	0	0
Urine obtained by catheterization five hours after injection	2,700,000	770.000	......	1,300,000	0
	B. coli.				
Urine obtained by catheterization five minutes before injection (control).	1,600,000	11,000,000	11,000,000	83,000,000	0
Urine obtained by catheterization one hour after injection.	5,600,000	5,500,000	3,810,000	7,700,000	0
Urine obtained by catheterization three hours after injection.	1,590,000	1,800,000	3,600,000	......	0

[1] Specimens obtained by catheterization, before injection and one, three, and five hours after injection, and inoculated with Staphylococcus aureus or B. coli.

The urine after administration of gentian-violet intravenously became markedly antiseptic for Staphylococcus aureus and moderately so for B. coli. The drug showed bacteriostatic action on B. coli, but was not bactericidal. In the specimens taken one and three hours after injection, the urine was bactericidal for Staphylococcus aureus, killing all the organisms during a twenty-four-hour exposure period.

Gentian-violet was first employed by us[1] as an intravenous germicide July 12, 1923 in the following case:

Case: Ureteral calculus; Staphylococcus aureus urinary infection; intravenous injection of gentian-violet; sterilization.

J. D. G., aged forty-seven years, admitted B. U. I. June 29, 1923. Diagnosis of calculus of the left ureter just above bladder was made and ureteral dilations and injections of oil, etc., were employed with the hope of causing the stone to pass. During this treatment patient developed an infection of left ureter and kidney with Staphylococcus aureus. On July 12, 1923 he received gentian-violet, 1 per cent. solution, 50 c.c. (7 mg./kg.) intravenously. Except for slight uneasiness in the abdomen patient had no reaction. Pulse, temperature, and respiration remained normal. No nausea, vomiting, or diarrhea, but the skin became very blue. This subsided within six hours. Urine voided one hour after injection had marked violet tinge. Colorimetric tests showed gentian-violet present in dilution of 1 : 50,000. Specimen one hour later contained drug in dilution of 1 : 100,000. A trace of the drug was present at the end of twenty-four hours. Cultures taken from urine several days later showed a complete sterilization, no organisms being present.

The second case in which gentian-violet was employed intravenously was a case of staphylococcus septicemia in the Harriet Lane Home, service of Dr. Howland.

Case: Infant with staphylococcus septicemia and multiple abscesses; gentian-violet intravenously; sterilization of blood and cure of abscesses.

Patient, fifteen months old, admitted with severe dysentery and otitis media. Later developed multiple large staphylococcic abscesses, and blood-culture showed Staphylococcus aureus. "His condition had gradually grown worse; temperature had ranged from 101° to 103° F.—had finally reached 106° F. He was apparently moribund. Staphylococcus aureus had been demonstrated in two cultures made during two days preceding the first injection (August 29th). There were about 10 colonies per cubic centimeter of blood. Three injections of a 0.25 per cent. aqueous solution of gentian-violet were given at twenty-four-hour intervals. The first 5 mg./kg., the second and third, 4 mg./kg. The child, whose condition was desperate at time of injection of gentian-violet, gradually improved. He gained in weight, the abscesses healed, and he was discharged from the hospital entirely well."

Our next case was the following:

Case: Staphylococcus septicemia with multiple osteomyelitis; gentian-violet, 5 mg./kg.; blood sterilized; recovery.

Boy, aged six, admitted September 18, 1923, to the service of Dr. J. M. T. Finney. Diagnosis: General septicemia following multiple osteomyelitis. "During first five days child became progressively worse and was practically moribund, with temperature of 106° F. Acute osteomyelitis of tibia, fibula, radius, ulna, and humerus present. Blood-culture showed Staphylococcus aureus. Multiple incisions were made and cultures from osteomyelitis showed Staphylococcus aureus. At 8 P. M. September 23d temperature 106.3° F., and as a last resort he was given gentian-violet intravenously, 5 mg./kg. by Dr. Rienhoff. Temperature fell at once to 101° F., patient became conscious, and improved steadily. Blood-cultures taken two days later were

[1] Young and Hill: The Treatment of Septicemia and Local Infections, Journal of the American Medical Association, 1924, lxxxii, 669–675.

sterile." Patient ultimately made an excellent recovery after two additional injections. These cases we reported at a meeting of the New York State Medical Society, Buffalo, October 4, 1923.

Since this report we have used gentian-violet in numerous cases in which there was staphylococcus infection present. These cases were urinary, general and local infections, and in almost all cases the results were excellent. In some cases of general septicemia due to staphylococcus the patient has died, and it is our impression that in some instances gentian-violet is not as effective as mercurochrome as an intravenous germicide. It is certainly not nearly so effective against other bacteria. Against streptococcus and Colon bacillus mercurochrome is much to be preferred. In the presence of staphylococcic infections it is now our practice to give mercurochrome first and if there is marked gastro-intestinal reaction, to use gentian-violet which has no such effect, then to repeat mercurochrome if necessary. It is possible that gentian-violet, if used in large doses, has a more irritating effect upon the kidneys than mercurochrome. In 1 case of pyelonephritis we have seen persistent albumen and casts for a time after its repeated use. It also seems to reduce the number of leukocytes in the blood, which is not the case with mercurochrome. Gentian-violet is sometimes followed by a feeling of suffocation and weakening of the pulse associated with decline in blood-pressure, symptoms which, however, rapidly disappear, especially if stimulative treatment is given.

Results Obtained by Intravenous Injections of Gentian-violet.—In an effort to come to definite conclusions as to the value of gentian-violet we have assembled all the cases which we have had in our own clinic or which were reported to us personally or found in the literature. These cases which are given in detail in Tables 25 and 26 may be summarized as follows:

One very interesting case of viridans endocarditis (A) with septicemia which recovered is recorded.[1] This is certainly a very rare accomplishment. Six cases of puerperal septicemia (B) recovered, and in each case the improvement, including drop in temperature, followed so rapidly after the injection that it seems warranted to attribute the recovery to the drug. We have cited one case of septicemia and phlebitis (C) of the left leg and thigh which showed immediate improvement and finally recovered. Shallenberger[2] reports 7 similar cases of phlebitis in which excellent results were obtained with gentian-violet intravenously, the dosage being 5 mg./kg., $\frac{1}{2}$ per cent. solution being employed. In a subsequent report he[3] gives additional interesting cases. There are 5 cases of septicemia with abscesses (D). Two patients died and 3 recovered, 2 being reported as extraordinary cures of almost moribund patients. Two cases of septicemia with osteomyelitis (E) comprise one remarkable recovery and one with no improvement. Two postoperative septicemias (F) were both treated unsuccessfully, although in one case the blood was sterilized. In the 2 cases of septicemia following trauma (G) one recovered and the other did not. We know of a number of other cases of septicemia in which gentian-violet was used without success, and our opinion is to date that as a rule it is not as successful as mercurochrome, which, we believe, should always be used first even in Gram-positive coccus infections. The 4 cases of infections of the urinary tract (H) were immediately improved as a result of intravenous injections,

[1] Major, R. H.: Journal of the American Medical Association, 1925, lxxxiv, 278, 279.
[2] Piedmont Hospital Bulletin, 1924.
[3] Shallenberger, W. F.: Surgery, Gynecology, and Obstetrics, 1924, xxxix, 292, 299.

TABLE 26

CASES OF SEPTICEMIA TREATED INTRAVENOUSLY WITH GENTIAN-VIOLET

Group.	Case No.	Diagnosis.	Blood. Culture.	Number of injections.	Treatment. Dosage.	Results.
A. Endocarditis.	G-31[1]	Subacute.	Strept. viridans.	4	5 mg./kg.	Immediate improvement. Recovery.
B. Septicemia, puerperal.	G-7	Puerperal, T. 105° F., W. B. C., 10,500.	Staph. aureus.	1	10 c.c., 1 per cent.	Drop in T. Recovery.
	G-24[3]	Puerperal, delirious, T. 105° F., W. B. C., 28,000.	....	2	15 and 10 c.c.	Immediate improvement. Recovery.
	G-25[3]	Puerperal, after incomplete abortion, T. 100° to 103° F.	....	2	10 and 10 c.c.	Drop in T. Recovery.
	G-26[3]	Puerperal, delirious, T. 104° F.	Strept. hemol.	2	10 and 10 c.c.	Immediate improvement. Recovery.
	G-30[3]	Puerperal, T. 103° F.	....	3	10, 10, and 15 c.c.	Drop in T. Recovery.
	G-32[2]	Puerperal, T. 104° F.	....	3	32 c.c., ?, ?.	Drop in T. Recovery.
C. Septicemia with phlebitis.	G-22	Left leg and thigh.	Staph. aureus.	1	20 c.c., 1 per cent.	Immediate improvement. Recovery.
D. Septicemia with abscesses.	G-2	Age fifteen months, almost moribund, multiple abscesses. T. 106° F., W. B. C., 22,000.	Staph. aureus.	3	5, 4, and 4 mg./kg.	Blood sterilized. Gradual recovery.
	G-4	Palmar abscess, diabetes mellitus.	Staph. aureus.	1	5 mg./kg.	Immediate improvement. Recovery.
	G-9	Abscess of right hip, Staph. aureus from pus.	....	3	?	Unimproved.
	G-11	Almost moribund, blood infection after opening of carbuncle.	Staph. aureus, hemolytic.	1	30 c.c., 1 per cent.	Unimproved.
	G-23[3]	Abscess around gall-bladder, drainage.	B. coli, Strept.	5	40 c.c., 1 per cent.; 100, 90, 90, and 90 c.c., ½ per cent.	"Some improvement, decreased drainage and exudate, Recovery."
E. Septicemia with osteomyelitis.	G-3	Almost moribund, T. 106.3° F.	Staph. aureus.	2	5 and 5 mg./kg.	Blood sterilized. Recovery.
	G-10	....	Staph. aureus.	1	?	Unimproved.
F. Septicemia, postoperative.	G-8	After mastoidectomy.	Strept. mucosus.	3	?	Immediate improvement. Blood sterilized. Died later. Pneumothorax.
	G-13	General peritonitis, acute gangrenous appendicitis, appendectomy, hemol. Staph. albus in drainage.	....	3	52, 57, and 60 c.c., ½ per cent.	Failed.
G. Septicemia, miscellaneous.	G-28[3]	After trauma.	....	1	15 c.c.	Immediate improvement. Recovery.
	G-2	Probably after trauma, incontinence of urine.	Staph. aureus hemol.	1	100 c.c., ½ per cent.	Unimproved.

[1] Major, R. H.: Journal of the American Medical Association, 1925, lxxxiv, 278, 279.   [2] Shallenberger, W. F.: Piedmont Hospital Bulletin, 1924.
[3] Mooser and Monroe: Medical Journal and Record, 1924, cxix, 58–60.

TABLE 26 (continued)

CASES (NOT SEPTICEMIA) TREATED WITH GENTIAN-VIOLET INTRAVENOUSLY

Group.	Case No.	Diagnosis.	Culture.	Treatment. Number of injections.	Dosage.	Results.
H. Urinary infections.	G-1	With ureteral calculus.	Staph. aureus in urine.	1	7 mg./kg.	Immediate improvement. Urine sterilized.
	G-5	Cystitis, prostatitis, urethritis.	Staph. and Strept. in urine.	1	40 c.c., 1 per cent.	Immediate improvement. Staph. killed. Strept. persisted. Recovery.
	G-19	Gangrenous tuberculous cystitis, resection and marsupialization.	Gram Diplococcus in pus.	1	40 c.c., 1 per cent.	Immediate improvement. Recovery.
	G-29	Nephritis after otitis media. Lung abscess.	Strept. in urine.	4	10 c.c.	Immediate improvement. Recovery.
I. Phlebitis.	G-34[1]	Para-III, pain in groin, thigh, and calf of leg, starting tenth day after delivery. T. 100° to 103° F.	....	2	30 c.c., 1 per cent.	Immediate improvement. Drop in T. Recovery.
	G-35[1]	Para-VI, drainage of breast abscess, followed by phlebitis of left leg.	Sterile.	1	30 c.c., 1 per cent.	Immediate improvement. Recovery.
	G-36[1]	Phlebitis after hysterectomy, T. 102° F., complete thrombosis of the right saphenous vein; bilateral infection.	....	2	30 c.c., 1 per cent.	Immediate improvement. Recovery.
	G-37[1]	Phlebitis of left leg following appendectomy.	....	1	20 c.c., ½ per cent.	Immediate improvement. Recovery.
	G-38[1]	Para-I, phlebitis after Cesarean section.	....	2	30 and 40 c.c., ½ per cent.	Immediate improvement. Recovery.
J. Miscellaneous infections.	G-6 G-14	Lung abscess. Acute appendicitis, peritonitis, liver abscess.	Gram cocci in sputum. Gram cocci and bacilli, Ps. pyocyanea and B. acidi-lactici.	2 1	5 and 5 mg./kg. 15 c.c., 1 per cent.	Failed. Immediate improvement. Recovery after drainage of liver abscess.
	G-15	Acute perforated appendix.	Staph. albus.	1	30 c.c., ½ per cent.	Immediate improvement. Recovery.
	G-16	Acute multiple osteomyelitis.	Staph.	2	20 c.c., ½ per cent.	Immediate improvement. Recovery.
	G-17	Subacute osteomyelitis, right femur.	Staph. albus hemol.	4	16, 16, 16, and 15 c.c.	Immediate improvement. Recovery.
	G-18	Fracture of femur and humerus.	Gram coccus in wounds.	1	55 c.c., ½ per cent.	Immediate improvement. Recovery.
	G-27	Trauma of hand, lymphangitis, amputation.	Strept. in wound.	2	10 and 10 c.c.	Immediate improvement. Recovery.
	G-20	Massive empyema after tonsillectomy; too sick for operation, bronchial fistula, ulcerative stomatitis, intestinal ulcers.	....	5	40 c.c., ½ per cent., 100, 90, 90, 90 c.c., ¼ per cent.	"Some improvement." Decreased drainage and exudate. Recovery.
	G-21	Tuberculosis of right knee, multiple abscesses.	Staph. aureus in pus.	4	30, 25, 28 c.c., 1 per cent.; 50 c.c., ½ per cent.	Secondary infection controlled. Tuberculosis not affected.

[1] Shallenberger, W. F.: Surgery, Gynecology, and Obstetrics, 1924, xxxix, 291, 292.

and in 2 of the cases the lives of the patients were apparently saved by the use of the drug. Among the 9 cases of miscellaneous infections (I) recorded, all but 2 recovered.

Analyzing these cases bacteriologically we find that of the 13 cases in which a non-hemolytic staphylococcus was present, 11 were improved and 2 failed. Of 3 cases infected with hemolytic staphylococcus, however, 1 was improved and 2 failed. One case infected with Streptococcus viridans and one with Streptococcus hemolyticus both recovered, and 5 cases of unclassified streptococcus infection also recovered. Of 5 cases of unclassified Gram-positive cocci, 4 were improved and 1 failed. It is interesting to note that in 1 case of cystitis infected with both staphylococcus and streptococcus the staphylococcus was eliminated by gentian-violet, but the streptococcus persisted.

Conclusions.—A fair statement of our experience with gentian-violet to date would seem to be as follows: This drug is not as satisfactory as mercurochrome even in the majority of cases of Gram-positive coccus infections. Mercurochrome should usually be employed first and repeated at intervals of two or three days in doses up to 5 milligrams per kilogram until improvement is effected or complications, such as stomatitis, which would interfere with further use of the drug, come on. Gentian-violet may then be used with the hope of effecting a result in Gram-positive coccus infections, more particularly staphylococci. The recoveries recorded in streptococcus septicemias and one case of Streptococcus viridans endocarditis are notable cases. The use of gentian-violet as an intravenous germicide, which was first brought out in this clinic, is undoubtedly an addition of considerable value, especially when taken in conjunction with mercurochrome.

Between the two great progress has been made in finding chemicals which will produce a therapia sterilisans magna against both general, local, and urinary infections.

Crystal Violet.—Experiments in our laboratories seem to indicate that crystal violet alone is an even better germicide than gentian-violet. The drug, however, is slightly more irritating and in one of our cases was followed by very marked lymphangitis of the arm and shoulder. In other cases there has been a slight phlebitis at the point of injection. Both gentian-violet and crystal violet should be used in weak solutions, preferably 0.25 per cent., and injected slowly. Dosage of 5 mg.-kg. is usually sufficient, but as much as 8 or even 10 may be given, preferably in divided doses four to six hours apart. In this way a longer retention of the drug in the blood-stream can be maintained.

Novarsenobenzol.—This drug is a condensation product of the salvarsan base with sodium formaldehyd sulphoxylate. The presence of the formaldehyd radicle is of great interest in view of its marked action in urinary infections, but the amount of formaldehyd which might be liberated from a therapeutic dose is very small in comparison, for example, with urotropin. Old salvarsan has been shown by Allison[1] to have a bactericidal action in vitro and in the blood of animals against streptococci, so that the action may be an arsenic action. On the other hand, Gross[2] states that old salvarsan is without action in pyelitis.

Certain observations by Gross[3] and Kall[4] indicated that neosalvarsan in-

[1] Journal of Medical Research, 1918, xxxviii (new series xxxiii), 55–67.
[2] Wiener Klinische Wochenschrift, 1917, xxx, 1381–1384.
[3] Ibid.   [4] Münchener Medizinische Wochenschrift, 1920, lxvii, 541–544.

travenously had a curative action in pyelitis, while in France Janet and Levy-Bing used it successfully in a case of gonorrheal arthritis. Studies in our clinic, controlled by bacteriologic work, show that this drug is undoubtedly of great value, and that its action is almost specific against staphylococci,[1] while streptococci and bacilli usually remain unaffected. In a series of 11 cases of staphylococcus pyelitis, mostly chronic cases, which resisted other forms of treatment, 7 became sterile after intravenous novarsenobenzol and remained so. Similar success was obtained in 2 of 3 cases of staphylococcus cystitis and prostatitis. Only 1 case in 6 of colon group pyelitis became sterile. The urine following these injections shows definite bacteriostatic power against staphylococci, none against the colon group.

The Flavins.—Acriflavin (the trypaflavin of Ehrlich) and proflavin have been used intravenously. Browning first called attention to the germicidal prop-. erties of these drugs against bacteria. E. G. Davis[2] included them in his list of 204 dyes studied in this clinic for antiseptic properties, and produced germicidal urine three and six hours after intravenous injection of 10 mg. per kilogram in rabbits. He was also able to obtain germicidal urine in a few experimental injections of small amounts in man. The effect is increased in alkaline urine.

Davis has recently shown that acriflavin in the form of enteric coated pills may be given by mouth and have a distinct bacteriostatic, if not germicidal, effect in the urine. He has reported a series of interesting experiments on animals and also clinical cases.[3]

In Germany intravenous injections have been tried for pyelitis and acute gonorrhea, with favorable results in the former and unfavorable in the latter. Full clinical trials have not yet been made, principally because the many specimens of the flavins available from different manufacturers vary widely in activity and in toxicity. There is, however, reason to think that these drugs may prove to be very valuable.

Chlormercury Fluorescin.—This drug has been shown by Davis, White, and Rosen[4] to be capable of producing germicidal urine in animals after intravenous injection. No clinical observations have been made.

A number of other drugs have been tried, without marked effect. Among them may be mentioned collargol and electrargol, with which a few successes have been reported from Germany, and urotropin, which gives no better results on intravenous injection than by mouth.

One may recall the various successful specific intravenous treatments of other diseases, namely, the *arsenobenzols* and *mercurials* in syphilis and yaws, quinin in malaria, tryparsimide and Bayer's "205" in trypanosomiasis, and experimental injections of chinin derivatives in pneumococcus infections.

A recent addition to this type of therapy is the successful use of *antimony* compounds,[5] especially tartar emetic, in the treatment of granuloma inguinale, and also bilharziosis by intravenous injection. It is obvious that this is another example of specific drug action, whether the organism concerned in granuloma

---

[1] Young: Urinary Antiseptics, Journal of Urology, 1924, xi, 19–27.
[2] American Journal of the Medical Sciences, 1921, clxi, 251–267.
[3] Journal of Urology, 1924, xi, 29–38.
[4] Ibid., 1918, ii, 277–297.
[5] Aragão and Vianna: Memorias do Instituto Oswaldo Cruz, 1913, v, 221–238.

inguinale be a Leishmania, as described by Donovan,[1] or an encapsulated Gram-negative bacillus, as described by Randall.[2]

We have not yet learned to connect accurately chemical structure with germicidal activity, but the evidence is incontrovertible that drugs of comparatively simple structure may have sufficient specific affinity for certain micro-organisms to enable them to be used therapeutically without harm to the body tissues. Mercurochrome, gentian-violet, and novarsenobenzol have already much increased our effective measures against urinary infections. Without doubt, other, perhaps even better, drugs will appear later. Renewed interest in this subject is our aim, but we would caution against the intravenous use in human subjects of any new drugs before full studies of toxicity by competent workers.

INTERNAL USE OF ANTISEPTICS BY INUNCTION.—Aside from Credé's original idea of introducing by inunction enough silver through the skin to cure infections, and the ancient treatment of gonorrhea by mercurial inunction, based on the idea that it was identical with syphilis, this route has not been used. Credé obtained no success.

INTERNAL USE OF ANTISEPTICS BY MOUTH.—*Urotropin* is usually given by mouth. Comment has been made above on its utility. *Mercurochrome* and *acriflavin* have been tried in this way, with some encouraging experimental results, but in general it is more difficult to secure an effective concentration in the urine than with intravenous injection.

In a study of mercurochrome by mouth we have administered the drug to animals and patients in salol-coated pills[3] and have shown definitely that the intestinal flora is modified and the bacterial count reduced by this form of administration sufficiently to justify further studies. Not only is it effective in normal feces, but also in intestinal infections due to typhoid and dysentery group bacilli and pathogenic protozoa. In a dosage of 900 mg. of mercurochrome daily the urine shows colorimetrically a dilution of between 1 : 15,000 and 1 : 40,000. At this strength the urine is bacteriostatic; stools become deeply stained, almost brick red in color, and the bacterial count is often greatly reduced.

As many infections of the urinary tract are supposed to be due to colitis and other chronic inflammatory conditions of the intestinal tract, it seems evident that the use of mercurochrome by mouth may prove of considerable value.

Other studies made in our laboratories by Hill and Scott[4] show that mercurochrome is eliminated through the bile in bactericidal strength. By inserting a drainage-tube into the gall-bladder of a rabbit and then administering mercurochrome intravenously it was found that the drug appeared in the bile about fifteen minutes after injection and in concentrations as high as 1 : 5000. It was often bactericidal to B. coli, B. typhosus, and Staphylococcus aureus. Moreover, it was possible to sterilize the bile in rabbits which had been experimentally infected with B. typhosus by direct inoculation of the gall-bladder.

In a limited number of clinical cases mercurochrome, both intravenously and orally, has been shown to be of value in cholecystitis and in multiple abscesses of the liver.

[1] Indian Medical Gazette, 1905, xxxix, 414.
[2] Surgery, Gynecology, and Obstetrics, 1922, xxxiv, 717–739.
[3] Young, Scott, and Hill: Journal of Urology, 1924, xii, 237–242.
[4] Archives of Internal Medicine, 1925, xxxv, 503–515.

The experiences to date are too small to warrant any sweeping deductions, but seem to indicate that valuable results may be obtained in both biliary and gastro-intestinal infections with mercurochrome, both intravenously and orally.

Hexylresorcinol.—This drug was prepared by Treat Johnson and has been studied clinically by Leonard at this hospital. It is given by mouth in doses of 0.3 to 0.6 gm. t. i. d., and may be continued over long periods without any toxic effects. Although largely broken down in the body, enough is excreted in the urine to make it bactericidal. According to Leonard[1] its effectiveness depends not only upon the species of organism present, but also on the extent of the infection. Thus, while cures of infections with staphylococcus, streptococcus, and pyocyaneus have been produced, colon group infections in which more than 500,000 organisms per cubic centimeter are present are resistant. Our own experience with this drug is small, but we have seen sterilization follow its use in some cases. This is another drug offering promise for the future in the treatment of urinary infections by mouth.

LOCAL USE OF ANTISEPTICS.—*Bichlorid of Mercury.*—Bichlorid has had some use in wound dressings, but is apt to be absorbed and give symptoms of mercurial poisoning. It has been more widely employed in irrigations of 1 : 20,000 and weaker for irrigation of the bladder and urethra, as well as for skin sterilization and in the treatment of syphilis. Bichlorid of mercury is toxic, irritating, and a protein precipitant, and it is our opinion that in spite of its high antiseptic power, it should be generally abandoned in medicine and surgery.

Silver Nitrate.—As has been shown, solutions of the lunar caustic were very early used in local infections. Recent studies have shown that it has high germicidal value, but that (1) it is immediately precipitated in the form of the inactive silver chlorid, if any chlorids are present, as for example in the urine, and (2) it is very irritant and precipitates protein. Its precipitation by chlorids makes its action in the urinary tract only momentary, while its irritant character contraindicates its use in some instances, but enhances its value in others. After pelvic lavage with silver nitrate solutions the mucosa is found congested, the epithelium desquamated, and a polymorphonuclear exudate is present.[2] This active inflammation may aid in eliminating a mild infection, and many clinical reports would seem to bear out this assumption. Silver nitrate substance or strong solutions are used for cauterizing granulations, polyps, etc., of the posterior urethra. This drug should, therefore, be reserved for those cases where the irritant or caustic effect is desired, since, if this is not the case, we now have other drugs of equal germicidal power, whose action is more prolonged, and which are not irritating.

Potassium Permanganate.—This substance is rapidly reduced to the inactive manganese dioxid in the presence of organic material, setting free "nascent" oxygen. It is during this reduction that the germicidal action occurs. If much nonbacterial organic matter is present, as blood, pus, etc., the reduction is quickly completed and there is no more bactericidal power. At best the bactericidal power is not high, but on account of the blandness of this drug, and its cleansing power, it has become a prime favorite for irrigations of the bladder and urethra in strengths of 1 : 4000 or 1 : 5000. Where strong bactericidal power is desired, other drugs should be used.

[1] Journal of the American Medical Association, 1924, lxxxiii, 2005–2011.
[2] O'Conor: Journal of the American Medical Association, 1921, lxxvii, 1088–1093.

Phenol.—Carbolic acid was much used in wounds following the work of Lister, and has been recommended for urethral injections and bladder irrigations. As a germicide its activity is almost nil in any strengths in which it can be used without harming tissue, and it may be disregarded. Its principal use is in concentrated form for its caustic effect, as to destroy the epithelium in tuberculous ureters or vasa. Rovsing[1] also recommends it in fairly strong solutions (up to 5 per cent.) for its anesthetic effects in tuberculous cystitis. We have seen cases greatly benefited by vesical instillations of 50 c.c. of a 6 per cent. solution. Guaiacol and tricresol are slightly more active than phenol, but still very weak germicides.

Calomel is used only in the form of a 30 per cent. ointment as a prophylactic against syphilis. Its effectiveness for this purpose was shown by Metchnikoff.

Potassium Mercuric Iodid.—This double salt was investigated by MacFarlane, who showed that its bactericidal power is practically the same as that of bichlorid of mercury, while it is much less irritating and does not precipitate protein. It may be used for irrigations at a strength of 1 : 5000 to 10,000. Its high germicidal value has been confirmed by us.[2] Cunningham, Graves, and Davis[3] have recommended solutions of this substance, with an excess of potassium iodid, as a pyelographic medium possessing also antiseptic properties. Dissolved in 85 per cent. acetone solution in a strength of 1 per cent. it makes an excellent skin disinfectant for operations.

Mercury oxycyanid is also a valuable germicide, and does not precipitate protein. Either of these two substances may well replace bichlorid for skin sterilization, etc., and also for certain irrigations (1 : 10,000). Mercury oxycyanid does not corrode metal instruments, and is probably the most suitable substance for sterilizing baths for sounds, dilators, cystoscopes, catheters, etc.

Argyrol, Protargol, Collargol (Silvol, Cargentos, etc.).—All of these drugs consist of finely divided metallic silver in colloidal suspension, with a protective colloid in the form of some albuminous substance to maintain the suspension. They are comparatively non-irritating, do not precipitate protein, and have very definite germicidal value. Apparently they do not penetrate living tissues well. They are used only in mucous membrane infections. While the germicidal activity is not as great as that of some recent drugs, the colloidal silver preparations are very popular, and will no doubt continue in wide use. The following percentages are employed:

	Per cent.
Collargol	0.5—1.0
Protargol	0.5—2
Argyrol	5 —15

The germicidal effects of boric acid and of the various astringent drugs is neglibible. (Zinc chlorid, acetate, sulphate, lead acetate, aluminum acetate.)

Mercurochrome.—In this drug mercury was joined to a dye molecule with the idea of producing a substance at once germicidal and penetrating. It does penetrate into the mucosa, even as much as 2 mm., and has powerful germicidal properties. In view of these facts, the results in acute gonorrhea have been disappointing, indicating that the infection is too deep seated in many cases even for

[1] Die Blasenentzündungen, Berlin, 1910.
[2] Davis and Swartz: Journal of Urology, 1921, v, 235–248.
[3] Journal of Urology, 1923, x, 255–260.

this penetrating agent. Recent studies seem to show that such cases may be advantageously treated by intravenous and local injections of mercurochrome simultaneously. On the other hand, good results have been obtained in cases of chronic urethritis, prostatitis, cystitis and pyelitis, and also in infected wounds and ulcers. It has also found use in the eye, ear, nose and throat, in dentistry, and as a general skin antiseptic after cuts, burns, etc. The intravenous use has been described. The solution used is usually 1 per cent. For continued usage in the male urethra $\frac{1}{2}$ or even $\frac{1}{4}$ per cent. may be preferable. In women Brady has employed 20 per cent. solutions, in the form of vaginal tampons, with good results.

Recently mercurochrome has been used as a preoperative skin disinfectant because of its great germicidal value, its lack of irritation, and its power of penetration. Scott and Hill[1] have shown that for this purpose it may be prepared advantageously with the addition of alcohol and acetone. This is done by dissolving 2 grams of mercurochrome in 35 c.c. of distilled water, to which solution are added 55 c.c. of 95 per cent. ethyl alcohol and 10 c.c. of acetone. In this way a quickly drying preparation is obtained which has been shown to sterilize the skin rapidly, to be non-irritating, and to penetrate the skin fully as well as picric acid and better than kalmerid or tincture of iodin. Traut[2] has confirmed these penetration studies, finding that this solution of mercurochrome penetrates the hair follicles and the deeper layers of the corium.

Meroxyl.—The sodium salt of 2-4 dihydroxy 3-5 di- (hydroxymercuri) benzophenone 2 sulphonic acid. This substance is a powerful germicide, markedly stronger than mercurochrome. It is practically colorless. It is slightly more toxic and slightly more irritant than mercurochrome. It is very useful as a wound dressing, and may be used in wet compresses. It also excels as a germicidal irrigation for bladder and urethra, to prevent infection after instrumentation.[3] Using an apparatus for gradual deflation of the dilated bladder, it is possible to keep the urine uninfected, even in the presence of a retained catheter, by free use of meroxyl solution. For urethral injections meroxyl may be used in 1 : 500 solution, for irrigations 1 : 1000 or 1 : 2000. It should be freshly prepared every day.

Methylene-blue has been given by mouth as a urinary antiseptic, but its efficiency is often nil. In vesical irritation it is frequently of distinct use as a sedative.

In Germany combinations of acriflavin and of methylene-blue with silver have been made (argoflavin and argochrome). Little is known about these compounds, but apparently no striking results have been obtained.

Gentian-violet, as has been shown above, has a specific action on the staphylococci. It has been found to have excellent effects in local infections with these organisms, such as pyelitis, cystitis, chronic urethritis and prostatitis, furuncles, etc. Its value in intravenous use has been discussed. It is used in the renal pelvis and urethra in strengths of 1 per cent. or more. Crystal violet is the active component of gentian-violet and recent tests in our laboratory indicate that this substance may prove to be superior for local and intravenous use.

Acid fuchsin has been recommended for local use in urinary infections, but clinical and laboratory tests in our clinic have failed to bear out the claims made.

Dakin's Solution, Eusol, Dichloramin-T, Chlorazene.—The chlorin antiseptics

---

[1] Journal of Urology, July, 1925.

[2] Personal Communication from Dr. Herbert Traut, Baltimore, Md.

[3] Young, White, Hill, and Davis: Surgery, Gynecology, and Obstetrics, 1923, xxxvi, 508–525.

are, generally speaking, too irritant for successful use in the interior of the urinary system. They are, however, invaluable in infected wounds, especially those associated with necrosis and fetid discharges. They are utilized according to the principles of Carrel and Dakin. One may especially mention the wounds following urinary extravasation, where the chlorin antiseptics are practically indispensable. After necrotic tissue has disappeared from a wound, and clean granulations are present, another antiseptic, such as one of the organic mercurials, may be substituted with advantage, thus avoiding maceration and irritation of the surrounding skin.

Iodoform has little germicidal action and a strong and disagreeable odor, and may cause serious intoxication when absorbed, as from wound surfaces. It may be classed among the non-essential drugs.

Soap (sodium oleate) has been shown here to be actively bactericidal for pneumococcus, gonococcus, and Treponema pallidum, and to prevent chancroidal infection. When present in sublethal concentrations it affects the pneumococcus and gonococcus, so that they are more easily killed by other germicides. On the other hand, soap is entirely inactive against colon group bacilli and staphylococcus.[1]

Soap is very useful as an addition to other drugs in venereal prophylaxis, since alone it is lethal for gonococcus and Treponema pallidum, and will prevent chancroidal infection. Since very weak solutions are effective in increasing the germicidal activity of other drugs against certain organisms, a little might well be added to solutions for application to external lesions, especially chancroids and syphilitic ulcers. On mucous membranes soap is irritating, so that it has not been possible, up to the present, to make use of it in the interior of the urinary tract. Berkeley and Bonney[2] find proflavin oleate useful in the treatment of wounds.

The vapors of *iodin, formalin,* and *ether* have been recommended in chronic, especially tuberculous, cystitis.

Mercurophen.—This mercury derivative of phenol, prepared by Schamberg, Kolmer, and Raiziss, is a powerful germicide, as will be seen by reference to the tables at the end of this section. Unlike mercurochrome and meroxyl, it is more active against the staphylococcus than against the colon group bacilli. It is, however, rather irritating, and has a definite toxicity, so that while it undoubtedly has a sphere of usefulness, it is not very suitable for infections in the urinary tract.

If used in large amounts over lengthy periods, especially in wounds or on raw surfaces, any of the mercurial drugs may be absorbed sufficiently to cause mercurial intoxication. Soreness of the gums and salivation will usually indicate this occurrence clearly enough.

Acriflavin, Proflavin.—The bactericidal properties of these drugs of the acridin series were first studied by Browning,[3] and utilized, mostly in infected wounds, during the Great War. The results were satisfactory. Davis and Harrel[4] first reported a series of cases of gonorrhea treated with acriflavin at this clinic. The drug has been found satisfactory for this purpose, but has not increased the percentage of cures in the striking way that was at first hoped for. It is also useful for irrigations of the bladder and renal pelvis, and its possible intravenous use

[1] Davis and Swartz: Journal of Urology, 1920, iv, 409–418.
[2] British Medical Journal, 1919, i, 152–153.
[3] Browning, Gulbransen, and Thornton: British Medical Journal, 1917, ii, 70–75.
[4] Journal of Urology, 1918, ii, 257–276.

has been discussed. Browning states that the activity of acriflavin and proflavin is not decreased in pus or serum (though there is perhaps some doubt about this), and Davis[1] has shown that they are markedly more active in alkaline than in acid urine.

Acriflavin is used in the urethra in strengths of 1 : 4000 to 1 : 8000 (preferably the latter).

Acid.—It has been found that the application of acid is very useful in certain kinds of infection. Local infections with the Bacillus pyocyaneus (Pseudomonas pyocyanea), or wounds infected with that organism, are best treated by the application of dilute solution of acetic acid with or without other antiseptics. If other antiseptics are used they must be selected so as to be compatible with the acid. The specific sort of wound infection characterized by a fetid odor and gangrenous condition of the wound surfaces, and, in wounds involving a urinary fistula, ammoniacal urine, yields readily when the wound is made neutral or slightly acid by the addition of an acid solution. For this purpose we have found acetic acid best suited. It is to be applied in such strength that the object of neutralizing the urine is attained regardless of the quantity required. This can best be done by using gradually increasing strengths and testing the discharge from the wound after each application. The applications must, of course, be frequent.

As cited elsewhere, wounds infected with the Corynebacterium Thompsonii, which are characterized by a severe slough, alkaline in reaction, are quickly cured by 2 per cent. acetic acid irrigations.

Summary.—The following tables give the results of our bacteriologic researches on the germicidal powers, under various circumstances, of a number of drugs.[2]

TABLE 27

BACTERICIDAL VALUE OF DRUGS AGAINST BACILLUS COLI IN SERUM AND SALT SOLUTION

Drug.	Strength injectable in urethra.	Serum 50 per cent.				Sodium chlorid solution.			
		Killing strength 1 minute.	Therapeutic factor —1 minute.	Killing strength 1 hour.	Therapeutic factor —1 hour.	Killing strength 1 minute.	Therapeutic factor —1 minute.	Killing strength 1 hour.	Therapeutic factor —1 hour.
Phenol	1 : 50	1 : 100	2	1 : 200	4	1 : 100	.2	1 : 500	10
Potassium permanganate	1 : 2000	1 : 200	0.1	1 : 200	0.1	1 : 10,000	5	1 : 20,000	100
Mercuric chlorid	1 : 20,000	1 : 10,000	0.5	1 : 30,000	1.5	1 : 80,000	4	1 : 1,000,000	50
Argyrol	1 : 20	1 : 100 fails	....	1 : 200	10	1 : 100 fails	..	?	?
Protargol	1 : 50	1 : 200 fails	....	1 : 1000	20	1 : 200 fails	..	1 : 8000	160
Silver nitrate	1 : 5000	1 : 10,000	2	1 : 10,000	2	1 : 10,000	2	1 : 10,000	2
Acriflavin	1 : 1000	1 : 200 fails	....	1 : 200 fails	...	1 : 200 fails	..	1 : 4000	4
Flumerin	1 : 100	1 : 100 fails	....	1 : 100 fails	...	1 : 100 fails	..	1 : 8000	80
Mercurophen	1 : 4000	1 : 1000	0.25	1 : 10,000	2.5	?	..	?	
Mercurochrome	1 : 100	1 : 200	2	1 : 600	6	1 : 200	2	1 : 200,000	2000
Meroxyl	1 : 200	1 : 10,000	50	1 : 20,000	100	1 : 10,000	50	1 : 200,000	1000

Table 27 gives the bactericidal value of various drugs against the colon bacillus in 50 per cent. serum and in salt solution. In this table we have included columns which show as follows: Column 1 gives the strength of the drug which can ordinarily be injected into the urethra with impunity. This may be taken as a fair index of what strength may be employed upon other mucous surfaces, but it is well

[1] Journal of Urology, 1921, v, 215–233.

[2] Young, White, Hill, and Davis: Surgery, Gynecology, and Obstetrics, 1923, xxxvi, 508–521.

known that the nose and throat will tolerate far greater strengths than the urethra, and we may add that it is possible to use some of these drugs for one or two applications in much stronger solutions than are here given.

Column 2 shows the germicidal value of the drug, the strength at which its solution kills or fails to kill in one minute. From these two columns a therapeutic factor is derived which indicates the presumptive curative value of the drug when used in dilutions which are commonly employed or may be used for limited periods without injury or pain. This therapeutic factor gives an interesting forecast of the practical value of the drug in treatment, so far as can be deduced from laboratory experiments. It will be noticed that while bichlorid of mercury will kill the colon bacillus at a strength of 1 : 10,000 in one minute, it cannot be used as an irrigation stronger than 1 : 20,000 in the urethra (and generally much weaker than this). Therefore its therapeutic factor (which is derived by dividing the killing strength by the usable dilution) is less than 1 (0.5).

In the other columns the same factor is worked out in serum for the one-hour tests, and in salt solution for one-minute and one-hour tests. Four columns of therapeutic factors are therefore presented which show graphically the value of eleven different antiseptics for different lengths of time, in salt solution or serum. It is thus possible to get an idea of the value of the drug for the conditions met with clinically. A survey of the columns giving the therapeutic factor for one minute in serum shows that meroxyl is twenty-five times as effective as any other drug. In fact, nitrate of silver, mercurochrome, and carbolic acid are the only 3 which approach within one-twenty-fifth of the value of meroxyl according to this factor in the short exposure of one minute in serum. At the end of an hour the difference is not so great, and argyrol and protargol approach to within one-fifth or one-tenth of the value of meroxyl. In the case of permanganate of potash and nitrate of silver in the presence of serum the effect of the drug is no greater in one hour than at the end of a minute. In other words, the chemical reaction between the serum and drug neutralizes the action of the antiseptic almost at once.

The next two columns of factors which give the therapeutic value of the drug in salt solution are not nearly so valuable, as the conditions present do not approximate those found in the body. In salt solution all antiseptics are more active, as a result of being freed from the inhibiting action of serum. For example, the albumin in serum reduces potassium permanganate to manganese oxid, which is inert. In the case of silver nitrate the chlorids in the serum precipitate the silver at once as insoluble silver chlorid, but this is true also in salt solution, so that the results with nitrate of silver are the same in serum and in salt solution, with a very low therapeutic factor, viz., 2, in each.

In salt solution meroxyl again shows its superiority both for one- and sixty-minute tests over all drugs except mercurochrome, which equals it in sixty-minute tests. Owing to the great penetration of the stain and its lasting effect, after several days, mercurochrome is probably more valuable as an antiseptic than meroxyl in certain cases, especially in those cases such as external wounds, skin surfaces, and glandular organs where penetration and prolonged action are desirable.

Table 28 is similar in every respect for the same drugs tested against Staphylococcus pyogenes aureus, and the results obtained are very similar to those mentioned above for the colon bacillus. It is evident, however, that meroxyl is proportionately more powerful against the colon bacillus than against the staphyl-

TABLE 28

BACTERICIDAL VALUE OF DRUGS AGAINST STAPHYLOCOCCUS AUREUS IN SERUM AND SALT SOLUTION

Drug.	Strength injectable in urethra.	Serum 50 per cent.				Sodium chlorid solution.			
		Killing strength 1 minute.	Therapeutic factor —1 minute.	Killing strength 1 hour.	Therapeutic factor —1 hour.	Killing strength 1 minute.	Therapeutic factor —1 minute.	Killing strength 1 hour.	Therapeutic factor —1 hour.
Phenol	1 : 50	1 : 100 fails	....	1 : 100	2	1 : 100 fails	...	1 : 400	8
Potassium permanganate	1 : 2000	1 : 100	0.05	1 : 100	0.05	1 : 1000	0.5	1 : 100,000	50
Mercuric chlorid	1 : 20,000	1 : 3000	0.15	1 : 9000	0.45	1 : 40,000	2	1 : 1,000,000	50
Argyrol	5%	1 : 100 fails	....	1 : 100	5	1 : 100 fails	...	1 : 10,000	500
Protargol	2%	1 : 200 fails	....	1 : 900	18	1 : 200 fails	...	1 : 1000	200
Silver nitrate	1 : 5000	1 : 3000	0.6	1 : 3000	0.6	1 : 4000	0.8	1 : 4000	0.8
Acriflavin	1 : 1000	1 : 200 fails	....	1 : 200 fails	.....	1 : 200 fails	...	1 : 3000	0.75
Flumerin	1 : 100	1 : 100 fails	....	1 : 100 fails	.....	1 : 100 fails	...	1 : 5000	50
Mercurophen	1 : 4000	1 : 10,000	2.5	1 : 30,000	7.5	?	...	?	
Mercurochrome	1 : 100	1 : 90	0.9	1 : 200	2	1 : 100	1	1 : 70,000	700
Meroxyl	1 : 200	1 : 600	3	1 : 2000	10	1 : 600	3	1 : 400,000	2000

ococcus. It is noteworthy here that next to meroxyl, mercurophen is the most active antiseptic in serum for one-minute exposures with the staphylococcus, and next in order is mercurochrome. But here again the question of permanent and lasting effect is not shown by the tables, and this, after all, is one of the most important questions in practical application of antiseptics to wound surfaces and deep mucous cavities and in the treatment of glandular organs where absorption and deep penetration are desirable.

TABLE 29

BACTERICIDAL VALUE OF DRUGS AGAINST THE GONOCOCCUS IN WEAK SERUM

Drug.	Strength injectable in urethra.	Killing strength 20 minutes.	Therapeutic factor 20 minutes.	Killing strength 5 minutes.	Therapeutic factor 5 minutes.
Meroxyl	1 : 200	1 : 80,000	400	1 : 40,000	200
Potassium mercury iodid	1 : 1000	1 : 40,000	40		
Mercurophen	1 : 4000	1 : 40,000	10		
Mercurochrome	1 : 100	1 : 16,000	160	1 : 4000	40
Acriflavin	1 : 1000	1 : 5000	5		
Chlorazéne	1 : 400	1 : 3200	8		
Potassium permanganate	1 : 2000	1 : 2000	1		
Argyrol	5%	1 : 800	40		
Cargentos	5%	1 : 800	40		
Silvol	5%	1 : 400	20		
Protargol	2%	1 : 400	8		
Phenol	2%	1 : 200	4		
Boric acid		2% fails			
Zinc sulphate		1% fails			

The gonococcus tests were made by the Swartz and Davis[1] method, which they describe briefly as follows:

One c.c. of the emulsion is pipetted into a centrifuge tube of diluted drug. The tube is placed in the water-bath at 37.5° C. for eighteen minutes. At the end of this time, it is centrif-

[1] The Action on the Gonococcus of Various Drugs Commonly Used in the Prophylaxis and Treatment of Gonorrhea, Journal of Urology, 1921, v, 235–247.

uged at high speed for two minutes. The supernatant fluid is poured off, and a quantity of salt solution pipetted in. This makes the complete time of action of the drug twenty minutes. The tube is then spun a second time and the wash fluid poured off. The gonococci settle readily in the centrifuge tube and form a compact mass at the tip of the tube, which can be transferred almost *en masse* to a tube of fresh media. This is corked and incubated, as described by Swartz. It is our custom to inoculate after seven days all tubes upon which no growth has occurred with fresh cultures of gonococci. If they develop, we assume that enough of the drug has not been carried over to the test medium to prevent growth. All final growths are examined microscopically with the Gram stain.

The five-minute gonococcus tests were made by the same method. The results of the meroxyl gonococcus tests are expressed in Table 29 where, with the exception of the acriflavin, mercurophen, and meroxyl tests, the figures of Davis and Swartz are quoted.[1]

On analyzing Table 29, it is proper to state that the technic of carrying out bacteriologic and germicidal tests upon the gonococcus is far more difficult than with the organisms previously mentioned. The gonococcus being a much more delicate organism, the conditions of the experiment have to be made somewhat different and the antiseptics are subjected to contact with a greater number of organisms.[2] Owing to the necessity of separating the organisms in the centrifuge, it is impossible to obtain one-minute tests and the five- and twenty-minute exposures are therefore adopted. Here again the therapeutic factor has been worked out and again meroxyl is shown to be far more germicidal than all the others; the next in order being mercurochrome. Argyrol shows a very high therapeutic factor, owing to the fact that it can be used in high concentration, and the same is true of some of the other silver compounds, although their killing strength is low. The question arises, however, whether these colloidal drugs existing as suspensions of comparatively large particles have as great penetration as the other aqueous solutions, particularly those which have the character of stains, as acriflavin and mercurochrome. The high therapeutic value of potassium mercuric iodid is of interest. While most of these drugs produce little or no irritation at the strength mentioned, practical experience shows that all urethral injections and irrigations should be used fairly dilute; *e. g.*, while acriflavin can be used at the strength of 1 : 1000 without much irritation, E. G. Davis recommends that it be used in a strength of 1 : 8000.

Methods.—The various methods of utilizing antiseptics may be grouped as follows:

Internal:
    Intravenously.
    By mouth.
    (By inunction.)
External:
    Irrigation.
        At intervals.
        Constant.

[1] Action of Mercurochrome 220 on the Gonococcus, Journal of the American Medical Association, 1921, lxxvi, 844–846.

[2] Davis, D. M., and Swartz, E. O.: The Testing of Germicidal Substances Against the Gonococcus, Journal of Infectious Diseases, 1920, xxvii, 501–601.

Simple application.

As solution.

As ointment or paste.

Instillation (bladder).

Injection (urethra, seminal vesicle, renal pelvis).

Infumation (injection of gas).

The methods of internal administration have already been discussed.

Constant *irrigation* of external *wounds* is accomplished by the method of Carrel, using the small tubes currently known as "*Dakin* tubes." Superficial wounds may be treated by keeping the dressings constantly in a moist condition. It is now possible to maintain a constant irrigation of the bladder[1] described elsewhere. Some urologists use a double-flow catheter for the same purpose. In the kidney pelvis two small catheters are sometimes left in situ for the purpose of constant irrigation, one serving for inflow and the other for outflow. When two-way catheters are employed, with the solution flowing in under constant pressure, great care must be exercised, first, to maintain constantly a free outflow, and, second, to be sure that no wound of the cavity concerned exists, so that extravasation can occur. The second caution also applies to freshly made surgical wounds, when if the end of the irrigation tube is pressed against the tissues, infiltration beyond the confines of the wound may occur. These methods of constant irrigation are the most successful, as under ideal conditions they maintain constantly an effective concentration of the antiseptic substance in all parts of the cavity or wound concerned. If the substance is so chosen as to be potent bactericidally, and to do no harm to the tissues or leukocytes, splendid results are often obtained.

Where constant irrigation is impracticable, solutions may be *injected* at intervals. This may be done, in the case of wounds, through tubes placed in them, or by flowing the antiseptic over the wound surface from a syringe.

In the *bladder*, one may give these periodic irrigations through a catheter, or simply by employing a conical nozzle applied to the urethral meatus. In the latter case, one first washes out the anterior urethra a few times, and then allows the solution, under a head of about 6 feet or more, to flow back against the external sphincter. The patient is instructed to attempt to void, or relax, whereupon the sphincter opens and the solution flows back into the bladder. This may be repeated as often as desired, the patient voiding between times to empty the bladder. Here the choice of an antiseptic which is not irritating or otherwise deleterious to the tissues is important, since to approach the ideal of constant irrigation, and to allow the germicide to act completely, the irrigations should be repeated as frequently as possible when a germicidal effect is hoped for.

Since the fluid introduced by the non-instrumental irrigation flows through the urethra, this method is also used in the treatment of infections of the *urethra* and *prostate*.

Simple application of a solution requires no discussion; it is poured, swabbed, or sprayed on the area to be treated. In the case of silver nitrate, a small "stick" of the lunar caustic may be applied directly to the affected area. Ointments or pastes may have an oily, gummy, or soapy base. Ointments of vaselin, lanolin, or lard are often useful, and substances insoluble in oil may be suspended in them

[1] Shaw and Young: Journal of Urology, 1924, xi, 373–394.

as fine particles or as concentrated aqueous solutions. Ointments of mercurochrome and meroxyl have been found to have good results in superficial wounds. Pastes made with colloid bases, such as gum tragacanth or gum arabic are theoretically superior for water-soluble substances, but are inconvenient in that they are so subject to drying. Aluminium hydroxid (permutit) has been used as a magma for antiseptics for local and intra-urethral application. Berkeley, Bonney, and Browning recommend proflavin oleate for wounds, as this soapy mass is slowly soluble, and maintains an effective concentration of the antiseptic in contact with the wound surface. A paste of some sort would seem to be desirable for intra-urethral application in order to obtain constant action, but none has as yet come into general use.

Instillations of more concentrated solutions into the bladder, to be retained as long as possible, may be made, like irrigations, through a catheter, or through the urethra with a blunt-nozzle syringe. The sphincter tone should be overcome by gentle, persistent pressure, rather than by suddenly exerted force.

Technic of Urinary Tract Injections.—Injections are made as follows: Renal pelvis, by a small syringe attached to a urethral catheter, never using more than 3 to 5 c.c.; urethra, posterior, through a catheter or by a Keyes-Ultzmann instillator, which is simply a syringe with a small silver catheter attached; anterior, by means of a blunt-nozzle syringe (such injections can also be made to reach the posterior urethra); seminal vesicle, through small ejaculatory duct catheters, inserted with the aid of an endoscope, or by means of vasotomy, with a syringe and needle. Antiseptics placed in the posterior urethra may penetrate the prostatic ducts, especially if the prostate has just been massaged. We have devised an instrument consisting of a small catheter with two inflatable balloons, one to close the vesical orifice, the other to close the membranous urethra. With this device in place, one can inject fluid into the posterior urethra with considerable force, and probably cause it to ascend the prostatic ducts for some distance. After all injections, the antiseptic solution should be retained in place as long as possible. Another principle is that the solution should be as concentrated as possible without harm to the tissues, to obtain maximum effect.

Infumation with vapors of iodin, ether, and formalin has been recommended.[1]

The accompanying table gives, in briefest possible form, the antiseptic drugs, and the form of administration, which may be considered as really useful in urinary infections. In our opinion the many substances omitted from this table are of no proved value, and may well be ignored, at least until additional proof of their effectiveness appears.

We are now able to select our treatment, to a certain extent, according to the character of the micro-organisms present, and this, of course, necessitates bacteriologic study of the cases. One may look forward to an era of specific therapy, when it is to be hoped the long, arduous courses of treatment will be eliminated or materially shortened.

Ideally, we should be able to select a drug with specific action on the organism causing the disease, and with a minimum destructive action on tissues. With such a drug at hand, two further principles govern the treatment: first, to use the drug in the strongest solution that will not harm the tissues, and, second, to apply it

[1] Farnarier: Archives Urologiques de la Clinique de Necker, 1914, i, 353–375. Vernier: Journal de Medicine et de Chirurgie Pratique, 1913, lxxxiv, 913–924.

so that it will act as nearly continually as possible. Following these principles success will often be obtained in a short time.

If success is not obtained, however, the treatment should be interrupted: first, because we know, if the treatment has been intensive to the limit, that nothing can be gained by its continuance; and, second, that the micro-organisms may develop an abnormal resistance to the drug employed. This has been definitely proved for mercurochrome. The procedure then is to change quickly to another suitable drug, the action of which may be favored by the effects of the first which are still present. Another possibility lies in combined therapy, of two or more suitably chosen drugs. This method has not as yet been thoroughly worked out.

The following list of drugs and other closely allied therapeutic procedures is given for quick reference.

General

(a) Local anesthetics: Procain (1 to 4 per cent. urethral injection); benzyl alcohol (1 to 4 per cent.).

(b) External antiseptics: Soap and hot water; mercuric chlorid, alcohol; tincture of iodin; potassium mercuric iodid (kalmerid); mercurochrome-acetone-alcohol.

(c) Lubricants: Liquid petrolatum; glycerin; tragacanth paste (KY); petrolatum; olive oil.

(d) Coagulants, styptics: Epinephrin; silver nitrate; copper sulphate; horse serum; blood transfusion; cephalin.

External Infections (Balanitis, Ulcers, Chancroids, Buboes, Chancres)

1. Washes: Boric acid; potassium permanganate, silver nitrate, mercuric chlorid, mercurochrome, copper sulphate, phenol, Rosenwald's solution, meroxyl.
2. Dusting powders: Lycopodium, boric acid, iodoform (rarely), calomel.
3. Ointments: Boric acid; mercurochrome; zinc oxid; ammoniated mercury; balsam of Peru; scarlet R.
4. Caustics: Silver nitrate; phenol; nitric acid; copper sulphate; cautery; fulguration.
5. Wet dressings: Saline (chancres until discovery of spirochetes)—later mercurochrome; hot meroxyl, bichlorid of mercury, magnesium sulphate, boric acid.

Infections of Genito-urinary Tract

1. Urethritis: (a) Acute (anterior and posterior, prostatitis, vesiculitis, epididymitis).
   1. Diluents: Internal antiseptics; water forced, sodium bicarbonate; potassium citrate and hyoscyamus; santal oil; hexamethylenamin (?).
   2. Injections: Argyrol; protargol; acriflavin; mercurochrome; colloidal silver oxid, meroxyl, etc.; silver nitrate (later).
   3. Irrigations: Potassium permanganate; mercuric chlorid; silver nitrate; acriflavin; mercurochrome; mercuric oxycyanid; meroxyl.
   4. Antispasmodics: Hyoscyamus; belladonna; extract of opium (suppositories); morphin, papaverin.
   5. Heat: Stupes; hot-water bag to perineum; hot rectal douches; hot sitz baths, etc.

6. Cold: Ice applied to external genitalia or perineum, or ice-water by two-way rectal douche.

(b) Chronic.

1. Same drugs as above, according to circumstances.

2. Instrumentation: Urethroscopic applications (silver nitrate, stick or in solution); instillations of silver nitrate 1 to 5 per cent.

3. Mercurochrome, 1 per cent., after massage of vesicles and prostate and cleansing irrigation.

2. Prostatitis, vesiculitis: (a) Acute, as above, 1 (a), as circumstances may require, with rest in bed and frequent cold rectal irrigations.

(b) Chronic, as above, 1 (b); also injections of vas deferens and vesicles through vasotomy or urethroscope with protargol, argyrol, collargol, or mercurochrome.

(c) Tuberculous: Injection (after epididymectomy) through vas; phenol (pure); iodoform oil; gomenol.

3. Cystitis:

(a) Acute:

1. Internally; potassium citrate; hyoscyamus (if painful); if not painful, reduced water, sodium benzoate, and hexamethylenamin; acriflavin; mercurochrome; gentian-violet; novarsenobenzol; hexylresorcinol.

2. Irrigations: Salt solution; boric acid; potassium permanganate; mercuric chlorid; silver nitrate; mercurochrome; meroxyl; acriflavin.

3. Injections and instillations: Silver nitrate; mercuric chlorid; argyrol; protargol; mercurochrome, acetic acid.

(b) Subacute: Same as above, more vigorously, to sterilize bladder; yeast; Bulgara tablets; B. acidophilus (instilled).

(c) Chronic: Same as above, more vigorously, to sterilize bladder; yeast; Bulgara tablets; B. acidophilus (instilled).

(d) Ulcerative and interstitial: Cystoscopic applications; silver nitrate; phenol; cautery; hydraulic dilation; fulguration; excision.

(e) Tuberculous: Gomenol; phenol (6 per cent. injection); iodin (gas); mercurochrome (1 per cent. injection); fulguration.

4. Pyelitis:

(a) Acute, febrile: Forced water (internal); sodium bicarbonate (sometimes alkalies forced, especially in children).

(b) Acute, afebrile:

1. Water reduced (internal); acids forced (sodium benzoate; sodium acid phosphate); hexamethylenamin (60 to 90 grains each day); mercurochrome, hexylresorcinol, acriflavin (by mouth); mercurochrome, neo-arsphenamin (intravenously).

2. Pelvic lavage: Silver nitrate (1 to 5 per cent.); mercurochrome (1 to 5 per cent.); meroxyl (1 : 500).

3. Pyelogram: Thorium nitrate (15 per cent.); sodium iodid (15 per cent.).

(c) Pyelonephritis: Same as (b) 1 and 2, as circumstances may require; nephrectomy if unilateral.

    (*d*) Ureteritis: Same as (*b*) 1 and 2, as circumstances may require; with dilation of strictures, if present, using bougies and paraffin bulbs.

5. Kidney, hematuria:

    1. Internal: Horse serum; blood transfusion; calcium chlorid; gelatin; ergot, etc.

    2. Pelvic lavage: Silver nitrate (1 to 5 per cent.); epinephrin (1 to 5 per cent.).

    3. Pyelogram: Thorium nitrate (15 per cent.); sodium bromid (15 per cent.); sodium iodid, to exclude neoplasm, stone, or tuberculosis.

SPECIAL CONSIDERATIONS

Before beginning treatment the case should have been thoroughly studied in clinic and laboratory. Until the type of organism, character of lesion, extent of invasion (kidney, bladder, prostate, vesicles, or urethra), presence of complicating local conditions (obstruction, stricture, stone, ulcer, tumor, etc.), and the general condition of the patient (focal infections outside the urinary tract) are adequately known, intelligent treatment cannot be instituted.

Focal Infections.—As these are responsible for many urinary infections, careful preliminary study of teeth, tonsils, sinuses, ears, respiratory and gastro-intestinal tracts should be made. If definite suppurative processes are discovered, they should receive energetic treatment. In many cases operative intervention is required and some urologists insist on removal of infected tonsils, adenoids, and teeth before attempting urologic treatment. Unfortunately, it is not always certain that the urinary infection has come from the remote focal infection under suspicion. Hundreds of such operations have been performed without facilitating the cure of the urinary infection or the nephritis.

This being the case, and especially since the advent of several valuable new germicides (acriflavin, mercurochrome, meroxyl, gentian-violet, etc.) it may often be well to see, first, what can be accomplished by some of these, either used locally, injected *in situ*, or introduced intravenously. The coccus infections are more apt to come from foci in the head (tonsils, sinuses, teeth) and bacilliary infections from the gastro-intestinal tract (colitis, etc.). Often no focal infection can be found.

Another potent factor in urinary infections is obstruction to the urinary tract. The methods employed in combating such conditions are described elsewhere, but no hope of permanent cure can be expected unless the obstruction is removed and free drainage of the ureter and kidney pelvis is obtained.

Granted, therefore, that everything has been done to discover and cure any outside focus of infection or local obstruction, what shall be done to cure the urinary infection? That depends on its location, character, and extent.

Kidney Infections.—In cases where the pelvis alone is involved (chronic pyelitis) lavage through a ureter catheter may be very efficacious. One per cent. nitrate of silver is most popular and sometimes gives startling cures after one or two treatments. Often it has to be repeated once or twice a week for months. Nitrate of silver is precipitated upon the mucous membrane, does not penetrate, and is painful. It is irritating and causes a cellular reaction which is supposed to be very beneficial in throwing off the infection. Occasionally 3 or even 5 per cent. solutions of silver nitrate have been employed with good result, but the reactions may be very severe.

Where silver nitrate fails other drugs may be employed. By referring to the section on germicides, the germicidal value of various antiseptics in solutions of normal salt, blood-serum (50 per cent.), and urine may be compared. Those of practical value are mercurochrome, meroxyl, acriflavin, gentian-violet, acid fuchsin, and argyrol. One advantage of the dyes is their penetration. Thus mercurochrome has been shown to penetrate quickly to the cortex of the kidney, while silver nitrate remained upon the surface of the pelvic mucosa.[1]

Mercurochrome is more efficacious for nearly all infections, while gentian-violet is a remarkable germicide for certain Gram-positive staphylococci. Of the two, mercurochrome is the better general germicide. Both may be introduced into the renal pelvis in solutions of from 1 to 5 per cent. without injury.

Meroxyl is a more powerful germicide, and also does not coagulate albumin or urine, but not being a stain it probably does not penetrate as deeply. A 1 per cent. solution is occasionally followed by a rapid sterilization of the urine, both in bacillary and coccus infections.

Occasional good results have also been reported from argyrol, acid fuchsin, and other drugs, but there are many failures from all forms of treatment. This is due to various factors, viz., reinfection from an outside focus, depth of infection in the kidney or submucosa of renal pelvis, obstructive conditions interfering with free drainage.

Simple *pyelitis* should be treated by attacking the primary focus, instituting appropriate internal treatment: water, acids, or alkalies, internal antiseptics (urotropin, mercurochrome, novarsenobenzol, gentian-violet) and lavage through ureter catheterization. The treatment employed will depend considerably on the nature of the infection, the character of the lesion, the symptoms present, and the results obtained. In young children, and occasionally in pregnant women, a simple pyelitis due to colon bacillus will often clear up promptly under the use of a large quantity of alkalies (sodium bicarbonate, 15 to 30 gr., four times a day). If the patient has been on this treatment for a time without results, occasionally the sudden change to a hyperacid treatment will effect a prompt cure (sodium benzoate or acid sodium phosphate). Along with the acid treatment urotropin, 60 to 90 gr. daily, may be employed with good results.

In adults where the foregoing treatment has not succeeded, pelvic lavage, beginning with 1 per cent. nitrate of silver, or if more reaction is desired, 3 to 5 per cent. nitrate of silver, should be tried. With stronger injections it is usually desirable to wait several days before giving further treatments, which will have to be regulated considerably by the amount of reaction which is produced by the treatment. Some patients suffer considerably and even have violent pain and considerable shock. Others have very little reaction and treatments may be repeated two or three times a week.

Leonard has shown that when, by means of pelvic lavage, the number of B. coli are greatly reduced, internal treatment with hexylresorcinol by mouth will often end in a speedy sterilization of the urine. Mercurochrome may also be used in a similar way. Some cases may indeed be treated entirely by intravenous medication. The course of treatment for pyelitis is often very protracted and discouraging, particularly because the infection is apt to recur even when the primary focus in the tonsils, teeth, etc., has been removed.

[1] O'Conor: Journal of the American Medical Association, 1921, lxxvii, 1088–1093.

Heitz-Boyer[1] and others have strongly advised the use of intestinal antisepsis to combat the primary source of infection from the intestine. Mercurochrome by mouth has also been advised for a similar reason.[2] It has been shown that patients may take it in capsules, each containing mercurochrome 100 mg., t. i. d., and that this dose may be gradually increased, until in three or four days the patient is taking 3 capsules three times a day. Treatment may be continued ten to fourteen days without much discomfort, but should then be discontinued for several days. The effect of this internal medication is to reduce the bactericidal count in the feces. The bile becomes strongly antiseptic.

A few cases of pyelitis of the colon bacillus type have already been cured by the oral administration of mercurochrome alone. Further experiments are necessary to determine what the effect of these oral intestinal antiseptics may be.

Pyelonephritis.—As remarked above the kidney is usually involved in cases of pyelitis and the probable reason for the difficulty in obtaining sterilization in these cases is due to this fact. It has been shown that mercurochrome injected into the pelvis penetrates rapidly through the tubules and cortical substance to the periphery of the kidney, but this is apparently not sufficient to cure many of these cases.

The treatment is much the same whether nephritis be present or not, and, in fact, the only method of determining positively, as remarked before, is by careful functional tests and blood studies.

Pyelitis with obstruction demands appropriate treatment for the relief or cure of the obstruction. If there be a definite ureteral stricture present dilations should be carried out, but as these cases are often associated with peri-ureteral inflammation or adhesions, operation may be necessary to obtain a cure. Where the obstruction is due to bands of fascia, aberrant blood-vessels, unduly mobile kidneys with kinking in certain positions, etc., appropriate operative treatment, described elsewhere, should be carried out. Calculi in the pelvis or ureter may not only cause obstruction, but sufficient irritation to keep up the infection. In certain cases it may be desirable to give the patient either internal treatment or pelvic lavage before operating to remove a calculus, but, as a rule, little can be accomplished by preliminary treatment and the operation should be done without undue delay.

If dilation is to be done, it should be thorough—to at least No. 11 or 13 F. Hunner uses bulbs as large as 6 mm. in diameter. The same principles apply as in urethral stricture.

Pyelitis is sometimes kept up by a renal fistula which may persist after perinephric abscess or operation upon kidney or ureter. Not infrequently the persistence of a fistula is an indication that obstruction to the pelvis or ureter is present. Occasionally a stone is the cause of the fistula and appropriate operative treatment for these conditions will be required before the fistula will close and the urinary infection can be cleared up.

Pyonephrosis, if accompanied with very great destruction of the kidney, generally requires nephrectomy, but where the disease is bilateral or where the condition of the patient is such that a major operation cannot be considered, palliative therapy will have to be employed. The principles above outlined may be fol-

---

[1] Journal Medical Français, 1922, xi, 178–212.

[2] Young, Scott, and Hill: Journal of Urology, 1924, xii, 237–242.

lowed. In such cases the physician may well try intravenous germicides. One of our cases[1] in which the patient was desperately ill following excision of a carcinoma of the bladder, a pyonephrosis was combatted, and finally cured, by the intravenous administration of germicides (mercurochrome and gentian-violet). Ureteral dilation may be helpful.

Perinephric abscess is often associated with pelvic or renal infections and generally demands prompt operative relief, with drainage of the abscess and removal of the kidney, if the conditions warrant. If the kidney is only slightly involved and the function fairly good, drainage may alone be required. In such cases, where the condition of the patient will not permit operation, here again intravenous therapy may be employed successfully. A remarkable case in which an extensive perirenal, retroperitoneal abscess was present and disappeared promptly after the intravenous injection of 34 c.c. of 1 per cent. mercurochrome has been reported.[2] Another case of acute perinephric infection, due to the staphylococcus (as shown by aspiration) disappeared promptly after 28 c.c. of 1 per cent. mercurochrome intravenously.

Conclusions.—The treatment of renal, perirenal, and pelvic infections requires a most thorough study of the case, and very persistent, and gradually varied treatment. No one method is suitable to every case and those which are remarkably efficacious against a certain organism will, in another case, in which apparently the same organism is present, be utterly useless. No cases tax the resourcefulness of the urologist more than these, but great progress has been made in recent years and these cases which were previously treated successfully by operation (generally nephrectomy) are now rarely treated except by non-operative procedures.

Surgical treatment has been proposed for a number of different forms *of renal infections.* Some surgeons, more enthusiastic than others, have considered as infections certain conditions of doubtful etiology, namely nephralgia, which has been called "nephritis with pain," and the so-called essential hematuria, or "nephritis with hemorrhage." The procedures utilized have been puncture, nephrotomy, pyelotomy, capsulotomy, capsulectomy or decapsulation, nephrolysis (freeing the kidney of adhesions), sympathectomy, and nephrectomy, and various combinations of these.

Pousson[3] divides the cases into the following groups:

Acute nephritis:

Toxic (bichlorid, turpentine, etc.).

Bacterial (surgical kidney, Brewer's acute unilateral nephritis, carbuncle of the kidney, etc.).

Acute Bright's disease.

Other acute nephritides, which may be toxic or bacterial (scarlatinal, syphilitic, eclampsia, etc.).

Chronic nephritis:

Bacterial (chronic pyelonephritis).

Under this heading are included varieties with pain (nephralgia) and with hemorrhage (idiopathic hematuria).

Chronic Bright's disease.

[1] Young and Hill: Journal of the American Medical Association, 1924, lxxxii, 669–675.
[2] Young: Johns Hopkins Hospital Bulletin, 1924, xxxv, 14–16.
[3] Encyclopædie Française d'Urologie, 1914, ii, 227–304.

Acute Toxic Nephritis.—Decapsulation has been done in many cases of mercury bichlorid poisoning, supplemented in some instances by nephrotomy and drainage. There is much dispute as to whether any good has been accomplished. In some of the fatal cases a temporary increase, quantitatively, in the urinary output followed the operation. According to Klose[1] this diuresis has occurred in more than half of his collected cases. Rollwage[2] makes the most sensible suggestion—that since there is so much doubt about the utility of the operation, future decapsulations should be done on one side only, so that the effects may be compared at autopsy, in case of death, with the other undisturbed kidney. In general, it may be said that no definite proof of the value of this procedure has been brought forward. The diuresis which follows it may justify its use in certain desperate cases, but no great hopes should be pinned to it.

Acute Bacterial Nephritis.—Here the chief indication for operation is in unilateral cases, a type first brought to attention by Brewer. He recommended nephrectomy, but others have shown that decapsulation, accompanied by nephrotomy with drainage, also produces excellent results. Pousson believes that success is more likely in hematogenous than in ascending infections. The indications are fever, increasing pyuria, severe hematuria, oliguria, and especially severe localized pain. The pain is usually found to accompany a tense, congested kidney, and is relieved by slitting the capsule. One should try to operate before abscess formation takes place. These unilateral cases are rare, but operation is often a life-saving procedure for them. It is important to make sure that the other kidney is sound by catheterization, even though the patient is quite ill. If suppuration has occurred before operation, nephrectomy may be necessary. In a few cases of localized abscesses, resection has been carried out.

Acute Bright's Disease.—Operation has been recommended in the acute crises. Pousson has collected the statistics of 116 cases so operated on. In 24, the intervention was in the early stages. Of these, 8 are *dead*. Five of the 8 showed temporary improvement. Sixteen *lived*, 2 showing very great improvement, 5 great improvement, 5 some improvement, and 4 no improvement. In 92 cases, the intervention was three months or more after the onset. Twenty-five are *dead*, of which 22 showed temporary improvement. Sixty-seven *lived*, 8 being apparently cured, 11 showing very great improvement, 34 marked improvement, 18 slight improvement, and 7 no improvement. Of the 8 apparently cured, 2 had been followed eight years, 1, seven years, and 1, four years. The operations performed were decapsulation, nephrotomy, and decapsulation followed by wrapping the kidney in peritoneum or omentum. It would seem that some such procedure is justified in cases where medical treatment fails to arrest the downward progress.

Other Acute Nephritides.—Similar operations have been done in scarlatinal and the so-called syphilitic nephritis. The remarks in the preceding paragraph apply here also. McIntosh[3] reports a case of severe syphilitic nephritis, which showed a large tense white kidney. The capsule retracted when incised, the parenchyma bulging out. Following decapsulation there was an immediate marked increase in the volume and specific gravity of the urine, the blood urea fell to normal

---

[1] Beiträge zür Klinische Chirurgie, 1922, cxxv, 459–468.

[2] Mitteilungen aus der Grenzgebiete der Medizin und Chirurgie, 1921–22, xxxiv, 374–392.

[3] Medical Journal of Australia, 1922, i, 668–670.

in two weeks, and recovery ensued. Fairchild[1] has collected a series of 92 cases of eclampsia treated by decapsulation. Sixty-two recovered, 32 died, and since the mortality rate of all cases of eclampsia is about 31 per cent., he concludes that the value of surgical treatment in this disease is very doubtful. Certain surgeons, however, report individual cases which seem very favorable. Cholmogoroff[2] reports a case of eclampsia which recovered as a decapsulation was about to be done, and observes justly that had the operation been performed the recovery would undoubtedly have been imputed to it.

Chronic Pyelonephritis and Chronic Bright's Disease.—These conditions may well be considered together. According to Fairchild, Reginald Harrison, of London, in 1878[3] was the first to attempt the surgical relief of nephritis by incising the kidney. Le Dentu, of Paris, in 1881 was the first to confine the incision to the capsule, splitting it from end to end. It was Edebohls,[4] however, in 1898, who advocated complete stripping of the capsule, and brought this operation to the attention of the entire medical world. His assumption was that the tissues surrounding the decapsulated kidney would reunite with it, and that new and more abundant vascular connections would be present in these adhesions. His first case was in a woman with albuminuria and casts from one kidney, which was also movable. Cure was complete after decapsulation and fixation of the kidney. There is some doubt that this case represented true Bright's disease. A large number of studies have been made on animals, practically all of which show that a new capsule forms after decapsulation, and that it is no more vascular than the original one. At first it is very thick, but later becomes thinner.

Clinical experiences have been many, but there is still little convincing evidence of a curative effect. Kelly decapsulated one kidney in a case where the divided function had previously been studied. Later examinations and ureteral catheterizations showed no change, for better or worse, in the kidney which had been operated on. Unless new and convincing evidence can be brought forward, the operation will probably have to be abandoned as ineffective. We have had little success with decapsulation.

On the assumption that idiopathic or "essential hematuria" is a hemorrhagic nephritis, operation has been recommended for this condition. Pousson advises nephrotomy and drainage. Others have done decapsulation. Since many of these cases can be relieved without operation, surgical interference should be a last resort. The most valuable non-surgical methods are intrapelvic lavages with adrenalin (3 c.c. of a 1 : 1000 solution) and silver nitrate (1, 2, or even 5 per cent.). Horse-serum may be given subcutaneously. If a nephrotomy is done, it should be in cases where the bleeding is quite serious, and should be wide enough to permit a search for a localized pelvic lesion—papilloma, varix, etc.—which may be treated by cauterization. In extreme cases nephrectomy may be necessary to save life.

In the same way "nephralgia" has been thought due to nephritis. Nephrotomy, decapsulation, and nephrolysis have been advised. On the basis that it is a neuralgia, the French surgeons denude the vessels of the pedicle, in order to divide all the nerves of the kidney—sympathectomy. We have found the "nephrolysis"

[1] Journal of the American Medical Association, 1912, lix, 2234–2237 (Lit.).
[2] Zentralblatt für Gynäkologie, 1910, xxxiv (2), 947–949.
[3] Lancet, 1896, i, 18–20.
[4] Medical News, 1899, lxxiv, 481–483.

of Rovsing, in which the kidney is merely freed from the surrounding tissues and dropped back, a very satisfactory procedure. It is necessary to free the kidney to carry out sympathectomy, and we have found the additional section of the nerves unnecessary. Possibly the nephrolysis is what cures in sympathectomy.

In *résumé*, then, we may say that decapsulation has been proposed on two bases: (1) To allow new vascular connections with the kidney to form, and (2) to relieve internal pressure of the kidney. The first-named object is probably not accomplished, the second can be sought only when the condition of the kidney is congested or edematous. In such cases, if properly selected, pain is relieved and increased flow of urine is usually observed. As to the ultimate results, however, little that is definite can be said. The most striking results are those in which suppuration has really begun, and which may for that reason be classified among the "surgical kidneys."

Bladder Infections.—Much that has been said above applies to the treatment of infections of the lower urinary tract. In cases of cystitis, after identifying the bacteria present, cystoscopy should be done to search for pathologic conditions of the bladder, prostate, and urethra, and to determine the character of cystitis present.

If prostatic obstruction, cellules or diverticula, calculi, tumors, ulcers, urethral stricture, prostatitis, etc., are present, little can be expected of treatment of the infection, until these conditions are corrected. Appropriate surgery is, therefore, the first indication in such cases.

The use of drugs by mouth or intravenously, as above outlined, should be considered. The near future will probably see a scientific basis for the selection of the germicide to be employed.

Water, in large amounts, is often of great value in washing the bladder clean, inhibiting bacterial growth and lessening the inflammation and irritation of the mucous membranes.

Local treatment varies according to the inflammatory process and symptoms present. In very irritable cases—with pain, frequency of urination and dysuria, or even strangury—rest, alkaline water, the tincture of hyoscyamus and potassium citrate mixture, hot applications or sitz-baths, etc., may be helpful.

Later vesical irrigations, silver nitrate 1 : 10,000 to 1 : 5000, permanganate of potash 1 : 6000, may be useful. The newer antiseptics, acriflavin 1 : 8000, meroxyl 1 : 1000, mercurochrome $\frac{1}{2}$ per cent. (as injection), mercurophen 1 : 10,000, and gentian-violet 1 : 500 may be used according to the nature of the infection and pathologic condition present.

Nitrate of silver is valuable, but is irritating, and should be followed by boric acid or other mild irrigations.

The dyes should be allowed to remain in the bladder as long as possible, so as to get penetration and, if possible, to kill the bacteria *in situ*. We have occasionally seen mercurochrome sterilize cases of chronic cystitis in three or four treatments (1 per cent. solution, retained each time two or three hours).

Acute gonorrheal cystitis is almost always associated with acute prostatitis or posterior urethritis, and is usually only a trigonitis, or at most a cystitis colli, in which the major part of the bladder is free from inflammation. In the acute stage, rest, the drinking of water in large amounts, and the use of bland diuretics or santal is about all the treatment that is required. When the symptoms are so acute as to produce strangury, associated with very frequent urination, pain, and sometimes hematuria, large doses of opiates or other sedatives may be required and the use of hot rectal douches or, sometimes, ice-water douches may be of value. With the subsidence of the acute stages of the prostatic inflammation the bladder symptoms usually disappear. A general gonorrheal cystitis does occur, but rarely, and chronic cystitis due solely to the gonococcus has only been described once.[1]

Non-gonorrheal Infections of the Bladder.—In the first stages there is usually a bacteriuria present, in which the urine may still be clear and the bacteria found only on microscopic examination. This may persist without the development of pus-cells, the bladder fluid acting as a culture-medium. In such cases active antiseptic treatment will often clear up the infection promptly.

Where pyuria has come on, a definite diagnosis of inflammation (cystitis) is made and energetic treatment undertaken, in which the rules previously laid down are to be followed, both as regards internal treatment and local bladder irrigations and instillations. No one antiseptic is universally successful and it is well to try them seriatim.

Where the cystitis becomes acute in its symptoms, and is associated with irritation, frequency of urination, pain, and possibly hematuria, rest in bed and the usual methods to make the urine bland may be employed until the acute symptoms disappear, after which active antiseptic treatment may be carried out.

When the cystitis has become chronic, nitrate of silver as an irrigation (1 : 5000 to 1 : 10,000) or as an instillation (1 per cent., 1 to 3 c.c.) may be of great value. The irritation and congestion produced may be very helpful in clearing up the infection, but, as a rule, this treatment should be followed up by other mild antiseptic irrigations and instillations, among which may be mentioned mercurochrome 1 per cent, meroxyl 1 : 2000, acriflavin 1 : 6000 or 8000, argyrol 1 per cent., etc.

Ulcerative cystitis may be benefited by instillations of nitrate of silver or carbolic acid 6 per cent., but local treatment through the cystoscope (local applications of nitrate of silver or electrical fulguration) may be necessary.

Where the lesions are *encrusted with urinary salts*, irrigations or cystoscopic methods to clean off the lesion should be carried out. If the urine is alkaline, sodium benzoate or acid sodium phosphate by mouth to acidify the urine may be used. Caulk[2] recommends frequent injections of suspensions of Bacillus acidophilus in the bladder in these cases. Acetic acid 1 per cent. is very effective.

Exfoliative cystitis may be caused by retaining very strong solutions of permanganate of potash. Dawson[3] has shown in one of our cases that the superficial epithelial layer of the bladder mucosa was exfoliated after retaining a solution of permanagnate of potash, used in the treatment of gonorrheal urethritis. In some cases of exfoliative cystitis a large part of the vesical mucous membrane has come away without operative intervention. In other cases suprapubic drainage has been required.

Leukoplakia, if localized, may be treated by local applications or fulguration. Radium applications may be also tried.

Submucous cystitis is very frequently associated with sterile urine and treatment is indicated principally on account of frequent and painful urination. Forcible

[1] Young: The Gonococcus, Johns Hopkins Hospital Reports, 1900, xi, 679–707.

[2] Cabot's Modern Urology, 1924, ii, 89–143.

[3] Johns Hopkins Hospital Bulletin, 1898, ix, 155–159.

distention of the bladder, which breaks up the fibrous contracture in the region of the submucous fibrosis and produces an increased blood-supply, will often be of great value in mild cases. The irrigating jar should be at least 6 feet, but not over 8 feet, above the level of the bladder. By means of twice daily overdistention of the bladder by hydraulic pressure, the capacity may be greatly increased and these cases ultimately cured. In some instances considerable hematuria is pro-

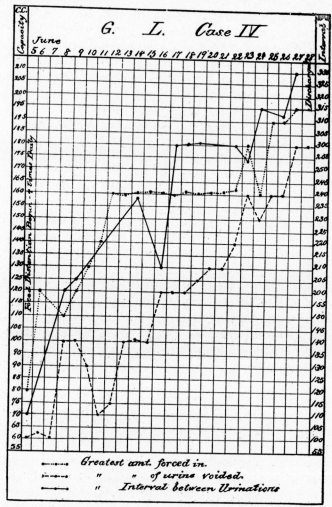

Fig. 115.—Contracture of the bladder treated by hydraulic distention. Amount voided, 60 c.c., at intervals of one hundred ten minutes; bladder capacity, 80 c.c. Under hydraulic dilatations, in twenty-two days, bladder dilated to 195 c.c.; amount voided, 180 c.c., at intervals of three hundred thirty minutes.

duced and the frequency and dysuria may for a time be increased. Many patients cannot tolerate this treatment and are, in fact, made worse under it, but in some cases excellent results are obtained by persistence in frequent vesical dilations by hydraulic pressure.

In some of the cases in which the bladder capacity has been greatly reduced a progressive increase in the capacity may be secured. Interesting cases of this type were cited by us[1] in a paper in 1898 in which the use of hydraulic dilation in genito-urinary practice was brought out. One of these, a patient with cystitis of many years' duration, voided urine every ten minutes during the night and day, and had a bladder capacity of only 15 c.c. Under forcible dilation, with weak bichlorid solutions, the capacity of the bladder was gradually increased, the interval between urination lengthened, and the amount of urine voided increased until, finally, in about six weeks' time, the patient had a bladder capacity of 260 c.c. and was able to retain urine for four hours. He was then discharged from the hospital and continued his treatment at home, finally dilating his bladder up to 460 c.c., and having an interval of urination of five or six hours. The chart (Fig. 115) graphically shows the remarkable progress made in another case of contracture.

This treatment has been employed in numerous cases since that time. Many of these cases were associated with submucous cystitis or interstitial ulceration and fibrosis and were either greatly benefited or permanently cured. The lesion producing the symptoms was recognized, and frequently described in cystoscopic notes, but no special name was given to it. Some cases of submucous cystitis do not tolerate the treatment above outlined and for these, local applications, preferably electric fulguration through the cystoscope, may be tried, followed by vesical lavage and ultimately forcible dilatation by hydraulic pressure. Nitrate of silver may also be applied with benefit through a ureter catheter cystocope to local ulcerative lesions, but in many cases operative intervention is required. It is here that the work of Hunner has been of very great value. After operative excision (the technic of which is described elsewhere, see Chapter XVI) vesical lavage and dilatation are usually necessary in order to restore the bladder to its proper capacity and to combat infection. In many cases after operation the disease recurs and cystoscopy may show similar lesions on subsequent examinations. In a few instances the suprapubic operation has been repeated, but we prefer to try local measures, fulguration, local applications, hydraulic dilation, antiseptic treatment, etc. It has recently been reported to us that cases of submucous cystitis have been cured by intravenous mercurochrome.

Although the subject of submucous cystitis has received considerable attention in the literature in recent months, there is still much to be learned in regard to the etiology, pathology, and treatment, which at best, is not very satisfactory.

Case of submucous cystitis seen first in 1904, and persisting after Bottini operation and, subsequently, perineal prostatectomy.

B. U. I. No. 741. E. B., aged fifty-five years. Admitted October 10, 1904, complaining of difficulty of urination and irritation in the bladder. Complains greatly of pain at the end of micturition.

Examination showed the prostate slightly enlarged. No residual urine. Bladder capacity, 250 c.c. Marked pain when the bladder becomes full and on emptying bladder through catheter. The cystoscope shows a small median bar. The bladder is negative everywhere except on the anterior wall. The following note was made at this time. "Over the anterior surface of the bladder are scattered several irregular areas which are very red in color, roughly granular of surface, sharply contrasted with, and elevated slightly above the surrounding mucosa, which is pale in color. At the margins of these areas the vessels are greatly injected. These areas are confluent with each other in an irregular way, the general direction of some of them being transverse and others longitudinal, and they cover an area about 3 cm. in diameter on the anterior wall of the bladder. There are no ulcerations to be seen and no septa or prominent trabeculæ in this region. The anterior limits of the area occupied by these lesions is apparently about

[1] Young: Johns Hopkins Hospital Bulletin, 1898, ix, 100–113.

2 cm. back of the prostatic orifice. The posterior and lateral walls of the bladder showed none of these irregular areas. There was no stone present." [Remark, 1925: The above description, written in October, 1904, is a very accurate description of the condition that we now recognize as submucous or interstitial cystitis.] The urine was negative for bacteria and only an occasional leukocyte was present. The prostatic secretion contained only a few leukocytes. Tubercle bacilli were carefully sought for in both urine and prostatic secretion and none found. The patient was given hydraulic dilatations of the bladder, but without benefit. It was impossible to dilate the bladder by hydraulic pressure, and as there were evidences of obstruction present in the form of median bar, on November 12th, a Bottini was done under ether; one posterior cut and one through the right lateral lobe with Young's four-bladed Bottini instrument, blade No. 2, 2 cm. being employed.

During the next year the patient was treated by hydraulic distentions and the bladder capacity increased to 360 c.c. As a result of the Bottini and this treatment he was greatly improved, and occasionally held urine for four hours, and eventually six hours. The next year, however, the irritation and frequency of urination returned.

In 1907 a cystoscopic examination showed 25 c.c. residual urine, and a definite median prostatic lobe. On the anterior wall of the bladder the same dark red, irregular, confluent areas were seen.

On November 8, 1907, perineal prostatectomy was done, and June 17, 1909, examination showed no residual urine, but the bladder capacity was 100 c.c., very irritable, and very spasmodic, and on the anterior wall several areas, deep red in color, which had been seen five years before, were still present.

Cystoscopy in 1910 showed eight small red, elevated, areas grouped in the shape of a horseshoe along the anterior wall of the bladder, and also along the lateral aspect. The rest of the bladder was negative. January 16, 1911, Letter: Urination still frequent, eight to ten times at night, pain on voiding.

Remark: Here, then, is a case of submucous or interstitial cystitis which was seen first in 1904, and was followed for seven years; was not cured by removal of an obstructing median bar by a Bottini operation; nor by prostatectomy, when, several years later, the prostate had become enlarged and obstructive. The lesion was recognized as probably the cause of the irritable bladder, and he was treated by hydraulic pressure which, for a time, was quite effective, but apparently the condition returned worse than ever. Such cases we would now treat by resection.

Contracture of the Bladder.—As above described this condition not infrequently complicates or follows submucous cystitis. In other cases it is due primarily to muscular hypertrophy associated with obstruction to urination, generally, however, complicated with chronic inflammation and infiltration of the submucous and muscular tissues.

The treatment indicated is to remove all causative factors, to combat inflammation, to dilate the bladder by hydraulic pressure or otherwise, according to the principles laid down above.

The question of ureteral reflux or regurgitation of fluid from the bladder into the ureters when forcible dilatation of the bladder by hydraulic pressure is carried out, was considered in detail in our first paper on this subject. It was shown apparently conclusively, that it did not occur under the circumstances in which the treatment was employed. These preliminary experiments have been confirmed by various authors and, although it has been shown that reflux may occur under certain circumstances, it is not when the bladder is rapidly and forcibly distended with fluid as advised in the treatment of these cases, unless the ureteral orifices are patent as a result of chronic inflammation, in which case ureteritis and pyelitis are always present. Before beginning treatment we determine by cystogram whether reflux into the ureters and kidney pelves occurs during the treatment by hydraulic dilatation. An excess of pain, followed by fever and tenderness in the region of the kidney and especially a fall in the phthalein test, will usually show that reflux has occurred. In very rare instances we have seen definite traumatism and perhaps partial or complete rupture produced by very forcible distention (with the irrigating tanks suspended at a very high elevation, 10 to 12 feet above the bladder). In none of these cases, however, were the ultimate results serious, the tenderness, pain, fever, etc., disappearing after appropriate rest, etc.

Hour-glass bladder occasionally follows chronic cystitis, but generally when associated with obstruction and most often accompanied by hypertrophy of the trigone. With the relief of the obstruction as a result of prostatectomy or operations upon strictures of the urethra, the vesical symptoms may improve or disappear. In some cases operative treatment is required. Division of the constricting ring, sometimes enlarged by plastic closure after the Heinecke-Mikulicz principle, may be required. The technic is described elsewhere. Following operation intravesical lavage and dilatations by hydraulic pressure are often necessary to complete the cure.

Pericystitis is so rarely met with and presents so few intravesical lesions that the treatment requires but brief reference. In the more acute stages when swelling, pain, tenderness, muscle spasm are present, the bladder symptoms—frequent and painful urination—are best treated by rest along with hot applications to the abdomen. Should the infection progress to abscess formation or extravasation of urine, early operative intervention is required. When the condition becomes chronic with or without operation, the inflammatory process may involve the bladder wall sufficiently to produce irritation, contracture, or submucous inflammatory lesions, the treatment of which has been described before.

Urethral, Prostatic, and Vesicular Infections.—*Urethral infections*, acute and chronic, are most often the result of gonococcus infections. Were we dealing with a superficial infection of a simple tube, destruction of the infecting bacteria and cure of the inflammation would be simple enough. Unfortunately, the infection lies deep in the tubules and glands of the mucosa and submucosa as well as the deep para-urethral ducts and Cowper's glands (occasionally). The minute size of these ducts, occluded by inflammation, makes penetration by germicidal solutions well nigh impossible. This accounts for the difficulty in curing gonorrhea.

Mercurochrome, on account of its penetrating qualities, seems to be of positive value, particularly in subacute and chronic cases. Nitrate of silver (1 : 5000 as an irrigation or 1 to 5 per cent., as an instillation of a few drops) is also of great value in chronic cases, on account of its cauterizing effect on old inflammatory areas, as well as the reaction it produces.

Other agents—acriflavin 1 : 5000, mercurophen 1 : 6000, argyrol 1 to 5 per cent., protargol 1 to 2 per cent., permanganate of potash 1 : 4000 to 1 : 10,000 may all be useful in certain cases.

By diligent treatment and persistence almost all cases of chronic urethritis may be cured. But the urologist must not call a case well until gonococci are not to be found in urethral or prostatic secretion or in the shreds, which should, if present, be few in number and composed mostly of epithelial cells. Otherwise treatment should be continued.

The presence of pus-cells in considerable number in urethral and prostatic secretion, even though stained slides and cultures show no bacteria (much less gonococci) should warrant withholding the assurance of a cure, with the hope of ultimately reducing the leukocytes to a small proportion of the cells present.

Urethritis—Gonorrheal, Acute.—When a patient is seen within a very short time after the inception of the disease (from a few hours to a day after the discharge is first noticed) strenuous efforts may be made to arrest, or abort, the disease by means of urethral injections. For this purpose many antiseptics are occasionally effectual. The most commonly employed are argyrol (5 per cent.) and protargol 2 per cent., but acriflavin 1 : 4000, mercurochrome or meroxyl 1 per cent., and mercurophen 1 : 4000 have been effective in a limited number of cases. It is preferable to give two or three, or possibly four injections, during the first twenty-four hours. Each should be retained in the urethra as long as possible. The patient meanwhile drinks water in very large quantities (6000 to 10,000 c.c. daily). Such treatment is not infrequently rewarded by a complete disappearance of the gonococci in a few hours, and where this is maintained the vigorous antiseptic treatment may be stopped on the second or third day, the water cure being continued. Simple non-irritating injections or irrigations may then be employed and if the gonococci do not reappear, the treatment may be stopped within a few days. Careful observations should be made to be sure that there is no recurrence.

As a rule, a patient is seen too late for the above-mentioned treatment to be of value, or the disease has already assumed such an acutely inflammatory character that it is evident that the bacteria have penetrated well beneath the surface of the urethra, beyond the reach of strong germicides. In such cases mild injections, supplemented with the water cure, may be employed. Argyrol is the most popular, but acriflavin, mercurochrome, meroxyl, etc., may also be employed in weak solutions, preferably twice daily.

The treatment should be controlled with careful examinations of the urine, voided in three glasses, and as soon as a cloudy third glass, or other signs and symptoms of involvement of the deep urethra or prostate come on, treatment should be appropriately modified at once. When the disease becomes subacute or has a tendency to become chronic, nitrate of silver may be employed either as an irrigation or occasionally as a fairly strong injection ($\frac{1}{2}$ per cent.) with the object of inciting cellular reaction which will have a curative effect. When the gonococci are absent and only a mucoid discharge persists, the use of bougies to detect strictured areas, or the passage of sounds which will thoroughly dilate the urethra, and upon which massage can be carried out to facilitate the absorption of peri-urethral infiltration, may be employed.

Not infrequently it will be necessary to desist from all treatment before a final complete disappearance of urethral discharge and shreds in the urine.

Posterior urethritis occurs in a large percentage of the cases, variously estimated at between 50 and 85 per cent. When the invasion of the posterior urethra is ushered in with frequency of urination, pain and discomfort in the perineum, bladder, and rectum, it is usually wise to stop all treatment, put the patient in bed, if possible, force water by mouth, give alkaline drinks, and await the subsidence of the acute symptoms. Sometimes hot rectal douches, given several times daily through a two-way rectal irrigator, may be of value.

If the disease continues and the prostate becomes markedly involved, urination may become so frequent or painful that complete retention may finally supervene. To induce urination the following methods may be tried: irrigation of the anterior urethra with a warm, mild, antiseptic solution; high enemata; the passage of filiforms gently into the deep urethra; the application of hot water-bags to the abdomen and perineum; a large dose of morphin or other sedative.

Not infrequently one or several of these methods may be effectual in restoring voluntary urination, but where everything fails, the question arises as to whether it is wise to pass a catheter. A small rubber catheter may often be passed without more than slight injury to the acutely inflamed prostatic mucous membrane, but it is sometimes better to aspirate the bladder suprapubically with a small needle, to which a suction syringe may be attached. The details of this technic are given elsewhere. We have had cases of acute gonorrheal prostatitis in which repeated aspirations (6 to 10) were necessary before normal urination was established. Other cases have been treated with a small rubber catheter, but generally had a more prolonged period before micturition returned.

In those rare instances in which the bladder is involved, it is either trigonitis or, at most, a cystitis colli. No special treatment is required. These conditions soon disappear.

The invasion of the posterior urethra is usually associated with only a mild involvement of the prostate. The treatment to be employed is usually intravesical irrigations of mild antiseptics of which permanganate of potash (1 : 6000 or 8000) is the most popular. These are forced in by hydraulic pressure by means of a blunt nozzle without the use of a catheter. Acriflavin 1 : 8000, meroxyl 1 : 1000, or injections with a bulb syringe of $\frac{1}{2}$ to 1 per cent. mercurochrome may be employed, often with splendid results. As the disease becomes less acute weak solutions of nitrate of silver (1 : 7000) as irrigations, or instillations of 1 to 2 c.c. of a 1 per cent. solution of nitrate of silver, with the Keyes syringe, may be necessary to effect a cure.

Complications due to the involvement of the various glandular adnexa of the urethra, unfortunately, occur with great frequence. Among these may be mentioned infection of the para-urethral ducts, the glands of Littré, of Cowper, the peribulbar glands, the ducts and glands of the prostate, the utricle, the ejaculatory ducts, seminal vesicles, ampullæ, vasa deferentia, epididymes and possibly the testes. Each of these may bring on a change in the character of the disease and its symptoms. It is this deep invasion of glandular structures, drained only by minute ducts and impossible to reach by antiseptic treatment, that makes the final cure of acute or chronic gonorrheal infections so difficult.

The surface may be benefited by urethral lavage and irrigations and the deeper lesions may be reached by a penetrating germicide such as mercurochrome.

If the inflammation goes on to abscess formation in any of these structures it may rupture either into the urethra or form subcutaneous collections of pus, which may rupture spontaneously, but require drainage by operation when discovered. Fortunately, such is rare.

Involvement of the prostatic ducts and glands is best treated by rectal irrigations of hot water, although some prefer them ice cold. The same is true for acute *seminal vesiculitis* and *ampullitis*.

After the acute stage of infection in the prostate, seminal vesicles, and ampullæ has subsided, and gonococci and shreds are absent from the urethral discharge no treatment should be used for a time. Later, gentle pressure upon the vesicles, ampullæ, and prostatic lobes may be employed to hasten the dispersion of the disease. Such emptying should be followed by injections of 1 per cent. mercuro-chrome, or other penetrating dye-stuff, into the posterior urethra. Such measures are usually reserved until the case has become distinctly chronic in type.

Acute vasitis is generally ushered in by pain in the groin and is usually followed by *epididymitis*. The use of ice in the groin and upon the epididymis is the accepted method for the treatment of such cases. The scrotum should be elevated and the patient kept quiet on his back in bed. In a number of cases sodium iodid injected intravenously (10 c.c. of a 10 per cent. solution) has been employed in this clinic with success. In some instances the disappearance of pain and swelling have been remarkably prompt. Hypodermic injections of antimeningococcus serum have produced some startling results. It is probable that intravenous therapy may be used with increased frequency in such cases in the future. Luys and others have employed the direct injection of electrargon or other colloidal silver preparations into the substance of the inflamed epididymis, while Hagner has championed early epididymotomy with multiple puncture of the inflamed epididymis. He has been followed by numerous surgeons and the literature now contains a vast array of cases which have been treated in this way. There is undoubtedly a rapid dis-appearance of pain and discomfort after the operation, but there is still a question whether the ultimate results are better and whether the convalescence is markedly shortened by the resort to operative intervention. Most cases of acute gonorrheal epididymitis subside spontaneously after a certain period of time. Nodules usually persist in the epididymis and sterility may occur regardless of the treatment employed.

Orchitis may rarely occur, always in conjunction with epididymitis. In most cases the diagnosis of orchitis is erroneous and due to the fact that the testicle is obscured by the greatly enlarged epididymis.

Acute gonococcus abscesses may occur anywhere along the urinary tract (or else-where) as a complication of acute gonorrhea. They may appear as peri-urethral, peri-bulbar, perineal, prostatic, or perivesicular, perirectal, perivesical, retroperitoneal, epididymal, or testicular. It is possible that with the development of intravenous therapy these may eventually be satisfactorily combated without operation, but at present incision and drainage, sufficiently early to prevent urinary extravasation or serious complications, including septicemia, etc., should be carried out. Perineal, prostatic, and vesicular abscesses should be opened through the perineum. We do not recommend breaking into a prostatic abscess from the urethra with a sound. Incision through the rectum is inexcusable.

Urethritis—Gonorrheal, Chronic.—Unfortunately, regardless of the treatment employed, a fairly large percentage of cases of gonorrheal urethritis become chronic. As stated before, this is manifested by the persistence of a glairy discharge or gluing at the meatus, by pus shreds in the urine, leukocytes in large number in the secre-tion obtained from the prostate, seminal vesicles, and ampullæ by massage, or by the microscopic study of secretion obtained from urethral ducts, glands, utricle, or ejaculatory ducts through the endoscope. The treatment to be employed will depend largely upon the extent of the lesion, the regions involved, and complica-tions present. In simple subacute or chronic anterior gonorrheal urethritis or "gleet," use of irrigations, injections, bougies, sounds, massage, and endoscopic treatments may be employed seriatim. In these chronic cases nitrate of silver is of the greatest value, either as an irrigation or as an instillation or local application through the urethroscope. If polyps, granulations, or other proliferative lesions are present, fulguration or diathermy, using a very small current of high voltage and low amperage, is often the treatment of choice. An open endoscope or a urethroscope of the MacCarthy type can be used. The penetrating germicides—acriflavin, mercurochrome, and meroxyl—may also be employed with great benefit. The use of sounds, dilators, massage, etc., is often essential. Treatment should not be too vigorous and there should be intervals of rest in order that the best results may be obtained. Not infrequently irritation and inflammation are kept up by harsh and long-continued treatment and it is only necessary to provide rest to obtain a prompt cure. It is not always possible to obtain a *restituo ad integram*. Shreds in the urine may persist for a long time, but if they contain few pus-cells and no gonococci, their presence need give little concern. It is essential that all strictures and areas of peri-urethral infiltration should be cured in order to prevent a recurrence of the disease.

Chronic Posterior Urethritis.—In rare instances this may be confined to the prostatic urethra where it is usually associated with involvement of the verumontanum. In such cases posterior irrigations and injections may be employed with good effect. Occasional urethroscopic applications to the verumontanum, if this is found enlarged, congested or covered with granulations, should be made. Similar pathologic conditions may be found elsewhere in the posterior urethra and at the vesical neck. Occasionally fulguration through the urethroscope may be the most effectual method of dealing with these pathologic conditions. One should use a spark of high voltage and very low amperage, to avoid sloughs and subsequent stricture formation. The open endoscope, or a specially designed urethroscope, like the MacCarthy, may be used with advantage.

Treatment of Prostatic Cysts.—Non-operative: This has been employed only once—by Kornfeld, who in 1902 ruptured a large obstructive cyst of the prostate by rectal massage. The cyst could be palpated by rectum and on very vigorous pressure it was felt to give away and the fluid escaped from the urethra, followed by micturition and complete relief of the obstruction. All other methods of treatment have been operative and may be divided as follows:

1. By suprapubic cystotomy: (*a*) Excision intact—this has been done in 3 cases: 1. Young, 1912, enucleation of a cyst 2 cm. in diameter. 2. Hottinger, cyst size of cherry. 3. Lower, 1915, cyst size of thumb.

(*b*) Excision of ruptured sac, 3 cases: Abbe, Bosch, and Van Houtum Aekhorn.

(*c*) Excision of ruptured cyst with cautery, 2 cases: Burkhart and A. Cabot.

(*d*) Ruptured cyst destroyed with curet, 1 case: Behrend.

2. By suprapubic prostatectomy, 1 case by Thompson Walker. Hypertrophied prostate and cyst removed together.

3. By perineal prostactectomy, 1 case, Frontz; cyst removed with prostate.

4. Removal by operative cystoscope: (*a*) By Young's cystoscopic rongeur (Fig. 117), 2 cases; Young, 1913; (*b*) by fulguration with ureter catheterizing cystoscope, 3 cases (Fig. 118); Young, 1921,[1] Wesson,[2] 1921 and 1923; (*c*) with Nitze cystoscopic cautery, 4 cases; Meyer, 1916, 3 cases, Wesson, 1924, 1 case. (*d*) By Bottini cautery incisor, 1 case; Legueu and Verliac, 1910.

Résumé: As noted above, the literature now contains 21 cases in which obstructive retention cysts at the prostatic orifice have been removed by operation. As

---

[1] Keen's Surgery, 1921, viii, 530–534.   [2] Journal of Urology, 1925, xiii, 605–632.

noted above 4 of these cases are from this clinic and comprise the first cases in which the cyst has been removed intact by suprapubic operation and in which the cysto-

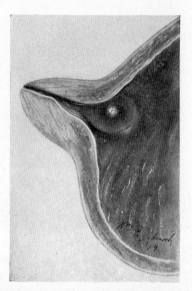

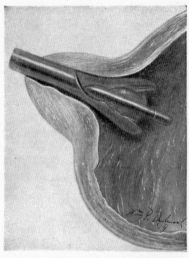

FIG. 116.—Cyst of the prostate. Sagittal section showing thin-walled cyst springing from the prostate at the vesical orifice.

FIG. 117.—Removal of cyst of prostate projecting into bladder with Young's cystoscopic rongeur.

scopic rongeur and fulguration have been employed to destroy cysts through the urethra. There have been no deaths from any of the operative procedures, but

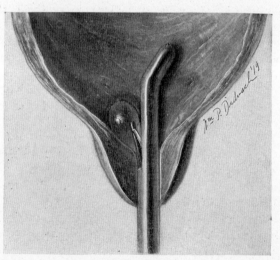

FIG. 118.—Cyst of the prostate. Sagittal section showing operative cystoscope in place, with fulgurating wire held against the cyst by the elevator, ready to commence destruction of the cyst by fulguration.

from our experience we would unhesitatingly say that a suprapubic operation is entirely unnecessary and that fulguration by means of a ureter catheterizing cystoscope is the simplest method and entirely satisfactory. The removal of the

PLATE VI

CYSTS AND EDEMA OF PROSTATIC ORIFICE AND BLADDER

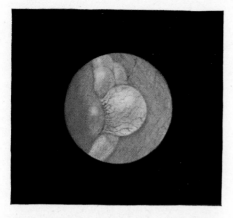

A. Cyst and edematous swellings on hypertrophied lateral lobe. B. U. I. 11,121.

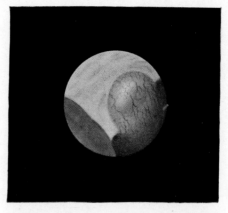

B. Single cyst of prostatic margin, bilateral hypertrophy. B. U. I. 8438.

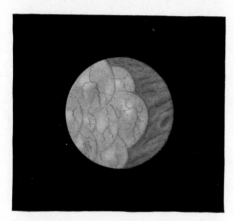

C. Mass of cysts filled with clear fluid covering hypertrophied prostatic lobe. B. U. I. 11,352.

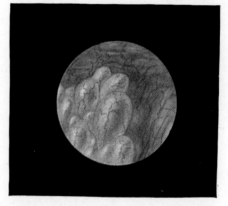

D. Multiple cystic polyps of trigone, median portion of prostate and floor of urethra; treated by fulguration. B. U. I. 9676.

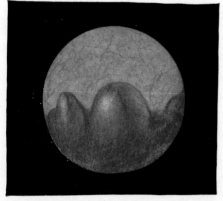

E. Edematous congested mucous membrane at prostatic orifice. Marked congestion of bladder mucosa. B. U. I. 9174.

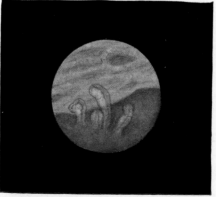

F. Edematous polyps at prostatic margin, treated by fulguration. B. U. I. 10,887.

cyst by means of our cystoscopic rongeur is more radical and generally satisfactory, but in 1 case was followed by considerable bleeding, requiring suprapubic operation, at which a spurting artery was found in the wound at the site of the removal. By means of fulguration or the cautery it should have been possible to stop this hemorrhage, and thus avoid a suprapubic drainage. Fulguration, however, is in our opinion entirely satisfactory, though it should be repeated until the sac is completely destroyed and removed. Owing to the fact that the sac is sometimes multilocular, several applications of high frequency cauterization may be necessary before the fluid is completely evacuated.

We are of the opinion that the small number of cases to be found in the literature is not a correct index of the frequency of this condition. Although only 9 cases have been reported in America, we are confident that the disease is much more common and that careful cystoscopic examination will reveal many obstructive

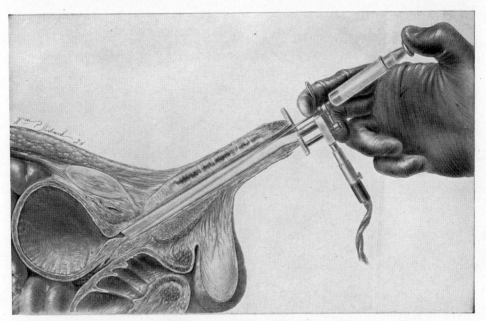

Fig. 119.—Injection of ejaculatory duct, vesicle, and vas through Young's urethroscope.

cysts in cases in which frequency and difficulty of urination are present in young men without palpable enlargement of the prostate by rectum. Careful cystoscopy and the detection of a translucent globular enlargement at the prostatic orifice will make the diagnosis positive.

In most cases of chronic urethritis the prostate is involved, and *chronic prostatitis*, generally associated with *seminal vesiculitis*, is present to keep up the inflammatory process. As remarked before, the diagnosis is made by careful rectal palpation, the expression of secretion from the prostate, vesicles, and ampullæ, and microscopic examination of fresh specimens. Massage or stripping is the most important therapeutic method to be employed in these cases. (The technic is described elsewhere.) It should be done with care so as to avoid injury to the inflamed region and also excoriation of the rectum. Intervals of two to four days are usually appropriate. The urethra may be emptied of the secretion either by urinating or lavage, after which it is usually desirable to inject some penetrating antiseptic into the deep urethra by means of a Keyes syringe, or a simple rubber bulb syringe. We usually employ 1 per cent. mercurochrome, injecting 5 to 10 c.c. into the deep urethra after massage, and not infrequently find the pus-cells stained two or three days later when expressed by massage. The seminal vesicles and ampullæ may be reached by injection through the ejaculatory ducts (Figs. 119, 120). Vesiculograms show it is easy to fill these structures by the endoscopic technic above described.

Belfield, Thomas, and others have highly recommended the injection of argyrol, etc., by means of vasotomy in the groin, and Cumming and Glenn[1] have recommended the use of 1 per cent. mercurochrome for the same purpose. Recent studies by Brams[2] have shown that these mild solutions may produce obliteration in the vas deferens and it seems now that all endovasal injections will have to be carried out with great care. Ross[3] takes issue with Brams and cites 4 cases in

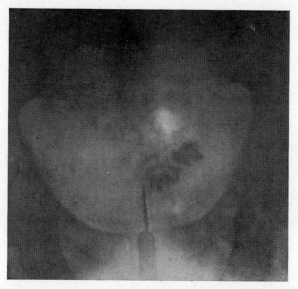

Fig. 120.—Vesiculogram made by injecting the left seminal vesicle with thorium. The vesicle is well filled and shows but slight distortion. B. U. I. x-Ray 2489.

which spermatozoa were present after double vasotomy and injections of 5 per cent. collargol. Statistics undoubtedly prove that when antiseptic fluids are injected by either of these methods into the seminal vesicles, vasa, and ampullæ, they remain present for a long period, being very slowly eliminated through the ejaculatory ducts. Many remarkable cures of long-standing chronic infections have been reported. With the injections introduced through the ejaculatory ducts, as we have described, there is the advantage that the ejaculatory ducts can subsequently be probed and dilated should stricture occur. This cannot be done when the injection has been made through a vasotomy in the groin or scrotum.

Seminal vesiculotomy is indicated in acute abscess, in certain chronic infections

[1] Journal of Urology, 1921, v, 43–61.

[2] Ibid., 1923, x, 393–404.

[3] Ibid., 1924, xii, 135–138.

of the seminal vesicles and ampullæ, in certain cases of chronic irritation of the bladder and prostate, and in certain cases of recurrent epididymitis. The seminal vesicles may be reached by simple incision with blunt dissection of the tissues to one side of the rectum as has been carried out by Fuller. We prefer an open operation with technic similar to that employed in exposing the prostate in perineal prostatectomy. As a rule, we make use of the long prostatic tractor, as fully depicted in the description of the operation for tuberculosis of seminal tract. The posterior surface of the prostate and seminal vesicles covered by the anterior layer of Denonvilliers' fascia is brought well into view and whatever operation is indicated may be carried out. In case of abscess the incision should be wide and directed over the most prominent and dependent portion, with the object of securing adequate drainage. If both vesicles are involved, it is usually well to strip back the fascia of Denonvilliers, opening it by means of an incision in the form of an inverted crescent. The vesicles may be simply incised and along with them the ampullæ should always be incised and drained. Owing to the multisaccular condition of the vesicles, we usually prefer to remove the posterior surface so as to open widely the cells and cavities, that more thorough drainage may be obtained. This drainage should be secured by the use of rubber tubes which are left in place for a prolonged period in order to insure a sinus tract which will continue to drain until the infection has completely disappeared. In some cases in which very extensive rheumatic foci, arthritis, or other serious general complications are present, it is well to take no chances with an inadequate operation, but to remove one or both vesicles completely. If the patient is quite old and the ampullæ are considerably involved, it may also be desirable to do ampullectomy as well as double seminal vesiculectomy. In one of our cases with very severe multiple arthritis in which drainage alone was provided, there was a complete return of the arthritis several months later, and the patient was only cured by a second operation in which seminal vesiculectomy was carried out. Even where both vesicles and both ampullæ are completely excised the patient may have fairly satisfactory coitus, as we have shown in several tuberculous cases.

The results obtained by vesiculotomy or vesiculectomy are often immediately brilliant. We have seen some of the most extraordinary chronic joint infections disappear like magic, but, unfortunately, in many cases the results are not so satisfactory, and in some cases entirely disappointing. Fuller has reported the most extensive series of cases, with a large percentage of cures of chronic rheumatic conditions. The results have not always been so brilliant. This is probably due to the fact that in many desperate cases where every other means had been attempted to cure disabling multiple joint infections, the seminal vesicles which were shown to be chronically inflamed were removed as a last resort.

It is evident from the failures which we have had that the seminal vesicles are often not the cause of such conditions, even though no other focus can be found, and rectal examination shows definite chronic prostatitis and seminal vesiculitis, but even though there may be failures, the condition of these patients is often so desperate that one is justified in attempting to obtain a cure by vesiculotomy. Intravenous mercurochrome often gives wonderful results in vesiculitis.

Strictures of the ejaculatory ducts have generally been denied or discounted in the literature. In a long series of endoscopic studies we have been surprised to find that this condition is not extremely uncommon and that it can be readily detected by the use of small, blunt, conical dilators introduced through the ure-throscope.   The presence of a stricture is shown not only in the difficulty of push-ing the probe upward, but also in the gripping or hanging which is present when one starts to withdraw the probe.   In a few cases great improvement of symptoms has followed endoscopic ejaculatory duct dilations repeated sufficiently often.

The treatment of *disorders of the sexual function* is often a difficult problem. When the local findings are slight or negative, the case is essentially a mental one. If the mental condition is not serious, the urologist can easily apply the necessary words of reassurance and confidence.   The investigation of the patient's sexual life will give opportunity for advice on the correction of unsuitable conditions. If the patient worries about old venereal disease, a statement of the facts of his present condition is in order.   If he worries about masturbation, the urologist should not hesitate to inform him that legends about the physical harm done by masturbation are exaggerated.   Frequent masturbation often causes congestive phenomena in the prostate, verumontanum, and posterior urethra, and there may be precocious ejaculation, imperfect erections, and less desire.   If the patient has this habit, it should, of course, be discouraged, but it is very important to avoid the familiar effort to frighten the patient by exaggerated accounts of its evil results.   The harm resulting from such a course is likely to be much greater than that from the masturbation.   Since excessive masturbation is the result of mental abnormality and not the cause of it, it is necessary to help the underlying neurosis as well as to stop the masturbation in order to obtain satisfactory results. Often the entire life of the patient must be altered, especial effort being made to overcome habits of solitude.   It is better not to use fear as a therapeutic agent.

If worry, depression, and impotence continue in spite of all efforts, the wise course is to turn the patient over to a psychiatrist.   Urologists may well study a little psychology, normal and abnormal, as suits their individual tastes, since these cases usually consult them first.   If this is done, more may be attempted by the urologist himself in the way of mental diagnosis and treatment.

Where definite local disease is present, and the sexual symptoms not dispro-portionate, local treatment should be at once started, according to the indications given by the examination.   No trouble is to be expected in these cases.

In the remainder of the cases, where local disease and disproportionate sexual symptoms are combined, the psychic disorder may be much more serious and important than the physical.   If this seems to the urologist to be the case, the recommendations of a psychiatrist are followed as to whether or no local treatment should be given.   If the local disease is most important, local treatment may be begun at once.   If the sexual symptoms do not disappear as the local lesions clear up, the mental features must be given attention, and we should especially avoid too long-continued series of treatments, which serve to fix the attention of the patient cn his genitalia, discourage his early hopes, and encourage delusional ideas.

Sexual abnormalities, especially excessive ungratified excitement, masturba-tion, and withdrawal, induce a chronic congestion of all the internal genitalia, which is really only an exaggeration of a normal phenomenon.   This congestion gives rise to pictures of redness and swelling in the verumontanum, posterior urethra, and even the trigone, which are often quite characteristic (Pelouze[1]), and which should not be mistaken for real inflammatory lesions.   It is our opinion

[1] Journal of Urology, 1924, xii, 77–82.

that prolonged courses of local treatment (cauterization, irrigations, etc.), are too often given these patients, the result being that the patient is made worse, and the doctor's reputation suffers. It is distinctly worth while to make the effort to get to the bottom of these unfortunate cases, and a little time devoted to a careful and sympathetic study of the intimate details of a patient's sexual and other problems will often reward the urologist with a brilliant success in an otherwise hopeless case, or enable him to turn over at once into the proper hands a case hopelessly mentally disordered. Aphrodisiacs and gland extracts are often helpful.

Vasitis of chronic character may manifest itself at either end, the ampulla being the most common seat of chronic inflammation requiring treatment which is the same as that above described for the seminal vesicle. At the distal end of the vas next to the epididymis little can be accomplished in the way of treatment except by operation. The intervening portions of the vas may be thickened and occasionally nodular and sometimes are painful, but no satisfactory treatment has, to our knowledge, been devised.

Epididymal Infections.—*Chronic epididymitis*, resulting from gonococcus infections, is fairly common. In most cases the disease after a time assumes a chronic fibrous character, gives little or no pain, and is finally associated with no escape of pus through the vas into the urethra. In other cases chronic posterior urethritis may be kept up by the chronic epididymitis. Painful areas are not uncommon in the postgonorrheal epididymis and not infrequently small cysts are found either in the epididymis itself or between the epididymis and the testicle, occasionally associated with adhesions or fibrous bands to the testicle and tunica vaginalis, which cause pain. This is particularly true when a hydrocele comes on, the accumulation of fluid leading to traction upon the adhesions which may be constantly painful and very distressing. In such cases operative intervention is desirable with separation of the adhesions or, if need be, epididymectomy. The fibrous changes in the epididymis may cause complete obliteration of the seminal ducts and sterility results. If the disease is bilateral, spermatoza may be completely prevented from gaining entrance into the urethra and such cases present the hopeless picture of childless marriages, which lead to such great unhappiness. The operative attack upon these conditions by epididymovasostomy is the only treatment of any value and, unfortunately, even this fails in the large majority of cases. The technic is described elsewhere. (For Acute Epididymitis, see p. 270.)

Testicular Infections.—The *testis* is rarely involved in gonococcus infections, but the great swelling of the epididymis which occurs may cause the region of the testicle to be so obscured that it is thought to be involved and as a result a diagnosis of orchitis is erroneously made. The *diagnosis of orchitis* or *epididymo-orchitis should rarely be made* in simple gonococcus infections. When it occurs the treatment is the same as that for epididymitis, viz., rest in bed, elevation upon a pad, application of an ice-bag, and the use of sedatives to relieve pain. Where a definite abscess is present operation is indicated.

CHAPTER IV

UROGENITAL INFECTIONS AND INFESTATIONS: TUBERCULOSIS

PATHOLOGY

Mode of Infection.—The primary focus in cases of urogenital tuberculosis is often in regions quite remote. The tubercle bacillus (Mycobacterium tuberculosis, S. A. B.) may enter along lymphatics or by the blood-stream from either the respiratory or the alimentary tracts, or even from the tonsils and glands of the neck. The original focus of infection often subsides, and may be discovered only at autopsy, and then found to be fibrotic or "arrested." In a large percentage of the cases of renal or seminal tract tuberculosis definite involvement of the lungs or pleura is present (40 per cent. in a recent report, and 28 per cent. in the statistics of this chapter).

Once settled in some portion of the urogenital tract, tuberculosis generally *spreads progressively to other parts of the tract.* If it begins in the kidney it may remain localized for a long time, but eventually the ureter and bladder may become involved, and in time the prostate, seminal vesicles, vasa deferentia, and epididymes may be affected. The urethra is remarkably resistant to the tubercle bacillus, which may pass through it in large quantities for years without producing clinically recognizable lesions. Even in extensive vesical and prostatic tuberculosis the urethra is generally found uninvolved. When the seminal vesicles or prostate form the initial point of attack the line of extension is usually along the cord to the epididymis, which is reached either by the lymphatics accompanying the vas or by the lumen of the vas itself. The globus minor of the epididymis is thus usually involved first, as shown by MacFarlane Walker,[1] ultimately the rest of the epididymis, and, very late, the testicle.

Many writers have held that the globus major of the epididymis is usually the site of primary attack, the tubercle bacillus coming by way of the blood-stream, but recent studies seem to show that tuberculosis of the epididymis is generally preceded either by tuberculosis of the seminal vesicles or of the kidney, the path of invasion being along the vas from the seminal vesicle, prostate, or urinary tract. In a series of 222 cases seen by us the vesicles were found definitely involved in 185, 83 per cent. In 47 of these cases the epididymis was not involved. Primary tuberculosis of the prostate does occur—but very rarely. We have one such case,[2] and a few cases are to be found in the literature. In one postmortem we found advanced tuberculosis of the prostate, without involvement of vesicles, epididymes, or kidneys, but with extensive pulmonary and peritoneal tuberculosis. The kidney often becomes involved subsequently to tuberculosis of the seminal tract, the route of infection being possibly along the peri-ureteral and retroperitoneal system of lymphatics. It may, however, be blood borne, and usually the exact

[1] Lancet, 1913, i, 435–440.
[2] Scott, W. W.: Journal of Urology, 1925, xii, 515–526.

path remains in doubt. The reader is referred to Chapter III for a detailed discussion of the modes of infection in the urogenital tract.

There is little or no evidence to show that a tuberculous infection does ascend by the lumen of the ureter from the bladder to the kidney. Baumgarten[1] held that it was impossible for bacteria to travel against secretion streams. There is, however, much more evidence to support the idea of an infection ascending from the seminal vesicles to the epididymes, and we know that extension from the epididymis to the testis can take place. Whether the extension along the vas deferens occurs through the lumen or through the surrounding lymphatics is still a moot point. MacFarlane Walker[2] holds that tubercle bacilli reach the epididymis from the seminal vesicle by way of the lymphatics of the vas and cord.

We had occasion in 1922[3] to review carefully the literature on this subject, and also a series of 86 cases of genital tuberculosis from the Johns Hopkins Hospital. The studies of MacFarlane Walker were most convincing as to the possibility of extension by way of the lymphatics of the vas from the urethra, prostate, and seminal vesicles to the epididymis. Clinical studies from all parts of the world support the view that tuberculosis of the epididymis is not independent, but coexistent with a focus elsewhere in the genital tract (i. e., seminal vesicles or prostate), since secondary involvement of the opposite epididymis, even after the originally diseased epididymis has been removed, is so common. For example, Barney[4] showed that the opposite epididymis was attacked within six months in 26.5 per cent. of his cases, Keyes[5] in 7 cases of 10, within two years, Boguljüboff, in 137 cases of 166 (82 per cent.) within fourteen months. Clinical studies reveal palpable lesions in the vesicles in most cases (see the tables at the end of this section, p. 300). We concluded[6] at that time "that infection of the epididymis takes place in tuberculosis, as in gonorrhea, by means of the cord and not by the blood-stream. That cases of hematogenous infection occur cannot be denied, but they are few in number." We have seen no reason to change our views since.

The fact that such extensions do occur, however, is of great importance, since they teach, first, the desirability of removing every focus from the urogenital tract; and, secondly, that so long as an active focus persists anywhere in the body, the prognosis after any sort of operation on the urogenital tract is measurably worse than in uncomplicated cases. Urogenital tuberculosis may occur at any age, but is very rare both in the young and in the aged. Our cases have fallen between twenty and sixty years of age and the majority of them are in middle life, between twenty-five and forty-five.

The thorough study of George Walker[7] should also be consulted concerning tuberculous urogenital infections.

Prevalence.—The prevalence of genito-urinary tuberculosis is difficult to determine. Whereas involvement of the epididymis or testis is generally noted at once, disease of the prostate, vesicles, and kidneys is often unrecognized. In

[1] Archiv für Klinische Chirurgie, 1901, lxiii, 1019–1026.

[2] Lancet, 1913, i, 435–440.

[3] Young: Archives of Surgery, 1922, iv, 334–419 (Lit.).

[4] Cabot's Modern Urology, 1924, i, 532–579. Excellent review of the literature.

[5] Annals of Surgery, 1907, xlv, 918–937.

[6] Young: Archives of Surgery, 1922, iv, 334–419 (Lit.).

[7] Johns Hopkins Hospital Reports, 1911, xvi, 1–222.

the sanatoria for tuberculosis pulmonary cases are almost exclusively taken, and as climate is not supposed to benefit tuberculosis of the genito-urinary tract, these are rarely found in such institutions except as a complication of lung cases. We have, therefore, no accurate statistics as to the proportion of all tuberculous patients having urogenital involvement. Table 36 (page 305) shows how long these cases often go unrecognized, and no doubt many are never diagnosed.

A personal study of records in six sanatoria, largely reserved for tuberculous cases and in fact almost specializing on cases of lung tuberculosis, revealed 65 cases of genito-urinary tuberculosis. The genital examinations were rarely thorough and the condition of the prostate and seminal vesicles was usually not noted. Cystoscopy and ureter catheterization were done in only 3 cases, although pyuria was not infrequently noted in the histories. But even with the records incomplete, they were sufficient to show that when the genital or the urinary tract became involved the prognosis was very bad and that most of the patients died.

The records are as follows: Number of cases, 65, all with lung tuberculosis in some form, but many classed as favorable cases on entrance. Seminal tract involved, 50; epididymis, single 37, double 13; testicle, single 18, double 9; prostate, 11; seminal vesicles, 7. Kidneys, 17 cases.

Operations performed: Epididymectomy, 3; castration, 17; nephrectomy, 4. Immediate result: Improved, 11; prognosis good, 11; bad, 21; not noted in others. Ultimate result: Only 1 is said to be well. Twenty-three had died when last heard of (35 percent.).

In one sanatorium where the ultimate result of all cases is known, all patients with renal tuberculosis (6) are dead. Among 21 cases of tuberculosis of the seminal tract 14 are dead, 1 in hospital, 1 recently discharged; 4 are alive after one to four years, and 1 after ten years. Among the 25 cases the fatalities are already 20, or 80 per cent. Another striking thing shown by these records is the continued progress of the disease after castration, deaths from renal and meningeal tuberculosis being recorded in numerous instances. At this sanatorium the records show that about 68 per cent. of the total hospital cases are arrested or cured. This high percentage of cures is in marked contrast to the 80 per cent. fatalities presented by cases with genito-urinary involvement and shows that a radical operative attack should be adopted to combat the present bad results.

Kidney.—In the urinary tract, the organ first affected is by far most frequently the kidney, with involvement of the remainder of the tract secondary thereto.

The original infection is *practically always confined to one kidney*, and this has been considered as an argument in favor of the "embolic" theory of transmission. According to this, the infection arrives as a coherent mass of bacilli or infected blood clot. A simple diffuse infection of the blood-stream should theoretically lead to a greater proportion of bilateral infections. When the opposite kidney is involved, it is usually *late*, leaving a period of months or years during which nephrectomy on the affected side will have a curative effect. The lesion occurs with equal frequence on either side. (See Table 33.) The two kidneys are equally affected in miliary tuberculosis.

The lesion in the kidney may be principally pelvic, or may originate in the cortical portion, or it may be disseminated everywhere, as in miliary tuberculosis.

In a few cases a true acute *tuberculous nephritis* has been found (Fig. 121); the

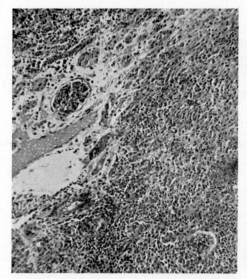

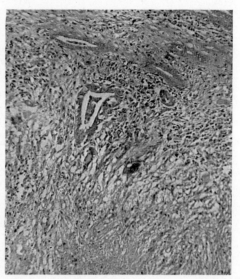

Fig. 121.—Acute tuberculosis of the kidney, showing edema, congestion, and cellular infiltration, mostly round-cells, but a few polymorphonuclears. There are a few small areas of beginning necrosis with nuclear fragmentation. B. U. I. Path. 2465.

Fig. 122.—Chronic tuberculosis of kidney, showing marked fibrosis with separation and compression of renal tubules. At the bottom of the picture is seen an edge of an area of caseation surrounded by typical zone of fibrous tissue, epithelioid and round-cells. B. U. I. Path. 2267.

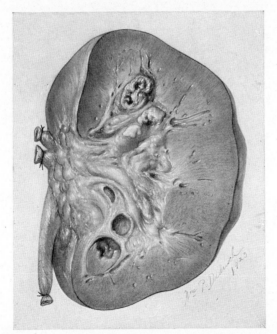

Fig. 123.—Nephrectomy for tuberculosis. The lesion is confined to upper and lower calyces, showing typical irregular enlargement of calyx. Cortex not involved. This kidney appeared normal until section after removal. Left testicle previously removed. Right epididymis, both seminal vesicles tuberculous. Epididymectomy. Subsequently pleural effusion, swollen joints. B. U. I. 5637.

kidney being enlarged, engorged, and edematous. The earliest beginning tubercles are seen and the exudate is principally polymorphonuclear.

The more common lesion is localized, in the *pelvic* or *pyramidal* portions of the kidney, and occasionally in the *cortex*. Tubercles, single or coalescent (Fig. 122), are surrounded by varying quantities of fibrous tissue. Central caseation occurs, and it is typical for this to involve the *calyx*, so that its tip becomes enlarged, irregular, and surrounded by tuberculous tissue (Fig. 123). By a continuation of this process, the entire kidney may be eventually involved, and converted into a series of *abscess* cavities with firm fibrous walls. In the course of this process secondary infection with pyogenic organisms may occur, or scar tissue may cause obstruction of the pelvis or ureter, with consequent hydronephrotic changes. The deposition of calcareous particles in the caseous material and in the walls of the cavities is common, and sometimes true calculi form in the pelvic spaces. Extension or per-

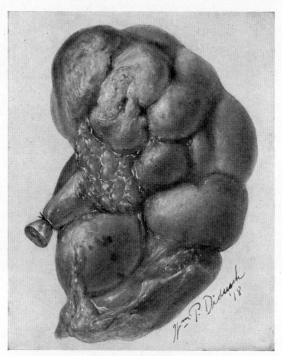

FIG. 124.—Specimen of tuberculous pyonephrosis with markedly thickened ureter, removed at operation. B. U. I. 6967.

foration to the outside of the kidney with *perinephric inflammation, abscess,* or *sinus* may occur.

After complete destruction of the secreting parenchyma, especially if the ureter is occluded, the process may become completely caseous (Fig. 129), quiescent, and fibrotic, often with blocking of the ureter, a condition which is known as *auto-nephrectomy*.

If there is obstruction of the ureter, the changes of *hydronephrosis* may be superimposed. The contents of the sac often becomes purulent from the tuberculous process, giving rise to tuberculous *pyonephrosis* (Figs. 124, 125, 127). In late stages of renal tuberculosis the term "pyronephrosis" is also applied to conditions in which large caseous abscesses of the calyces coalesce in the interior of the kidney, converting it into a sac. This is commoner than a true tuberculous pyonephrosis, although it may also be combind with an obstructive dilatation of the pelvis.

Since involvement of the pelvis is so common, it may happen that in early cases no lesions are visible on the outer surface of the kidney. It is, therefore, most important to make the diagnosis before operation, and never to rely on an "exploratory" operation, in which the kidney may appear normal (Figs. 123, 126).

Tuberculous abscesses in the kidney may discharge only periodically into the pelvis, as is often the case also in the lungs. Pus and tubercle bacilli may, therefore, be absent, from time to time, even for long periods, from the urine just as from the sputum. For this reason, the urine must be examined repeatedly and patiently in cases of suspected renal tuberculosis.

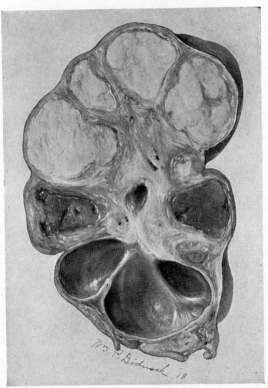

Fig. 125.—Longitudinal section of tuberculous pyonephrosis specimen removed at operation. This is the same case as the preceding picture. B. U. I. 6967.

Microscopically, renal tuberculosis does not differ from tuberculosis elsewhere in the body. The tubercle, the pathologic unit, is exactly the same. The fibrotic process surrounding the tubercles may spread over a great part of the kidney and add much to the functional destruction. In microscopic sections it is easy to miss a few small tubercles in large areas of this fibrotic tissue, everywhere beset with lymphocytic infiltration and remnants of kidney architecture.

When both kidneys are involved, the lesion is usually much more advanced in one than in the other.

Secondary involvement of the genital tract is by no means uncommon, although it has never been emphasized in the literature. In a series of 65 primary nephrecto-

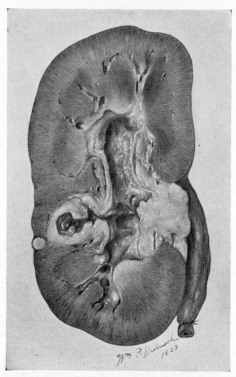

Fig. 126.—Specimen of tuberculosis of kidney removed at operation. In this case the lesion was small and scarcely appeared on the surface, except at one small spot which was not noticeable until the kidney was split. B. U. I. 11,394.

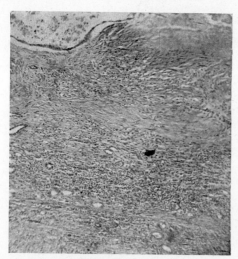

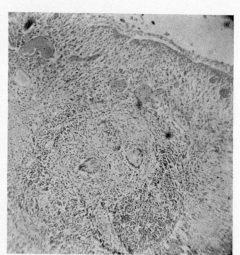

Fig. 127.—Tuberculous pyonephrosis, showing typical infiltration and fibrosis in the medulla and a caseous tubercle on the pelvic surface, with the necrotic area involving the pelvic epithelium and communicating with the pelvic cavity. B. U. I. Path. 4590.

Fig. 128.—Tuberculosis of the ureter, showing multiple conglomerate tuberculosis in the submucosa. Marked thickening of the wall of the ureter. B. U. I. Path. 4525.

mies, invasion of the genital tract, usually first observed by the patient in the epididymis, was noted subsequent to the operation in 17, or 26.1 per cent. In another series of 47 cases, however, where operative treatment of genital tuberculosis accompanied or preceded the nephrectomy, only one recurrence in the genital tract was observed. Early and complete diagnosis and operation are the only means of avoiding these complications. In the light of recent studies we believe that many of these patients had involvement of the seminal vesicles before nephrectomy was done.

Ureter.—It commonly occurs that the products of tuberculous inflammation passing down the ureter set up a non-specific inflammation there. This form tends to heal if the active focus in the kidney is removed. In later stages, however, true tubercles are found (Fig. 128), and the ureteral lumen is

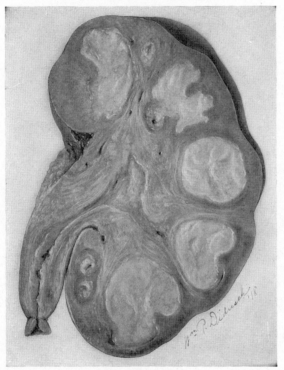

Fig. 129.—Tuberculosis of kidney and ureter. Extensive caseation, almost autonephrectomy. Ureter greatly thickened.

thickened, distorted by ulceration, and constricted by scarring. Strictures and even obliteration occur. Rarely, the ureter itself becomes the seat of active independent tuberculosis, which may persist after nephrectomy. Sometimes the ureter is greatly shortened so that the corresponding corner of the trigone may be drawn out through the ureteral orifices, as first described in one of our cases[1] (page 288). The lower end is usually involved first.

The ureter may be involved in a tuberculous process beginning outside the urinary tract, as in the pelvic bones, vertebræ, retroperitoneal glands, and directly by invasion from a tuberculous seminal vesicle or vas deferens. In only 3 of

[1] Young: Changes in the Trigone due to Tuberculosis of the Kidney, Ureter, and Bladder, Surgery, Gynecology, and Obstetrics, 1918, xxvi, 608–615.

112 cases in which nephrectomies were carried out was it thought necessary to do ureterectomy, and in only 1 case afterward.

Bladder.—Involvement of the bladder in tuberculosis is usually *secondary* to that of the kidney. Since in many cases of vesical tuberculosis no tubercle bacilli can be demonstrated in the urine, or even in pieces of excised bladder wall, some authors have suggested that the lesion may be caused not by bacilli, but by their products, in the nature of endo- or exotoxins. This question, however, is of minor importance, the really significant thing being that the bladder inflammation is usually of a peculiar, superficial, or catarrhal nature, without tubercles, and comparable only to some conditions found in the ureter and upper respiratory tract. These lesions usually begin in the neighborhood of the ureteral orifice of the affected side, and are characterized by reddening and edema of the mucosa. Later, they may spread to other parts of the bladder, but commonly remain more pronounced at the base.

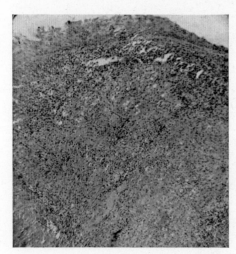 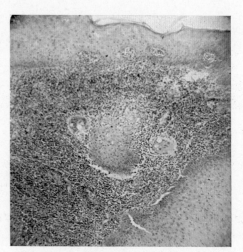

Fig. 130.—Tuberculosis of the bladder. This section shows true tubercle formation in the submucosa of the bladder, different from the superficial catarrhal inflammation often seen and less likely to clear up after removal of a tuberculous focus in the kidney. B. U. I. Path. 2428.

Fig. 131.—Tubercles in the wall of an old chronic suprapubic urinary fistula. Fistula has become epithelialized. In the subepithelial tissue there is marked round-cell infiltration with multiple tubercles. Such fistulæ seldom heal spontaneously. B. U. I. Path. 4009.

Eventually, a shallow ulceration, with an indolent, hemorrhagic base, appears, and even at this stage the microscope fails to reveal tubercles. There is an infiltration, essentially lymphocytic, involving the mucosa and submucosa, but penetrating usually only slightly into the muscularis. It is, however, sufficient to decrease markedly the elasticity of the bladder and increase its sensitiveness, so that frequency and pain are characteristic accompaniments. Secondary infection with pyogenic organisms, increasing the polymorphonuclear exudate, is common. This type of lesion tends to heal spontaneously when the focus in the kidney is removed by nephrectomy or otherwise (as by autonephrectomy).

In cases of long standing, however, true *tubercles* may develop in the bladder wall, and the lesion become thereby independent (Fig. 130). When this happens, the lesions become extensive and severe, bladder symptoms persist after nephrectomy, and the infection may spread to the urethra, prostate, etc. In such cases the tubercles can sometimes be seen cystoscopically. *Direct extension* may occur to the perivesical tissues, adjacent coils of intestine, seminal vesicles, prostate, or rectum, and abscesses and fistulæ (Fig. 131) may develop.

In severe lesions of the base of the bladder the ulcers may undermine the edges of the *trigone*, so that they stand up prominently, and may even cause obstruc-

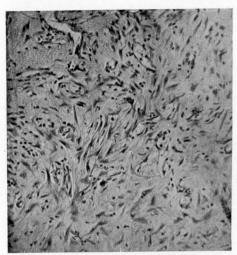
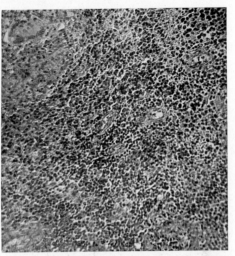

FIG. 132.—Section showing organized granulation tissue around a sinus of long standing (non-tuberculous). B. U. I. Path. 4094.

FIG. 133.—Section of tuberculous granulation tissue from suprapubic fistula. The infiltrating cells are largely round and plasma cells. There are a few small areas of necrosis not associated with polymorphonuclears. In the upper corner is a typical tubercle with giant-cell, although this is not always seen and a diagnosis of tuberculosis can be made without it. B. U. I. Path. 3642.

tion at the vesical orifice. We have observed 4 cases in which the trigone with its muscle was dissected quite free from the remainder of the bladder wall except at

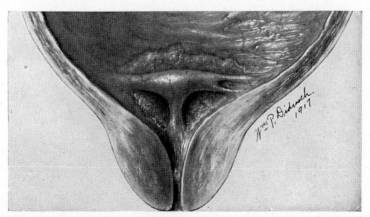

FIG. 134.—Trigonal bridge caused by tuberculous dissection. Trigone attached at three corners, undermined elsewhere. B. U. I. 3565.

its three corners, where it still remained attached (Fig. 134).[1] These cases are of such interest that we will quote from this article at length:

[1] Young: Surgery, Gynecology, and Obstetrics, 1918, xxvi, 608–615.

These cases appear to me to represent three progressive stages:

1. *Elevation* of the trigone (due to traction of a shortened tuberculous ureter) with pouch formation behind and to the outer side (Cases 1 and 2).

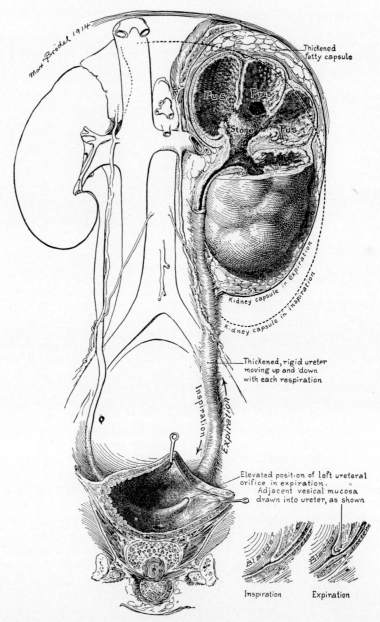

Fig. 135.—Conditions as found at operation, large pus kidney, adherent to diaphragm, short thick ureter drawing left corner of trigone up into orifice, to- and fro- movement on ascent and descent of diaphragm. B. U. I. 3890.

2. *Ulceration* of depressed portions of the bladder leading to complete undermining of the elevated trigone which thus forms a bridge of healthy tissue (mucous membrane and trigonal muscle) across the new-formed tuberculous cavity (Case 3).

3. *Healing* (after nephrectomy) of the subtrigonal tuberculosis, leaving the separated trigone

as a bridge with fairly healthy mucosa beneath it. It seems very evident that tuberculosis not only may produce marked thickening but also shortening of the ureter. This, in turn, may make traction upon the vesical end of the ureter and trigone, leading to invagination of the ureteral margin and elevation of the trigone on that side, leaving the bladder depressed around it. Tubercle bacilli coming from the ureter naturally find easy lodgment in these vesical pouches, while the greatly elevated ureteral ridge and trigone remain uninvolved. Ulceration in the pouches leads to undermining of the trigone from the bladder, a condition which the anatomists have shown us to be possible, as the trigone is separated from and superimposed on the bladder muscle in that region (Fig. 1). The movement of the ureter, synchronous with respiration (described in Case 1) is surely due to adhesions between the kidney and diaphragm: on expiration the diaphragm goes upward and the trigone is drawn upward with it by the adherent kidney and short thickened ureter. On inspiration the diaphragm and kidney allow the ureter and trigone to descend. The orifice, being surrounded by vesical mucosa, remains more or less stationary, while the trigonal ridge plays back and forth like a piston-rod in the invaginated ureteral orifice (Fig. 135). It is strange that this occurrence has never been noted before.

It is interesting to note the changes in micturition which occur as a result of these transformations of the trigone. Urination is apparently normal as long as the trigone is not detached, and the bladder has not become tuberculous. (In one case the trigone was much elevated, drawn to the left by a shortened ureter, with deep pouches behind and externally. Micturition was normal.)

When the trigone becomes pathologically dissected free from the bladder muscle, and even after new mucous membrane has formed beneath it, obstruction is present. (In another case 100 c.c. residual urine was present.) This was apparently not much improved by removal of the "floating trigone," as the patient continued to have residual urine and complained of having to strain to urinate nine months afterward. This brings up the question of the part taken by the trigone in the act of urination. It seems to me to indicate that one function of the trigone is to pull open the internal sphincter of the bladder. I have long held to this view, as I have frequently observed during cystoscopy, that if violent desire to urinate came on, the trigone would contract greatly and the prostatic orifice would open widely, the median (posterior) portion being apparently drawn backward by the muscle-fibers which run from the trigone down into the posterior urethra, and which were seen to contract violently. The opening of the internal sphincter during urination will have to be viewed, therefore, not as an inhibitory action, as heretofore, but as a result of the contraction of the powerful trigonal muscle which passes in the form of an arc through a weaker muscle of circular shape (the vesical sphincter) and pulls it open when it contracts.

It is abundantly demonstrated by these cases that tuberculosis of the kidney may lead to great shortening of the ureter, resulting in traction on and marked elevation of the trigone, and invagination of the ureteral ridge into the ureter; that tuberculous ulceration may then produce an undermining of this elevated trigone and finally complete separation of the trigone from the bladder beneath except at the three corners (where the trigone is continuous with the ureteral muscle above and the urethral muscle below); that after nephrectomy healing of the vesical tuberculosis may leave this "trigonal bridge" with new mucous membrane beneath it except at the three corners where the "bridge" is attached and gets its blood supply.

In another case (B. U. I. 12,564) with a greatly shortened thickened ureter the tuberculous kidney was not adherent above, and did not draw the trigone upward, but rather the kidney itself was drawn down until the ureter was only one-half normal length.

In chronic cases polypoid masses of granulation tissue simulating, to cystoscopic examination, neoplasms may occur.

While we are not prepared to say that urogenital tuberculosis may not begin in the bladder, it is certainly very rare, and cases described as such might be explained as due to a localized renal lesion discharging its products into the bladder only at intervals.

The bladder may also be involved by *direct extension* from the seminal vesicle or prostate, but less frequently than from the kidney. We have seen several cases of extensive tuberculosis of the seminal vesicles in which the base of the bladder was ulcerated. At times the seminal vesicles discharge into the bladder. Tuberculosis of the bones, etc., may invade the bladder. In some of these cases communication between the bladder and other pre-existing lesions may cause extensive and complicated systems of urinary fistulæ reaching to great distances from the bladder.

Urethra.—Tuberculous involvement of the urethra usually occurs later, and is absent in many cases where bladder or prostatic lesions are well developed. Definite evidence of tuberculous involvement of the urethra was noted in 9 of our cases, 2.6 per cent. Pathologically, it is a *chronic urethritis*, with ulceration and a ten-

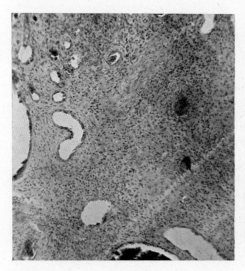 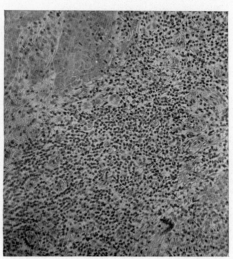

Fig. 136.—Tuberculosis of the urethra involving the corpus spongiosum. The vascular sinuses are seen separated by a tremendously thickened stroma in which there are multiple tubercles with round-cell infiltration, fibrosis, and giant-cells. B. U. I. Path. 1767.

Fig. 137.—Tuberculosis of the penis. The lesion is located in the skin and resembles other cutaneous tuberculous ulcers. A tubercle with epithelioid cells and a giant-cell is seen just beneath the cutaneous epithelium. B. U. I. Path. 4124.

dency to *stricture* formation. This last may be a serious complication in a case of urogenital tuberculosis, since it demands intervention of some sort. The stricture recurs after sounding or internal urethrotomy. A number of cases are reported in which rapid dissemination, with miliary tuberculosis, followed these procedures. Peri-urethral inflammation (Fig. 136) and abscess may occur, with fistula formation. These fistulæ are extremely persistent. If there is involvement of the prostate, cicatricial contractures of the vesical orifice may occur.

Penis.—Tuberculosis of the penis is more properly in the realm of skin tuberculosis, and usually does not occur in connection with urogenital tuberculosis, except when tuberculous ulcers and granulomata appear around the external orifices of sinuses in the penis, as they may also do in the perineum and scrotum. These are rare and only occurred four times in our 342 cases of urogenital tuberculosis. When tuberculosis is primary in the penis, it appears as a small papule which soon ulcerates—similar, in fact, to a chancre, except that it is more indolent and seldom shows any tendency to heal, often resisting treatment for years. It grows slowly, the ulcer having a grayish base and somewhat undermined indurated edges. There may be destruction of tissue, with fistulous opening into the urethra. The lesion, while rare, should be kept in mind in all cases of extremely resistant genital ulcers. Its nature can usually be determined by a section made from the edge (Fig. 137).[1]

Prostate.—In prostatic tuberculosis the tubercles are usually confined to the neighborhood of the ejaculatory ducts, from which the spread is by the posterior lobe to the dorsal portions of the lateral lobes, the median lobe being less frequently involved. The vesicles are almost always tuberculous in such cases, and if only one vesicle is affected, the prostatic lesions are usually confined to the same side, or at least more pronounced there. There is little reason to doubt that this patho-

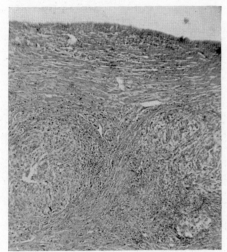

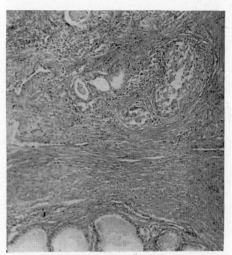

FIG. 138.—Section from the edge of a specimen removed by prostatectomy for benign prostatic hypertrophy, showing two very definite fibroid tubercles. B. U. I. 11,683.

FIG. 139.—Section from a specimen removed by prostatectomy for benign prostatic hypertrophy, showing benign hypertrophy below and tuberculosis above. In this specimen the tuberculosis was confined to one small portion and had not been detected before operation. B. U. I. 11,683.

logic picture usually represents an infection descending from the vesicle to the prostate. In a series of 15 cases of genital tuberculosis operated on radically in our clinic, there were 7 cases in which one vesicle was not removed. The other vesicle in these cases, and both vesicles in all the other cases, were definitely tuberculous, with fibroid and caseous tubercles, with one exception. In this case the right vesicle was tuberculous, and the left vesicle was very scarred and fibrous, although no definite tubercles were seen. It is probable that this represented an old tuberculous process, as the left epididymis was also diseased. In other words, there was no case in which the vesicles were not diseased, and in no case in which the epididymis was involved did the vesicle on the same side fail to be involved. In 2 cases in which the vesicle and epididymis of one side, being apparently normal, were left *in situ*, both became tuberculous at a later date. The prostate was found involved in all but 1 of the 24 radical operations and both lobes of the prostate

[1] Wilson and Warthin: Annals of Surgery, 1912, lv, 305–313.

were removed in 18 cases, one lobe only in 5 cases, and no lobes in 1. This patient is still suffering from bladder symptoms.

In a few cases no lesions are demonstrable except in the prostate. In our series there was only 1 case of pure prostatic tuberculosis among those proved by operation or autopsy (Figs. 138 and 139).[1] In this case benign prostatic hypertrophy was also present. The patient (B. U. I. 11,683) died and a complete autopsy demonstrated the absence of any other urogenital lesion. Scott, from his study of the literature, feels that only 7 other cases are acceptable, of which only 4 were proved by autopsy.

Microscopically, prostatic tuberculosis presents little of note. The tubercles often lie in the *stroma* (Figs. 140, 141), suggesting that lymphatics play a rôle in the progress of the disease. One sometimes sees early tubercles within *acini* just

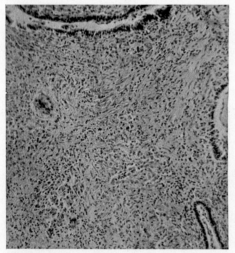
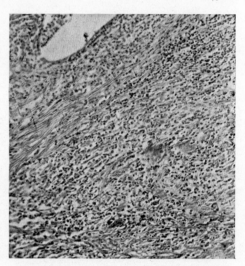

Fig. 140.—Tuberculosis of the prostate where the tubercle formation is seen to be confined to the stroma. B. U. I. Path. 4094.

Fig. 141.—Another example of the interstitial type of tuberculosis of the prostate. This section is particularly interesting since in other parts of the same prostate there are found benign hypertrophy and carcinoma of the prostate (see Fig. 407). B. U. I. Path. 3086.

beneath the epithelium (Fig. 142), so that the spread within the organ may also be by way of the tubules of the prostate, as George Walker[2] believes.

We have had 2 cases of prostatic hypertrophy in which a small area of tuberculosis was present in the posterior lamella of the prostate (Fig. 143), and also a case of tuberculosis combined with cancer and hypertrophy of the prostate (Figs. 141 and 407).

From the prostate *the infection may escape into the perineal tissues*, giving rise to induration and abscess formation. Rupture may occur in the perineum, giving rise usually to a *urinary fistula*. The rectum may be involved, with the possible consequence of *recto-urethral fistula*. These tuberculous urinary fistulæ are most persistent, and are among the most distressing consequences of the disease.

Seminal Vesicle.—There is reason to believe that the *seminal vesicles can be infected by tuberculosis in three ways, i. e.,* from the blood-stream, by descending

[1] Scott, W. W.: Journal of Urology, 1924, xii, 515–526.
[2] Johns Hopkins Hospital Reports, 1911, xvi, 1–222.

infection from the epididymis, and by ascending infection by the ejaculatory duct and prostate in urinary tuberculosis. None of these paths can be proved categorically, but the possibility of any of them must be considered in each case. In this connection it is interesting that in our series of 222 cases of genital tuberculosis there was combined epididymal and seminal vesicular involvement in 139 cases, 62 per cent., the vesicles alone were involved in 47 cases, while in 37 cases of epididymal involvement there was no demonstrable lesion of the vesicles. The vesicles were, therefore, involved in at least 83 per cent. of the cases, and very probably in nearly all. Some of our recent radical operations have shown a seminal vesicle to be tuberculous which was recorded as normal on rectal examination. The proportion of cases in which the vesicles are involved is, therefore, in all probability, higher than 83 per cent. That urinary infection plays a rôle is suggested by the fact that in only 15 of the 37 epididymis cases was renal tuberculosis present,

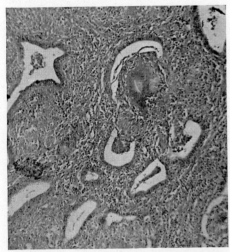

FIG. 142.—Tuberculosis of the prostate. There is generalized round-cell infiltration and slight fibrosis, but the tubercle is seen developing just beneath the epithelium of an acinus and pushing into its lumen. B. U. I. Path. 3390.

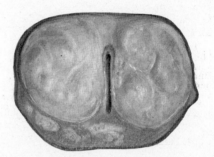

FIG. 143.—Specimen of prostate removed at operation. The prostate is very hard and irregular and the clinical diagnosis was carcinoma of the prostate. Radical removal of the entire prostate and seminal vesicles was carried out. Examination of the specimen showed benign prostatic hypertrophy of the lateral lobes, while the posterior lamella was grossly tuberculous, as shown. This is an example of an error which may easily arise when there is no involvement of the epididymes or seminal vesicles to indicate tuberculosis. B. U. I. 8150.

while it occurred in 31 of the 47 seminal vesicle cases. The combined cases were equally divided, 68 with kidney involvement, and 70 without.

The important fact, however, is that *the vesicles are involved more often than the epididymes* in genital tuberculosis, and, therefore, treatment for this condition directed at the epididymis alone cannot possibly be satisfactory. It is also certain that the vesicles are not infrequently extensively involved before the epididymes are attacked. On the other hand, long-standing tuberculosis of the seminal vesicles may show only slight changes (hardly more than seen in chronic vesiculitis) on rectal examination, and the prostate may show almost no palpable abnormality in the proximity of tuberculosis of the vesicle.

By whatever path the vesicles may be infected, the pathologic picture is essentially the same. Specimens showing a superficial or catarrhal inflammation of a sort which might be expected to clear up after removal of an original focus in the epididymis are very rare (Fig. 144). The anatomical structure of the vesicle does not favor such an inflammation. Its cavities are extremely complicated and convoluted, and, therefore, readily occluded by edema or fibrosis. There is, of

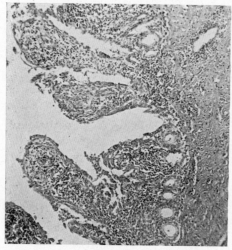

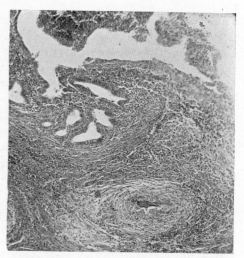

Fig. 144.—A very early and superficial stage of tuberculosis of the seminal vesicle. Trabeculæ are thickened and club shaped due to edema and round-cell infiltration. The lumen is dilated with a purulent secretion. The muscular coat of the vesicle, however, is normal. This resembles the superficial inflammation seen in the bladder and might clear up after the removal of the tuberculous epididymis, but it is an extremely rare finding. This is the only case we have seen. B. U. I. Path. 4723.

Fig. 145.—The more usual picture in tuberculosis of the vesicle. A moderately advanced stage. The epithelium is preserved, the lumen is dilated with a purulent secretion, the muscular coat is infiltrated and thickened, and there are definite fibroid and caseous submucosal tubercles. B. U. I. Path. 3390.

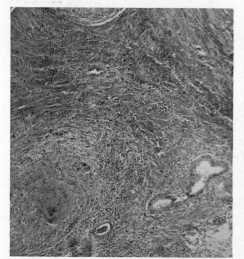

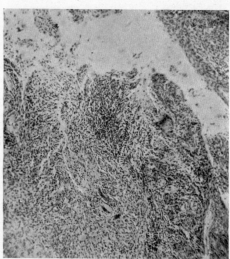

Fig. 146.—A somewhat higher magnification showing definite fibroid tubercle with epithelioid and giant-cells deep within the muscular coat of the vesicle. B. U. I. Path. 3390.

Fig. 147.—Tuberculosis of the seminal vesicle similar to the foregoing except that the cellular infiltration is more marked and there is extensive desquamation of the epithelium. B. U. I. Path. 4094.

course, a slow current through the ampulla, but this is not true of the vesicle proper, which is a blind sac, and both are dependent for drainage upon the minute ejaculatory duct. Tuberculosis of the seminal vesicles is, therefore, almost always a true chronic granulomatous lesion. Multiple or conglomerate tubercles are present,

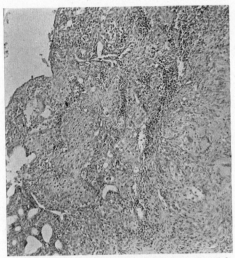

FIG. 148.—Tuberculosis of the seminal vesicle showing multiple conglomerate tubules throughout the entire depth of the wall of the vesicle, although the vesicular epithelium is still preserved. B. U. I. Path. 3482.

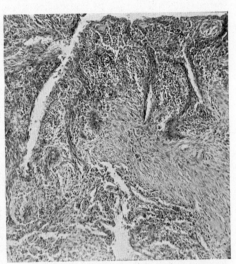

FIG. 149.—Advanced and chronic tuberculosis of the seminal vesicle. Here the fibrosis is more marked; the cellular infiltration less marked. The epithelium is partially preserved. Tubercles are found in the submucosa and muscular coat. B. U. I. Path. 4422.

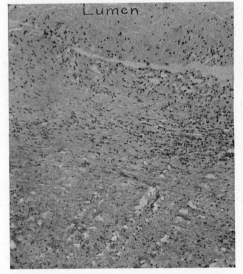

FIG. 150.—Tuberculosis of the seminal vesicle showing very marked fibrosis and thickening of the wall, and complete destruction of the vesicular epithelium, so that the lumen is transformed into a sort of tuberculous abscess. B. U. I. Path. 4917.

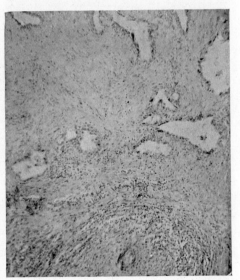

FIG. 151.—Tuberculosis of the seminal vesicle showing a fibrous tubercle which has developed in the stroma of the vesicle apparently without reference to the epithelial lined spaces. The crypts seen in the upper part are apparently normal except for the marked thickening of the interstitial tissue between them. B. U. I. Path. 4233.

often with extensive caseation, always with distortion or destruction of the vesicular architecture (Figs. 145–151). In many cases this destruction is so complete that no trace remains, and one could not identify, microscopically, the organ from which the specimen came. In a few cases we have seen early lesions, with intense round-cell infiltration of the entire organ, and dozens of early tubercles, still without caseous centers. In a few other cases of definite genital tuberculosis, where no tubercles were found in the sections of vesicle examined, the organ showed extensive scarring and distortion and a heavy round-cell infiltration. In only one case was the lesion superficial, without caseation or fibrosis (Fig. 144). In this case the epididymis was tuberculous, and the vesicle was distended with pus.

By coalescence of caseous tubercles the vesicle may be transformed into what is practically a single *abscess* (Fig. 150). The process may extend into the surrounding *retrovesical tissues*, with scarring or cold abscess formation. The scarring may involve the *ureter* and cause *stricture*. Perforation into the *bladder* may occur, and more rarely into the *rectum*, since Denonvillier's fascia (see p. 156) lies between the vesicles and the rectum. In case of both of these events in the same case there will be *rectovesical fistula*.

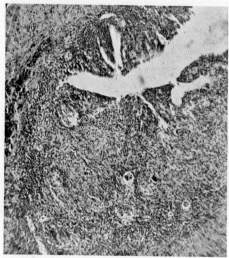

FIG. 152.—Chronic fibrous tuberculosis of the vas deferens showing multiple conglomerate submucosal tubercles. B. U. I. Path. 4754.

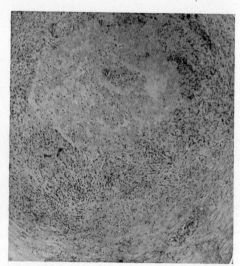

FIG. 153.—Another form of tuberculosis of the vas deferens showing a more superficial, acute, and destructive process with less fibrosis. B. U. I. Path. 4821.

Simmonds[1] describes a lesion in which, the epididymis being involved, the seminal vesicle is filled with purulent material containing myriads of tubercle bacilli, the walls showing little or no change, like our case figured above.

There is usually some degree of prostatic involvement in all cases of seminal vesicle tuberculosis.

Vas Deferens.—A study of the vas deferens in tuberculosis does not throw light on the course followed by the infection in the genital tract. Sometimes no involvement will be found in cases where both epididymis and vesicle are affected. In other cases involvement will be confined to one end of the vas (usually the ampullar end), or it may be tuberculous throughout its extent. In a careful study of the specimens from radical operations done in this clinic both vesicle and epididymis were tuberculous in all; the vas was generally involved in various places

[1] Aschoff's Pathologische Anatomie, 1909, ii, 549 et seq.

(Figs. 152, 153), though we found long stretches which were normal in almost every vas. In two it was apparently normal throughout. In one case, already mentioned, the prostate and ampulla were tuberculous, and the epididymis normal. Tubercles and caseous nodules in the vas and invading surrounding structures in the cord or inguinal canal are sometimes seen. In other cases the tissues of the cord show a marked chronic inflammatory reaction without any evidence of active tuberculosis in the vas or around it. A very thick dense "vas," felt on examination, often proves to be a normal sized vas surrounded by marked inflammatory fibrosis. Whether this perivesical inflammation is due to involvement of the lymphatics coming from the seminal vesicles, as contended by MacFarlane Walker, is as yet unknown.

Epididymis.—The epididymis, for purposes of description, is divided into the globus major, or head, the body, and the globus minor, or tail. *Early tuberculous lesions* are found most often in the globus minor, which is the beginning of the vas deferens. Tuberculosis of the epididymis is often represented in its early stages by a circumscribed *nodule*, which to examination is characterized by hardness and irregularity. The duct is occluded early. A more fulminant process produces greater swelling, with redness, heat, pain, etc., to indicate its acuteness, and frequently progresses rapidly to abscess formation. Most of our cases were seen late, but the globus minor was found involved, right 110, left 121; whereas the globus major was involved, right 77, left 95. These figures show the greater frequency of involvement of the globus minor and also the left side; the latter being true for the seminal vesicles.

On section it will be found that the lesions most frequently originate within

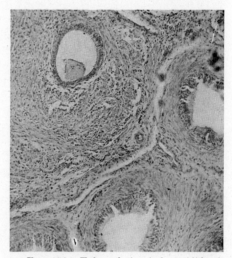

Fig. 154.—Tuberculosis of the epididymis showing tuberculous process located in the submucosa and entirely surrounding the lumen. Three adjoining lumina are unaffected. B. U. I. Path. 3430.

the ducts (Fig. 154), but may be confined to the stroma (Figs. 155, 156). As in the vesicle, however, distortion and obliteration of the architecture quickly follow, and one sees intense round-cell infiltration with varying degrees of fibrosis. In more *acute cases* the exudate may be partly polymorphonuclear, but the typical rounded areas, with circumferential zones of round and epithelioid cells, give the diagnosis. In later stages the architecture of the epididymis may have vanished completely. The process usually spreads until it involves the entire epididymis, but extension into the testis is much more uncommon.

Frequently the process extends beyond the bounds of the epididymis and involves the *areolar tissue of the scrotum*. The skin becomes adherent, and sooner or later rupture to the outside occurs, with formation of a *sinus* which shows little tendency to heal (Fig. 157). Rupture into the cavity of the tunica vaginalis is rare, but *hydrocele* with a thick-walled sac is sometimes seen. In certain cases the mass of inflammatory tissue becomes very large, and the entire scrotum honeycombed with sinuses. When the entire genital tract is involved it may happen, in exceedingly rare cases, that urine will come from scrotal sinuses. Processes in

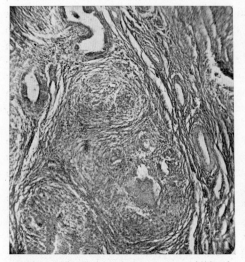 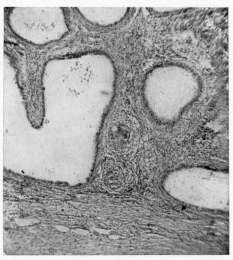

FIG. 155.—Tuberculosis of the epididymis showing multiple fibroid tubercles which have apparently developed within the lumen of the duct. There is also marked general fibrosis. B. U. I. Path. 4726.

FIG. 156.—Tuberculosis of the epididymis showing tubercles developing in the interstitial tissue, apparently without reference to the duct, and possibly originating in the lymphatics. B. U. I. Path. 4754.

the globus major may extend to the vas deferens by contiguity without involvement of the globus minor.

Testis.—Tuberculosis beginning in the testis is extremely rare, and such cases

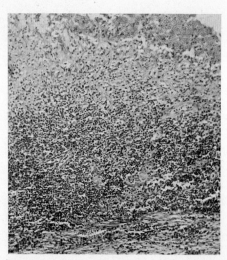

FIG. 157.—Granulation tissue lining a tuberculous abscess of the scrotum arising from tuberculosis of the epididymis. The characteristic zonate arrangement with necrotic material containing fragmented nuclei, but no or few polymorphonuclears is seen. B. U. I. Path. 3365.

as have been described are open to some doubt. We have never observed one. Mark[1] reports one in which the involvement of the epididymis was minimal. Practi-

[1] Journal of Urology, 1921, v, 171–176.

cally, one may say that testicular tuberculosis is always *secondary* to that of the *epididymis*. It commonly occurs only when the globus major is involved, and the route is by the tubuli recti. In many cases, however, the testis remains intact in the presence of very extensive tuberculosis of the epididymis. In our series of cases of genital tuberculosis the testis was involved in 8.3 per cent. only, and many of these were late cases. For this reason one should make very sure at operation that the testis really is involved before removing it, and an excision of that portion of the testis next to the epididymis will generally suffice. We have frequently seen great enlargement (3 to 4 cm.) of the epididymis with an abscess plastered against the posterior surface of the testis, but with no invasion of the testis proper.

When the testis is involved there are frequently seen tubercles beginning *within the tubules*, and it is probable that this is the method of spread in many

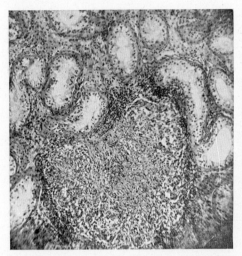
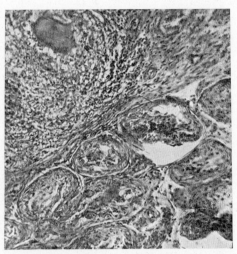

FIG. 158.—Tuberculosis of the testis. In this case the epididymis was heavily involved. The picture shows a single tubercle in the testicular tissue isolated and at some distance from the epididymis. The spread may have been intratubular or lymphatic. B. U. I. Path. 4530.

FIG. 159.—Tuberculosis of the testis. This picture shows the manner of direct spread from the epididymis through the interstitial tissue in the region of the tubuli recti. B. U. I. Path. 4726.

cases. In others, it is by way of the interstitial tissue (Figs. 158, 159). The testicular elements disappear, the elastic coats of the tubules persisting longest. In a narrow zone around the tuberculous portion there is round-cell infiltration, edema, and cessation of spermatogenesis. The interstitial cells are not spared. In the unaffected part of the testis, however, spermatogenesis goes on as usual.

In late stages the testis may be entirely destroyed, or may *rupture* and discharge its contents to the outside as a *fungus* or hernia testis.

The tendency of the testis to be involved late is fortunate, as it enables us, by dissecting the epididymis away, to preserve these organs so necessary for the welfare of the patient from an endocrine standpoint.

Peron and Galavielle[1] described a mechanism by which the tuberculous in-

[1] Quoted by Le Dentu and Delbet, Nouveau Traité de Chirurgie, 1916, xxxii (Maladies des Organes génitaux de l'Homme).

fection begins in the serous cavity of the tunica vaginalis, spreading secondarily to the testis and epididymis, as in glanders. Certain observations in guinea-pigs and infants point to the possibility of this route, but it is probably a very rare one.

The testis may be involved by extension from tuberculous peritonitis in *cryptorchidism*, or in cases of *congenital hernia*, with patent funicular process.

Distribution.—The following tables are given to show the distribution of the lesions in our series of 342 cases. From these it will be seen that in a large majority of cases a number of organs are involved, that extension to other parts of the urogenital tract are common, and that complete and early eradication of all possible foci is necessary to obtain the best results.

TABLE 30

DISTRIBUTION OF TUBERCULOSIS IN THE GENITAL TRACT

A. Epididymes and Seminal Vesicles. 222 cases.

Regions which the tuberculosis also involved.	No urinary involvement.	With right kidney and bladder.	With left kidney and bladder.	With bilateral kidney and bladder.	With bladder.	Total.
Right epididymis	3	1	1	1	0	6
Left epididymis	7	3	1	1	0	12
Bilateral epididymis	11	4	3	0	1	19
Right epididymis and right seminal vesicle	6	2	1	1	1	11
Right epididmyis and left seminal vesicle	0	0	1	0	0	1
Right epididymis and bilateral seminal vesicle	7	4	0	0	0	11
Left epididymis and right seminal vesicle	0	0	0	0	0	0
Left epididymis and left seminal vesicle	6	2	5	1	0	14
Left epididymis and bilateral seminal vesicle	9	3	3	2	1	18
Bilateral epididymis and right seminal vesicle	3	0	3	0	0	6
Bilateral epididymis and left seminal vesicle	4	1	2	2	0	9
Bilateral epididymis and bilateral seminal vesicle	31	14	10	11	2	68
Right seminal vesicle	1	2	3	0	1	7
Left seminal vesicle	1	2	3	2	2	10
Bilateral seminal vesicle	5	10	5	4	6	30
Total	94	48	41	25	14	222

SUMMARY

Epididymis and seminal vesicle cases with kidney involvement 114
Epididymis and seminal vesicle cases with doubtful kidney involvement 8
Epididymis and seminal vesicle cases without kidney involvement 100
Epididymis involved in 175
Seminal vesicles involved in... 185
Epididymes alone (or lesion in prostate or vesicles not recognized)..................... 37
Epididymes and seminal vesicles combined... 138
Seminal vesicles alone... 47
Total left epididymis 44   Total left seminal vesicle 34
Total right epididymis 29   Total right seminal vesicle 24
Total bilateral epididymis. 102   Total bilateral seminal vesicle.......... 127

TABLE 31

DISTRIBUTION OF TUBERCULOSIS IN GENITAL TRACT

B. Testes—Prostate. 191 cases

	No urinary involvement.	With right kidney and bladder.	With left kidney and bladder.	With bilateral kidney and bladder.	With bladder.	Total.
Right testis involved.................	9	0	2	0	0	11
Left testis involved..................	3	1	1	3	0	8
Prostate, with right seminal vesicle.....	8	4	5	0	1	18
Prostate, with left seminal vesicle......	12	5	9	6	2	34
Prostate, with bilateral seminal vesicle..	46	29	16	12	9	111
Prostate, with epididymis, without seminal vesicle......................	1	2	1	2	1	7
Prostate, without epididymis, or seminal vesicle...........................	5	6	8	0	1	20
Total of prostate cases...............	72	46	39	20	14	191

SUMMARY

Prostate cases with kidney involvement.................. 105
Prostate cases without kidney involvement............... 86
Prostate cases with other genital involvement............ 171   With kidney, 91; without, 80
Prostate cases without other genital involvement demonstrated....................................... 20   With kidney, 14; without, 6
Prostate cases without genital or kidney involvement demonstrated.. 6
Testis cases with kidney involvement, 7; without, 12; total, 19, which is 8⅓ per cent. of all genital cases.
In the 242 cases in both tables, pulmonary involvement was noted in 67 (27 per cent.).

TABLE 32

COMPARATIVE FREQUENCY OF INVOLVEMENT OF THE VARIOUS PORTIONS OF THE SEMINAL TRACT AND BLADDER IN 342 CASES OF UROGENITAL TUBERCULOSIS

Epididymes: { Globus minor, right 110, left 121
{ Globus major, right 77, left 95
Seminal vesicles...........right 147, left 162
Prostatic lobes.............right 177, left 174
Bladder: { Cystitis..........   182
{ Ulceration.......   61
Urethral involvement.......   9
Penile ulceration...........   4

Other statistics in our possession, given in the section on Treatment of Urogenital Tuberculosis, indicate plainly the *adverse effect of active lesions elsewhere in the body*. While it may be useless to cure urogenital tuberculosis if the patient is to die of tuberculosis elsewhere in the body, in many cases the removal of urogenital foci exercises a very beneficial effect on other foci of the disease. Great local benefit and relief of suffering may be obtained by operation, which is often maintained as long as the patient lives. Some apparently hopeless cases are "arrested." In solving this question each case must be considered individually, and much good judgment is called for. In general, one should seek a period of arrest,

TABLE 33

DISTRIBUTION OF URINARY TUBERCULOSIS IN RELATION TO TUBERCULOSIS OF THE SEMINAL TRACT

	Alone.	With bladder.	With bladder and prostate.	With bladder, prostate, and seminal vesicle.	With bladder, prostate, seminal vesicle, and epididymis.	With bladder, vesicles, and epididymis.	With bladder and epididymis.	With bladder, prostate, and epididymis.	Total.	With lung involvement.	With urethral involvement.
Right kidney	7	31	5	17	26	2	6	3	97	20	2
Left kidney	3	23	8	10	23	5	4	0	76	23	0
Bilateral kidney	0	7	1	4	15	3	1	1	32	17	2
Total	10	61	14	31	64	10	11	4	205	60	4

There were also 6 cases of bladder tuberculosis in which a renal lesion was not demonstrated.

TABLE 34

SUMMARY OF ALL CASES

Proved kidney cases with proved genital involvement.	128	Proved genital cases with proved kidney involvement.	128
Proved kidney cases with no genital involvement.	71	Proved genital cases with no kidney involvement.	108
Proved kidney cases with doubtful genital involvement.	6	Proved genital cases with doubtful kidney involvement.	6
Proved kidney cases, total.	205	Proved genital cases, total.	242
Doubtful kidney cases with proved genital involvement.	6	Doubtful genital cases with proved kidney involvement.	6
Doubtful kidney cases with doubtful genital involvement.	17	Doubtful genital cases with doubtful kidney involvement.	17
Doubtful kidney cases, total.	23	Doubtful genital cases, total.	23
Kidney cases, total.	228	Genital cases, total.	265

Total kidney cases.	228	Total genital cases.	265
Genital cases with no kidney involvement.	108	Kidney cases with no genital involvement.	71
Total.	336	Total.	336
Bladder cases.	6	Bladder cases.	6
Grand total.	342	Grand total.	342

"*Doubtful*" = data incomplete for location of lesion; always, however, good reason for diagnosis of tuberculosis. Bladder cases, no other involvement demonstrated, 6.

TABLE 35

DISTRIBUTION OF KNOWN RECURRENCE AFTER OPERATION, FROM GENITAL TO URINARY TRACT AND VICE VERSA

	Number of cases included.	Genital recurrences.	Kidney recurrences.
Radical operations, unilateral..........	7 } 24	3	0
Radical operations, bilateral...........	17	0	1
Epididymectomies, unilateral..........	75 } 98	25	Proved 10 / Probable 3
Epididymectomies, bilateral...........	23	1	4
Total genital operations...............	122	29	Proved 15 / Probable 3
Nephrectomies, primary...............	65	17	Proved 2 / Possible 7[1]

if that be possible, in the other lesions before attacking the urogenital tuberculosis. In certain cases, however, it seems that the only hope of betterment lies in taking rather desperate chances; one should be sure, in such cases, that there is at least some chance of improvement.

SYMPTOMS

General.—The most important general symptom of urogenital tuberculosis is *frequency of urination*, which was seen in 236 of our 342 cases. It indicates irritative changes in the bladder or posterior urethra, and may, therefore, appear in either genital or urinary tuberculosis. Associated with it there may be *dysuria*, *urgency*, and *difficulty*. Examination of the urine at the time these symptoms are first noted in cases of tuberculosis usually shows pus, although pyuria, as a symptom noted by the patient, is less frequent. It is probable that it often exists for considerable periods without being noticed. The second important symptom is *hematuria*, associated especially with renal tuberculosis. Most significant, however, is the *conjunction of the two*, and every medical student should be taught that when frequency and hematuria appear together out of a clear sky, tuberculosis should be most strongly suspected. Loss of weight is frequent enough to have definite significance, while chills, fever, and sweats were noted in 22.5 per cent. of all our cases.

Urinary Tract.—On the *renal* side *localized pain* and *renal colic* are about the only localizing symptoms. Diffuse pain was present in a little over one-third of our kidney cases, and colic in about one-fifth.

Genital Tract.—In the genital tract the first signal is usually a swelling of the epididymis, which is painful only in about one-half of the cases. The only symptom usually occurring from seminal vesicle involvement is perineal pain, which may equally well indicate prostatic or urethral lesions.

These are the commonest early symptoms. A study of the appended table of the duration of symptoms before treatment was instituted shows that by far too many of these cases go long unrecognized.

[1] There may have been other recurrences in opposite kidney in cases lost to view. See complete table of results under "Treatment."

TABLE 36

Duration of Symptoms Before Treatment in Urogenital Tuberculosis—Series of 317 Cases

0 to 1 week	4				
1 week to 1 month	12	0 to 6 months	83		
1 month to 6 months	67			0 to 1 year	139
6 months to 1 year	56	6 months to 1 year	56		
1 to 2 years	56				
2 to 3 years	30	1 to 5 years	117		
3 to 4 years	21				
4 to 5 years	10				
5 to 7½ years	19	5 to 10 years	41		
7½ to 10 years	22			Over 1 year	178
10 to 15 years	11				
15 to 20 years	6				
20 to 25 years	0	10 to 50 years	20		
25 to 30 years	1				
30 to 40 years	1				
40 to 50 years	1				

Over 2 years...................... 122
Over 5 years...................... 61

The *initial symptoms* in our series are shown in Table 37. It should be noted that in very many cases the frequency was followed almost immediately by hematuria.

TABLE 37

First Symptom Noted in Urogenital Tuberculosis—Series of 342 Cases

Frequency	84
Swelling in scrotum	62
Dysuria	49
Hematuria[1]	32
Pain in testicle	26
Diffuse renal pain	24
Renal colic	19
Pyuria[1]	16
Constant pain in bladder	10
Difficulty of urination	10
Pain in perineum	8
Swelling in perineum	6
Ulcer on penis	2
Pain in rectum	1
Urgency	1
Tenesmus	1
Urethral discharge[1]	1
Pain on coitus	1

The relative *frequency* of the various symptoms is best shown in Table 38. It may be commented that the pain in dysuria is often referred, as in other bladder conditions, to the end of the penis. Neglected epididymal tuberculosis, or that treated by simple incision, gives rise to many scrotal *sinuses*, which cause the patient to seek surgical assistance. Loss of sexual power, while not uncommon, is

[1] Includes only those cases where noted by patient himself before examination.

TABLE 38

OCCURRENCE OF SYMPTOMS OF UROGENITAL TUBERCULOSIS

In Series of 342 Cases.

Frequency of urination	236	Constant bladder pain		35
Hematuria[1]	177	Pain referred to penis		32
Painful urination	172	Pain in rectum		19
Scrotal swelling	143	Urethral discharge[1]		17
Pyuria[1]	119	Perineal swelling		11
Loss of weight	117	Pain on ejaculation or coitus		10
Diffuse renal pain	84	Passage of calculi		10
With radiation to groin	3	Spontaneous perineal urinary fistula		8
With radiation to shoulder	2	Spontaneous recto-urethral fistula		7
With reverse radiation	2	Tumor in kidney region		4
With radiation to umbilicus	1	Fistula in ano		3
Chills, fever, sweats	77	"Lumbago"		3
Pain in testicle	74	Pain in epigastrium		2
Spontaneous scrotal sinus	57	Pain in legs		2
Urinary	1	Hematospermia		2
Difficulty of urination	51	Ulcer on penis		2
Pain in perineum	47	Pain on erection		1
Urgency of urination	45	Pain in hip		1
Renal colic	43	Pain in groin		1
With radiation to groin	29	Pain in chest		1
With radiation to shoulder	0	Nausea and vomiting		1
With reverse radiation	6	Swelling in groin		1
With no radiation	8	Spontaneous sinus in groin		1
Loss of sexual power	42			
Partial	27			
Complete	15			
(Not affected, noted)	75			

usually a rather late manifestation. *Urethral discharge* may occur, and may be mistaken for acute or chronic gonorrhea. Perineal swelling indicates extension from prostate or urethra, and often goes on to abscess formation and rupture, in which case a urinary *fistula* is very apt to follow. Since, as we have seen, calculi may form in tuberculous kidneys, the appearance of a small stone does not necessarily explain the symptoms or rule out tuberculosis. It was noted in 10 of our cases. Hematospermia is less common than one would expect, but may easily go unnoticed.

TABLE 39

FEATURES IN HISTORIES OF UROGENITAL TUBERCULOSIS—IN SERIES OF 342 CASES

Family history positive	70
Family history negative	219
Family history not noted	13
History of injury	12
To testes	6
Instrumental	1
To body (falls, etc.)	5
Present illness began with pregnancy	1
History pointing to pulmonary tuberculosis	66
History pointing to bone tuberculosis	27
History pointing to gland tuberculosis	7
History pointing to skin tuberculosis	1
Persistent sinuses and fistulæ, postoperative	55
Scrotal, non-urinary	17
Scrotal, urinary	3
Perineal, non-urinary	3
Perineal, urinary	11
Renal, non-urinary	4
Renal, urinary	1
Suprapubic, urinary	12
Vesicoperineal fistula	2
Recto-urethral fistula	2

[1] Includes only those cases where noted by patient himself before examination.

A positive *family history* is suggestive, but in a majority of our cases it was not elicited. Injury to the testes had been noted in only a few cases, and cannot, therefore, be considered a very important factor. The history of *pulmonary tuberculosis* is important, and is strong presumptive evidence of a tuberculous origin for urogenital symptoms. This is also true for other forms of tuberculosis, as bone involvement, especially Pott's disease.

DIAGNOSIS

After the alert physician has had his suspicions aroused by a symptom-complex suggesting tuberculosis, there are certain simple diagnostic measures to be applied. While they may fix the diagnosis at once, they are quite often equivocal, and in such cases the utmost skill may be required to reach a definite conclusion. As we have seen how important it is to neglect no focus in the urogenital tract, a *complete examination* should be made in every case to locate every lesion. It is especially important in cases of genital tuberculosis to rule out the *kidneys*.

The first step is a careful examination of the *urine*. The one indubitable proof of tuberculosis is the discovery of *tubercle bacilli*, and pains must, therefore, be taken to exclude the smegma bacillus from the specimen. To do this catheteriz-

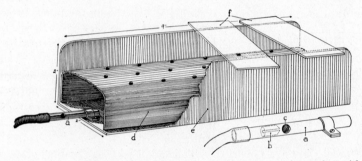

Fig. 160.—Device with burner for heating slides with carbolfuchsin or other stains without boiling, breaking, or spilling.

ation is not necessary, as shown by Young and Churchman,[1] but the meatus and glans should be carefully cleansed with alcohol. Following this the urethra is irrigated with sterile water or antiseptic solution, and the last part of the urine voided in a sterile test-tube and taken for study. It has been shown that this technique always excludes the smegma bacillus. The urine should be centrifugalized at high speed, preferably for an hour. If very large quantities of pus, mucus, and débris are present, it is advisable to digest the specimen with antiformin for twenty-four hours. The sediment is spread on slides, fixed, and stained by any one of the standard methods. Soaking the slide in dilute carbolfuchsin solution over night instead of heating for a few minutes will save many cracked slides and soiled hands and clothes. The simple apparatus (Fig. 160) described by Elvers[2] of this clinic is very satisfactory and saves time. Prolonged and patient search and frequently repeated examination are often necessary to discover the bacilli. If they are not found, urinary sediment is injected intraperitoneally in a guinea-pig. This is the most delicate test we have. Three or four weeks, however, are required for the development of unmistakable lesions.

[1] American Journal of the Medical Sciences, 1905, cxxx, 52–75.
[2] Johns Hopkins Hospital Bulletin, 1924, xxxv, 94, 95.

Aside from the tubercle bacillus itself, the presence of *pus without other organisms* is of most importance. In a large majority of the other cases of pyuria the causative cocci or bacilli will be seen in the pus. Pus without organisms is, therefore, strong presumptive evidence of the presence of tuberculosis. The presence of other organisms, however, does not rule out tuberculosis, as secondary infection is not infrequent.

Prostatic secretion, obtained with similar precautions, should be studied with the same ends in view. The glans and urethra are first cleaned and a specimen of urine obtained. The patient then bends forward, a gloved finger is inserted into the rectum, and secretion from vesicles and prostate forced by massage into the prostatic urethra, and from there successively into the bulbous and the penile urethra, where it appears at the meatus, and drops into a sterile tube held beneath by an assistant or the patient.

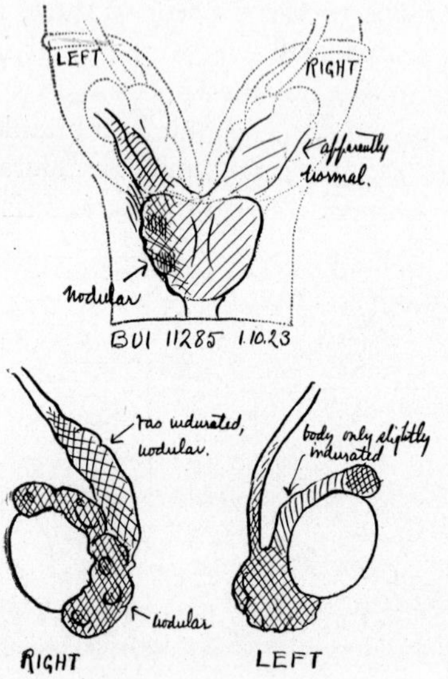

For the *genital tract*, one begins by a thorough examination of the *external genitalia*.

The urinary meatus may, in rare instances, show *ulceration*, or *periurethral thickening* may also be palpated along the upper urethra. Generally, however, even when tuberculous pus has been voided through the urethra for years, no evidence of erosion is made out. But occasionally one may find a *urethral discharge* which is not gonorrheal in character. A study of our cases shows that a history of treatment for supposed chronic gonorrhea is not so rare (5 per cent.).

The *scrotal contents* are much more frequently involved. If the skin of the scrotum shows evidence of inflammatory infiltration—*redness, thickening, adhesions*—to epididymis or tunica vaginalis—and particularly if a suppurative *sinus* is present, one should suspect tuberculosis. Sometimes tubercle bacilli may be found in the secretion.

Fig. 161.—Rectal and scrotal findings in a case of bilateral genital tuberculosis. While the epididymes are both markedly involved, the prostate is very little involved on the right. The nodularity of the left lobe of the prostate is distinctive. This patient also had bilateral renal tuberculosis and did well under medical treatment. (Tuberculin and fresh air.)

The findings in tuberculosis of the *epididymis* are very variable. Not infrequently the involvement is ushered in by *acute swelling*, with marked enlargement and pain, which may involve only the globus minor or the entire epididymis. Such cases are often accompanied by acute *hydrocele*, so that the intrascrotal swelling is great, forming a large ovoid tender mass, hot to the touch, which may closely simulate a gonococcal infection. After the acute symptoms, swelling, pain, etc., have subsided, a moderately enlarged, hard, and sometimes nodular epididymis remains.

In most cases one finds, in the early stages, an enlargement of a *portion* of the epididymis, which is very hard, sometimes irregular or even nodular, and rarely quite tender or painful. The globus minor is probably involved with greater frequency, though it may often begin in the globus major. The body and eventually all of the epididymis is involved as the diseased area increases (Fig. 161).

In some cases areas of focal suppuration or caseation *fluctuation* may be recognized. These are generally associated with invasion of the subcutaneous tissues.

These areas of fluctuation are usually not to be mistaken for cysts, which are smooth, ovoid, often pedunculated, or found springing from an otherwise normal epididymis, generally the globus major.

Chronic induration of the epididymis, left after gonococcal inflammation, tends to decrease, and finally results in a hard, nodular, painless epididymis, which does not simulate an active tuberculous process. In some cases, however, tuberculous epididymitis may be so "inactive" and so "fibrous" as to make diagnosis difficult. It is here that rectal examination of prostate and vesicles is so helpful.

Some degree of hydrocele is common, and if at all marked will prevent palpation of the testis. The globus minor and body of the epididymis, however, will always be found outside of the sac, since they are not surrounded by the tunica vaginalis. The globus major, which lies within the tunica vaginalis, if only slightly enlarged may be concealed by a hydrocele. If large it is usually palpable outside of the sac. In case of doubt it may be advisable to remove the fluid by tapping to permit closer study, but it is better not to do this unless necessary, especially if testicular neoplasm is suspected.

Early involvement of the *testis* cannot usually be made out, since the affected region may be concealed by the enlarged epididymis, but in later stages *irregularity, areas of induration*, and *adhesions* can be felt. The testis, if involved, is generally indurated in the upper posterior portion *adjacent to the globus major*.

The history, subsequent course, and other findings (induration or enlargement of vesicles and prostate, pyuria) give the diagnosis, but if still doubtful, aspiration of the epididymis will generally give enough fluid for microscopic examination and detection of the tubercle bacillus. The *vas deferens* should be outlined as far up as possible. When it is involved it is enlarged and indurated, and while it may occasionally be smooth, the characteristic sign is an *irregularity*, occasionally described as resembling a string of beads.

Charts and sketches of the findings are very valuable, as they contribute to accuracy and are useful for comparison at later stages and for record. A few of these are shown in Figs. 162–165.

The *seminal vesicles, prostate*, and *membranous urethra* are studied by *rectal examination*. Here again sketches are recommended. *Induration* and *irregularity* are again the characteristic findings, together with varying degrees of *enlargement*. Adhesions are usually present. The induration produced is nodular and firmer than that found in ordinary vesiculitis and prostatitis, and is sometimes hard enough to be confused with that of prostatic carcinoma. In fact, it is often difficult to differentiate between chronic and tuberculous seminal vesiculitis, and we have seen 2 cases diagnosed as carcinoma of the prostate. The *age* of the patient, the *history*, the *findings elsewhere*, and study of the *urine* and *prostatic secretion* will usually clear up the diagnosis. In the *prostate* discrete nodules may be found or the entire organ be enlarged, indurated, and irregular. *Abscess* formation is rare, but may occur, and very extensive invasions of pelvic structures may be found. Rectal, recto-urethral, or rectovesical *fistulæ* may be palpated and located by probing or shadowgrams. In *urethral* involvement irregularity, induration, and adhesions may be felt, and extensive fistulous tracts of perineum, scrotum, and even buttocks, known as the "watering-pot perineum," are seen.

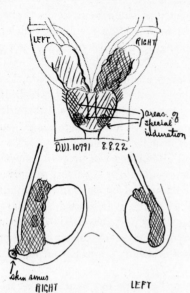

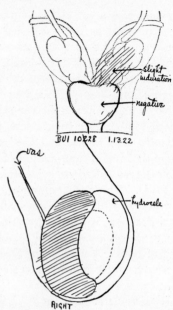

FIG. 162.—Rectal and scrotal findings in a case of bilateral genital tuberculosis. Note the irregular nodular character of the prostate. Swelling of left testicle began two years previously. Patient also had acute gonorrheal urethritis. Treatment was by double epididymectomy.

FIG. 163.—Rectal and scrotal findings in a case of genital tuberculosis. Note that the vas is normal, prostate negative, but that a slight induration is present in the right seminal vesicle. Epididymectomy was done. A later stage of this case is shown in the following diagram.

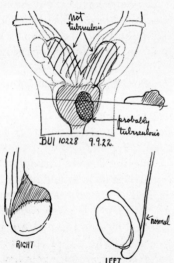

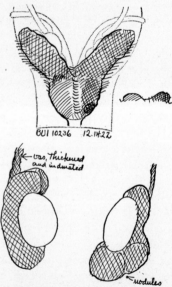

FIG. 164.—Rectal and scrotal finding in a case of genital tuberculosis. The hardness and irregularity of the nodule in the prostate are distinctive. The diagram was made after a right epididymectomy had been done, the mass shown having recurred after operation. Radical removal of the seminal vesicles, part of the prostate, both vasa, and the left epididymis was then done. Patient had also had previously a nephrectomy. Following the operation tuberculosis of hip developed and patient was still in bed, but without urinary symptoms.

FIG. 165.—Rectal and scrotal findings in a case of bilateral genital tuberculosis. The entire tract is seen to be involved on both sides. Patient's history extended over three years, with swelling of the testicle and later painful and frequent urination. Double epididymectomy and later left nephrectomy were done. Patient had pulmonary tuberculosis and developed tuberculosis of the spine with psoas abscess. Died in hospital.

PLATE VII

ULCERS OF THE BLADDER

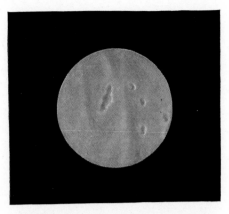

A. Multiple small tuberculous ulcers in hyper-
emic bladder wall. B. U. I. 8542.

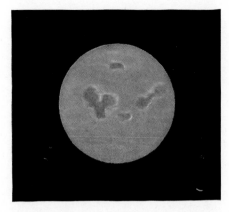

B. Same case (A). Larger, more confluent
ulcers. B. U. I. 8542.

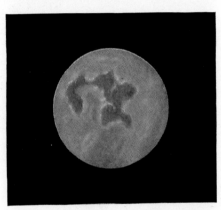

C. Same case. Deep, very confluent, large,
tuberculous ulcers. B. U. I. 8542.

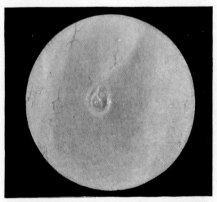

D. More chronic tuberculous ulcer; bladder pale; granulation tissue filling center of
ulcer. B. U. I. 6795.

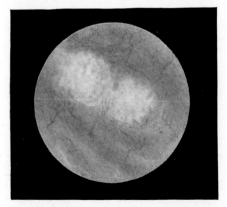

E. Exudate and necrosis produced by extensive fulguration and destruction of benign
papilloma of bladder. B. U. I. 7092.

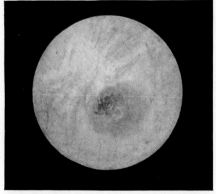

F. Small tuberculous ulcer of bladder and
large cicatrix of healed ulcer following nephrectomy for tuberculosis. B. U. I. 3120.

Sinuses should be investigated, the secretion stained for tubercle bacilli, and scrapings taken for microscopic study. This is important, as it is *practically useless to attempt to close tuberculous sinuses or fistulæ* by operation. Suspected recto-urethral or other fistulæ can be investigated by injecting a dye, such as gentian-violet or mercurochrome, in the rectum or elsewhere as indicated, and by watching for its appearance in the urine.

Radiographs: Plain *x*-rays of the entire urogenital tract should be taken. An enlargement or irregularity of the kidney may be shown by the plain *x*-ray. Caseous areas are often seen and sometimes a thick fibrous or caseous ureter is well shown. Lesions in the vesicles may be visible.

Cystoscopy: When the cystoscope is introduced one first observes the bladder. The milder degrees of *catarrhal tuberculous cystitis* present no characteristic appearance. There is a diffuse or spotty reddening, often most pronounced about the ureter of the affected kidney. The *base* of the bladder is most involved, and occasionally the lesion is symmetrical even in unilateral tuberculosis. In later stages *ulceration* occurs. The ulcers may be small or large, single or multiple, but when large are usually irregular in outline (serpiginous). There are often tags of mucosa and polypoid masses of granulation tissue, with adherent mucus, slough, or blood-clot, so that the picture may suggest vesical neoplasm. Since the lesion usually begins and is most pronounced about the ureteral meatus, this orifice is often concealed in these later stages. It may be found in many cases by probing or by observing the source of the stream of blue-stained urine after injection of indigo-carmin. In advanced cases the bladder is extremely *contracted*, irritable, and tender, so that general or sacral anesthesia may be necessary for the examination. The ureteral meatus is sometimes strictured by scar tissue.

After careful study of the bladder the *ureters* should be *catheterized*, preferably with catheters large enough to fill the ureteral lumen completely. After introduction of ureteral catheters the *urine* should be collected in sterile test-tubes and a *phenolsulphonephthalein* test done. It is best not to take a pyelogram unless necessary for diagnosis. The microscopic study of the kidney urine and the functional tests will usually give not only the diagnosis, but the information which is required before operative treatment. In a few difficult cases, however, the pyelogram is of distinct help.

If the total phthalein has been normal, it is evidence that one kidney is healthy, and we may find the divided function from the sound side about twice normal. In early cases, however, where the lesion is small, the affected kidney may still show a normal or only slightly decreased function. If the total phthalein is subnormal one may expect to find bilateral involvement, but the examination should be made carefully, since one kidney may be injured by some other process than tuberculosis, or occasionally the renal function may be depressed reflexly in the healthy kidney as a result of the tuberculous disease of its fellow.

The divided urines should be caught in sterile tubes and carefully examined, as sometimes pus and tubercle bacilli are found when they have been absent from the voided urine. This may well be due to the mechanical removal by the ureteral catheter. Before removal of the ureteral catheter an injection of some mild antiseptic should be made (1 : 1000 nitrate of silver or 1 : 500 meroxyl).

The pyelogram will generally show the typical *erosion, irregularity,* and *enlargement* of affected calices (Figs. 166, 167). It also discloses calculi, hydronephrosis, and hydro-ureter, and gives an idea of the location and nature of the *obstruction.* Such obstruction may be due especially to stones or to cicatricial or inflammatory strictures of the ureter. The latter may be due to lesions arising outside it, as in the tip of the seminal vesicle. Rectal examination will help to confirm this finding.

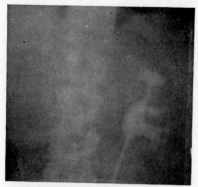

FIG. 166.—Pyelogram showing little if any change in the lower and middle calyces, but marked dilatation and irregularity of the upper calyx. Although this patient was treated for a long time for chronic pyelitis the appearance of this calyx is very suggestive of tuberculosis. B. U. I. *x*-Ray 2628.

If the examination of the kidneys is negative on one occasion, *it does not necessarily rule out tuberculosis,* as we have seen that the discharge of tubercle bacilli and pus may be intermittent, and if reason for suspicion still exists, the examination must be repeated.

The plain *x*-ray is of assistance, especially in advanced lesions. Here calcareous deposits give shadows, which are typically irregular and spotty and lack the density of those from solid calculi (Fig. 168). The entire kidney may be outlined by such shadows where destruction is extensive,[1] and they may be present when the urine is clear in cases where the ureter is occluded. Involvement of the ureter may be indicated by an irregular, ragged outline of the ureteral shadow (Fig. 169).

If, after repeated trials, ureteral catheterization is impossible, conclusions must be drawn from the total phthalein, from the urine examination, and from ureteral

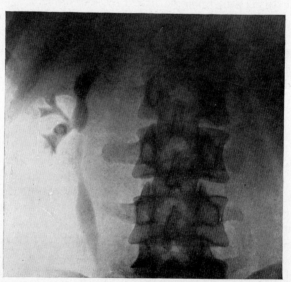

FIG. 167.—Pyelogram of a case of tuberculosis of the right kidney. Changes are seen only in the upper calyx, which is slightly dilated and irregular. B. U. I. *x*-Ray 2618.

meatoscopy with indigocarmin. Such cases are usually well advanced, and will show secretion of this dye from one side only. In any case the disparity between

[1] Colston and Waters: Johns Hopkins Hospital Bulletin, 1919, xxx, 268–271 (Lit.).

the two sides will readily be seen.   If the total phthalein is consistently low, however, one may safely assume a bilateral lesion or nephritis, and refrain from operation.

When genito-urinary tuberculosis is suspected a most exhaustive *general physical examination*, with study of the sputum, *x*-rays, etc., must be done, to determine the existence of active tuberculosis in the lungs or elsewhere in the body, and also to discover tenderness, muscle spasm, tumor, sinuses, etc., relating to the kidneys and ureters, and sometimes indicating hydronephrosis, pyonephrosis, or perirenal abscess.

Résumé.—A history of frequency of urination, irritation, hematuria coming on insidiously, especially in patients under fifty years of age, should be held suspicious of tuberculosis of the urogenital tract.   After careful study of scrotum, prostate and vesicles, the urine and plain *x*-ray plates, cystoscopy should be carried out,

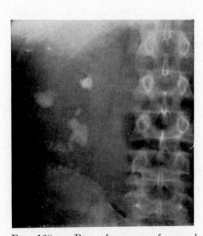 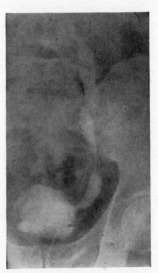

Fig. 168.—*x*-Ray of a case of very large tuberculous pyonephrosis with multiple stone formation.   The outline of the greatly enlarged kidney is well seen.   The patient refused operation.   B. U. I. *x*-Ray 4949.

Fig. 169.—Case of extensive tuberculosis of the bladder, kidneys, and ureters.   This picture shows distortion of the bladder and ureter with multiple strictures of the latter.   Ureteral reflux was present in this case.   B. U. I. *x*-Ray 3352.

ulcerations in the bladder sought for, and the ureters catheterized, urine examined. function tests, and pyelogram on suspected side (or both if advisable) taken.   If it is impossible to find tubercle bacilli, the diagnosis of tuberculosis may still be made from the findings in epididymis, seminal vesicle, bladder, or kidney (by cystoscope, function tests, and pyelograms).   The history of or presence of lung tuberculosis is strong presumptive evidence of urogenital tuberculosis in the presence of symptoms referable to the urinary or genital tracts.   The presence of pyuria, when no organisms can be cultured from the urine, is strong presumptive evidence of tuberculosis.

TREATMENT

Operation.—This has been placed first because a radical excision should be carried out whenever possible.   Our statistics show that operative is far more satisfactory than non-operative therapy except in tuberculosis of the bladder and of the ureter.

Tuberculosis of the Kidney.—*Nephrectomy* should be done.   The accepted method is through a curved, muscle-cutting, extraperitoneal incision in the side. The wound should be large enough to give a good exposure so that the kidney can be freed, the ureter isolated and divided and the vascular pedicle clamped triply, divided, and the stump doubly ligated.   The kidney should be removed with as little pressure and traumatism as possible.   The details of technic are given else-where.   Some authors have urged the importance of removing the fatty capsule, which is sometimes involved, along with the kidney, but this is not always possible. The adrenal is rarely seen and almost never excised, even partially, unless found to be diseased.   The ureter need not be removed unless found to be extensively diseased.   When it is only slightly or moderately enlarged and indurated, the disease in the ureter either disappears or is arrested after the flow through it of tuberculous pus and urine ceases with nephrectomy.

The injection of pure *carbolic* into the ureter is, we believe, valuable in sterilizing the ureter, destroying its epithelium, and leading to an early resorption of inflam-matory changes.   Where a very large, indurated or nodular ureter is found, *ureter-ectomy*, as complete as possible, is to be done, if conditions warrant.   By careful blunt dissection the ureter can often be followed to its insertion into the bladder and excised, leaving only the terminal 2 or 3 cm.   In some cases the adhesions to seminal vesicle, vas, rectum, and pelvic cellular tissues are so great that the point of division is necessarily remote from the bladder.   In such cases the terminal portion of the ureter may drain tuberculous pus into the deep pelvic wound and be a source of danger, and we have seen miliary tuberculosis of the wound occur and cause a fatal ending.

It is, therefore, safer to leave the ureter to conduct the pus within it down to the bladder or up to the loin wound, trusting to the carbolization or subsequent antiseptic treatment (local injections of mercurochrome 1 per cent. into the sinus from above, or into the ureter through a ureter catheter through a cystoscope) eventually to close the sinus.

In the female the terminal portion of the ureter may be excised through the vagina, as shown by Kelly and others.   As stated above, this is generally undesir-able and rarely necessary.

The diagnosis of tuberculosis of the kidney or the desirability of carrying out nephrectomy should not be made at operation—but *beforehand*.   Not infrequently, when exposed on the operating table, the kidney looks so nearly normal as to give no indication of the tuberculous process within.   To do a nephrotomy for diagnosis is unpardonable.

The operation of nephrectomy in tuberculosis is one of the most satisfactory in surgery.   We have recently had a series of 111 consecutive cases without a death, and the results obtained are generally all that can be desired, unless other organs are involved.   The most remarkable disappearance of tuberculous lesions in the bladder and ureter occur after simple removal of the diseased kidney, likewise tuberculous processes in the deep urethra and prostate are "arrested."   The persistence of a sinus or urinary fistula in the loin is a disagreeable and not so infre-quent sequel, but rarely lasts a long time.   Antiseptic treatment or cauterization of the tract from above or below (ureter catheter) usually suffices, but secondary resection of the sinus or even the ureter may be required.

Nephrectomy is contraindicated in bilateral renal tuberculosis unless one side is giving great pain and the other side is but slightly involved, when it may sometimes be justifiable. We have usually found it disappointing.

Bidgood[1] has recently studied 89 cases of nephrectomy for tuberculosis in our series, and finds that in 16 (18 per cent.) the wound broke down after the operation. This complication has had little effect, apparently, on the ultimate results, but is a serious matter for the patient, since it incapacitates him for weeks or months after he would otherwise be well. In an analysis of these 16 cases it appears that no feature in the history or preoperative examination was related with the breaking down of the wound, and that it might occur after various methods of handling the ureter, including 1 case of complete ureterectomy. It was the lesion present in the kidney which was of greatest importance. All the cases of pyonephrosis in the series broke down, while no case of chronic fibroid tuberculosis did so. In the other cases breaking down, 8 had multiple abscesses, 1 acute tuberculous nephritis, and 4 large cavities. Of the 4 with cavitation (the most chronic sort of the 16) it was noted in 3 that some of the caseous material was spilled in the wound. We may say, therefore, that the cases likely to break down are those with acute tuberculosis, especially pyonephrosis, and those in which tuberculous pus is spilled in the wound. On the other hand, some cases of acute tuberculosis and some cases in which caseous material from old quiescent lesions is spilled heal *per priman*. In addition, it is impossible to predict from the examination what kind of lesion will be found at operation.

The breaking down occurs during the third week, a time at which the chromic catgut sutures may be assumed to have been absorbed. If left alone, healing occurs by granulation, but may be very slow, occupying many months (up to two years). The non-union is due to an actual tuberculous infection of the wound, as shown by microscopic studies. In addition, healing is not accelerated even if the wound is kept free of other organisms by irrigations with Dakin's solution, meroxyl, etc.

Stimulation with iodoform, balsam of Peru, ultraviolet rays, etc., has been used, with but slight evidence of favorable effect. Two cases (B. U. I. 11,983 and B. U. I. 11,392) were treated by a thorough débridement of the wounds by sharp dissection after disinfection by lengthy Carrel-Dakin and mercurochrome treatment, followed by immediate suture with silver wire, using no catgut. In each case a very small sinus persisted at the lower angle of the wound, indicating that in these patients who may be expected to be soon out of bed this is the point of election for drainage. This procedure undoubtedly saved the patients a great deal of time, and is to be recommended.

In bilateral renal tuberculosis non-surgical methods are necessary. These are discussed elsewhere. Only under the rarest circumstances should nephrectomy be done when the other kidney is tuberculous.

Tuberculosis of the Ureter.—This is secondary to renal tuberculosis, and, as stated above, disappears after nephrectomy in all but exceptionally severe cases. Ureterectomy may be carried out by enlarging the extraperitoneal wound employed in nephrectomy. Some surgeons have advised a second incision for the removal of the lower segment of the ureter after the kidney and upper portion have been freed, but it can be done through a single incision. In only 4 of our 112 cases of nephrectomy was ureterectomy done; in 3 simultaneously and in 1

[1] Journal of the American Medical Association, 1924, lxxxiii, 1573–1577.

subsequent to nephrectomy. Postoperative ureterectomy may be required to cure persistent ureteral fistula (see Operative Chapter).

Tuberculosis of the Bladder.—Here non-operative treatment should be followed to the exclusion of all operative methods if possible. Of prime importance is it to remove the *source* of infection (kidney, prostate, or vesicles), after which the vesical ulceration will usually disappear promptly. It is remarkable how extensive serpiginous ulcers often clear up after nephrectomy without other treatment. Sometimes intravesical injections and irrigations may be of value: *e. g.*, carbolic acid, 6 per cent., 30 c.c. injected every four to six days (Rovsing's method); instillations daily of mercurochrome 1 per cent. and retained as long as possible; nitrate of silver 1 per cent., 5 c.c. once a week.

Farnarier[1] has recommended the use of iodin vapor, and has published an ingenious apparatus for introducing it into the bladder. Vernier[2] uses ether vapor in the same way, while others recommend the introduction of sterile air. Good results have been reported, but other methods are usually sufficient.

Gomenol 20 per cent., in a medium of oil, sometimes is very effective in relieving pain, spasm, and great frequency of urination. It is injected by a Keyes-Ultzmann syringe. Methylene-blue, administered orally, also gives surprising relief in such cases at times.

More radical is the use of cystoscopic fulguration, which is often very effective in destroying a tuberculous ulcer and inducing healing.

Occasionally irritation of the prostatic urethra may require relief by instillations of a few drops of 5 per cent. silver nitrate or gomenol. If a contracture of the vesical orifice is present, a punch operation, preferably with a cautery blade, may be necessary to give free micturition.

If it can be proved, as, for example, by obtaining pus and tubercle bacilli from the remaining ureter on the side where nephrectomy has been done, that there is a definite tuberculous focus in the ureter, it may become necessary, in very rare cases, to remove the ureter in order to obtain healing of the bladder.

In a few cases the bladder lesions apparently become sufficiently deeply rooted so that they are self-sustaining, and then the bladder symptoms persist after nephrectomy. In addition to the discomfort caused by this condition, it sometimes happens that the scarring around the ureteral orifice of the healthy ureter will cause a contracture, with resulting hydro-ureter, hydronephrosis, and renal insufficiency. Hinman[3] has treated two such cases by transplanting the dilated ureter into the rectum, obtaining complete relief in both instances, with marked improvement in the renal function. One of these patients is still living and in good health four years after the operation.

Suprapubic cystotomy should be avoided at all hazards, as it usually means a permanent fistula and a source of unending trouble. In very rare cases, with extreme pain and irritation, it is necessary to drain the bladder, at which time the ulcerations may be cauterized or fulgurated as thoroughly as possible. But, as remarked above, after nephrectomy or seminal vesiculectomy the secondary vesical

---

[1] Archives Urologiques de la Clinique de Necker, 1914, i, 353–375 (Lit.). See also Normand: Journal d'Urologie, 1914, v, 271–289.

[2] Journal de Médécine et de Chirurgie Pratique, 1913, lxxxiv, 913–924.

[3] Personal communication.

lesions usually disappear and bladder symptoms ameliorate sufficiently to restore comfort and fairly normal micturition.

Tuberculosis of the urethra is rare except as a late complication of urinary or seminal tuberculosis. It disappears usually when the higher source of suppuration is removed. At most, mild injections are required—argyrol, boric acid, mercurochrome, etc.—unless stricture is present. In such cases dilation is to be preferred to external urethrotomy, as miliary tuberculosis may follow internal urethrotomy or even dilation.

Tuberculosis of the Seminal Tract.—As set forth at length above, our studies seem to prove conclusively that, whereas the epididymis attracts most attention, and gives more pronounced symptoms, especially at the outset, the seminal vesicles are, in fact, the primary and principal seat of the tuberculous process. It is not surprising, therefore, to find in an exhaustive review of the surgical literature that the results obtained by simple removal of the external focus by epididymectomy or castration are very bad. We have pointed out these facts in several papers on the subject, and have been amazed at the tenacity with which our confrères have clung to procedures which are manifestly incomplete and unradical, and demonstrably poor as to results.

In a recent paper[1] our position was set forth as follows:

"The preceding statistics seem, therefore, to show conclusively that in the great majority of cases the primary involvement is in the seminal vesicles (or prostate), from which the epididymes or testicles are subsequently involved, the external disease being bilateral in from 30 to 50 per cent. of the cases. In a probably larger percentage of the cases the involvement of the seminal vesicles is bilateral (61 per cent. of my cases in series B and probably higher). The disease reaches the epididymis generally by the lymphatics of the cord from the seminal vesicles and first involves generally the globus minor. It is probably erroneous to suppose that primary tuberculosis of the epididymis often occurs. It probably seldom occurs through blood-stream infections, as so often asserted. The seminal vesicles are not only the primary focus from which the epididymes are involved, but from which also the prostate, bladder, and the kidneys in many cases are involved. In fact, tuberculosis in the region of the prostate and vesicles is far more dangerous to the entire human organism than tuberculosis of the epididymes, and is probably responsible for the fearful mortality which is variously estimated at from 27 to 60 per cent. in cases of genital tuberculosis. Therefore, it is the duty of the surgeon to attack the most dangerous focus of involvement, namely, that of the vesicles and prostate. In tuberculosis of the seminal tract in the great majority of cases radical operation not only should be the operation of choice but also should be practically imperative. A realization of the bad results obtained by epididymectomy or castration led me in 1913 to devise the radical operation described herewith."

The *radical operation* is described in another chapter. It suffices here to say that the seminal vesicles, ampullæ, and both lateral lobes of the prostate are removed through the perineum, after which the epididymis and vas are extracted through the groin. As experience has increased it has become evident: 1, that in tuberculosis of the epididymis, where there is involvement of vesicle or prostate, removal through the perineum of both vesicles, ampullæ of the vasa, and the lateral

[1] Young: The Radical Cure of Seminal Tuberculosis, Archives of Surgery, 1922, iv, 334–419.

lobes of the prostate is indicated at the same time that the epididymis and vas deferens are removed completely.

2. That where only one vesicle is removed the chance of involvement of the remaining epididymis is almost as great as after simple epididymectomy.

3. That the entire involvement can be radically removed—epididymis, vasa, ampullæ, seminal vesicles, and lateral prostatic lobes—without opening the urinary tract; that micturition returns to normal, and even coitus is generally only slightly impaired (ejaculated fluid being much less in amount).

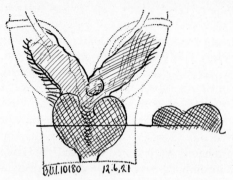

4. That the operation, *per se*, is not dangerous, even where nephrectomy is also necessary to eradicate the entire urogenital involvement. Figures 170–172 indicate the findings before and after operation in a typical case.

Epididymectomy.—This operation, which was brought out by Bardenheuer in 1887, consists in a careful dissection of the epididymis and vas, leaving the testicle with its blood supply intact. The introduction of this

Fig. 170.—Extensive involvement of the entire prostate and both seminal vesicles in a case of genital tuberculosis. Note the adhesions along the left seminal vesicle and the nodule in the intravesicular region. Prostate itself is not markedly nodular.

operative procedure so long ago should have put an end to the unnecessary removal of testicles which is, alas, the common practice among surgeons the world over to this very day.

As pointed out in the pathologic discussion, one of the most remarkable facts in pathology is the relative immunity of the testis to tuberculosis—even in the

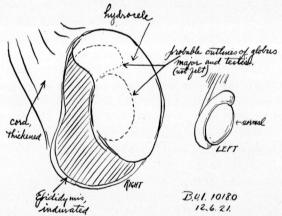

Fig. 171.—Scrotal findings in the same case shown in the preceding diagram. The cord is much thickened, the epididymis tremendously enlarged and indurated, but not especially nodular. A hydrocele conceals the testis.

presence of a long-standing extensive process in the epididymis immediately adjacent, and one of the most interesting niceties of surgical technic is the ease with which a large tuberculous epididymis may be dissected free from the testis without injuring its blood and nerve supply, thus leaving it to continue to function as an important gland of internal secretion.

Even where a small portion of the testis is involved it is usually possible, by means of a cautery resection, to preserve the remainder of the testis. This should always be attempted in young men who have already lost the other testis through castration.

Castration, until recent years the universally practised procedure in "genital tuberculosis," is generally unjustifiable. When, however, one testicle is manifestly tuberculous, castration should usually be done unless a partial resection offers chance of success. The presence of sinuses or extensive scrotal involvement necessarily require excision of sufficient scrotal tissues to effect a cure.

The *handling of the vas* depends upon whether the seminal vesicles and ampullæ have been removed at the same sitting. If so, every effort should be made to extract the entire vas deferens so as to remove the whole infected tract. If it is impossible to free the vas (generally in its deeper retrovesical portion), one may either use forceful traction, hoping thus to remove all the vas through the groin incision, or deliberately leave the vas to drain out in the groin. The latter plan is the safer procedure in such cases, as we have seen deep-seated tuberculous abscesses come on after von Büngner's forcible divulsion, which operation had left behind a portion of the vas.

When, in performing the radical operation, the vas breaks, and a portion is left behind the bladder, one should keep a tube in the perineal wound to drain the distal end of the remaining vas for ten days or more. If the break occurs in the inguinal canal or just above it, a small rubber drain should be left in the groin.

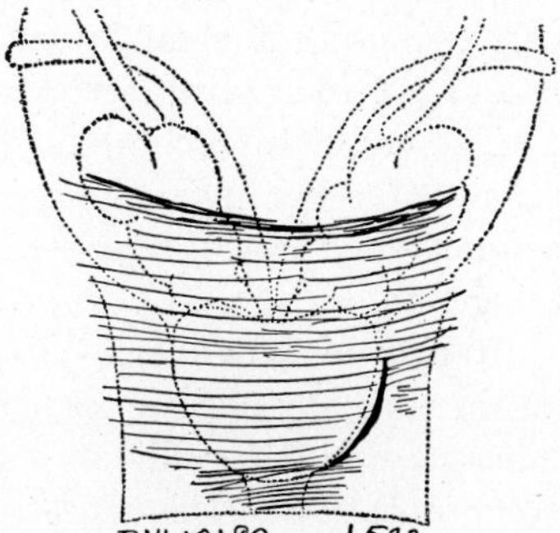

When the radical operation is not carried out the vas should not be divulsed, but should be injected with pure carbolic (1 or 2 c.c.) and then brought out in the groin and sutured to the skin for drainage and, if possible, further injections. Some prefer to ligate at the external inguinal

BUI.10180   1.5.22

FIG. 172.—Rectal findings after bilateral seminal vesiculectomy and partial prostatectomy in the same case shown in the preceding figures. The shelf indicated in the upper part demarcates accurately the extent of the operative wound. The scar tissue resulting from the operation conceals the prostate entirely except at its lower right border.

ring, and bury the stump. The recurrence of fistulas in the scrotal wound attests the incompleteness of such procedures.

Non-operative Treatment.—*Climatic* and *general treatment* of tuberculosis of the urogenital tract is to be used where the extent of the disease or the condition of the patient does not warrant radical operative procedures, *e. g.*, in bilateral renal tuberculosis, vesical tuberculosis, prostatic and vesicular tuberculosis with extensive fistulæ (perineal, rectal, vesical), extensive tuberculosis of other viscera (lungs, pleura, peritoneum, etc.), great general weakness of patient.

The mere presence of a tuberculous process in the lungs or pleura does not contraindicate a radical operation in urogenital tuberculosis under spinal or epidural anesthesia if the general condition of the patient warrants it (general anesthesia should never be used). But where radical operation is contraindicated, as outlined above, much may be accomplished by sanatorial treatment. In an exhaustive study of the work of several large sanatoria in Colorado we were amazed to find some remarkable cures or arrestations in a few cases of very extensive urogenital and pulmonary tuberculosis. The usual regimen—rest, forced feeding, fresh air, etc.—were employed, but the most effective curative agent was heliotherapy. One case of lung tuberculosis with involvement of both kidneys, epididymes, and seminal vesicles had progressed so remarkably as to be apparently well. In the epididymes only fibrous cords remained, and the urine was practically normal.

The marvelous effect of the sun's rays in a dry climate in cases of "surgical tuberculosis" is to be seen at the Fitz Simmons U. S. General Hospital at Denver, where extensive tuberculous disease of bones and joints, cold abscesses, fistulas, and large ulcerative processes are seen to clear up under heliotherapy, rest, fresh air, and forced feeding. Where the patient is unable to take institutional treatment in a dry sunshiny climate, such as Colorado, New Mexico, Arizona, or Texas, the "alpine lamp" treatment will give almost identical results.

But the mortality in pulmonary cases which are complicated with urogenital tuberculosis remains very high, and where it is possible to remove a tuberculous kidney, epididymis, and seminal vesicles under procain (local, spinal, caudal, or paravertebral) it should undoubtedly be done. The pulmonary or other deep lesions are then given a chance to get well.

The use of tuberculin has been very disappointing in our hands (see Table 43, page 334). We have seen one early kidney case, which might have been cured by nephrectomy, die of a generalized tuberculosis after a most thorough course of tuberculin.

Results of Treatment.—In the following pages will be found a summary showing in their details the results of treatment of our series of cases of urogenital tuberculosis. Since this series reaches back almost twenty-five years it comprises every variation of the operative treatment of this disease.

NEPHRECTOMY, PRIMARY, NO SEMINAL TRACT INVOLVEMENT AT TIME OF OPERATION.—Sixty-five cases. Of these, 30 cases are *well* at last report; namely, over five years, 11; four to five years, 2; three to four years, 1; two to three years, 4; one to two years, 3; less than one year, 9. *Of these 30 cases, 23 had bladder symptoms before operation and have been completely relieved.*

Twelve cases are reported as *improved* after the operation, but *bladder symptoms are still present* in some degree, there being, however, no indication of any further spread of the disease. These cases have been followed over five years, 2; four to five years, 1; three to four years, 1; one to two years, 2; under one year, 6. Of these 12 cases, 4 complain of frequency, pain, and occasional hematuria; 7, frequency and turbid urine; and the twelfth has an extremely contracted bladder and suprapubic fistula, otherwise he is in good health. Four cases are reported *unimproved* followed three to four years, 1 (great frequency, tenesmus, hematuria); one to two years, 2 (frequency and hematuria; great frequency and hematuria); 1 case is reported alive, but with *recurrence in the opposite kidney.*

A further group of 14 cases are *living* after a *recurrence of the disease in the epididymis* at some time after nephrectomy (21.5 per cent.). Of these, 4 had no operation upon the epididymis. Of the others, 9 had epididymectomy and 1 castration, and 4 of them subsequently became well, while in the others the disease has spread to other organs. It is further noted that of these 14 cases in which the disease spread to the epididymis, 5 had pulmonary tuberculosis at the time of nephrectomy and 2 had bone tuberculosis. In none were the prostate and seminal vesicles noted as involved before the nephrectomy. Nine cases, however, were examined at the Brady Clinic before the secondary operation on the epididymis, and in 8 of them the prostate or seminal vesicles or both were found to be involved, in 1 "suspected areas" of induration were present, while in none was rectal examination still negative. In 6 of the 14 cases not only one but both epididymes became involved, and of these 6, all showed positive findings in the prostate and seminal vesicles. Of the 8 cases in which the opposite epididymis has not become involved, in only 2 has the patient been followed more than one year.

Two patients are *dead* following *recurrence of the disease in the genital tract.* (I), B. U. I. 5194. This patient had a cystotomy after the nephrectomy on account of persistent bladder tuberculosis. The trigone was divided. Symptoms continued, and three years after the nephrectomy, the genital tract having become involved, the seminal vesicle and epididymis of one side were removed at another clinic. Although much improved, pyuria continued, and he died five years later, probably with involvement of the other kidney. (II), B. U. I. 6449. The genital tract became involved nine months after nephrectomy, and the patient had, successively, epididymectomy, orchidectomy (same side), and epididymectomy on the opposite side. Two years later internal urethrotomy was done for tuberculous stricture of the urethra. The patient died two weeks later of miliary tuberculosis and autopsy showed that the remaining kidney was tuberculous.

One patient is *dead* of *pulmonary tuberculosis* (B. U. I. 10,834). This patient had pulmonary tuberculosis and tuberculosis of the hip before nephrectomy. He died fifteen months later of pulmonary tuberculosis.

One patient *died* after operation in the hospital (B. U. I. 11,436), a child thirteen years old. Although symptoms had been present only six weeks, the kidney was found to be extremely adherent and almost impossible to free, the operation being an exceedingly difficult one. The pleura was accidently opened, and in treating the pedicle, it was so short and fibrous that it was thought necessary to insert sutures to secure the vessels. The operation lasted two hours and the patient was much shocked. He died twenty-seven hours later. Autopsy showed that sutures had passed through the wall of the vena cava, but there was no thrombus about them. There was a pneumothorax and death had apparently been from operative shock. This is our only death in the hospital following nephrectomy for tuberculosis (125 cases).

NEPHRECTOMY CASES IN WHICH INVOLVEMENT OF THE SEMINAL TRACT WAS NOTED BEFORE OPERATION.—(a) Nephrectomy: *Epididymis involved, no note of involvement of the seminal vesicles,* 4 cases. One patient is *well* twelve years after operation. The epididymal involvement was very slight.

The other 3 are living and *improved*, but with bladder symptoms of some degree still present (five years, one year, ten months).

(b) Nephrectomy: *Seminal vesicles involved, epididymis not involved,* 10 cases. Of these, 4 are reported *well* (ten years, three and a half years, one year, one month). All 4 had bladder symptoms before operation which have disappeared since. Four are *improved*, bladder symptoms of some degree still being present (seven years, four years, fourteen months, ten months). One is living with *recurrence of tuberculosis in the opposite kidney*, symptoms of which began five years after nephrectomy. One patient is still living after a spread of the disease in the genital tract requiring, successively, epididymectomies on each side. Now, three years later, he has frequency, pyuria, and pain in the region of the remaining kidney.

In this group of 10 cases the epididymis has become involved in only 1, although the seminal vesicles were apparently tuberculous before the nephrectomy. Seven have been followed over one year. This seems to indicate that when the renal focus is removed, seminal vesicle tuberculosis, if not accompanied by epididymal tuberculosis, may sometimes be arrested and give no further symptoms. In all of these cases, however, the involvement of the seminal vesicles was slight.

(c) Nephrectomy: *Epididymis and seminal vesicles both involved,* 7 cases. (No operation was done on the epididymis or seminal vesicles in these cases.) Only 1 (B. U. I. 4752) is reported *well* (three years). The other 6 cases, 4 of which have been followed more than one year, are all *unimproved,* all having severe bladder symptoms. Three have recto-urethral fistula, all of which came on spontaneously after nephrectomy. The nephrectomy wound is still open in 2 cases and 1 has bone tuberculosis. In only one of these patients was pulmonary tuberculosis noted before nephrectomy, and radical seminal tract operation could probably have been performed satisfactorily in each case and the evident bad results avoided. The prognosis is bad in all but 1. The progress of the disease may be slow, as shown by one of the patients with recto-urethral fistula, who has lived eight years since the nephrectomy.

(d) Nephrectomy: *Epididymis or seminal vesicles involved. Unilateral epididymectomy performed within a short time of nephrectomy,* 7 cases. Three are reported *well* (ten years, seven years, sixteen months). In 2 of these the seminal vesicle was noted as involved. Three cases are *unimproved.* In 1 the kidney wound is open seven months after operation. In 1 the bladder symptoms are present two years after the operation and he states that he is "worse." In the third there is *recurrence in the opposite kidney and in the larynx* six months after operation. The 2 latter patients had pulmonary tuberculosis before nephrectomy. One is *dead.* He was reported as well eleven and a half years after nephrectomy. The other kidney then became involved and the patient died six months later of uremia. This case shows the fallacy of considering a patient well in whom any tuberculous focus has been left *in situ.*

(e) Nephrectomy: *Epididymis or seminal vesicles involved; bilateral epididymectomy done within a short time of nephrectomy,* 4 cases. One case is reported as *improved,* with pulmonary tuberculosis being arrested and the bladder symptoms less marked three and a half years after operation. Two cases are reported as *unimproved.* (1) B. U. I. 3597 has frequency, burning, and hematuria. General condition worse four years after operation. (2) B. U. I. 8971 has pyuria, burning, tenesmus, and great frequency three and a half years after operation. One patient (B. U. I. 6364) is *dead.* This patient was symptomatically well four and a half years after operation. At rectal examination it was noted that the seminal vesicles and prostate were "much improved." One year later, however, there was urinary suppression on account of a stone in the remaining ureter. The stone was removed and the patient died of uremia five and a half years after the primary nephrectomy. Autopsy showed the remaining kidney almost destroyed by tuberculosis; another instance of the evil results likely to follow in cases where a tuberculous focus is left *in situ.* It should be noted that none of the cases in this group is reported as well.

(f) Nephrectomy: *Seminal vesicles and epididymes involved. Radical operation for tuberculosis of the seminal tract done within a short time of nephrectomy,* 3 cases. *Two of these cases are greatly improved or well.* (1) B. U. I. 8707. Bilateral radical removal of lateral portions of prostate, seminal vesicles, vasa, and epididymes was done two and a half months before the nephrectomy. Two years later there was a contracture of the vesical orifice causing a residual urine of 75 c.c. Cautery punch operation was performed. Three years after punch operation general condition is good. There is no pain, but some frequency of urination still persists (followed five years). (2) B. U. I. 10,840. Bilateral radical removal of the lateral lobes of the prostate, vesicles, vasa, and epididymes was done two and a half months before the nephrectomy. Pulmonary tuberculosis was present before operation. One year eight months after operation patient is in excellent condition and following his usual occupation of riding master.

In 1 case (B. U. I. 7933) there is *little if any improvement*. In this patient symptoms of renal tuberculosis were present for two years before operation and of epididymal tuberculosis eighteen months before operation. Bilateral radical removal of the prostate, vesicles, vasa, and epididymes was done four months after the nephrectomy. Report two and a half years after operation shows a good local result with no sinuses or fistulæ, but the general condition is not good and there is still marked urinary frequency. Pulmonary tuberculosis was present before operation.

These cases are examples of what can be accomplished in extensive tuberculous involvement with pulmonary complication by radical excision of all the foci in both urinary and seminal tracts.

NEPHRECTOMY SECONDARY TO OTHER OPERATIONS FOR TUBERCULOSIS ELSEWHERE IN THE UROGENITAL TRACT.—(*a*) *Nephrectomy following epididymectomy or castration on one side*, 5 cases. Two cases are reported *well* (nine years and four years after nephrectomy). One case is reported *improved* two years after nephrectomy—"well, except frequent urination." Two cases are reported *dead* (eighteen months and sixteen months after nephrectomy). Both died of uremia, indicating spread to the opposite kidney. The spread to the kidney occurred fifteen years, nine years, seven years, three years, and one year after the original operation on the epididymis. The seminal vesicles were involved in all 5. This again shows the possibility of a later spread of tuberculosis in cases where foci are permitted to remain *in situ*.

(*b*) *Nephrectomy following epididymectomy or castration on both sides*, 5 cases. Two cases are reported *well* (four years, eight months). One case is reported *improved* one year after nephrectomy, there being no urinary symptoms, and the general condition being good except for a tuberculous lesion in the finger. One case is *unimproved*, with severe bladder symptoms, including great frequency, eight months after nephrectomy.

One case (B. U. I. 10,236) is *dead* two months after nephrectomy. Autopsy showed tuberculosis of lungs, spine, and seminal vesicles.

In these cases the tuberculosis of the kidney developed thirteen years, five years, two years, one year, and ten months after the original operation on the epididymis. The seminal vesicles were involved in all these cases, indicating again the possibility of a later spread due to organisms if any tuberculous focus is allowed to remain *in situ*.

(*c*) *Nephrectomy following radical operation on the seminal tract*, 2 cases. Both of these are reported as *well* two and a half years and two years after nephrectomy. In 1 case (B. U. I. 3515) only one seminal vesicle was removed. Tubercle bacilli had been found in the urine from one kidney in this case previous to the radical operation, but since this finding could not be repeated and there were no symptoms, the kidney was not removed. Kidney symptoms occurred seven years later, at which time nephrectomy was done. In the other case (B. U. I. 9523) renal involvement occurred six years after a bilateral excision of the seminal tract. Nephrectomy was done at that time. This is the only case in which the spread to the kidney has occurred after a complete bilateral radical excision of the seminal tract for tuberculosis. In the other case it is highly probable that the renal tuberculosis was present before the radical operation was done.

Ultimate Results in Nephrectomy Cases.—In studying the ultimate results of the cases in which nephrectomy was done the following figures are arrived at. These results indicate the present condition in each case, including those where other operations were done besides nephrectomy. For example, if a case developed seminal tract tuberculosis several years after nephrectomy and became well after a radical excision of the seminal tract, he would be noted in this tabulation as ultimately well, regardless of the fact that he had a recurrence in the seminal tract at one time.

TABLE 40

RESULTS OF NEPHRECTOMY FOR TUBERCULOSIS Per cent.

Total cases...	112
Well...	53 (47.5)
Improved...	24 (21)
Unimproved, bladder symptoms still present........................	18 (16)
Unimproved, recurrence in the opposite kidney.....................	4 (3.5)
Unimproved, recurrence in the epididymis, but no operation........	4 (3.5)
Total unimproved..	26 (23)
Dead of tuberculosis since leaving hospital.........................	8 (7)
Dead, operative..	1 (0.89)
Total now dead..	9 (8)

Of the 53 patients who are well, 17 have been followed five years or more; four years, 5 cases; three years, 5 cases; two years, 8 cases; one year, 6 cases; under one year, 12 cases.

Of those improved, 5 have been followed five years or more; four years, 2 cases; three years, 3 cases; two years, none; one to two years, 6; less than one year, 8.

Of the 8 who died of tuberculosis, 3 have lived more than five years; three years, 1; one to two years, 3; less than one year, 2.

It is of interest to know what degree of healing of cystitis and vesical ulcerations may take place after nephrectomy. The following table includes 50 cases reported well after nephrectomy; that is, of course, with no bladder symptoms.

TABLE 41

No bladder symptoms before operation........................	9
Of these, normal bladder on cystoscopy...................	4
No cystoscopic note.......................................	4
"Slight cystitis"..	1
Cases with bladder symptoms, but with bladder normal on cystoscopy..	2
(In each case slight frequency was the only bladder symptom.)	
Cases with bladder symptoms which cleared up after operation..	41
Of these, cystoscopy before operation showed:	
Cystitis...	18
Cystitis and ulcers......................................	17
Normal bladder..	2
No cystoscopic note......................................	4

Only 4 cases were cystoscoped after operation.   The findings were:

1. Ulcers seen three years after operation, treated with 20 per cent. silver nitrate and fulguration, no ulcers seen one year later.
2. Ulcer seen three months after operation, no subsequent cystoscopies.
3. Small ulcers seen one year after nephrectomy.   No later notes.
4. Several cystoscopies, large ulcer gradually healed after operation (within eighteen months), no treatment.

EPIDIDYMECTOMY, NO URINARY INVOLVEMENT, UNILATERAL.—Thirty-eight cases.

Well, without further operation, 5 cases. Five years, 1; four years, 1; two years, 1; one year, 1; less than one year, 1.   In 3 of the cases the seminal vesicles were positive, 1 negative, 1 doubtful before operation.   No notes as to present condition of vesicles.

Improved, but no definite spread, 2 cases.   One case in which seminal vesicles were doubtful was followed for two years.   One case in which seminal vesicles were positive was followed for six months.

Unimproved, 3 cases.   One case, seminal vesicles positive, followed for seven years, now has perineal fistula, frequency, and pyuria.   One case, seminal vesicles not noted, followed for two years, now has frequency and dysuria.   One case, seminal vesicles negative, followed for one and a half years, now has hematuria and frequency.

Alive, with recurrence in the opposite epididymis.   Fourteen cases.   Of these, in 2 the seminal vesicles were noted as negative before operation, in 1 the seminal vesicles were noted as doubtful before operation, and in 5 the seminal vesicles were noted as positive before operation.   Ultimate result: 12 had operations on the second tuberculous epididymis; 2 radical operations (epididymis and seminal vesicle, bilateral); 1 now well after three years; 1 improved after eight years; 10 had epididymectomy, of these, 4 are well for more than five years, 1 is well for one year, 1 is well for less than one year, 1 is improved less than one year, 1 is unimproved less than one year, 1 recurrence in kidney three years; 2 had no second operation.

Alive, with recurrence in kidney.   Three cases.   All had nephrectomy.   Now all are well, nine, four, and two years (the last case has slight frequency).

Dead, recurrence opposite epididymis, 1 case.   Epididymectomy, five months later, radical seminal vesiculectomy.   Died five months after epididymectomy, one week after radical seminal vesiculectomy and epididymectomy (miliary).

Dead, recurrence, kidney.   Two cases.   One case died nine years after epididymectomy, two years after nephrectomy, of tuberculosis of other kidney.   The other case died two and a half years after epididymectomy, eighteen months after nephrectomy, of uremia.

Dead, recurrence to prostate and seminal vesicles.   One case.   Abscess of seminal vesicle was incised and drained; died one year later of tuberculous peritonitis.

Dead, pulmonary tuberculosis.   Three cases (four years, two years, one year). In 2 on admission seminal vesicles were positives for tuberculosis; negative in 1.

Dead, bone tuberculosis.   One case.   Seminal vesicles were involved before operation.   Patient lived eight months.

Dead, cause unknown.   Three cases (seven years, 1 year, 10 months).   Of these, in 2 the seminal vesicles were positive for tuberculosis; in 1 negative.

Résumé of 38 cases of unilateral epididymectomy without urinary involvement. Dead, 11 cases, 29 per cent. Of those alive, 5 have been followed less than one year. Well on last report, five years or more, 6 cases; four years, 2 cases; three years, 1 case; two years, 2 cases; one year, 2 cases; less than one year, 3 cases; total, 16, or 42 per cent. Well over one year, 13, or 38 per cent. Improved, 5, or 13 per cent. Not improved, 6, or 16 per cent. Of the 16 cases classed as well, all but 5 required other operations after the primary epididymectomy, viz.: Nephrectomy 4, epididymectomy, 7; radical seminal tract, 1. In 15 (40 per cent.) we know that the opposite epididymis became involved subsequently.

Remark: These figures are overwhelming proof of the incompleteness of epididymectomy even in favorable cases such as these in which the urinary tract was not involved.

Epididymectomy, No Urinary Involvement, Bilateral.—Sixteen cases.

Well, without further operation, 5 cases. Over five years, 3; over 1 year, 1; under one year, 1. Of these 5 cases the seminal vesicles were involved in 2, doubtful in 2, negative in 1.

Improved, 1 case.

Not heard from, 1 case.

Alive, with recurrence in kidney, 3 cases. Of these, 2 had nephrectomy (1 reported well; 1 improved); 1 had no operation, now reported unimproved.

Alive, with recurrence in the seminal tract, 1 case. Orchidectomy performed, now well seven years later.

Totalizing, there are now well 7 cases (1 after subsequent nephrectomy, 1 after orchidectomy). Well, 43 per cent. Well over five years, 3, or 18 per cent.; over one year, 6, or 38 per cent. Improved, 2, or 13 per cent. Unimproved, 1, or 6 per cent. Not heard from, 1, or 6 per cent. Dead, 5, or 31 per cent. (recurrence, seminal vesicles, kidney, spine, lung, 1; recurrence, pulmonary, spine, and knee, 1; recurrence, seminal vesicles and pulmonary, 1). One-fourth of the cases had recurrences to the kidney.

Epididymectomy, Cases in which Urinary Involvement was Present.— (a) *Epididymectomy, unilateral, and nephrectomy,* 7 cases. On admission all these cases had involvement of both seminal and urinary tracts.

Well, 3 (five years, 2; one year, 1), 43 per cent. (over five years, 2, or 28 per cent.).

Improved, 1 (seven months).

Unimproved, 1 (two years).

Alive, recurrence in opposite kidney, 1 (six months).

Dead, cause unknown, 1 (14 per cent.) (well eleven years; died, hematuria, one year later).

(b) *Epididymectomy, bilateral, with nephrectomy,* 4 cases. On admission both epididymes and one kidney were involved.

Well, five years, 1 (25 per cent.).

Improved, three and a half years, 1 (25 per cent.).

Unimproved, four and three years, 2 (50 per cent.).

(c) *Unilateral epididymectomy. One kidney involved on admission, but nephrectomy not performed,* 3 cases.

Dead, 3 (three and a half years, nine months, nine months). The seminal vesicles were involved on admission in all 3 cases.

(d) *Bilateral epididymectomy—one kidney involved on admission, but nephrectomy not performed*, 2 cases.   In both the seminal vesicles were involved.

Both *died* (five months and three years later).

The 5 cases mentioned in the last two groups illustrate the paramount importance of symptoms referable to the kidney in urogenital tuberculosis, and the necessity of nephrectomy as early as possible.   When these cases are compared with others in which both lungs and kidneys were involved, but in which a primary nephrectomy followed by a radical removal of the seminal tract was carried out, one must be impressed with the importance of early complete removal.

EPIDIDYMECTOMY, SECONDARY TO OTHER OPERATIONS FOR TUBERCULOSIS ELSEWHERE IN THE UROGENITAL TRACT.—(a) *Epididymectomy after epididymectomy*, 9 cases.

Well, 5 (sixteen years, eight years, eight years, seven years, seven months); *improved*, 1; *unimproved*, 1; *recurrence* in kidney, 1; *dead*, renal tuberculosis, 1 case.

Of these 9 cases, in which one epididymis was involved after epididymectomy on the opposite side, the seminal vesicles were found involved in 6 cases, doubtful in 2, negative in 1.   In 1 case the seminal vesicles found involved before operation are now, after twelve years, negative on examination.

(b) *Epididymectomy after unilateral seminal vesiculectomy and epididymectomy*, 3 cases.

In these 3 cases one epididymis and one seminal vesicle were thought to be the sole involvement.   Two cases recurred in the opposite epididymis within one year and one within two years.   Two died of pre-existent pulmonary tuberculosis two and ten months after the last epididymectomy.   The other patient left the hospital well, but has not been heard from.   These cases have shown us the necessity of removing both seminal vesicles (and ampullæ) in all cases in which the radical operation is performed.   When this has been done the second epididymis has never become involved in any of our cases.

(c) *Epididymectomy following nephrectomy*, 12 cases.   These patients had tuberculosis of one kidney, treated by nephrectomy, and subsequently an epididymis became involved.   In 5 cases only one epididymis became involved.   In all of these the seminal vesicles were found indurated before epididymectomy, and in 3 of these a positive diagnosis of tuberculosis of the vesicles was made.   In 7 cases both epididymes were tuberculous, and in 5 of these the seminal vesicles were noted as involved.   In 1 of these cases the seminal vesicles were found involved before nephrectomy, after which both epididymes became involved.   The results are: Well, 2 (six years, two years); improved, 2 (three years, two months); unimproved, tuberculosis present in urogenital tract, 6 (six years, one year, six months, five months, five months, two months).   Dead, with recurrence in remaining kidney, 1 (two years).

Remark: In 10 of the 12 cases of this group the seminal vesicles were involved along with the epididymis.   In only 1 did the epididymis apparently become involved after nephrectomy without the seminal vesicles being involved.

Final Summary: Results of Epididymectomy, 85 cases.   This represents all cases in the files of the Brady Urological Institute to August, 1923, of cases of genital tuberculosis treated by epididymectomy, and gives the final result observed even where other operations were necessary to obtain a cure.

TABLE 42

Total number of cases.. 85
Reported "well".. 30 (34 per cent.)
"Improved"... 12 (14 "   )
Not improved.. 18 (21 "   )

    (a) Urinary tuberculosis, probably kidney............................ 5
    (b) Urinary tuberculosis, probably prostate or seminal vesicles........ 2
    (c) Urinary tuberculosis, doubtful origin........................... 4
    (d) Positive, prostate and seminal vesicles.......................... 3
    (e) Scrotal tuberculosis... 1
    (f) Recurrence other epididymis, no operation...................... 2
    (g) Pulmonary tuberculosis.. 1

Dead.. 25 (29 per cent.)

    (a) Recurrence other epididymis................................... 1
    (b) Recurrence kidney.. 4
    (c) Recurrence prostate and seminal vesicles....................... 1
    (d) Recurrence pulmonary... 8
    (e) Recurrence bone tuberculosis.................................. 1
    (f) Dead, cause unknown.. 5
    (g) Dead, pre-existent renal tuberculosis.......................... 5

COMPLETE (BILATERAL) RADICAL REMOVAL OF THE SEMINAL TRACT.—Seventeen cases. In these both seminal vesicles and both ampullæ were removed, in 14 with the prostatic lateral lobes and with one or both epididymes (in all but 1 case in which neither epididymis was involved). We have analyzed these cases according to tuberculous involvement of other organs as follows:

(a) *Cases with lung tuberculosis present on admission,* 6 cases. In 3 of these the kidneys were also involved and nephrectomies were done preliminary to radical operation. All 3 patients are alive. One still has bladder symptoms, but no fistulæ, now two and a half years since operation. One is practically well, lung tuberculosis arrested, slight frequency of urination, no pain. The third has a sinus (not urinary), but the lung tuberculosis is apparently arrested. In 1 case bone tuberculosis was present in addition to the lungs (B. U. I. 8729). This patient was greatly improved, married, lived two years. He died of tuberculosis of lungs, meninges, spine, and hip. Urogenital tract negative. In 1 case (B. U. I. 11,566) the lungs alone were involved with seminal vesicles and epididymis. He is in a sanatorium and now much improved since radical operation fifteen months ago. B. U. I. 10,434 came from a sanatorium with active pulmonary tuberculosis, marked dysuria, involvement of both seminal vesicles and prostate, but not of epididymes (Fig. 173). He survived the radical operation, but died three months later; autopsy showed tuberculous lungs and peritonitis; kidneys and epididymes negative; bladder tuberculosis and fistula.

Résumé: In these 6 cases of lung tuberculosis, all with the seminal tract involved, with renal tuberculosis present in 3 cases, and multiple bone involvement in another, there have only been 2 deaths. These cases, which exemplify the worst type, show what may be accomplished by radical excision of the seminal tract involvement.

(b) *Cases with renal tuberculosis* at or before radical operation, 5 cases. Three of these patients had pulmonary tuberculosis also on admission. In 2 cases the nephrectomy was done before the radical operation and in 1 afterward. In 1 case (B. U. I. 7933) frequency, urgency, and pain on urination, which were marked before operation, are still present. Radical operation has apparently been successful, no fistulæ are present, and his general condition is excellent. In the other 2 cases the results have been excellent. One (B. U. I. 9352) reports himself practically well, followed eighteen months. The third (B. U. I. 10,840), also followed eighteen months, is well, with a urinary fistula through which a few drops escape with urination. These cases represent very "bad risks." B. U. I. 8707 had a radical operation followed, three months later, by nephrectomy. Result excellent, except difficulty and frequency of urination, due to a bar, with residual urine, 75 c.c. Punch operation done, with much improvement. Now, three years later, condition excellent, "sexual powers normal," and this after bilateral removal of both seminal vesicles, lateral lobes of prostate, vasa, and epididymes! B. U. I. 5430 is in fair general condition after nephrectomy, unilateral epididymectomy, and radical operation three years later, the other epididymis being also removed. Case followed three years, no fistula.

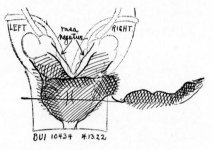

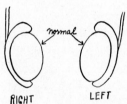

Remark: To have lost none of these 5 complicated cases is an indication of the value of radical surgery in urogenital tuberculosis.

(c) *Cases with tuberculosis confined to the seminal tract. Radical operation, 9 cases.* These cases were much less severe than the previous groups, but 1 patient (B. U. I. 10,717) died of miliary tuberculosis two weeks after operation. Two patients left the hospital, 1 (B. U. I. 4322) with a perineal urinary fistula which was present before operation, and the other well (B. U. I. 10,180). Neither has answered letters. One patient (B. U. I. 4330) is well with the exception of a vesical urinary fistula, now eight years since operation. Five patients are well: B. U. I. 9523, eight years; B. U. I. 8486, three and a half years; B. U. I. 8970, three

FIG. 173.—Rectal findings in a case of tuberculosis of the prostate and left seminal vesicle. The patient had severe pulmonary tuberculosis of long standing. There was also vesical tuberculosis with severe urinary symptoms. The vasa, epididymes, and kidney were found negative on repeated examination. Seminal vesiculectomy and partial prostatectomy were done. The patient died, however, of pulmonary tuberculosis and tuberculous peritonitis. Autopsy proved the absence of all other urogenital involvement.

years; B. U. I. 8524, three years; B. U. I. 9463, one year after radical operation. B. U. I. 9523 came back with renal tuberculosis six years after the radical seminal tract operation. (Scrotal and rectal examinations negative.) Nephrectomy; now well two and a half years later. B. U. I. 8486, who had had considerable portions of the lateral lobes of the prostate removed (Fig. 175) at the radical operation, came back, two years later, with marked adenomatous enlargement of the periurethral glands of the prostate causing obstruction to urination, and was cured by suprapubic prostatectomy. There was one small area of tuberculosis in the center of a hypertrophied lobe. He is well two years after the prostatectomy.

Summarizing the 17 cases in which the complete radical operation was done all are alive, at last report, except 3, viz.: One who died of miliary tuberculosis two weeks after operation (making the operative mortality 5.9 per cent.); 1 who died three months after operation of pulmonary and peritoneal tuberculosis, and 1 who died two years after operation of extensive tuberculosis of lungs, meninges, spine, and hip. One patient has pyuria and pain in the remaining kidney. One

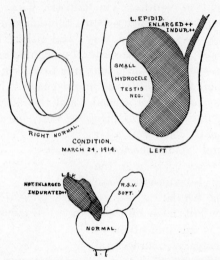

FIG. 174.—Scrotal and prostatic charts showing extensive tuberculosis of left epididymis, vas, vesicle, and ejaculatory duct. Prostate, right vas, and right epididymis negative. B. U. I. 3515.

patient with marked vesical tuberculosis before operation, still has great frequency of urination. Of the remaining 12 cases, 10 have excellent results, and 2 have not been followed. In none of the cases did a remaining epididymis become in-

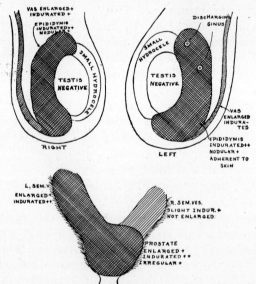

FIG. 175.—Extensive involvement of epididymes, vasa, vesicles, and prostate. Testicles not involved. B. U. I. 8486.

volved after removal of both seminal vesicles. Among these 17 cases there were 6 with pulmonary, 5 with kidney, and 1 with multiple bone tuberculosis.

UNILATERAL RADICAL OPERATION.—Seven cases. In these cases only 1 seminal vesicle was removed along with vas and epididymis and sometimes a portion of the prostate. In 3 cases (B. U. I. 3632, B. U. I. 4158, B. U. I. 8712) the opposite epididymis became involved (42 per cent.), and 2 of these died, after the secondary epididymectomy, of pulmonary tuberculosis. These cases show the necessity of bilateral seminal vesiculectomy and ampullectomy. Two other patients (B. U. I. 3515, B. U. I. 8561) had renal tuberculosis before the seminal tract operation. One has been cured by nephrectomy (two years) and in the other the renal tuberculosis was bilateral and he lived nineteen months. Four patients are well (B. U. I. 3515, nine years; B. U. I. 3632, two years; B. U. I. 4980, eight years; B. U. I. 8681, three years). Four of these 7 cases had severe complications (pulmonary 2, renal 2, and 3 are now dead one, one, and one and a half years after operation). These results are not as good as after the bilateral vesicle operation, and possibly two of the deaths, which occurred after secondary epididymectomy,

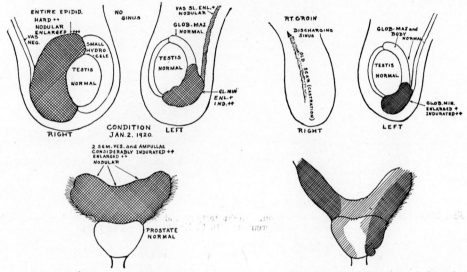

FIG. 176.—Clinical charts before operation. Testes and prostate negative. Rest of seminal tract extensively involved. B. U. I. 7933.

FIG. 177.—Scrotal and rectal charts before operation. Right testicle and epididymis absent. Left globus minor greatly enlarged and indurated. Both seminal vesicles and both lobes of prostate, especially right, tuberculous. B. U. I. 8526.

might have been prevented by a primary bilateral vesiculectomy, instead of unilateral, as done. Figures 174–177 show the extent of invasion in some of the cases operated upon.

Summary: Radical excision of seminal tract, 24 cases. Operative deaths, 1; mortality, 4 per cent. Alive and apparently cured of genital tuberculosis, 13 (54 per cent.). Three are alive, but cannot be called well; 2 of them having bladder symptoms and 1 a vesical urinary fistula (12.5 per cent.). Two have not been followed; both were improved on discharge (8 per cent.). During the nine years 5 have died, all of tuberculosis (3 after unilateral, 43 per cent., and 2 after bilateral vesiculectomy, 7.8 per cent.). Only 1 patient has a troublesome urinary fistula. Three have prostatic fistulæ from which a few drops of urine escape during urination. We consider these safety exits, which usually heal as soon as the tuberculosis is completely arrested.

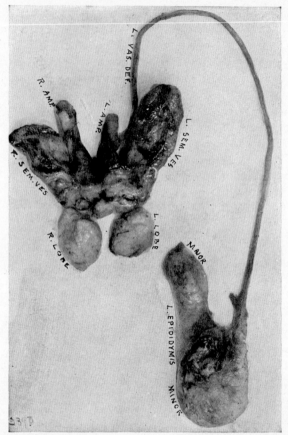

Fig. 178.—Specimen removed at operation. Right testicle and vas had previously been removed. The entire tract was tuberculous. B. U. I. 8526. (See Fig. 177.)

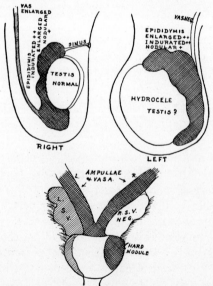

Fig. 179.—Clinical charts showing extensive involvement of epididymes, ampullæ, and prostate. B. U. I. 8561.

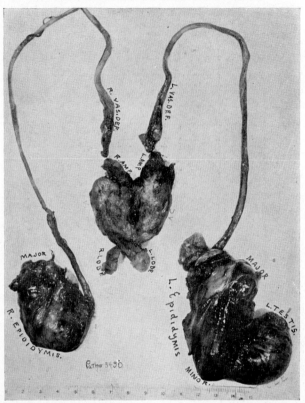

FIG. 180.—Operative specimen. Left testis, epididymis, vas, seminal vesicle, and lobe of prostate removed. Right testis preserved, Epididymis, vas, vesicle, and right lobe of prostate removed. B. U. I. 8561. (See Fig. 179.)

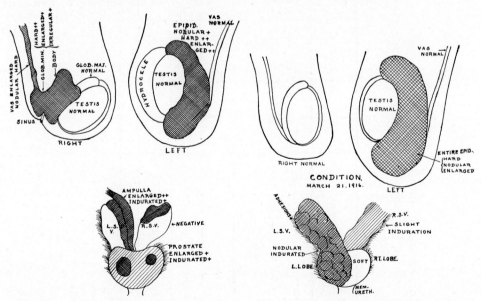

FIG. 181.—Scrotal and prostatic charts before operation. Note extensive involvement of epididymes with testes normal. B. U. I. 8707.

FIG. 182.—Prostatic and scrotal charts before operation. B. U. I. 4980.

In comparison with the above results of operative treatment, the accompanying table, showing 47 cases of urogenital tuberculosis which, for various reasons, were not operated upon, is of interest:

TABLE 43

Region involved.	Well.	Improved.	Unimproved.	Worse.	Dead, urogenital tuberculosis.	Dead, pulmonary or general tuberculosis.	Dead, cause unknown.	Total.
Genital tract	4 (22 years, 17 years, 5 years, 9 years.)	2 (7 years, 17 months.)	4 (3 years, 5 months, 8 years, 3 years.)	2 (6 months, 1 year.)	....	3 (6 years, 1 month, 2 weeks.)	2 (survival not known.)	17
Kidney, unilateral	....	2 (5 years, 2 months.)	....	2 (4 years, 1½ years.)	3 (4 months, 2 years, 15 years.)	1 (4 years.)	....	8
Kidney, bilateral	....	2 (21 months, 6 years.)	....	....	2 (1 year, 6 years.)	....	....	4
Genital tract and kidney, unilateral	....	2 (15 years, 4 months.)	2 (1½ years, 15 months.)	1 (6 months.)	....	2 (1 month, 8 months.)	1 (3 months.)	8
Genital tract and kidney, bilateral	....	1 (6 months.)	3 (5 months, 1 month, 1 year.)	....	3 (6 years, 8 years, 3 months.)	2 (11 years, 1½ years.)	1 (2 years.)	10
Total	4	9	9	5	8	8	4	47

Of the 4 cases reported well, all had no renal involvement, and all have been followed five years or more. Of the 9 cases reported improved, only 2 have been followed more than five years. Of the 47 cases, 34 are unimproved, worse, or dead (72 per cent.). Many of these cases received tuberculin treatment. While this table indicates that a certain small proportion of cases of urogenital tuberculosis may recover spontaneously or be arrested for a long time, it is a striking evidence of the hopeless inferiority of non-operative treatment in general. Total known mortality, 42.5 per cent.

CHAPTER V

UROGENITAL INFECTIONS AND INFESTATIONS: SYPHILIS, MYCOSES, AND PARASITIC DISEASES

SYPHILIS

SINCE syphilis is now well known to be a general disease, we shall consider only its local manifestations in the urogenital tract, in much the same manner as those of tuberculosis.

Kidney.—*Syphilis of the kidney* has been the subject of much discussion. There can be no doubt that *gumma of the kidney* and congenital or *fetal syphilitic nephritis* represent actual infection of the renal substance by the Treponema pallidum. In regard, however, to the disease known ordinarily as *syphilitic nephritis* diverse opinions have been expressed. The condition is characterized by edema, with abundant albumen and casts in the urine. In the blood the retention of chlorids is more marked than that of nitrogen. The kidney is found to be enlarged, pale, and opaque, the consistence softer than normal. The cortex is thickened and the striations obscured. Microscopically, one sees the picture of tubular nephritis with intense cloudy swelling of the epithelium of the convoluted tubules, some of the cells being degenerated and desquamated. The glomeruli are intact. The French authors describe certain cases in which some interstitial proliferation and desquamation of the glomerular epithelium were also observed. Spirochetes have not been demonstrated in these kidneys. Munk[1] maintains that the lesion is a true syphilitic infection, and has demonstrated in frozen sections that most of the vacuoles appearing in the swollen epithelial cells in ordinary preparations are really occupied by lipoid substances which stain with fat-soluble pigments. Further, many of these globules are doubly refracting, as shown under the polarizing microscope, and similar doubly refracting globules can be found free in the urine or in the casts. Stengel and Austin[2] have found the lipoid globules constant in nephritic patients with syphilis, but have also discovered them in 5 of 14 non-syphilitic cases. MacNider[3] has demonstrated similar lipoid globules in the epithelium of normal kidneys and shows that they are increased in chronic inflammations. It seems, therefore, that the specific syphilitic character of this nephritis is by no means proved, and we may continue to regard it as a toxic manifestation. This also explains satisfactorily the marked improvement in symptoms, with disappearance of albumen, casts, and edema, often noted after antisyphilitic treatment.

Clinically, the condition is usually seen in the secondary stage of syphilis, but may occur somewhat later. It is probably quite frequent, though often of slight degree. Gaucher[4] found albuminuria in one-third of his syphilitic cases. The *symptoms* are, as above stated, edema, especially of the face, weakness, and anemia.

[1] Zeitschrift für Klinische Medizin, 1913, lxxviii, 1–52 (Lit.).

[2] American Journal of the Medical Sciences, 1915, cxlix, 12–17.

[3] Journal of Pharmacology and Experimental Therapeutics, 1921, xvii, 289–322.

[4] Encyclopædie Française d'Urologie, 1914, iii, 183–226.

Headache, diarrhea, and drowsiness, so characteristic of the nitrogen-retention type of uremia, are usually in the background, but may be added in the later stages in severe cases. In the *urine* are found large quantities of albumen and hyaline and granular casts, which may contain the lipoid globules. *Hematuria* may occur. There is often an *oliguria;* in extreme cases, *anuria.* *Therapeutically* the presence of this type of nephritis should not be allowed to deter one from treating the syphilis, as it is the only hope of improving the condition. The arsenicals are preferable, but while mercury should be used with some caution, it is not contraindicated. If the damage is not too extensive, or secondary infection present, the nephritis will usually clear up concomitantly with the other manifestations of the disease. In some cases, however, it passes into a chronic nephritis.

Gaucher speaks of a *diffuse chronic syphilitic nephritis* in which the pathologic picture is like that of other chronic diffuse nephritis. The evidence upon which these conditions are ascribed to syphilis seems somewhat slight, principally a positive Wassermann, other evidences of syphilis, or a favorable response to antisyphilitic treatment.

Gumma of the kidney[1] occurs in the tertiary stage of the disease as do gummata elsewhere. This is, of course, a true syphilitic infection and the treponema may be found in the tissues. Gumma is usually multiple, but may be single, and arises within the kidney proper. The disease is almost always unilateral. The gross and microscopic pictures are those typical of gumma elsewhere, as described in the subsequent paragraphs on Syphilis of the Testis. There are infiltration and fibrosis of the neighboring kidney tissue. On healing, these lesions leave a characteristic contracted scar. Since both active gummata and the scars of healed lesions are but rarely found at autopsy, we may conclude that gumma of the kidney is rare.

Confusion with tuberculosis may, however, easily occur both in the gross and microscopically, so that the lesion may sometimes be missed. Contracted scars may equally well be ascribed to healed infarcts.

Clinically, small gummata are symptomless. Rupture of softened lesions into the pelvis is possible, but, being accompanied by no pain, is likely to go unnoticed. Most of our information as to the symptomatology and evolution is derived from cases in which the process was extensive, producing a palpably enlarged kidney. In these cases pain was usually present, and often edema, suggesting perinephric inflammation. The urine contained pus, albumen, and often much epithelium. In such cases operation has usually been done, disclosing kidneys irregularly scarred, containing necrotic areas and surrounded by edema. Microscopic sections were characteristic of gumma. In some cases the diagnosis has been made at operation, and the kidney left in place. In such cases later disappearance of the tumor, the albuminuria, and the pyuria under antisyphilic treatment has been observed. If the destruction of renal tissue is extensive, uremia may supervene.

In *congenital syphilis* the kidneys may be affected. The lesion is usually an *interstitial nephritis*, with fibrosis having a generally perivascular arrangement, and deposits of lymphocytes. The glomeruli are involved. Spirochetes are present in large numbers. The kidney is white, firm, and irregular. It may be larger or smaller than normal, depending on the extent of the infiltration. The clinical aspects are uncertain, since the observations have all been made at autopsy,

[1] Gaucher and Druelle: Encyclopædie Française d'Urologie, 1914, iii, 183–226 (Lit.).

and there are usually numerous other lesions of the disease elsewhere in the body. *Gummata* have also been found in the kidneys of congenitally syphilitic infants.

In old, chronic, and especially in untreated syphilis *amyloidosis* of the kidney, as of other organs, may develop.

Various observers have reported the discovery of treponemata in the urine of syphilitics, especially those cases with acute nephritis. In view of the facts that spiral organisms often occur on the external genitalia, and that spiral structures which are not treponemata may be found in the kidneys and in tube casts, these reports must be taken with reserve.

The treatment of syphilis of the kidney is little different from that described elsewhere for the general treatment of syphilis. It is, of course, of primary importance to determine that the renal lesion is due to the treponema, and not to previous treatment, arsenical or mercurial. A careful study of the history of the case, and observation and hygienic treatment for a sufficient period of time during which a chemical nephritis will probably improve, should be carried out. Sometimes it is impossible to be sure, and treatment should, therefore, be begun cautiously, with small doses of neo-arsphenamin (10 or 15 centigrams).

Mercurials (preferably flumerin) and potassium iodid may also be used separately or combined, sometimes with excellent results.

When it is demonstrated that the drug used is well borne, and improvement of the urine is observed, one may increase the dosage (cautiously) until a thorough course has been given.

In many cases it is remarkable how rapidly a syphilitic albuminuria will disappear under treatment, even when symptoms of serious nephritis have been present. In the regulation of the treatment frequent urinalysis and renal function tests—phthalein and blood urea—are of great importance.

Bladder.—There is still, unfortunately, a great deal of confusion concerning syphilitic lesions of the bladder. Gaucher, in the Encyclopædie Française d'Urologie, has collected 34 cases described as syphilis of the bladder, and Corbus, in Cabot's Modern Urology, describes 45, 30 of which are not included in Gaucher's collection. These cases include some in which ulcers and granulomatous tumors were found at autopsy in patients with other lesions of syphilis, and a larger number in which lesions of various sorts observed cystoscopically healed under antisyphilitic treatment. Of the few operated on, in only 2 were microscopic descriptions given, and in neither of these were treponemata demonstrated.

While there is no reason why syphilis should not localize in the bladder, and while quite possibly some of these cases were true syphilitic lesions, yet it cannot be said that any one of them is categorically proved. It must be remembered that any sort of a condition can exist in a person with a positive Wassermann or evidence of more active syphilis, and that in many such cases there are coexistent gonorrheal lesions of the urethra, or of the prostate and vesicles in males. Some of the cases described were in tabetics, in whom the bladder is particularly subject to secondary infection. Finally, we now know that some of the drugs employed in the treatment of syphilis, especially neo-arsphenamin (novarsenobenzol) and intravenous mercurials, are excellent remedies against ordinary coccal or bacillary infections of the urinary tract. (See the section on Antiseptics under Infections of the Urogenital Tract.) The fact that a bladder lesion disappears after such treatment, therefore, is in no sense a proof of its syphilitic nature. These considerations should lead us to be very critical of cases diagnosed as syphilis of the bladder, and it is to be hoped that in the future careful study of such cases will disclose the presence of the Treponema pallidum and place the sujbect on a firm basis.

In the descriptions usually given secondary and tertiary lesions are described. Patients in the *secondary* or eruptive stage of the disease have sometimes shown bladder lesions described as: (1) Multiple small rounded erythematous spots, with some general congestion of the bladder; (2) small, slightly elevated, usually yellowish papules, with red halo of congestion, and (3) small, shallow ulcers, with slightly elevated edges and halo of inflammation, often said to resemble mucous patches. These ulcers may well be a later stage of the papules mentioned above. Denslow and Corbus each describe edematous papillary or vegetating syphiloma of the secondary stage. In Corbus' case the bladder was markedly indurated on vaginal palpation, and cystotomy showed the entire vesical wall to be diffusely indurated. That bladder lesions are not constant or even frequent in secondary syphilis was shown by Levy and Zimmerman,[1] who examined cystoscopically 25 patients in the secondary stage, selected at random at the Brady Clinic, and found the bladder normal in all.

As *tertiary* syphilis, the lesion oftenest described is an ulcer, usually single, with elevated, indurated edge, and indolent base, sometimes covered by a purulent membrane. In other cases intravesical projections, either papillary, villous, or smooth and rounded, have been mentioned. In some cases coming to autopsy extensive necrosis of apparently gummatous masses has been observed, involving the surrounding tissues and leading sometimes to fistulæ between the bladder and the rectum, sigmoid, small intestine, or vagina.

The *symptoms* described in the cases reported are mainly those of bladder irritation—painful and frequent urination. In addition, there was often hematuria, and pyuria was common. It is evident that there is nothing characteristic about the symptoms.

On *examination*, the cystoscopic lesions described above have been found, and, in addition, a history of syphilis, a positive Wassermann, a secondary eruption, or other evidences of syphilis. Yet in a few cases, even in the absence of all of these, the diagnosis of syphilis has been made because the lesions healed after antisyphilitic treatment. This is probably an error. It is impossible to make definite statements about the diagnosis of bladder syphilis, since so much of the available data is from cases where the diagnosis was doubtful. Careful study will serve to eliminate many cases as possibilities. The descriptions of many cases are such that a differentiation from tuberculosis seems difficult. The finding of tubercle bacilli will resolve these doubts, and they should be sought diligently. Bacteriolgoic studies should always be made. Thus, if staphylococci are found in the urine, we should not be surprised to see the bladder lesions clear up under neo-arsphenamin. A few cases have been described in which the same drug apparently caused the disappearance of bacillary lesions (colon group).

Other cases appear to be scarcely distinguishable cystoscopically from neoplasms. These cases will often be subjected to radium, fulguration, etc., and the diagnosis may be very difficult. A microscopic section, if obtainable, may solve the problem by showing neoplasm. If negative, it is of no value, as biopsies from tumor cases

[1] Journal of Urology, 1919, iii, 407–410.

often show no tumor cells. If a suspicion of syphilis arises, any therapeutic test employed should be intensive and of short durtion, as delay may be very harmful if the lesion is really a tumor.

Question may also arise in cases of solitary ulcer (Fenwick) or interstitial (submucous) cystitis. For the diagnosis of these lesions the reader is referred to the paragraphs on those subjects under Infections of the Bladder.

In general, all patients should be subjected to the Wassermann test, always remembering that a positive test does not rule out any other disease. If any suspicion of a syphilitic origin of the bladder lesion arises it is well to rule it out, but if that cannot be done, one should hesitate long before making a positive diagnosis. It is to be hoped that in the future some completely proved cases of vesical syphilis may appear to add to our knowledge on the subject.

The *treatment* is that of syphilis in general.

Urethra.—Primary syphilis of the urethra is not extremely rare. Among 1187 cases of chancre collected by Fournier[1] and Jullien,[2] 34 were endo-urethral, while 121 involved the meatus. Chancre of the meatus is ordinarily considered along with chancre of the urethra, but since it is exposed to view, as are the ordinary chancres, it falls in an entirely different category of interest, and we shall include it with chancre of the penis. The important fact about endo-urethral chancre is that it is concealed from view, and, therefore, very liable to escape diagnosis.

The location of *chancres of the urethra* is practically always in the fossa navicularis, that is, within 1 cm. of the meatus. Sometimes they can be seen by spreading apart the lips of the meatus. If of large size, the proximal border may well extend farther along the urethra than 1 cm. Only a very few cases are reported in which the lesion lay deeper in the urethra, and Gaucher is inclined to attribute these instances to the use of contaminated sounds or other instruments.

Why intra-urethral chancre should occur at all is an interesting subject. Experimental evidence that an abrasion of some sort is necessary before syphilitic infection can take place is very strong. The organism of syphilis, being motile, is better able to ascend the urethra than is the gonococcus, but if the lesions depend on the motility of the organism, one would expect to find them at various points along the anterior urethra, instead of all in its terminal centimeter. Long-pointed syringes and fellatio have been suggested as possible traumatic agents.

Microscopically, these chancres are like the external ones, to be described in the paragraphs on Primary Syphilis of the Penis.

In the gross they are usually not recognized until ulceration and induration have occurred, when palpation reveals a *mass* along the balanic urethra. The *induration* is very firm. There may be some inflammatory reaction about the mass, so that it is somewhat obscured by *edema*. With the endoscope an *ulcerated* area with indurated edges can be seen. Sometimes the edges are sufficiently proliferated to encroach on the urethral lumen. The base of the ulcer is indolent and may have a pyogenic membrane, but is seldom frankly purulent.

In later stages the picture depends upon whether necrosis or fibrosis dominates the scene. If necrosis is conspicuous, *fistula* may occur, or, if pyogenic organisms escape through the defect made by the chancre, there may be periurethral *abscess.*

[1] Traité de la Syphilis, Paris, 1901.
[2] Traité pratique des Maladies Vénériennes, Paris, 1879.

In any event, fibrotic changes are likely to occur eventually, especially in un-treated cases, as a result of which the urethra is distorted and in some cases *stric-tured*. Since most cases of this sort are complicated by chronic urethritis, gonor-rheal or non-specific, the exact etiology of a given stricture is often obscure. When really due to the syphilitic lesion we must assume, as in gonorrheal stricture, that all or most of the circumference of the lumen has been involved. These strictures are characterized by the location—the terminal 1 or $1\frac{1}{2}$ cm. of the urethra—and by their similarity to traumatic strictures in density and in tendency to recur rapidly after dilation.

The *symptoms* of intra-urethral chancre are few. The principal one is a *dis-charge*, coming on from two to four weeks after exposure, and which is watery or only slightly turbid, and moderate in quantity. There may be some pain or irrita-tion at the time of voiding, and the patient may note the induration in the balanic urethra. Slight *bleeding* may occur, especially after instrumentation or palpation. *Secondary eruptions* occur in due course.

The *diagnosis* of urethral chancre is often missed, and the urologist must always be on the watch for it. In uncomplicated cases the character of the discharge and the incubation time will arouse suspicion, and the discovery of the *Treponema pallidum* in the secretion obtained from within the urethra by a platinum loop fixes the diagnosis. Often, however, the lesion is complicated by pre-existing acute or chronic gonorrhea, balanic chancroids, or phimosis. Where *acute gonorrhea* is present, the lesion often goes unnoticed, unfortunately, by both patient and physician until the secondary eruption appears. If the induration is felt, it may be taken for a periurethral inflammatory focus. This is the more likely when there is edema about the chancre, with congestion and local heat. Unretractable phimosis, especially if there is balanoposthitis and edema of the prepuce, makes it more difficult to palpate the chancre. In general, the chancre is distinguished by extreme firmness, which may be made out even in the midst of an area of edema, and by the absence of the tenderness which is usually so pronounced in periurethral inflammation. Urethral chancre is accompanied by an indolent, non-suppurative inflammation of the *inguinal lymph-nodes*, just as in the external forms. This is not a decisive feature, as secondary acute pyogenic adenitis may occur in any case. Vigilance alone can be relied upon to detect those endo-urethral chancres which occur in the course of a gonorrheal infection.

Secondary syphilis of the urethra is an uncertain quantity. Certain observers report mucous patches at the meatus, but we have little or no reliable data as to their occurrence in the deeper portions of the urethra. Ravogli[1] describes super-ficial ulcerations in the prostatic urethra.

In *tertiary syphilis* gummata may arise in the urethra or invade it from adja-cent parts. They usually involve the anterior urethra. Casper has observed one 8 cm. from the meatus. When arising in the urethra proper a cylindric in-duration may occur, causing urinary *obstruction*. When softening occurs, there may be a purulent *discharge* simulating gonorrhea. Necrotic gummata may serve as the starting-point for periurethral inflammation or urinary extravasation and *fistula* may occur. When extensive, great destruction may be caused, although this wide necrosis is usually associated with a phagedenic process due to secondary infection.

[1] The Urologic and Cutaneous Review, 1916, xx, 125.

The *diagnosis* of gummata of the urethra will usually depend largely on concomitant evidences of syphilis. The Wassermann test is valuable. Other conditions which may give similar pictures are chronic urethritis with periurethral inflammation and usually stricture, and the rare neoplasms of the urethra. While gumma does not cause an inguinal adenitis, this sign is not reliable, as inflammatory bubo from secondary infection may occur.

The treatment should be thorough and in accordance with the principles laid down for the general treatment of syphilis.

Penis.—The most important manifestations of syphilis in the penis are the primary lesion or *chancre*, and the tertiary lesion or *gumma*. These will be found described in the section on Ulcerative Lesions of the External Genitalia, where they are placed for convenience of reference.

In the *secondary* stage any of the skin lesions may occur on the penis as elsewhere. They need not be considered at length here. Mucous patches have been described on the glans and on the interior surface of the prepuce. The existence of similar lesions elsewhere should make the diagnosis easy.

Prostate.—The available data on syphilis of the prostate is well summarized by Druelle.[1] It must be admitted, after studying his article and those of Thompson,[2] Ravogli,[3] and Corbus,[4] that the pathologic and diagnostic criteria are very deficient.

The lesions described are shallow ulcers and granulations in the prostatic urethra in the secondary stage, and nodular enlargments in the prostate proper in the tertiary stage. Pathologic material was not available, as far as we can discover, in any case. The lesions disappeared or improved after antisyphilitic treatment. In a number of instances there were associated ulcerous lesions in the bladder. The same reservations must be made in regard to these cases as those mentioned in the section on Syphilis of the Bladder.

The *symptoms* mentioned are hematuria, pain, and urinary difficulty.

The *diagnosis* can scarcely be more than presumptive unless pathologic specimens are available showing treponemata or definite gummatous lesions. One should keep in mind the commoner lesions, especially prostatic hypertrophy, prostatic carcinoma, chronic prostatitis, and tuberculosis, in their less typical and often intermittent manifestations.

Testis.—The testis may be involved in *congenital syphilis*. Microscopically one sees an extensive interstitial round-cell *infiltration*, largely perivascular, followed later by an interstitial *fibrosis* which may lead to compression and later destruction of the tubules. This progress causes an enlargement of the infantile testis, but later, if the patient survives, the testis is *atrophic* and firm. Fundamentally, this picture is similar to the syphilitic fibrosis occurring later in life. The epididymis may be somewhat involved, showing a perivascular round-cell infiltration and some fibrosis without epithelial change. In certain cases, where the effects of hereditary syphilis do not make themselves felt until after childhood is passed, the lesions in the testis resemble those of adult acquired syphilis.

In the gross, the testis of the infant is *enlarged, smooth, firm,* and *painless.*

[1] Encyclopædie Française d'Urologie, 1923, Paris (Doin), vi, 426–436.
[2] American Journal of Syphilis, 1920, iv, 50–90.
[3] The Urologic and Cutaneous Review, 1916, xx, 125.
[4] Cabot's Modern Urology, 1924, i, 145–146.

The lesion is practically always *bilateral*. A moderate hydrocele is a common accompaniment. On cross-section the tissue is grayer and firmer than normal, it does not evert, and difficulty is encountered in teasing out the tubules with a forceps.

The *symptoms*, aside from the local enlargement, are of no importance unless the patient attains the age of puberty. He is then the victim of a double testicular atrophy, and if the process has not been arrested in its active stage, the fibrosis will have destroyed the interstitial as well as the spermatogenic cells and infantilism will result. It is quite possible that congenital syphilis may account for some of the cases of dystrophia adiposogenitalis (Fröhlich's syndrome).

The *diagnosis* is easy in cases with other manifestations of syphilis. Where these do not occur, the disease should be suspected in every infantile testicular enlargement. A Wassermann test should be made not only of the patient but also of both parents, and the history carefully investigated.

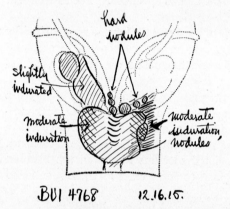

Fig. 183.—Irregular and indurated prostate with very marked adhesions and nodularity in the right side. Symptoms were swelling of the testicle for three months. (See the following diagram.) Following antisyphilitic treatment the scrotal mass decreased markedly in size and the patient became clinically well, but the nodules in the prostate were still present two years later. It is just possible that this represents syphilis of the prostate.

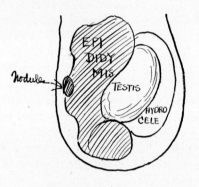

Fig. 184.—Markedly enlarged indurated and nodular epididymis in the same case shown in the preceding diagram. There is a small hydrocele and a small sinus over the nodule indicated. A diagnosis of syphilis was made because the lesion cleared up rapidly under antisyphilitic treatment. The diagram represents, however, a condition indistinguishable from tuberculosis.

In the *adult* syphilis ordinarily affects the testis only in the tertiary stage. Dron,[1] Balme,[2] and Cuilleret[3] describe an *epididymitis*, subacute or chronic, in the *secondary* stage, characterized by localized nodules, usually painless, in the globus minor or major. Michelson,[4] Lisser and Hinman[5] and Rolnick[6] have written more recently on this condition. One would have to rule out very carefully gonorrheal or non-specific epididymitis before making such a diagnosis. We have seen one doubtful case (Figs. 183, 184).

In the *tertiary* stage testicular orchitis appears as *gummata*, single or multiple,

[1] Archiv generale de médécine, 1853, 6th series, ii, 513–724.
[2] De l'épididymite syphilitique, Thèse de Paris, 1876.
[3] Étude sur l'épididymite syphilitique secondaire, Thèse de Lyon, 1890.
[4] Journal American Medical Association, 1919, lxxiii, 1431–1433.
[5] American Journal of Syphilis, 1918, ii, 465–471 (Lit.).
[6] Journal of Urology, 1924, xii, 147–152.

or as a diffuse *fibrosis*. Reclus[1] observed in many cases of syphilitic fibrosis testis small, almost pin-point gummata distributed through the lesion, and suggested that the condition should properly be called "sclerogummatous orchitis." Such pictures do occur, and probably indicate a close relation between the two processes, so that we should not be surprised to find these intermediate forms. While the scars from such tiny gummata would be inconspicuous, and one could not be sure that they had not previously been present, yet we usually see the fibrotic testis quite uniform on section, with no suggestion of focal lesions in it.

Syphilis of the testis occurs in about 1 or 2 per cent. of cases of syphilis.[2]

Gumma occurs in the testis proper, and practically always spares the epididymis —a sharp differentiation from tuberculosis. It is, perhaps, oftener single than multiple, but confluence of smaller gummata is common.

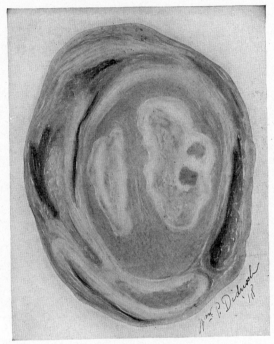

Fig. 185.—Specimen of gumma of the testis removed at operation. Note the great thickening of the testicular tunics and extremely irregular outlines of the necrotic areas in the testis. The epididymis, which is not shown, was not involved. B. U. I. 6803.

In the gross, one may see the unaffected part of the testicle normal or some-what fibrosed. The testis is increased in *size*, though with the smaller gummata this may be slight. Moderate *hydrocele* is common—a point of similarity with malignant tumors. If a small gumma is central the shape of the testis may be regular, but if it is larger, or near the surface, the organ will be *irregular* and *nodular*. On section, the gumma itself cuts with difficulty on account of the fibrous layer surrounding it. This fibrous layer is grayish and translucent. In the center there is usually an area of *necrosis*, which often differs from that of tuberculosis by an

[1] De la Syphilis du Testicule, Paris, 1882.

[2] Sebileau and Descomps: Maladies des Organes Genitaux de l'Homme, Nouveau Traité de Chirurgie, Paris, 1916, xxxii, 487.

outline which is totally irregular (Fig. 185), and different from the polycyclic outline seen in tuberculosis which is due to the coalescence of the roughly spherical tubercles. In certain cases the necrotic material is tenacious and slightly translucent; Sebileau and Descomps have graphically compared its appearance to that of the substance of a pineapple, with the more complete caseation of tuberculosis represented by that of a boiled chestnut. It is from this characteristic of the necrosis that the syphilitic lesion received its name of "gumma." The distinction is not absolutely reliable, however, as syphilitic necrosis is sometimes more complete and frankly caseous.

Microscopically, one sees a round-cell infiltration, often more marked in the regions of the blood-vessels. There is marked deposition of fibrous tissue; in the early stages fibroblasts are seen, while in the later stages hyalinization occurs.

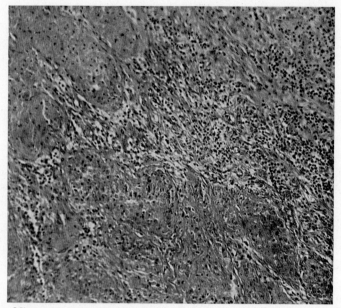

Fig. 186.—Microscopic section of gumma of the testis. Note the fibrosis and round-cell infiltration and also that the outlines of the seminiferous tubules are preserved, although their contents is completely degenerated. B. U. I. 2739.

The blood-vessels undergo intimal proliferation, hyalinization, and eventually the lumina are obliterated. The tubules are enclosed and compressed in this fibrous mass. The tubular wall thickens, undergoing itself a fibrous change like the stroma, and soon this thickened wall becomes hyalinized. Spermatogenesis persists for a time, but as the fibrosis advances, it ceases, and the tubules come to be lined with only a single layer of rather large, irregular cells with clear cytoplasm and moderate sized, round nuclei. These are thought to represent the Sertoli cells, the spermatocytes having completely disappeared. In the final stage this epithelium too vanishes, the entire tubule becomes a fibrous, hyaline cylinder of reduced diameter, and is eventually completely obliterated. Elastic tissue fibers from the tubular wall persist, even in an isolated condition, longer in syphilitic than in tuberculous lesions, but, as this is a relative matter, it is not particularly valuable in the differentiation. The interstitial cells are compressed and finally destroyed in the fibrotic change, but may last longer than the tubules, and always longer than the spermatogenic function.   The necrotic area often retains vaguely the outlines of the pre-existing cellular elements in a manner similar to that seen in the kidneys of corrosive sublimate poisoning (Fig. 186).   The chromatin seems to disappear completely, but this again is not constant, and one may see extensive karyorrhexis, with quantities of hematoxylin-staining nuclear dust, as is so common in tuberculous caseation.   In these cases remains of the architecture of the tissue is usually less noticeable, the degeneration of all elements being more nearly complete.

Secondary infection is not very rare, in which case polymorphonuclears are superadded to the round-cell infiltration, and may be present in large numbers in the necrotic area, or in certain peripheral portions of it, so that the picture approaches that of an abscess.

In general, we may say that syphilis is an infection producing a granulomatous reaction, but more chronic, as a rule, than tuberculosis, with more tendency to fibrosis and less tendency to necrosis.   These tendencies are probably to be ascribed to the greater chronicity, which allows the circulation of the affected area to survive longer.   In the same way the more bizarre forms of cellular change, as epithelioid cells and giant-cells, are much less common in syphilis than in tuberculosis, and zonate arrangements about the central point of the lesion are much less definite. It is possible, however, for any of these to occur.

In the testes which are the seat of syphilitic *fibrosis* the entire testis is involved in a fibrotic change, the microscopic features of which are the same as those described above for the peripheral layers of the gumma.   The relation between the two types is illustrated by the fact that fibrosis is seen along with every gumma, while apparently fibrosis may occur without any necrosis.   The difference then is one of degree, the fibrotic lesion being more indolent and more diffuse, but otherwise fundamentally similar.

While the entire testis is involved, the changes are usually more marked at first at the *hilus* and along the *septa*.   Thus tubules which are least affected are to be found in the central portions of the testicular compartments or lobules.   Later the entire organ is transformed into a mass like a fibroma, in which it may be difficult or impossible to find any trace of the original elements.

In the gross, the organ is *enlarged*, occasionally to as much as three times its original volume.   It is *firm, smooth,* and *rounded*.   There may be moderate *hydrocele,* or obliteration of the cavity of the tunica vaginalis.   On section, the organ is *firm* and rubbery.   The surface is flat, does not evert, and is grayish and translucent.   Where the transformation is incomplete, yellowish, opaque areas of surviving tubules may be seen between the thickened septa.   They do not tease out readily as do normal tubules.

In the final stages of the process the originally enlarged testis *contracts* again, until it may be markedly smaller than normal.   It is very firm, and irregularities may develop.   This change is marked by a disappearance of the leukocytic infiltration and of all original elements of the organ.   Its functions, both secretory and endocrine, are, of course, entirely suppressed.

While beginning, as a rule, on one side, syphilitic fibrosis not infrequently involves the other side later, unless arrested by treatment.

Complications are rare in fibrosis testis.   With gumma, however, the process may extend and involve the testicular tunics and scrotal tissues, finally ulcerating through to the outside. When this occurs, the remaining portions of the testis may evert through the sinus, forming a fungus or hernia testis, and leading to complete destruction of the organ. In such a case secondary infection, of course, occurs and helps in the destruction. Ulceration to the outside is, however, rare and late. Secondary infection of an unopened gumma may, however, occur, probably by way of the blood-stream. When this happens, edema, congestion, etc., appear, and the clinical picture of acute orchitis, with pain, fever, etc., is superadded.

The *epididymis* usually appears to be unaffected. Microscopically, however, one may see a slight degree of round-cell infiltration and fibrosis similar to that in the testis, only rarely sufficient to obstruct the duct. While gumma may involve the epididymis and destroy it, this event is remarkably uncommon. Delahaye[1] describes a tertiary syphilitic epididymis with intact testis, but this lesion is certainly so extremely rare that its existence must be open to doubt. Reclus enunciates as a practical law that "every time that the epididymis is affected by syphilis, the testis is more seriously involved."

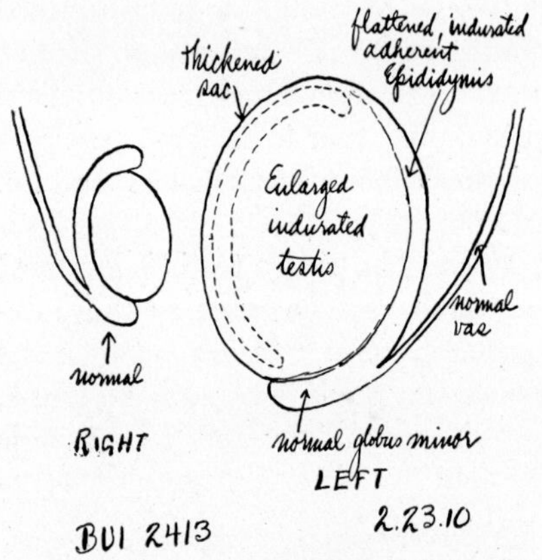

Fig. 187.—Scrotal findings in a case of syphilis of the testis. The vas is normal. Testis is symmetrically enlarged, indurated, not nodular. The epididymis can still be felt, not enlarged, but stretched over the surface of the testis. Rectal examination showed only slight induration of the prostate. Treatment by antisyphilitic medication.

The *symptoms of syphilitic orchitis* consist almost entirely of the local *enlargement*, as both fibrosis and gumma are usually painless. Secondary infection of gumma may cause pain, heat, swelling, and fever.

The *onset* is extremely insidious and the progress slow.

The *diagnosis* of syphilitic orchitis is often a matter of considerable difficulty. The lesions which come especially into question are malignant tumors and tuberculosis, while hydrocele and hematocele may also present problems.

In syphilitic fibrosis the patient usually comes in for enlargement of the testis. If this stage is passed, the atrophic testis usually gives no trouble, and is found only by accident or at autopsy.

The testis is enlarged, smooth, rounded, very firm, and has a feel described as "heavy," though this is doubtless due to lack of elasticity, since the specific gravities of solid tissues and fluid collections are practically the same. An important feature is lack of tenderness and absence of the normal testicular sensation on squeezing the testis. The testis may be somewhat flattened from side to side. Hydrocele may be present and is sometimes sufficient to prevent palpation of the testis. The condition of the epididymis is important, as in malignant tumors, since if it is normal tuberculosis is practically ruled out (Fig. 187).

In *gumma* the picture is practically the same except that the testis is apt to be irregular, even nodular, or it may be possible to palpate the hard, inelastic gumma within the testis. Again, the epididymis is uninvolved, but in most cases it is

[1] De l'épididymite syphilitique tertiare, Thèse de Lyon, 1895–96, No. 1104.

flattened out and adherent to the enlarged testis and its outlines cannot be made out (Figs. 188, 189).

The *history* is, of course, carefully investigated, inquiring particularly for the primary sore and secondary eruption, and the Wassermann test performed.

A positive Wassermann does not rule out *malignant tumor*. Indeed, the diagnostic criteria are inexact, and it will often be entirely impossible to make a positive diagnosis before operation. Nodularity and slow but steady growth are somewhat in favor of gumma, while, of course, a negative Wassermann is strongly in favor of neoplasm if the lesion is in the testis proper and the epididymis normal. If there is doubt, it is permissible to institute a short and intensive course of anti-syphilitic treatment for a period of not over one week. If no change occurs, it is better to operate, since the removal of a syphilitic testicle, doomed to destruc-

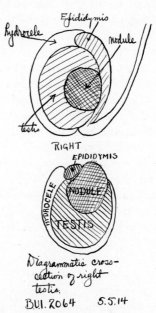

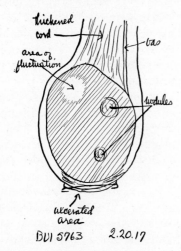

FIG. 188.—Scrotal findings in a case of gumma of the testis. The cord is thickened, but the vas is normal. The testis is markedly enlarged and the epididymis cannot be identified. Nodules and areas of softening are present. Also an ulceration. Rectal examination negative. Duration of swelling one year. Castration performed. Diagnosis confirmed microscopically.

FIG. 189.—Scrotal findings in a case of gumma of the testis. Vas and epididymis are normal. There is a slight hydrocele. The testis is enlarged, but the enlargement is due to a hard nodule growing in the region of the hilum. The remainder of the testis is of practically normal consistence. The lower figure shows how the findings can be more clearly indicated by making an imaginary cross-section. Rectal examination negative. No operation; diagnosis presumptive.

tion in great part or completely, can do no harm, while delay in the case of neoplasm may be fatal.

Since it is extremely rare for *tuberculosis* to arise in the testis, the condition of the epididymis will usually give the important clue. If the testis is approximately normal, with an enlarged, indurated, irregular epididymis, the case is probably one of tuberculosis. This conclusion is fortified if one finds similar indurated nodules in or general enlargement of the seminal vesicles and prostate, as these organs are ordinarily not affected by syphilis. Tuberculous lesions elsewhere in the body have the same significance. If the testis is involved, the concomitant enlargement of the epididymis speaks in favor of tuberculosis. Rarely the testis and epididymis may be converted into a mass of tuberculous tissue in which they cannot be separated by palpation, as in a case described by Hinman,[1] where such a mass was taken for malignant tumor. Similar confusion with syphilis might arise.

If *sinuses* are present the same diagnostic criteria apply if it is possible to palpate the scrotal contents. Often, however, edema and infiltration of the scrotal tissues prevent this. Tuberculosis is more apt to ulcerate than either gumma or neoplasm, and it may be possible to demonstrate the bacilli in the secretion from the sinus, but in case of doubt it is better to operate, as the organs are destroyed in any case. The operative specimen should be carefully examined as soon as removed, frozen sections being made, in order to be sure of the diagnosis before proceeding further.

Hydrocele may occasionally simulate syphilis, especially when tense, thick walled, and opaque, so that it will not transmit light. Inability to palpate the epididymis, or to pinch up the tunica vaginalis between the fingers, speak in favor of hydrocele. Hydrocele accompanying syphilis often makes palpation impossible. Here, as in the case of malignant tumors, it may in some cases be permissible to tap for diagnosis. It is better to avoid this if possible, however, as it is conceivable that the procedure might do harm in case a neoplasm were really present.

Hematocele is rare, but may be confusing. Here again, as in hydrocele, inability to palpate the epididymis suggests the filling of the cavity of the tunica vaginalis.

To recapitulate, it will usually be possible to diagnose tuberculosis with a good degree of certainty. In all other cases of testicular enlargement the best procedure is (1) with negative Wassermann, immediate operation, and (2) with positive Wassermann, an intensive seven-day course of antisyphilitic treatment, followed immediately, if this does not clear up the diagnosis, by operation.

Treatment.—Syphilis of the testis is usually successfully treated by means of antisyphilitic medication, which should be thorough and long continued. Potassium iodid may be given and seems in some cases to hasten the resolution of gummatous lesions. In the case of gumma there will in many cases be some doubt as to the diagnosis, and, as we have stated in the section on Tumors of the Testis, it may be wise in certain of these cases to perform orchidectomy, since a testis which is affected by gumma is no longer a useful organ. One should not neglect, however, in case the lesion is found by pathologic examination to be a gumma, to follow the operation by a thorough course of antisyphilitic treatment. In fibrosis of the testis antisyphilitic treatment arrests the process, but since the testis is the seat of a fibrous reaction no restitution to normal can be expected.

Among 12,500 cases in our records there have been 14 cases of gumma of the testis. Nine were treated by orchidectomy. Since these patients are usually from the lower walks of life, most of them failed to appear for antisyphilitic treatment after discharge from the hospital, and have not answered letters. One with generalized syphilis died soon after admission from "syphilitic" nephritis with uremia. Two report themselves well six years and four years, respectively, after orchidectomy. The rest were not followed.

ACTINOMYCOSIS

Actinomycosis is a common disease of cattle, usually manifested as the condition called "lumpy jaw" or "big jaw." Similar infections occasionally occur in man. The *bacteriology* of human actinomycosis is still very confused. The com-

---

[1] Cabot's Modern Urology, 1924, i, 580–609.

mittee on nomenclature of the Society of American Bacteriologists has decided to group in the genus Actinomyces all organisms of similar type, which include those formerly called "streptothrix." The name "streptothrix" is, therefore, to be abandoned, and with it the term "streptothricosis." There are no doubt numerous species of actinomyces, but their differentiation is incomplete and unsatisfactory. Bergey[1] lists 65 species, more or less completely described, but it seems likely that many of these are identical. Seven species are described as pathogenic for human beings, as follows:

TABLE 44

Actino-myces.	Bovis.	Hominis.	Maduræ.	Freeri.	Gedanensis.	Candidus.	Asteroides.
Source......	Cattle and human cases.	Human cases.	Ulcers of "madura foot."	Mycetoma.	Pulmonary lesions.	Pulmonary lesions.	Abscess or brain and lung.

Some of these may be identical; the Actinomyces bovis and Actinomyces hominis especially appear to be very similar.

No rigorous classification on bacteriologic grounds can, therefore, be attempted, and we shall confine ourselves to a description of the disease as it has been seen in the urogenital tract.

The ordinary habitat of actinomyces is in the soil and on various kinds of grasses and grains. It gains access to the bovine or human body, as a rule, through the buccal mucosa during the ingestion of food. Sixty per cent. of human cases are in the face or neck. Other portals of entry, as through wounds or scratches, or through the lungs, probably by inhalation, also come into question.

Actinomycosis is comparatively rare in human beings, and in human cases involvement of the urogenital tract is exceptional. Cecil and Hill[2] in 1922 were able to collect only 11 cases, including 1 of their own from our clinic, and excluding those in which the urogenital tract had been invaded by direct continuity from other organs. However, since of late years a number of cases of obscure pulmonary disease, resembling tuberculosis, has been found to be due to actinomyces, it may well be that urogenital infections are somewhat more common than has been realized. Not infrequently in renal infections giving the picture of tuberculosis it is impossible to demonstrate the tubercle bacillus. Some of these are possibly actinomyces infections.

Bacteriologically, Actinomyces bovis (the type organism) grows on most bacteriologic media, but best on media enriched with uncoagulated protein. The growth is slow, sometimes not appearing for one or two weeks. The colonies are rounded, convex, and dry. The color varies from buff to yellow, or in older cultures brown. The organism may survive for months or years in the dry state. Under the microscope one sees a fine, branching mycelium, which when young is uniformly Gram positive. Later small Gram-positive granules or pseudospores develop in the mycelial threads, the remainder of which becomes Gram negative. Finally the threads break up into short bacillus-like rods, sometimes Gram positive, sometimes Gram negative, and sometimes containing the granules mentioned above, and into small round coccus-like bodies, always Gram positive. The organism

[1] Manual of Determinative Bacteriology, 1923.
[2] Journal of the American Medical Association, 1922, lxxviii, 575–578.

may thus take the form of a *mycelium*, a *bacillus*, or a *coccus*, and if only the last two are found in a preparation, as in a urinary smear, the presence of a mycotic infection may not be suspected.

Pathologically, actinomyces produces a chronic granulomatous lesion which, in typical cases, is markedly more destructive and progressive than tuberculosis. In the gross, one sees at the outside of the lesion a very marked zone of fibrous reaction, within which is a softer zone of cellular infiltration, and at the center a necrotic area. The necrotic material is soft and semifluid, and takes on the character of frank pus from the participation of many polymorphonuclear cells in the reaction. Floating in the pus are tiny, opaque yellow bodies, pin-point in size, and described as resembling grains of iodoform powder. These are the "sulphur granules" characteristic of the disease.

Microscopically, the pus is typical, with many degenerated leukocytes. The sulphur granules in it, however, stand out conspicuously if properly stained.[1] They are about 100 to 500 micromillimeters in diameter, and are composed of a closely packed mass of mycelial threads. In ordinary hematoxylin and eosin sections they stain a uniform red and with the dry lens will be taken for bits of necrotic tissue. In a thin, well-stained section there may be seen radiating from the edge of this mass innumerable tiny club-shaped rods, with the enlargement at the peripheral end. The above-described picture is pathognomonic and cannot be mistaken for anything else.

The zone of cellular infiltration contains round-cells, but also very many polymorphonuclears and large phagocytes (macrophages). These cells seem to have little power to resist the growth of the fungus. The macrophages especially are destroyed by the advancing growth, the polymorphonuclears appearing to be spared, at least in a relative sense. The fibrous reaction in the outermost zone is of the ordinary type. Although well marked, it too in many instances seems unable to oppose an effective barrier to the progress of the disease.

In the gross, these destructive qualities are evidenced by *abscess* cavities, often multilocular or honeycombed, which invade all tissues with equal freedom. Extension from one organ to another, therefore, is frequent. When the fibrous reaction is pronounced, the lesions may resemble those of a fulminating tuberculosis, while in other cases the preponderance of destruction over reaction has given the naked eye appearance of a necrotizing malignant growth.

The above description is that of the usually recognized picture of "actinomycosis." There are, however, other lesions due to "actinomyces" (or streptothrix) which are more chronic and less destructive. They have been described especially in the lungs. In these cases the tissue reaction is more pronounced, and takes on a form practically indistinguishable from that seen in tuberculosis. Tubercles, epithelioid cells, giant-cells, and typical caseation are seen. On hasty examination the diagnosis of tuberculosis may even be made, but with special stains no tubercle bacilli can be demonstrated, while the mycelial networks will be seen in the central

---

[1] Actinomyces does not stain with hematoxylin. A section, either a paraffin section from which the paraffin has been removed, or a frozen section, should be lightly stained with anilin gentian-violet. It is then washed, counterstained with aqueous eosin, covered with anilin oil, and blotted. Repetition of this blotting process four or five times will dehydrate the section, and it may be mounted at once in balsam. The mycelial masses will stand out sharply, being stained a deep blue.

portions of the tubercles and other lesions.   It is at present impossible to say whether this more chronic picture represents a different form of the same disease, in which the reaction of the body is more effective, or whether it is due to an infection with a different species of actinomyces.   We have not found a description of such lesions in the urogenital tract, unless the cases of Reed[1] can be so considered, but we must certainly reckon with the possibility.   Wider use of bacterial stains in tissues would no doubt add much to our knowledge of mycotic infections.   Search should especially be made in those cases, apparently of tuberculosis, where the tubercle bacillus has not been demonstrated.   It is possible, however, for tuberculosis and actinomycosis to coexist.   In a case seen by us Hill recovered both Bacillus tuberculosis and Actinomyces bovis from a kidney removed for tuberculosis.

In the *urogenital tract* a few cases have been described as "primary," that is, no other focus could be demonstrated anywhere.   We must assume here as in tuberculosis that the organism has gained entrance to the body through a small and inconspicuous lesion, or that the original portal of entry is healed at the time of examination.   Ordinarily, the involvement of the urogenital tract is *secondary*, due to extension from some other organ, or *metastatic*, due to a blood-borne infection from some other lesion.   Metastatic involvement is perhaps the commonest, as the terminal stages of the disease are so often marked by a generalization throughout the body.   On the external genitalia actinomycosis may occur as on other skin surfaces, by direct infection, usually following a cut or abrasion.   Certain cases of prostatic actinomycosis with incomplete bacteriologic studies have been reported.

The data concerning urogenital actinomycosis without obvious infection elsewhere are best shown in the table of Hill and Cecil in a report from this clinic and reprinted on page 352.

Few *pathologic* reports are available.   In the *kidney* the findings have always been those of the acuter form of actinomycosis.   Where the lesion was of renal origin, the foci were usually multiple, and gave rise to an enlargement, with extensive destruction.   On section the picture recalled in some cases cavernocaseous tuberculosis, in another (Israel) a necrotic cancerous growth.   Where the involvement was by extension (autopsy specimens) the kidney was found destroyed by the advance of an actinomycotic abscess beginning in the liver, intestine, etc.   In all cases the microscopic picture was typical, and in most the sulphur granules were demonstrable.   In Israel's case there was a pelvic calculus, with actinomycotic granules as a nucleus.

That the *ureter* may be involved is indicated by the case of Kunith, where actinomycotic pus was found in the urine after nephrectomy.

The *bladder* may be infected from the kidney, in which case ulcers appear about the ureteral orifice.   In the majority of cases reported the bladder infection has been secondary, often to actinomycosis of the lower abdominal wall.   In other cases the rectum, appendix, uterus, or perineum were the primary foci.   Fistulæ are the rule in these cases.   In the extraordinary case of Poncet,[2] the patient, who had a perianal actinomycosis, apparently produced a superficial infection of his bladder by introducing a grain of wheat through the urethra.   There was no

---

[1] Contributions to the Science of Medicine, dedicated to William H. Welch, Johns Hopkins Press, Baltimore, 1900, 525–541.

[2] Quoted by Niçaise, Encyclopædie Française d'Urologie, 1921, iv, 605–612.

TABLE 45

SUMMARY OF CASES OF PRIMARY GENITO-URINARY ACTINOMYCOSIS FOUND IN AVAILABLE LITERATURE

Author.	Patient.	Diagnosis.	Actinomycosis recognized.	Organisms found.	Identity of organism.	Treatment.	Termination.
1. Poncet......	Not stated.	Cystitis.	At time of treatment.	In nodules in pus in urine.	"Actinomyces."	Not stated.	Not stated.
2. Stanton......	Man, aged fifty-three.	Cystitis; pyelonephritis.	Postmortem.	In kidney abscesses.	"Actinomyces."	Not stated.	Fatal.
3. Leger.........	Male.	Not stated.	Not stated.	Glans penis.	"Actinomyces."	Not stated.	Not stated.
4. Earl..........	Not stated.	Not made.	Postmortem.	Abscess of kidney and bladder; brain.	"Actinomyces."	Not stated.	Cerebral actinomycosis; fatal.
5. Kunith.......	Boy, aged four and three-quarter years.	Pyelonephritis.	Postoperatively.	In urine after operation and in kidney abscesses.	"Actinomyces."	Operative.	Recovery.
6. Cohn.........	Man, aged forty-six.	Pyelonephritis; prostatitis.	At time of treatment.	In urine and prostatic secretion.	"Actinomyces."	Not stated.	Not stated.
7. Kellock......	Female.	Probable tuberculosis of right kidney.	Postoperatively.	In kidney lesions.	"Actinomyces."	Operative; potassium iodid.	Recovery.
8. Eustace.......	Man, aged thirty-five.	Chronic inflammatory process; probably tuberculous.	Postoperatively.	In testicle and cord.	"Actinomyces bovis."	Operative; followed by KI, 5 grains three times a day for three months.	Recovery.
9. Israel........	Man, aged thirty-three.	1. Kidney stone. 2. Actinomycosis.	During treatment.	In exudate from fistula, and in urine.	"Actinomyces."	Operative.	Recovery.
10. Israel........	Woman, aged sixty.	Perinephritis.	After nephrectomy.	In kidney lesions.	"Actinomyces."	Operative.	Recovery.
11. Cecil and Hill.	Man, aged thirty-five.	Pyelonephritis, actinomycosis and Ps. pyocyaneus.	During treatment.	In urine.	"Actinomyces bovis."	Pelvic lavage, iodids.	Unimproved.
Summary.........	7 male. 2 female. 2 not stated. Age from four and three-quarter to sixty years.	2 cases, not made. 2 cases, probably tuberculosis. 1 case, perinephritis. 1 case, cystitis. 1 case, cystitis and pyelonephritis. 1 case, pyelonephritis and prostatitis. 1 case, kidney stone and actinomycosis. 1 case, actinomycosis and Ps. pyocyaneus.	4 during treatment. 4 postoperatively. 2 postmortem. 1 not stated.	3 in kidney lesions. 1 in kidney, bladder and brain lesions 1 in kidney lesions and urine. 2 in urine. 1 in urine and exudate from fistula. 1 in urine and prostatic secretion. 1 in glans penis. 1 in testicle and cord.	9 "Actinomyces." 2 "Actinomyces bovis."	3 operative. 2 operative and KI. 5 not stated. 1 local and KI.	5 recovery. 2 fatal. 3 not stated. 1 unimproved.

communication between the bladder and rectum, and the grain of wheat, surrounded by mycelium, had become the nucleus of a small calculus.

Eustace[1] reports a case in which the *testicle* and *cord* were involved and Leger[2] a case with a skin lesion on the *glans penis*.

It is not possible to make any definite statements about the *symptomatology* of urogenital actinomycosis. In some cases the symptom complex has apparently been identical with that of tuberculosis, while in other more fulminant cases the clinical story has been that of an acute inflammatory process (pyonephrosis, abscess of testicle).

As to the *diagnosis,* in only 4 of the purely urogenital cases has the diagnosis been made before pathologic material was available. In each of these the organism was found in the urine, and in 1 of them in the secretion from a fistula as well. Since, as stated above, the organism may assume bacillary or coccoid forms, the diagnosis can seldom be made definitely by microscopic examination. The presence of long filaments may arouse suspicion, but cultures alone can give positive evidence. It is important to incubate the cultures a long time, since, as we have seen, the actinomyces may not appear for as much as two weeks—a time when other organisms which may be present are dying out. The use of an acid (Ph 4.0–4.5) medium may be advantageous, since while inhibiting ordinary organisms it does not influence the growth of the usual species of actinomyces.

For the diagnosis of pathologic material, *cultures* and *special stains* are essential. It is quite possible that actinomyces may be present in certain cases apparently of tuberculosis, and if the case is in any way atypical, or if tubercle bacilli have not been demonstrated, search for actinomyces should be made by these methods.

In secondary involvements the diagnosis will usually be evident from the presence of other lesions. Here again tuberculosis comes in question, and actinomyces must be sought in the sputum, the feces, or the secretion of any ulcers, sinuses, or fistulæ which may exist.

The *treatment of actinomycosis* is unsatisfactory and the prognosis poor. The only medical treatment which has been recommended is the use of iodids in large quantities, which has brought about improvement in some instances.[3] Surgical treatment must be radical to be effective. Partial removal of an actinomycotic lesion is worse than useless. In a few cases of *renal actinomycosis*, "recovery" is reported after nephrectomy, but late reports are lacking. If no other organs are involved, this is certainly the method of choice. We have not, however, any data as to how often renal actinomycosis is bilateral, nor do we know whether the absence of actinomyces from the urine of the apparently sound kidney is reliable evidence of the absence of infection. It is probable that the principles governing the treatment of tuberculosis apply here. Intravenous mercurochrome is suggested.

Testicular actinomycosis is treated by excision according to the extent of the lesion. There is apparently good reason for being less conservative here than in tuberculosis, and removing the testis also unless the lesion can surely be entirely circumscribed by doing an epididymectomy.

[1] British Medical Journal, 1899, ii, 1704.

[2] Quoted by Rosenstein, Berliner Klinische Wochenschrift, 1918, lv, 114–117.

[3] Myers and Thienes: Journal of The American Medical Association, 1925, lxxxiv, 1985, 1986, recommend thymol and cinnamon oil, locally and internally.

OTHER MYCOSES

There is little literature on other mycoses of the urogenital tract. Reed[1] described kidney lesions, consisting mostly of masses of organisms, with little cellular reaction, due to what was designated "Bacillus pseudotuberculosis murium." This organism showed true branching. Castellani[2] states that he has seen in tropical countries various mycoses of the urogenital organs due to "fungi of the genera Nocardia, Aspergillus, and Cladosporium." Presumably most of these are of the external genitalia. In some there has been a profuse urethral discharge of a black color, due to the presence of Aspergillus fumigatus. Chute[3] reports a case of chronic cystitis, in which the bladder and voided urine contained large masses of Penicillium glaucum. Blastomycosis and coccidioidal granuloma may rarely, especially in generalized infections, affect the kidney.[4]

BILHARZIOSIS[5]

Bilharziosis is the invasion of the human body by trematode worms of the genus schistosomum. The parasite was first discovered by Bilharz in 1851, and has often been called "bilharzia"; hence the name bilharziosis. There are three species of schistosomum, respectively, the Schistosomum hæmatobium, the Schistosomum Mansoni, and the Schistosomum japonicum. It is the Schistosomum hæmatobium which Bilharz discovered, and which is principally concerned in urinary infestations.

The *parasite* is of the phylum Vermes, class Platyhelminths, order Trematodes, suborder Distomata, family Distomida, genus Schistosomum. All the species of this genus are characterized by a peculiar sort of symbiosis, in which the long, slender female is partly contained in a canal on the ventral surface of the shorter, broader male. This conjunction takes place in the body after sexual maturity is reached. The male of Schistosomum hæmatobium is 8 to 16 mm. long and 1 mm. broad. The body is flat, and for the posterior nine-tenths of its length the two edges are rolled over ventrally until they overlap, forming the gynecophoric canal.

The female is about 20 mm. long and 0.1 mm. in diameter. After copulation, the anterior portion of the female remains enclosed in the gynecophoric canal, the posterior extremity being free.

The *life history* of the parasite includes an obligate intermediate host. The ova are excreted mostly in the urine, and eventually die unless they fall in water. In water they develop quickly, setting free the free-swimming miracidium, which, in turn, dies in from twenty-four to forty-eight hours unless it finds a snail of a variety suitable to serve as intermediate host. Such varieties are the Bullinus contortus, Dybowski, Innesi, and africanus. Other snails are ignored by the miracidia, and they cannot infest man. Within the snail a sporocyst is formed

---

[1] Contributions to the Science of Medicine, dedicated to William H. Welch, Johns Hopkins Press, Baltimore, 1900, 525–541.

[2] Castellani and Chalmers: Manual of Tropical Medicine, New York, 3d ed., 1920.

[3] Boston Medical and Surgical Journal, 1911, clxiv, 420–422.

[4] Wright: Nelson's Loose Leaf Medicine, 1920, ii, 355–372.

[5] This section is based principally on the following authorities: Niçaise: Encyclopædie Française d'Urologie, 1924, iii, 124–126, and iv, 585–603. Castellani and Chalmers: Manual of Tropical Medicine, New York, 1920, 3d ed. Fantham, Stephens, and Theobald: The Animal Parasites of Man, New York, 1916. Thompson-Walker, Genito-urinary Surgery, New York, 1916.

in the liver, from which eventually the bisexual cercariæ or embryos are liberated. These also are free swimming, and infest man.

It was at first thought that the embryos were swallowed and made their way through the intestinal mucosa. Allen doubted this, and thought that they penetrated the mucosa of the prepuce, suggesting that circumcision would largely prevent infestation. Later investigations make it seem probable that the parasites can pass through any mucous membrane, and possibly even the skin; thus those taken into the mouth would penetrate the buccal or pharyngeal membranes before reaching the stomach, where they could not survive if the hydrochloric acid content were normal.

Within the body they are carried by the blood-stream to the portal system, where they remain until mating occurs. Since the males are more numerous than the females, some are unable to mate, and these remain in the portal system. The united pairs proceed actively against the blood-stream to the vesical veins. How and why they are able to do this, avoiding all other parts of the body, remains unexplained. Once in the small vesical veins, the females begin to lay eggs, which penetrate the vesical wall and eventually reach the cavity of the bladder, ready to renew the cycle.

In monkeys artificially infested, ova have been found in the urine within ten weeks of infestation. Ordinarily it is considered that three to six months elapse in the human before this takes place. With repeated reinfestations, the number of parasites living in the bladder wall increases, and upon their number depends the severity of the disease. Apparently their life in the adult stage is not over three or four years, as the disease may entirely disappear in that length of time in persons removed from all possibility of reinfestation.

Bilharziosis *is confined to certain countries.* In Egypt it is especially prevalent. In 1 case 79 per cent. of the boys in a rural school were found infested. The agricultural population is especially affected, as the methods in vogue there require much contact with water and damp soil. The disease is, however, found in all parts of Africa, including the Cape Colony. Cases have also been found in Siam, India, Mesopotamia, Madagascar, Greece, and Japan. The forms of schistosomiasis common in Japan (Schistosomum japonicum) and South America and the West Indies (Schistosomum Mansoni) do not ordinarily involve the urinary tract.

Urinary bilharziosis affects all *ages* and both *sexes.* It is very uncommon in the United States. There has never been a case at the Johns Hopkins Hospital.

The *pathology* in the bladder is that of a chronic infection, with granulomatous proliferation, and an epithelial hyperplasia which is apparently peculiar to this parasite and may go on to malignancy. The adult parasites in the venules, and the ova in the tissues may be seen in sections. Since each female lays numbers of eggs, one after another, they often occur in groups, and may be closely placed and very numerous. Surrounding the parasites and ova is a marked round-cell infiltration, with accompanying fibrous change. The mucosa may be much thickened, in small tubercle-like areas, or much more extensively. The *epithelium* usually shows proliferation, in the form of villous or papillomatous outgrowths, or of finger-like down growths. As the ova pass the epithelium, ulceration may occur. Stone formation may take place in the interstices of the ulcers, granulations, or papillomatous areas, leading to encrusted cystitis or vesical calculus.

Secondary infection is common in advanced cases, with the picture of acute and chronic cystitis. *Malignant changes* in the epithelial overgrowths, either papillary carcinoma or epithelioma, may occur in chronic cases. Many ova fail to reach the bladder cavity, die, and become encysted and later calcified.

In the *gross*, the bladder wall is thickened, and loses its elasticity, either in areas or diffusely. The surface lesions are best studied with the cystoscope. In early cases there is some general congestion, with local lesions representing the groups of ova near the surface. They consist of small rounded nodules with a yellowish cast, projecting above the surface and a millimeter or two in diameter. They are surrounded each by a small red halo of congestion. These are known as bilharzia nodules. These nodules may rupture, leaving small ragged ulcers. The ulcers may coalesce. Eventually the repetition of this process produces irregular, red masses of granulation tissue, in the midst of which a few bilharzia nodules may be seen. Sometimes typical papillomatous tumors are seen, even in the absence of any marked granulations or ulcers.

The bladder is usually the site of the lesions. The *urethra, ureter*, and more rarely, the *prostate, seminal vesicles*, and *renal pelvis* may be affected. The pathology is the same. Occasionally the parasites reach the rectum. Ruffer[1] has found unmistakable evidence of bilharzial disease in Egyptian mummies about three thousand years old, and in two of them the kidneys were involved.

In *advanced cases* the pathologic changes involve other organs. Thus the bladder may become adherent to the abdominal wall, the ova finally reach the surface, and ulceration occurs, with multiple sinuses and fistulæ over the lower abdomen. The same process may involve the perineum, and in advanced cases there are multitudes of infected sinuses and fistulæ, with inflammatory elephantiasis of the scrotum and penis.

Calculus formation and *infection* are common in advanced cases. Lesions in the urethra, ureter, or renal pelvis may produce urinary obstruction, resulting in hydronephrosis, pyelonephritis, or pyonephrosis as described elsewhere. The prostate and seminal vesicles may be affected, and ova have been found in the semen. Ova with surrounding tissue reaction have been found in the corpora cavernosa and corpus spongiosum, and involvements of the vagina and uterus have been reported. Madden describes hydrocele with ova in the fluid, and an ova-containing mass in the spermatic cord. Occasionally the parasites invade the rectal vessels, when ova and blood appear in the stools. Ova have also been found in the liver and lungs.

The *symptoms* of urinary bilharziosis consist at first of a painless, but rather constant *hematuria*. It should be noted, however, that individuals can have the disease and be excreting numerous ova in the urine without any symptoms whatever. Later *frequency* and *dysuria* supervene, associated with infiltration of the bladder wall. Genital hyperexcitability has been reported in involvement of the prostate and vesicles.

In later stages there are symptoms of severe vesical irritation—extreme frequency, constant pain, tenesmus. Anemia may result from the constant hemorrhage. Involvement of kidney and ureter cause renal pain and colic. If infection occurs, pyuria is added, and if the infection reaches the kidney, pain and fever indicate pyelonephritis. Urethral involvement causes difficulty or retention, and there is sometimes peri-urethral abscess or extravasation.

[1] British Medical Journal, 1910, i, 16.

Complications, especially *pyelonephritis*, *malignancy*, or *extravasation* may cause a fatal ending, but in cases not too advanced, if reinfestation is prevented, a gradual amelioration may be expected even in the absence of treatment.

In the *diagnosis*, especially of early cases, the examination of the *urine* is most important. There are usually red blood-cells and some mucus, but it may often be otherwise clear except for the *ova*. Before searching for ova the centrifugalized sediment should be obtained. The ova of Schistosomum hematobium are oval, being 120 to 190 μ long by 50 to 73 μ wide. There is a thin, elastic outer envelope, prolonged at one pole into a sharp-pointed spine about 12 μ long. Within, the ovum may be seen in various stages of development, sometimes displaying definite movements. The number of ova excreted may be enormous. Brault counted 4000 in one day, and calculated that one of his patients had voided 15,000,000 ova while under observation. The ova of Schistosomum Mansoni, with a lateral spine, is only occasionally found in the urine, while that of Schistosomum japonicum, with only a very tiny lateral protuberance, is even rarer. The *blood* shows in many cases a typical parasitic eosinophilia.

On *cystoscopic* examination, the early lesions are characteristic, but later, with severe cystitis, villous tumors, and calcareous deposits, nothing pathognomonic is seen. The lesions have been described above. In such cases one must keep in mind the possibility of *malignant* change, and watch closely for it during the period of improvement.

Rectal or *vaginal* examination will disclose induration of the bladder wall, if present.

The constant presence of ova in the urine makes the diagnosis simple, and it is only in regard to the detection of complications that the skill of the physician will be taxed. Fairley[1] has described a complement-fixation test, using an extract of the cercariæ of the infested snail as an antigen. There is little need for this test in the primary form of the disease, as the diagnosis is seldom in doubt.

In the *treatment of urinary bilharziosis* the parasite is attacked with *antimony*, which has a specific action against it. In the past methylene-blue, male fern, quinin, turpentine, emetin, and salvarsan were tried, but these have all been replaced by antimony.

The antimony is usually administered in the form of *tartar emetic*, but colloidal antimony, and more lately, sodium antimony thioglycollate and antimony thioglycollate triamide have been recommended. The latter two are reported by Randall, who believes that sodium antimony thioglycollate is probably less toxic than tartar emetic (sodium and potassium antimony tartrate). The tartar emetic is usually given *intravenously* in 1 per cent. solution, and the dose ranges from 0.02 to 0.15 gm. (The solution may be boiled for sterilization.) Occasionally doses as high as 0.2 gm. have been given, but they are not recommended. The first dose should be small (0.01–0.02 gm.) for two reasons, (1) idiosyncrasy may exist, and (2) the reaction is usually greatest with the first dose, diminishing with successive ones. Injections may be given daily, although every other day is perhaps safer, and are gradually increased to 0.12 or 0.15 gm. Courses of twelve to fifteen doses should be given, with intervening rest periods. Severe cases may require much treatment. Extravasation must be avoided, as the drug is very irritant.

The *reaction* to antimony may include headache, nausea and vomiting, and

[1] Journal of the Royal Army Medical Corps, 1919, xxxii, 243–267.

pain in the bones, and a frequent feature is cough, with feeling of tightness in the chest. The reaction is seldom alarming. In the presence of other diseases, especially of the heart and kidneys, and in old age, caution is necessary. The renal function should be followed, preferably by the phenolsulphonephthalein test, during the period of treatment.

The *results* from the antimony treatment are apparently much better than from any other. Death of the ova has been observed directly in the voided urine. In all cases, however, it is important to institute effective precautions against reinfestation. In poor people living in countries where the parasite is prevalent, this is difficult, but much may be accomplished by cleanliness attained with the assistance of boiled water, the use of proper water-proof foot-wear, and the drinking of boiled or filtered water. Fruits, and especially vegetables, should be eaten cooked.

Complications usually require surgical treatment, especially if the kidney is involved. Hydronephrosis and pyonephrosis must be treated exactly like similar conditions arising from other causes; the same is true of sinuses and fistulæ. In ureteral obstruction pyelostomy or nephrostomy may be done in the hope that the stricture will improve as a result of antimony treatment. Intravesical growths, villous or papillary, may be removed by fulguration. If malignancy occurs, it is treated according to the principles laid down in the section on Neoplasms of the Bladder. Stones are to be removed, preferably by lithotrity, as bladder fistulæ may not heal kindly.

Cystitis may be treated by any of the recognized methods. Irrigations of silver nitrate and quinin have been recommended. Discomfort may be decreased by making the urine alkaline with sodium bicarbonate. Excessive hemorrhage is combated by rest in bed and opium, and some have suggested instillations of adrenalin.

ECHINOCOCCUS DISEASE

Hydatid or echinococcus disease is caused by the platyhelminth Tænia echinococcus (dog tapeworm). This tapeworm is in its adult stage a parasite of the dog and wolf, though it has been found very occasionally in the cat and other carnivorous animals. Man shares with cattle, swine, sheep, and a number of other animals the honor of serving as intermediate host.

The adult *Tænia echinococcus*, which is only 4 or 5 mm. long, lives in the upper small intestine of the dog. The terminal segment, distended with ova, is shed from time to time. After expulsion with the feces, the structure of the segment disappears, leaving the ova. Herbivorous animals may eat directly infested grass, but in the case of man the infestation is usually water-borne, either by drinking-water, or by indirect contamination of vegetables or fruits which are eaten raw. Within the body the ovum is so perfectly adapted to its parasitic life that the digestive juices of the stomach and duodenum serve only to dissolve the resistant envelope and set the larva free to penetrate the intestinal wall. Further progress is usually by the portal system, the parasite often being arrested in the liver. If it passes the liver, it may stop in the lungs, but if it arrives in the left ventricle, it may then be carried by the arterial stream to any part of the body. Migration by way of the lymphatics and thoracic duct, as well as by direct passage through tissues, has been suggested. The portal route is the common one, however.

Niaçise,[1] in a study of nearly 10,000 cases of echinococcus disease, finds that the

[1] Encyclopædie Française d'Urologie, 1914, iii, 75–117 (Lit.).

liver is affected eight times as frequently as the lungs, and that these two organs are the usual seat of the disease, cysts elsewhere being greatly in the minority.

Once arrested, the larva commences to grow, and the form of this growth is one of the strangest in zoölogy. A small mass of cells is formed, which soon becomes cystic, consisting of a thin layer, or germinative membrane, composed of nucleated, apparently undifferentiated cells. These cells, however, secrete on the outer surface a substance which hardens into a chitinous membrane exactly like the chitinous exoskeleton of arthropods. This membrane is formed of thin lamellæ, but is otherwise homogeneous and structureless. Inside the cyst there are here and there small projections like grains of sand, which on section are found to be tiny "brood capsules," containing one or more scolices, or heads of the embryonic worms. Each scolex has four sucking-disks and a double circular row of the characteristic hooklets. The cyst enlarges slowly, the interior being filled with a water-clear, albumin-free fluid secreted by the parasite. While the parasite cannot advance beyond the scolex stage in the intermediate host, the cyst is apparently capable of giving rise to any number of scolices. The cyst may remain single, with numerous scolices on its interior, or the tiny daughter cysts above described may enlarge within the mother cyst. In this way, two, three, or even four generations may be represented by cysts, one within another in the manner of a Chinese box. The chitinous envelope is elastic and fairly tough, so that when such a mother cyst is opened, scores or hundreds of daughter cysts of all sizes may roll out, looking much like white grapes. Counts show that millions of scolices may arise from a single mother cyst, and probably therefore from a single larva.

The scolices are able to develop into adult tæniæ only when the flesh of an infested animal is eaten by a suitable host (dog or wolf). The usual cycle is between dogs and sheep, so that the human disease is commonest in localities where many sheep are raised, and among the shepherds. Examination of house dogs and city dogs shows that they are never infested unless they have access to an abattoir.

As to *distribution*, the disease is commonest in Iceland and Australia, but there have been many cases also in the Argentine Republic, Italy, Greece, North Africa, Russia, and certain parts of Germany. Lyon has collected 279 cases in the United States, and new ones are constantly being added.

Greenway[1] believes that the disease is increasing markedly in Argentina. He notes that the number of animals found infested in the abattoirs has risen in the last ten years from 5 to 15 per cent. for cattle, and from 5 to 30 per cent. for sheep.

All ages and both sexes are affected, but it is most frequent in middle age, and quite a large proportion of cases occurs in children.

Pathologically, the lesion consists of the parasitic cyst, which has been described above, and of a firm fibrous wall, derived from the host, which develops about the parasite as about any other foreign body. There is nothing characteristic about this fibrous membrane, although it has received such names as ectocyst, adventitia, etc. Peripherally, the fibrosis fades away gradually into the normal tissue of the surrounding organ.

It should be stated here that there is a special kind of echinococcus disease occurring only in the Bavarian Tyrol and Russia or in persons coming from those

[1] Semana Medicale, 1922, ii, 761.

regions. Melnikow-Raswedenkow[1] has reported 101 cases with pathologic examination, and believes that it is due to a different variety of parasite. In this form there are germinative cells outside as well as inside the chitinous membrane, and ovoid embryos develop as well as scolices. There is also a much more marked tissue reaction, leading to the formation of granulomatous tumors. The cysts are small, separate, and produce a spongy structure. There are no endogenous daughter cysts. Only one case of urogenital involvement with this form is reported, in which there were two walnut-sized masses in a kidney.[2] Lesions in the adrenal are also reported.[3]

Apparently the ordinary form of hydatid disease can occasionally give rise to external daughter cysts, but only in brain or bone.

Echinococcus cysts are harmless except as they (1) destroy organs by their growth, (2) press upon adjacent organs, causing obstruction, paralysis, etc., and (3) become infected, giving rise to extensive and deep-seated abscesses.

In the urogenital tract the two important locations of hydatid cysts are: (1) *In the kidney,* and (2) in the *retrovesical tissues.* Cases of cysts in the tissues of the cord and scrotum, and projecting into the bladder, have been reported, but are so extremely rare that they are practically negligible.

Kidney.—The parasite may go directly to the kidney (primary) or may reach it secondarily after rupture of a cyst elsewhere, either by the blood-stream or by implantation on the juxta-renal peritoneum. Kretschmer's[4] studies show that various observers find the kidney affected in from 0.021 to 5.4 per cent. of all cases of echinococcus disease. He has collected 18 cases of renal hydatid from the United States and Canada. Niçaise found 197 cases in the right kidney, 185 in the left kidney, and 12 with bilateral involvement. Among his 446 cases the existence of echinococcus cysts in other organs was noted in 58, and probably in numerous others were not noted.

The poles are oftenest affected by the *cyst.* The parasite is commonly arrested in the capillaries of the cortex. The subsequent events depend on the depth of the cyst. Oftenest it enlarges exteriorly, forming a sac springing from the kidney by a broad attachment, and adherent to the perirenal tissues. If deeper, it may push the kidney apart as it grows, even dividing it in two. Finally, if at the hilum it may grow within the kidney, distending it like a hydronephrosis until the thinned-out renal tissue comes to form part of the fibrous capsule of the cyst. In 20 of 446 cases, there were multiple mother cysts.

When the sac becomes extrarenal, *displacement of the kidney* is the rule. It occurs in a direction away from the location of the sac. In 219 of Niçaise's cases which were not operated on, the cyst *opened into the pelvis* in 120. When this occurs, the contents is usually evacuated through the ureter. Rarely rupture may occur into the pleura, intestine, or stomach. Pelvic rupture may be repeated several times, the cyst refilling with daughter cysts in the meanwhile.

Infection and *abscess formation* may rarely occur spontaneously, not infre-

[1] Beiträge zur Pathologischen Anatomie und Allgemeinen Pathologie, 4th Supplement-volume, 1901, 1–295.

[2] Sabolotnow: Tageblatt der Aertzegesellschaft an der Universität Kasan, 1897 (quoted by Melnikow-Raswedenkow).

[3] Huber: Deutsches Archiv für Klinische Medizin, 1881, xxix, 151–174 (26te Berichte des Naturhistorischen Verein in Augsburg).

[4] Surgery, Gynecology, and Obstetrics, 1923, xxxvi, 196–207.

quently following pelvic rupture, and usually after surgical opening, unless thorough removal is practised.

The remaining kidney tissue suffers from pressure, from interference with the blood-supply, from infection, and more rarely from pelvic or ureteral obstruction. Fibrosis and round-cell infiltration, especially in the vicinity of the cyst, are the rule.

The growth of the cyst is *slow*, and may extend over many years. The parasites may survive an indefinite time, as much as twenty years, but sometimes they die and the cyst contents degenerates and hardens, while the fibrous capsule may become calcified. In such cases the disease may never be noticed by the patient during life. The records of the Melbourne Hospital[1] indicate that about 30 per cent. of echinococcus infestations undergo spontaneous degeneration and natural cure. If the entire cyst membrane is extruded at the time of intrapelvic rupture, spontaneous cure may occur, but if any of the parasitic elements remain, it will refill.

The *symptoms* of renal hydatid disease are at first simply those of *renal tumor*. There is usually no pain, but it may be present in advanced cases, and a sensation of weight or dragging is not uncommon. There is no hematuria unless rupture occurs.

Rupture into the pelvis is accompanied by pain, renal colic due to the passage of the daughter cysts through the ureter, and occasionally hematuria. Absolutely characteristic is the voiding of these cysts, which usually alarms the patient thoroughly, and may be accompanied by difficult and painful urination. The urine is usually turbid.

Rupture into the peritoneum usually follows a traumatism of some sort. It is accompanied by great pain and marked collapse, due, according to Brieger, to a toxic substance in the cyst fluid. The intoxication includes often a characteristic general urticaria.

Infection of the cyst causes pain, fever, and leukocytosis. The symptoms may be very severe, due to the large area involved in good-sized cysts.

The *diagnosis* of *renal echinococcus* disease is difficult before rupture occurs. The *history*, including occupation, residence in infested localities, and association with dogs is important. Careful search should be made for *other localizations* of the disease, especially in the liver. The local examination of the kidney regions shows an enlargement, but nothing characteristic, except in those rare cases where a sort of thrill, due to friction among the daughter cysts, can be elicited by a sharp tap. The tumefaction is localized in the kidney as described in the sections on Malignant Neoplasms and Solitary Cysts of the Kidney.

Examination of the *blood* shows in about half the cases a marked eosinophilia—characteristic of all parasitic affections. The *urine* is negative. The *x-ray* shows only a shadow in the kidney region. The *pyelogram* rules out hydronephrosis and often shows compression or distortion of the pelvis as in solitary cyst or malignant tumor.

In countries where the disease is prevalent great efforts have been made to perfect *serologic methods* of diagnosis. Of these, the *complement-fixation* test of Ghedini and the *intradermal* test of Casoni may be mentioned. Fairley[2] has worked out the former in great detail. Fresh, clear, and sterile cyst fluid from the sheep is

---

[1] Fairley: Medical Journal of Australia, 1922, ix (1), 94–96.

[2] Quarterly Journal of Medicine, 1922, xv, 244–267.

usually employed as antigen, and the remainder of the test is exactly similar in technic to the Wassermann test, using heated serum. Others recommend unheated serum. The scolices, however, are rich in antigen, and an alcoholic extract made from the sediment of the fluid (which contains scolices) also gives a powerful antigen. Efforts are being made to produce a permanent preparation, which will be very useful in this country where, the cases being rare, the antigen is now never on hand when needed. The complement-fixation test is extremely valuable. At the Melbourne Hospital correct preoperative diagnoses were made in only 40.7 per cent. of cases before the test came in use, whereas in a series of 83 cases since its adoption, it was positive in 84.3 per cent. In patients above twenty years of age, the test is positive in close to 90 per cent., while the percentage of failure is greater in children. The cause of this is not known. The test becomes more strongly positive after operation or rupture of the cyst, due to diffusion of antigen in the body. After operation, the test usually becomes negative in less than twelve months, if all echinococcus material has been removed, and is, therefore, of value also in prognosis. It is absolutely specific, no positive reactions having occurred in normal individuals, or in those with bilharzia, ascaris, oxyuris, Tænia saginata, syphilis, or any other disease.

South American investigators have given attention to the *intradermal* test. Ithurrat and Calcagno,[1] using 0.2 to 0.6 c.c. of fresh, sterile cyst fluid, state that a positive local reaction will occur, usually within fifteen minutes, in 90 per cent., or better, of cases. Italian workers use cyst fluid sterilized with 5 per cent. of phenol, and state that in some cases a general reaction also is produced. Pontano[2] makes the injection subcutaneously. In this test, also, the production of a stable commercial antigen is awaited. If it is as specific as the Ghedini test, it is recommended by its greater simplicity.

After *rupture* into the pelvis, the diagnosis is greatly simplified. The pain and renal colic are accompanied by no hematuria, or by less than would be expected in the case of stone or neoplasm. In the turbid urine can be found the *hooklets* and sometimes complete scolices. *Daughter cysts* are usually passed sooner or later, and are quite unmistakable.

Diagnosis from other enlargements of the kidney, if we except hydronephrosis, is difficult before rupture. The serologic tests should be of great aid. *Tuberculosis* is detected by a careful study of the urine. Even if the tumefactions caused by hydatid cysts in other organs are found, the picture may suggest that of a *malignant tumor* with metastasis. The general condition of the patient, usually good in hydatid disease, may give a clue. Operation is indicated in all renal tumefactions, practically without exception, and we may apply this rule and explore the kidney even in the presence of masses elsewhere if there is any suspicion of hydatid disease.

Puncture has been generally discarded in the diagnosis and treatment of all kidney lesions. It is inadvisable in echinococcus cyst, since it very often leads to infection.

The *treatment of echinococcus disease of the kidney* is principally surgical. If the cyst ruptures into the pelvis and discharges its contents, the treatment may be expectant until signs of refilling appear. If operation is necessary, *nephrectomy* is the procedure of choice. *Resection* of small cysts with an adjoining portion of

[1] Semana Medicale, 1922, ii, 857–864.
[2] Policlinico, 1922, xxix, 335.

kidney has been practised successfully in a few instances. If nephrectomy is impossible, *marsupialization*, or suturing the edges of the sac to the skin, is to be done. This allows the contents to be thoroughly evacuated, irrigations can be carried out, and the tract heals, in favorable cases, from the bottom. Garcia[1] calls attention to the important fact that the parasite always reacts to any injury with a much increased proliferation. In addition, echinococcus disease is comparable to malignant new growth in that it is capable of local recurrence and distant metastasis. Complete removal without rupture of the cyst is, therefore, the rule whenever possible. In marsupialization, it has been recommended to suture the unopened sac to the skin edges, opening it with the cautery in twenty-four or forty-eight hours, after the wound tract is sealed. This prevents local implantation of scolices. The secondary operation should then be thorough, preferably under an anesthetic, so that the parasite or endocyst can be completely removed. Irrigations are then to be given, with weak iodin solution, mercurochrome, or some other harmless antiseptic.

All efforts to devise a drug treatment for echinococcus disease, either by mouth or intravenously, have been, up to the present time, entirely unsuccessful.

The presence of hyadtid cysts elsewhere in the body need not deter one from operating on the kidney. The others can be treated separately later, if necessary, or may never give any serious trouble.

Retrovesical.—The available data concerning pelvic or retrovesical echinococcus cysts has been collected by Deming,[2] who found 114 cases in the literature and added one of his own from our clinic. According to this, the condition is slightly less frequent than renal hydatid. One hundred and five cases collected by Jendy,[3] however, were from a series of 2729 cases of echinococcus disease, giving a percentage of 3.8. While rare, this condition is important in that it leads to very serious troubles. In 48 of the 114 cases, there was complete retention of urine. Of these 48, 41 were males and 7 females.

Three theories have been advanced to explain the pelvic location. Charcot suggested that it was secondary to liver involvement and Fagg added the idea that the scolex descended by gravity to the lowest point in the peritoneal cavity after rupture of a liver cyst. This theory, however, does not explain those cases where there were no cysts of the liver—which was true in 6 of the 19 in Deming's series which came to autopsy. Other theories are, that the parasites reach this region, as they do others, through the blood-stream, and, that they burrow directly in from the rectum.

The usual location is in the neighborhood of the *seminal vesicles* and *peritoneal cul de sac*. In women the cyst may be either in front of or behind the *uterus*. In a few cases there has been smooth muscle in the capsule of the cyst, suggesting that it arose in the rectal, vesical, or uterine wall.

The cyst may be simple or contain daughter cysts. Great sizes are reached, up to 8 or 10 inches in diameter. The effects are those of *pressure*. The *rectum* is flattened and may be obstructed. The *prostate, vesicles,* and *base of the bladder* are pushed forward, the *urethra* ultimately obstructed. Rarely the cyst may cause a

---

[1] Semana Medicale, 1922, ii, 741.

[2] Journal of Urology, 1923, x, 1–43.

[3] Contribution a l'étude du kyste hydatique retrovésicale chez l'homme, Thèse de Paris, 1912–13.

protuberance in the *ischiorectal fossa*. The *ureters* are pressed upon and obstructed, causing obstructive changes in the kidneys. The cyst, when large, rises out of the pelvis, and may encroach largely on the abdomen. *Rupture* may occur into the rectum, bladder, uterus, or vagina. *Infection* often follows rupture, and suppuration of a pelvic cyst is usually a serious matter, owing to its deep situation. Peritonitis not infrequently follows. Cystitis may complicate the obstruction.

The character of the obstruction depends largely on the location. If above the seminal vesicles, a large abdominal tumor may be produced without obstructive complications, but if at the level of the prostate, a cyst the size of the fist may cause complete urinary obstruction. Pelvic hydatids are usually single, but may be multiple.

The *symptoms* of pelvic echinococcus are typically those of obstruction, of the urethra or rectum, or both. The rectal obstruction is often noted first. Rupture has occurred in late cases, but usually after obstructive symptoms were manifest. In some cases without marked obstruction, the cyst has flattened the bladder to such an extent that its capacity was reduced and there was marked frequency of urination. In women the development of the cyst may rarely simulate pregnancy. If rupture occurs, typical daughter cysts are extruded. If infection occurs, there are pain, fever, and the other symptoms of pelvic abscess. Obstructive symptoms may be increased. Rupture of the abscess may occur, and in such cases the parasitic elements may be so much destroyed that they are overlooked in the pus.

The *diagnosis* is usually difficult. Since most of the patients are not of "the prostatic age," benign hypertrophy and carcinoma seldom come into question. The obstructive symptoms will indicate a thorough urologic examination. Rectal or vaginal examination discloses a *rounded*, usually *firm* and smooth *tumor* which is not tender. In the male it is usually located anterior to the rectum and above the prostate, which can often be delimited from the mass. This is important to rule out prostatic enlargements. The seminal vesicles are usually completely obscured. Fluctuation in the cyst is exceptional. The upper pole of the cyst may be felt suprapubically.

Urethral instrumentation is often difficult, owing to *displacement* or *distortion* of the urethra. *Cystoscopic* examination shows usually only the deformation of the bladder cavity. With obstruction there is residual urine. *Catheterization* will disclose whether the suprapubic tumor, if present, is a distended bladder or not.

In cases where the cyst presents suprapubically, it is usually, in the presence of urinary difficulty or retention, taken for a *distended bladder*. In such cases catheterization, when possible, discloses this error. When impossible, suprabubic puncture has sometimes been done, yielding not urine but *cyst fluid*. In other cases the catheter has been passed into the cyst, with the same results. The smooth, round tumor, suggesting a cyst, even though not fluctuant, has been punctured through the rectum in certain instances. All of these procedures, of course, are incorrect. The mistaken suprapubic puncture is probably unavoidable in some cases, but should always be preceded by a careful rectal examination. Where a definite infravesical tumor is present, puncture of the bladder can give only temporary relief at best. Rectal puncture is to be unqualifiedly condemned, regardless of what disease is present. Of 6 of Deming's series in which this was done, 4 died from the resulting infection.

The lesions coming most into question are *retrovesical sarcoma, cyst of the utricle* (Müllerian duct cyst), and *abscess* of the *prostate* or *seminal vesicles*. Only infected cysts suggest the last. Masses may be found in the liver, which, of course, does not rule out sarcoma. The only exploratory puncture justifiable is perineal puncture, provided it is made with strict asepsis, and provided the discovery of hydatid material is followed by immediate operation. If this is done, or if any cyst fluid becomes available in any way, its character is diagnostic. It is *water-clear*, of *low specific gravity*, and contains no *albumin*. No other cyst produces such a fluid. *Hooklets* or *scolices* may be found in it. The sediment should be used, as these elements are heavy and soon settle to the bottom. If the cyst is infected, hooklets may be found in the sedimented pus. In case of puncture, thorium, sodium iodid, or perhaps better the antiseptic medium of Cunningham, Graves, and Davis[1] may be injected and an *x*-ray taken (Fig. 190). This is especially valuable in the detection of multiple cysts. If antigen is available, the *serologic tests* described above simplify the diagnosis greatly.

If rupture occurs, the diagnosis is unescapable.

The *treatment* of *pelvic hydatid* is along the same principles as described for the kidney, with the addition of measures to relieve the urinary obstruction. Previous procedures based on incorrect diagnosis complicate the treatment. Total excision is rarely possible, and, therefore, *marsupialization* is the method of choice. This is best done suprapubically when possible, but if the cyst is low, the perineal route may be used. Every effort should be made to remove the parasitic material completely. If puncture has been made, through mistake or for diagnosis, operation should follow immediately. The urinary obstruction is usually relieved when the cyst is evacuated.

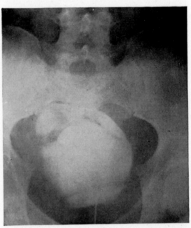

Fig. 190.—Shadowgram of a case of retrovesical echinococcus cyst obtained by filling the cyst with thorium through a needle inserted through the perineum. The cyst contents were purulent, owing to a previous puncture done elsewhere through the rectum. B. U. I. *x*-Ray 3040.

If not, a retention catheter or even surgical drainage is necessary. The urinary sinus in such cases should be made as far from the opening of the cyst as possible.

The complications to be feared are *infection* and *uremia*. Marsupialization provides drainage if infection be present. Uremia is combated by the usual procedures, and if ureteral obstruction persists, as indicated by anuria or polyuria of low specific gravity, nephrostomy may be necessary.

Another unfavorable possibility is the presence of *multiple cysts*. Exploration should be thorough, to disclose them if present. This is a strong point in favor of abdominal operation, as perineally it is scarcely possible to open, or even discover, any but the lowest of the cysts.

In Deming's series, 41 of the 48 were treated surgically. Of these, 14 died and 1 developed incontinence. Data on recurrence is lacking. Secondary infection following suprapubic or rectal puncture caused 40 per cent. of the deaths,

[1] Journal of Urology, 1923, x, 255–260. One gram of mercuric iodid is added to 3000 c.c. of 12 per cent. solution of sodium iodid. The double salt, potassium-mercuric iodid, which is strongly germicidal, is formed.

and in a number of cases unsuitable operations were performed because of faulty diagnosis. This emphasizes the importance of a correct diagnosis and suitable treatment in these cases.

OTHER ANIMAL PARASITES

Dichotophyme Renale.—This parasite (also called Dichotophyme gigas or Eustrongylus gigas) is a nematode worm of which the male is 14 to 35 cm. long and 4 to 6 mm. in diameter, the female 25 to 100 cm. long and 4 to 12 mm. in diameter. It resembles Ascaris closely, except for its size and red color. It occurs principally in the kidneys of carnivorous animals, but has been found in cattle. It is extremely rare in man, 6 cases according to Niçaise,[1] 12 cases according to Castellani.[2]

Since dogs cannot be infested by feeding the ova it is supposed that there is an intermediate host, but it has not as yet been identified. There is reason to suppose that it is a fish. The means by which the embryo reaches the kidney is uncertain. It may go directly, without entering the blood, since specimens have been found free in the peritoneal cavity. In the kidney, the parasite occupies the pelvis. There may be one, or as many as eight individuals. As they grow, the kidney is destroyed as by hydronephrosis. Infection sooner or later is the rule, producing a pyonephrosis. A worm may leave the kidney, as specimens have been found in the ureter and bladder and Moscato[3] describes a case in which the complete worm was passed per urethram, with relief of symptoms.

The *symptoms* are pain and hematuria, with those of pyonephrosis added if infection has occurred. One patient described by d'Aubinais[4] was conscious of the movements of the worm in his kidney.

The *diagnosis* is made by discovery of the ova, which are regularly in the urine. They are ovoid, with a thick capsule, 68 to 80 μ by 40 to 43 μ in size.

Nephrectomy would no doubt be the proper *treatment* if the other kidney were sound. It is possible that the parasite could be killed by intrapelvic injections, but it is doubtful if it would be expelled afterward.

Myiasis.[5]—This condition is caused by the larvæ of various flies (maggots) which ascend the urethra, and is commonest in paralytics. If there is sufficient expulsive force, they are usually expelled spontaneously, but in paralyzed bladders may set up or aggravate a cystitis. The diagnosis is made by examination of the urine and cystoscopy, the treatment is obvious.

There may also be a vaginal myiasis. In these cases it is to be suspected that pre-existent ulcerations have attracted the insects.

Various wounds and ulcerations may be invaded by maggots in hot weather.

Canthariasis.[6]—This is a similar condition due to invasion by larvæ of Coleoptera (beetles). Few cases are reported, and in them one suspects that the larvæ were introduced by the patient. They are treated like any other foreign body.

Dracunculus Medinensis.—The guinea-worm may occasionally be found be-

[1] Encyclopædie Française d'Urologie, 1914, iii, 126–129.

[2] Castellani and Chalmers: Manual of Tropical Medicine, New York, 3d ed., 1920.

[3] Quoted by Fantham, Stephens, and Theobald: The Animal Parasites of Man, New York, 1916.

[4] Journal de la Section de Médecine de la Société Académique du Département de la Loire, livraison cvi, Revue Médicale, 1846, 569 (quoted by Niçaise).

[5] Castellani and Chalmers: Manual of Tropical Medicine, New York, 3d ed., 1920.

[6] Ibid.

neath the skin of the scrotum, or even more rarely in the testis itself.   In the latter case the testis is destroyed.

Flukes.—Sparganum mansoni and Sparganum prolifer, flukes which occasionally infest man, have been found in a few cases in the kidney.

Platyhelminthes.—Tapeworm larvæ may occur in the urogenital system in general infestations.   The commonest variety is that of Tænia solium (Cysticercus cellulosæ).   It is probable that no symptoms would be caused unless, for example, the cyst happened to obstruct a ureter—a remote possibility.[1]

PROTOZOA

Amebæ.—Amebæ occur rarely in the urinary tract.   They have usually been identified as Loeschia histolytica (*Entamœba histolytica*).   While some cases have been those in which enterovesical fistula occurred in patients suffering from amebic dysentery, in others there was no such fistula.   Lesions may apparently be caused in the bladder, or the kidney itself may be involved, with the clinical picture of pyelitis or pyelonephritis.   The *diagnosis* could only be made by discovering the organisms in the urine; the *treatment* would be with emetin, as in amebic dysentery.   Dobell[2] gives an excellent critical review of the subject, and calls attention to the care which must be used in distinguishing certain cellular elements of infected urine from amebæ.

Ciliata: Trichomonas, Cercomonas, Prowazekia.—These and various other ciliata have been found in urethral discharges in tropical countries, but it is not known whether or not they are the cause thereof.

Coccidiosis.—This disease may affect the kidneys in animals, but does so extremely rarely in man.[3]

[1] A good account of animal parasites affecting the urogenital tract is given by Ransom, Nelson's Loose Leaf Medicine, New York, 1920, ii, 381–433.

[2] The Amœbæ Living in Man, New York, 1919, 125–129 (Lit.).

[3] Simon: Tice's Practice of Medicine, 1924, iv, 371–374.   Strong: Nelson's Loose Leaf Medicine, 1920, ii, 335–337.

CHAPTER VI

UROLITHIASIS

FORMATION

THE formation of stones in the urinary tract has long been a problem of the greatest interest and difficulty, both to pathologists and urologists. Since a large proportion of these stones have their origin in the kidney, the discussion of the general theories of stone formation will be taken up here, reserving only special considerations for the other urinary organs where lithiasis occurs.

While modern diagnostic methods have greatly improved the treatment of this condition, by enabling us to discover and remove calculi before they have caused great damage, yet the inability, from which we still suffer, surely to prevent recurrences makes the therapy of the disease unsatisfactory.

To understand the peculiar circumstances which surround the formation of a calculus, we must consider the chemical aspects of the urine. Among the substances which the kidney is called upon to excrete are some which are very slightly soluble in water, which is the urinary solvent. In this class the principal examples are uric acid and calcium oxalate. Other urinary constituents are somewhat more soluble, as the urates, with carbonates and phosphates following in ascending order, while such substances as urea, creatinin, and sodium chlorid are extremely soluble. The quantities of, for example, uric acid and calcium oxalate which must often be excreted daily from the body could not possibly be dissolved in a quantity of water equal to the average output of urine in twenty-four hours. It is evident, therefore, that some different mechanism comes into play here.

Everyone has noticed that not infrequently the voided urine contains a sediment composed of tiny crystals of uric acid, calcium oxalate, or the various phosphates already precipitated, yet many of these cases never show the slightest tendency toward stone formation. It is evident that a change in the urine which brings about a precipitation of such substances is not alone sufficient to cause the particles to cohere in the form of a stone.

What conditions are necessary for this? A great many theories have been put forward. Most of them have started with the idea that many substances exist in the urine in the form of supersaturated solutions. This phenomenon can be observed in simple watery solutions, and it is characteristic of it that if a small crystal of the substance in solution be inserted, it will immediately begin to grow by the deposition on it of that portion of the dissolved substance which is in excess over the true solubility. Upon this assumption, therefore, it has been thought that the existence of a nucleus is necessary for the formation of a stone. Similar conditions exist in the gallbladder, and here bacteria of various kinds have been found at the centers of gallstones. Acting on this hint, various investigators have found bacteria in the central portions of urinary stones. It has therefore been put forward that clumps of bacteria bits of mucus, mucopus, or desquamated epithelium, in general products of an inflammatory reaction, are the nuclei of all urinary stones not due to foreign bodies. Where stones exist in the absence of infection, it has been necessary to assume that a transitory inflammation, responsible for the inception of the stone, has since disappeared. The fact that the central portion of a stone often differs markedly from the peripheral portions has been held to support this theory.

These "nucleus" theories are, however, by no means satisfactory. In addition, they hold out little promise of practical therapy. Certain facts appear to be incompatible with them. In many stones it has been impossible to demonstrate any such nucleus. Many cases of extensive inflammation of portions of the urinary tract exist without any tendency to stone formation. "Nuclei" exist plentifully in many essentially normal patients, as desquamated epithelial cells, precipitated particles or crystals of urinary constituents, or, in case of mild renal disease, urinary casts, without any tendency to stone formation. Carnivorous animals show little tendency to stone formation, although their urine is habitually very concentrated. Pieces of urinary calculi placed in the bladders or kidney pelves of normal dogs do not grow, but may even decrease in size.

It has been shown by experiment that the urine does not follow accurately the laws of supersaturation in pure watery solution. Although a specimen of clear urine may contain many times the quantity of some constituent that could be dissolved in the same amount of water, yet the suspension of a crystal of the same substance in the urine does not lead to growth of the crystal. It is evident that the mere presence of a particle of any kind in the urine will not, in itself, cause the formation of a stone. The important element is some quality in the urine itself which causes it, in one case, to remain clear, in another, to deposit a fine sediment, and in a third, to form a stone.

In an effort to answer the many questions raised by these various observations, physical chemists have devoted much thought to the problem. Their findings can be no more than summarized here. At the beginning it should be noted that when the word "colloidal" is used it may have either of two connotations: (1) Crystalloids, which normally go into solution in water in a molecular solution, or ionized to a greater or less extent, may, under certain conditions, exist suspended in a fluid as small particles, the size of which may vary greatly, but which are always larger than a molecule. The crystalloid is then said to be in a state of "colloidal dispersion" or "colloidal suspension," which—and this is the important thing—is not inherent in the substance, but due to outside influences. (2) True colloids are those which always exist, in fluids, in a state of colloidal dispersion, and never ionize or go into molecular solution. This quality is inherent in the substances, and, while it may be altered in various ways by external influences, it is not dependent on them.

The fundamental discovery which has been made by physical chemists is that some of the urinary constituents exist in the urine normally in a state of colloidal dispersion. This explains why a specimen of clear urine may contain more, for example, uric acid or calcium oxalate than could be dissolved in the same quantity of water, and why urines "supersaturated" in this manner do not follow the same laws as supersaturated watery solutions.

The maintenance of this state of colloidal dispersion for substances which do not normally take that form is not due to the reaction of the urine, for changes in reaction do not affect it greatly. It appears to be due to what is known as the "protective action" of the true colloids of the urine. These true colloids are not albuminous in nature, and are present in all urines. They will not diffuse through a collodion membrane. Their nature is not thoroughly known, but certain workers have identified among them mucin, chondroitin-sulphuric acid, nucleic acid, "animal gum" or glycogen, and a nitrogen-containing complex carbohydrate. The quantity present is very small, but is increased in certain diseases, as pneumonia. The nature of the "protective action" is also not thoroughly known, but a familiar example of it is in the Lange colloidal-gold test for cerebrospinal fluid. An increase in certain colloids "protects" the colloidal gold, which otherwise goes on to an increase in the size of its particles, through various color changes to frank turbidity. The protective action does not depend on the quantity of true colloid present, but on its degree of dispersion and especially on its nature. Some colloids are much more active than others in this respect.

Another peculiarity of this action is that its greatest effect is seen on substances which are soluble with difficulty, while no effect is seen on easily soluble substances; in fact, their solubility is slightly lowered. Thus the true colloids of the urine have no effect of any moment on the urea, sodium chlorid, or creatinin present, and these substances are never seen in concretions, since they are very soluble, and depend for their solution on no special mechanism which is subject to derangement.

It has been further observed that where urates are held in colloidal suspension by the protective action of the true colloids, the particles gradually increase in size until until they are large enough to be visible under the ultramicroscope. The urine still remains macroscopically clear, and the addition of a urate crystal causes no precipitation. This state is quite different from a simple water solution of urate, since in such a solution the addition of acid causes precipitation, while the colloidal suspension of urates is most nearly stable at a slightly acid reaction. This is interesting in view of the fact that the normal urine is slightly acid. The condition is called by its discoverer[1] "intermediate droplet stabilization."

One more fact that should be noted is that in any solution or colloidal suspension the dissolved or suspended particles tend to accumulate at any point where the surface tension is increased. Normally the surface tension between the urine and the healthy urinary mucosa is practically zero. In contact with air, glass, foreign substances, etc., the surface tension is raised, and an accumulation takes place, illustrated by the "pellicle" which often forms when urine stands in contact with air.

What relation have these facts to urinary stone formation? It has been observed that when a solution containing a crystalloid urinary constituent and a very small quantity of a true colloid (fibrin, 0.07–0.1 per cent.) is so treated that both are precipitated simultaneously, a mass is formed. The colloid is in the form of a "clot" or "gel" and holds the particles of the crystalloid in its meshes. The "gel" then contracts, according to rule, and the end-result is a mass the shape and consistence of a urinary stone, having the same concentric layers and radial striation. (It should be stated here that "stones" comprised entirely of a true colloid are sometimes, very rarely, found; the so-called "albumen-stones" of the bladder or peritoneal cavity.) Many urinary stones contain, on analysis, varying quantities of organic material in addition to the principal constituent of the stone.

On the other hand, some stones contain only a single substance, and arise in

[1] Schade: Die Physikalische Chemie in der Inneren Medizin, 1920, 296–347.

individuals where no infection can be demonstrated, and where the entire urinary tract is to all appearances normal. A study of such stones shows that they are formed of the substance not in its normal crystalline form, but in a form erroneously called "atypical crystals" which is in reality the form taken by the substance when it collects by further agglutination or mutual coherence of the particles in the "intermediate droplet stabilization" suspension. Such concretions have been formed experimentally, and their formation, far from depending upon the simultaneous precipitation of the true colloids, cannot occur unless their precipitation is entirely prevented. Observations of this sort have given rise to the belief that the "protective action" of true colloids consists of a localized accumulation of the particles of the true colloid about the aggregations of the particles of the temporary colloid, forming a sort of membrane or pellicle which prevents further agglutination and consequent growth of the particles. This type of stone formation, then, would seem to depend on some influence which inhibits or overcomes the protective action of the true colloids, which, of course, are always present in urine. As we have seen, this might be a change in the state of dispersion of the true colloids, a change in their chemical nature, or a tremendous excess of the temporary colloid to a point where the protective action is insufficient. In favor of the last possibility are experiments where stones have been produced experimentally in animals by overloading the urine with some substance. Thus oxalate stones have been formed by injecting into the animal repeatedly large doses of calcium chlorid and a soluble oxalate, as sodium oxalate or butyl oxalate, simultaneously, but at different places, or oxamid stones by giving oxamid by mouth. Oxamid is a poorly soluble substance which is excreted unchanged by the kidney.

Changes in surface tension will also cause stones to form, as is seen in incrusted cystitis or when foreign bodies are present in the urinary tract. Since such stones are practically inevitably associated with infection, the mechanism of their primary formation is somewhat conjectural, but it is obvious that a foreign body collects calcareous material much more rapidly in some cases than in others, showing that the state of the urine has much to do with the process. It is further noteworthy that when the character of the foreign body is such that little or no increase of surface tension is caused, as, for example, a clean piece of pure paraffin, no stone formation occurs.

Experiments aiming to show the rôle of infection have been, as a rule, indecisive. Extensive chronic inflammations may exist without stone formation. Infection, however, undoubtedly has a great deal to do with the course and results of stone. The presence of a stone in the urinary tract usually, sooner or later, induces by its irritation an infection, presumably hematogenous. Under the influence of this change, in addition to changes in composition of the urine brought about by obstruction from the stone, the reaction of the urine may be altered and its true colloids much increased, so that a stone beginning by simple coherence of particles of a temporary colloid may have its outer layers of an entirely different composition, and put down according to the first mechanism described, i. e., simultaneous precipitation of true and temporary colloids.

Rosenow has reported experiments in which a focus of infection produced in the teeth of animals by streptococci obtained from the urine of patients with urinary calculi has caused similar calculi to appear in the kidneys of the animals. These experiments, extremely important in that they indicate that the conditions favoring stone formation are brought about by the specific action of certain organisms, have not at present been confirmed by other workers.

The importance of infection is, however, so obvious that every effort should be made to eliminate or prevent it in the urinary tract to forestall any stone formation to which it might give rise.

The modern ideas of stone formation have inspired some important therapeutic suggestions.

There is no reason why stones formed by simple agglutination of particles of a temporary colloid should not be reversible and resoluble, so that if the urine can be so diluted as to cause it to be unsaturated in the substance composing the stone, it should be slowly redissolved. Careful chemical examination of the urine will show whether it is overloaded with the substance in question, and if so, it should be possible to reduce it by managing the diet and increasing the fluid intake. True colloids when precipitated may be in reversible or irreversible form. If a stone has a colloidal "matrix" which is reversible, it should be possible, by properly altering the urine as to concentration, composition, reaction, etc., to cause the matrix to be redissolved. Experiments with such stones outside the body show that if the matrix is dissolved away, the crystalloid constituents of the stone do not cohere, but reduce themselves to a fine sediment. Such a process may account for the occasional spontaneous fracture of stones, or the reduction of a firm stone to a crumbly mass. If the matrix is irreversible, only some external influence could have any effect on it. On this theory it has been proposed to introduce into the bladder a proteolytic ferment such as trypsin, which in an alkaline urine should dissolve the matrix and allow the stone to crumble. A number of cases are on record where there was strong evidence of dissolution of stones, and spontaneous fracture is not infrequently seen. Klemperer[1] reports the solution of cystin stones after the ingestion of large quantities of sodium bicarbonate, and in a recent case of Crowell[2] a large renal cystin calculus was completely dissolved in this manner despite the presence of infection. It must be said that these suggestions, interesting and fundamental as they are, have not as yet been put to full and satisfactory test. Enough has been learned, however, to foster the hope that should these investigations be crowned with success, the treatment of urinary lithiasis will become almost entirely medical. It would be a great comfort to the urologist to be able to assure his patient, when operation became necessary, that no further formation of stone would take place.

COMPOSITION

In analyzing calculi, one distinguishes between the primary or original formation, and the more peripheral layers of secondary formation, which may be of quite different composition. The secondary formation often constitutes by far the greater part of the stone. To get an idea of the origin of the trouble, however, one should always know the nature of the primary nucleus. The secondary portion of the stone may contain several urinary constituents, and in addition foreign substances such as methylene-blue, when that drug has been given by mouth, silver compounds, mercurochrome, etc., which have been injected, and blood pigments

---

[1] Therapie der Gegenwart, 1914, xvi, 101–103.

[2] Transactions of the American Association of Genito-urinary Surgeons, 1923, xvi, 169–181. See also Harris: Surgery, Gynecology, and Obstetrics, 1924, xxxviii, 640–645 (Lit.).

consequent upon hemorrhage. The amount of albuminous substances may be increased by the presence of a purulent exudate. Stones colored by silver or hemoglobin may be almost black.

Ultzmann states that of 545 nuclei of calculi examined, 80.9 per cent. were composed of uric acid, 5.6 per cent. of calcium oxalate, 8.6 per cent. of phosphates of the alkaline earths, 1.4 per cent. of cystin, and 3.3 per cent. of some foreign body. The secondary formation, according to Hammarsten, most frequently consists largely of phosphates, and is a mixture of alkaline earth phosphates with triple phosphates. Often there is an admixture of some ammonium urate and calcium oxalate.

Uric Acid.—Pure uric acid stones are quite hard, and generally colored with variable shades of yellowish brown. They may be smooth, or show a surface covered by small, closely set, characteristic warty protuberances. These correspond in general contour to the agglomerations of colloidal uric acid.

Ammonium Urate.—The primary stones of this substance occur oftenest in young children. The color is a shade of yellow. They are characteristically soft and doughy and when dry tend to crumble easily.

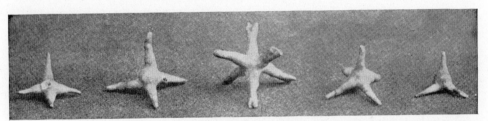

Fig. 191.—Five jackstone calculi removed from the bladder of a man aged eighty-four with prostatic hypertrophy and complete retention of urine. The large central calculus is in the form of a perfect jackstone with branches at right angles and of equal length (Halsted[1]).

Calcium Oxalate.—These stones are the hardest formed in human beings. They may be smooth, rough, or pronged, the so-called mulberry and the jackstone calculi (Fig. 191). The color is generally dark, but since they are apt, by their irregularity, to cause bleeding, it is occasionally almost black from blood pigment.

Phosphates.—Phosphate calculi are usually mixed with other substances. They are of moderate hardness. They contain mixtures of normal sodium, potassium, and calcium phosphates and triple phosphate. The color is light, but the stones are often discolored from various causes. In rare cases, stones of pure triple phosphate or mono-acid calcium phosphate may be found. These last are white.

Calcium Carbonate.—Herbivorous animals are prone to form calcium carbonate stones. In man they are comparatively infrequent. They are whitish in color and chalky in consistence.

The above-mentioned calculi all arrest the x-rays, and, therefore, throw shadows on the plates. The following forms throw no shadows, or less distinct ones, and, while comparatively infrequent, are important in that they may not be disclosed by roentgenographic examination.

Cystin.—These stones are of moderate hardness, may be smooth or rough, and have a yellow or yellowish-white color. They are the least uncommon of those

[1] Johns Hopkins Hospital Reports, 1900, ix, 1047–1059.

which cast a light shadow with the x-ray.   They occur only in patients with cystin-uria, which is a familial disease.   Large cystin stones are visible in roentgenograms.

Xanthin.—Xanthin stones are very rare.   They are of medium hardness, and appear somewhat waxy when rubbed.

Urostealith.—The composition of these stones is not entirely clear, but appears to be mostly of fatty acids and fat.   There is a suspicion that some of them are really foreign bodies, such as masses of paraffin or lard, which have been inserted in the bladder.   They are rare.

Cholesterin.—A few cases of pure cholesterin stones have been described.   They are rare.

Fibrin.—These are the "albumin stones" mentioned in the literature.   It is possible that they begin as blood-clots or masses of coagluated inflammatory exudate.   Rovsing believes that they are ordinary stones from which the mineral matter has been dissolved, leaving only the organic matrix.   They are exceedingly rare.   In a number of cases there have been described as "fibrin" stones certain soft, putty-like structures containing various quantities of urinary salts.   Some have felt that these merely represent cases where the true colloid "matrix" is in much greater abundance than usual.

Leucin stones are very rare.   They occur only in cases of leucinuria.   In a case of Pincoffs[1] there were a number of large concretions in the parenchyma, while all the convoluted tubules were filled with smaller masses of the same material.

For the detailed methods of analyzing stones chemically the reader is referred to the various works on chemistry and laboratory technic.

The deposition of urates and oxalates may occur in acid or alkaline urine, while the phosphates and carbonates are thrown down only in alkaline urine.   For this reason the occurrence of an infection with some organism, usually the Proteus, which splits urea, will change the mechanism of the process entirely, and from the time it occurs the outer coat or "secondary" layer of phosphates will begin to be formed.

PATHOLOGY

Kidney.—The great majority of all stones which do not arise upon foreign bodies and which are not in the nature of localized incrustations on an ulcerated surface, form originally in the calyces or pelvis of the kidney.   Since stone forma-tion is a slow process, and since stones begin as very small structures, the form of the urinary tract will have much to do with their subsequent history.   If the tract is everywhere quite normal, if there are no pockets, dependent sacs, or undue narrowings, if the muscular tissues are well developed, the tiny calculi will pass uninterruptedly out of the body.   Consequently, *retention* in any form is a most important factor.   If the stone is arrested at any point, it may lodge there and continue to grow.   A theory opposed to this is that the stone, in the beginning, adheres to the mucosa—presumably over a point of inflammation, and, therefore, is not free to pass out.   This has not been proved, but has been invoked in cases where, with stone in the kidney, there was no evidence of obstruction or sacculation to account for the retention of the stone.

If a stone passes out of the kidney it may still do harm, but the pathology of such conditions will be discussed under the sections on Calculi of the Ureter, Bladder, and Urethra.

[1] Personal communication.

If it is retained in the kidney, it may be due to a narrowing, congenital or inflammatory, of the ureteropelvic junction, or to external influences, such as nephroptosis, aberrant vessels, etc.

If it is true that stones are sometimes held in the pelvis by adhesion, they may grow to such a size that they cannot enter the ureter. Stones may be held in a calyx by an abnormally small orifice into the pelvis, or in one part of the pelvis by a constriction or hour-glass shape of the pelvis itself. If the lower portion of the pelvis is more dependent than normal, or if the ureter enters the pelvis unusually high, stones may remain by gravity at the inferior pole of the pelvis. It is questionable whether stones ever develop in the kidney tubules. They are sometimes seen apparently lying in the kidney substance, but this may be due to ulceration of a calyx. We once saw a case (B. U. I. 10,418) in which a solitary cortical cyst had developed behind a small stone, lying either in the renal substance or at the tip of the calyx. While it must have obstructed some tubules, yet it may not have arisen in the parenchyma.

It is a general truth concerning urinary calculi that they do not necessarily cause an obstruction at the point at which they are arrested. Variability in this regard brings about two radically different pictures in kidney stones. In one of them, the typical case shows a stone, which may be of quite small size, lying free in the pelvis, or impacted at the ureteropelvic junction. Such a stone may lie harmlessly in the most dependent portion of the pelvis, or it may cause any degree of obstruction. It thus often happens that a small stone in this manner causes the most extreme degree of renal destruction.

In the other picture, the stone, arrested at a constriction in the pelvis, or in the neck of a calyx, may grow to great size, following the general outlines of the pelvis, without causing marked obstruction. It may ultimately destroy the kidney by direct pressure of the stone itself. The condition may be painless in the absence of obstruction. In fairly numerous cases the first symptoms occur when the stone, by continuous growth, sends a process down the mouth of the ureter itself, causing obstruction. Such stones, forming more or less perfect casts of the pelvis, are known as "stag-horn" or "coral" calculi. If, however, the stone causes obstruction at its point of arrest, a local or partial hydronephrosis, involving only those calyces or parts of the pelvis cut off from the general pelvic cavity, occurs.

In general, then, and excluding the effects of infection, the extent of renal damage compared to the size of the stone depends wholly on whether or not obstruction has occurred.

If *obstruction* occurs the changes in the kidney are those which have been fully described under the heading of Hydronephrosis. *Infection* is so apt to occur when there is a stone in the kidney that it is difficult to know what proportion of cases are uninfected at the beginning. The statistics of any clinic would include many cases in which the infection was secondary. When infection occurs, its course is that described under Infections of the Kidney, except that the presence of the stone itself is a complication, which acts by pressure and local irritation in its own immediate vicinity. Therefore, in an infected stone case, ulceration of the mucosa is especially apt to occur at points adjacent to the stone. The rôle which infection plays in the further development of stones has already been discussed.

Where obstruction occurs late, as in the example previously mentioned, the development of hydronephrosis may be limited by scar tissue already laid down as the result of direct injury by the stone. If a stone causes a complete and sudden obstruction, the resulting hydronephrosis will be much smaller than that following partial or intermittent obstruction.

Where no obstruction occurs, the stone may grow until it fills the pelvis entirely. It encroaches upon the renal tissue, causing actual pressure necrosis and absorption. The parts first involved are the pelvis itself, the pyramids, and the lower portions of the vascular columns. The normal cells are replaced by fibrous tissue. Similar effects gradually make themselves felt in all parts of the kidney, and in addition the scarring of the peripelvic tissues infringes on both the blood-vessels and the collecting tubules. The nutrition of the kidney is, therefore, interfered with, and dilated tubules or retention cysts may be seen. Infection is the rule at some stage of this long-drawn-out process, and adds its destructive influence to those already mentioned.

It sometimes happens that a single calyx or a portion of the pelvis will be completely cut off by a septum of scar tissue, the result of irritation from the stone itself or infection. A hydronephrotic condition ensues in that part of the kidney isolated by the septum. That such an occurrence may possibly be due to the presence of stone and not to infection is suggested by a case reported by Kelly, in which the hydronephrotic portion of such a kidney was uninfected, while the remainder, containing the stone, was the seat of a severe pyelonephritis with abscesses.

The microscopic picture of such a "stone-kidney" is that of a chronic pyelonephritis, with scattered areas of fibrosis and round-cell infiltration which ultimately spread until they involve the whole kidney. In addition, one sees the direct encroachment, due probably to pressure necrosis, on the tissues near the pelvis, often with ulceration. If neither infection nor obstruction supervenes, the destruction may be well confined to the zone immediately adjacent to the pelvis, and the renal function surprisingly well preserved even in kidneys where the calculus is so large and complicated in form that its removal is impossible without the most extensive mutilation of the kidney.

Case: Very large stag-horn calculi in both kidneys.

B. U. I. 8479, age thirty-three. An interesting point in the history is that there was pneumonia at twenty-one, complicated by pulmonary abscess, which was operated upon and which caused a long illness. Symptoms began six months before admission, with fever, chills, and pain in the left kidney region. Examination showed pyuria and extensive bilateral kidney stones. The phthalein was 20 per cent. the first hour, 15 per cent. the second hour. Ureter catheterization showed that all of this was coming from the right side. Nephrotomy showed that the left kidney was the seat of a pyonephrosis, while the stones had almost destroyed the cortex. Although only one suture was taken, the hemorrhage being stopped by packing, no more than a trace of phthalein was ever recovered at any later time. Although the stones in the right kidney continued to grow, the function improved to as much as 30 per cent. in one hour, appearance time fifteen minutes. This improvement was maintained for one and a half years, with one period of hospital treatment by rest in bed and forced fluids. Pain in the right side then became more severe. Two years after the first operation examination showed the stones increased in size, the total phthalein, appearance twenty-three minutes, first hour 10 per cent., second hour 5 per cent. An effort to remove the stones proved fatal. Autopsy showed the left kidney reduced to a very small, thin lappet, while the right kidney, which had carried on the entire function for two years, had been made into a very thin sac by the enormous stones.

This progressive destruction is accompanied by the contraction characteristic of scar tissue so that the kidney, typical of non-obstructing stones, is a small, irregular contracted kidney. In some extreme cases the kidney is only a thin sheet of dense scar tissue in which no trace of tubules or glomeruli can be found, overlying a large stag-horn calculus. The fatty capsule is increased, and often woven through with many bands of scar tissue resulting from extension of an infective process to the perirenal tissues. Such a case may well be called a true "autonephrectomy" (Fig. 192). As a rule, however, unbearable symptoms supervene before this stage is reached. Often a stone involves only one or a few calices,

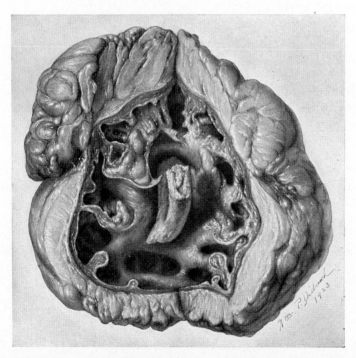

FIG. 192.—Nephrectomy. The kidney is extremely contracted and consists almost entirely of scar tissue. Pelvis is filled with a large calculus. The perirenal fat is indurated and increased in amount. Absolutely no symptoms until two months before operation when following an acute cold, pain in region of kidney came on. Pathologic condition evidently of much longer duration. B. U. I. 3836.

and exactly similar changes occur in its neighborhood, while the rest of the kidney remains essentially normal, except as it is influenced by intercurrent infection.

If the inflammation extends to the perirenal tissue by extension or by rupture of the capsule, and becomes more fulminant, a definite *perirenal abscess* (*q. v.*) may develop. This may point in the lumbar region, or may burrow in various other directions, as detailed in the section on Infections of the Kidney.

Case: *Long-standing complete destruction of kidney due to calculi.*

An interesting case was that of a young man who came here complaining of a sinus in the left lumbar region. He had had previous operation for supposed tuberculous disease of the lumbar spine, but the sinus simply discharged seropus. Cystoscopy was carried out as a routine measure; the right ureteral orifice was normal, but the left ureter was found not to function. The ridge was atrophic and there was no movement suggesting peristalsis. The orifice was extremely minute. x-Ray showed a fairly large group of stones in the region of left kidney and when nephrectomy was carried out the kidney was found to be a mere fibrous sac closely investing the calculi. The ureter was blocked. No urine was secreted.

It sometimes happens that a renal stone is extruded through the perforation in the kidney and comes to lie in the perirenal tissues. This is a very rare occurrence. Even more rarely, if the stone is single, the kidney may heal after this extrusion and resume its function. Such an extruded stone may remain *in situ* if the abscess heals, or be discharged through a spontaneous sinus or an operative wound. The presence of a stone, either inside or outside the kidney when a perinephric abscess has opened spontaneously or by simple incision, tends, like that of a foreign body, to keep up the inflammation. Such sinuses may, therefore, discharge pus for long periods—many years. In stone cases sinuses are perhaps more apt to become fistulæ than in other conditions since, if the stone has any obstructive action the urine must seek exit through the opening to the outside, and healing cannot occur. The rule that a urinary fistula above an obstruction cannot be expected to heal holds good throughout the entire urinary tract. If the extension of the inflammatory process to the perirenal tissues takes place by actual rupture of the capsule and cortex, and there is also obstruction from stone, urine will be mixed with the contents of the abscess. In that case, the inflammation will spread more rapidly, with necrosis and the severe toxic reaction common to all urinary extravasations.

The direction of spread follows the same rules as in perinephric abscess, and the tumefaction may, therefore, not be evident at the surface. If the extension is retroperitoneal and downward, it is sometimes first appreciated on rectal examination. Rupture into the peritoneum leads to general peritonitis.

In rare cases where extravasation takes place very slowly, there may develop an extrarenal urinary cyst.

It must always be kept in mind, however, that stone in the kidney is a destructive process, the destruction being hastened by infection. It is an important matter, therefore, to preserve to the patient every bit of functional renal tissue possible. The operation should be no more extensive than is absolutely necessary, and nephrectomy should not be done with a light heart, since we know that recurrence of stone in the opposite kidney may easily happen. This is especially true if the opposite kidney is already infected.

The following table shows the distribution of the stones in our series of 184 cases:

TABLE 46

	Single.	Multiple.	Number not stated.	Total.	Percentage.
Right..................	49	20	0	69⎫	71.7
Left..................	39	24	0	63⎬132	(unilateral)
Bilateral..............	1	30	0	31	17.0
Side not noted..........	0	1	20	21	
Total................	89	75	20	184	

Ureter.—The effects of a stone arrested at the ureteropelvic junction have already been described. If, however, a stone enters the ureter, it may pass through into the bladder, or be arrested at any point along the ureter. While it is in the ureter, it may or may not obstruct the flow of urine but usually does so. The obstruction may be complete or partial. A round, smooth stone is more apt to cause obstruction, while an irregular or spiculated one may allow more or less urine to pass. We have seen, in a child, a stone with a hole through the middle, like a bead. This, however, did cause obstruction, as shown by hydro-ureter and hydro-nephrosis. In another case a stone, about the length and thickness of a small cigar, had been lodged in the left ureter for years (ten years or more) and gave no symptoms. On removal it was found to be grooved, so that urine passed down unimpeded—this accounting for the absence of pain. Blood-clots from hemorrhage caused by the stone and edema of the mucosa may increase the obstruction.

The irritation from the obstruction, or from the stone itself, is very apt to cause renal colic. In rare cases, however, a stone may be extruded from the ureter without colic. The spasmodic contractions during colic must retain some semblance of order, as stones may be passed into the bladder during colic. The stone may exercise a certain dilating effect on the ureter, for after being arrested for a long time, it may be able to pass on. Stones may travel the length of the ureter in an hour or so, or may take as long, even, as six months. In a recent case a small stone blocked the ureter about 3 inches above the bladder and caused great pain. As soon as a catheter was passed to drain the kidney the pain ceased and did not recur in the three days during which the catheter remained in the ureter, which was thus distended by both stone and catheter at the point of lodgment. It is evident, therefore, that the pain is usually due to obstruction and the overdistention of the urinary tract above the stone, and not to pressure upon the ureteral wall by the stone or to spasm at that point.

If the stone is arrested, temporarily or permanently, this usually occurs at one of the normal constricted points of the ureter—opposite the iliac artery, at the mid-pelvic constriction, or in the intramural portion. A spiculated stone is more apt to be arrested at an unusual point. After arrest, the pathologic effects multiply. The effects of ureteral obstruction on the kidney, as we have seen, increase with time. Pressure from the stone injures the walls of the ureter, and infection may be present, and spread to the ureteral wall. The stone, being still bathed in urine, may continue to grow in size. The portion of the ureter above the stone may dilate, giving hydro-ureter. The obstruction may at any time become complete, or more nearly so.

The spread of infection to the ureteral wall may cause ulceration, and eventually scarring, with contraction and *stricture* formation, which may prevent a return to normal function even after the stone is removed. Extensive spread to the peri-ureteral tissues is rare.

Diffuse pain may be caused by pressure of the stone, either on the ureteral nerves or on those of contiguous structures, as the rectum, bladder, and seminal vesicle.

If arrested in the intramural portion of the ureter, the stone may ulcerate through the ureteral wall into the bladder.

Obstruction and colic may be caused by masses of crystals filling the ureter, or even the kidney pelvis, after intemperance in eating, with dehydration of the body.

Bladder.—Stones in the bladder may arise in that organ or be carried there from the kidneys. In very many cases of vesical calculus it is impossible to say where the stone has originated, though a history of previous renal colic may give a clue.

Immediately after a stone has been extruded from the ureter, the effects of its trauma will be visible at the ureteral orifice, which is surrounded by a halo of inflammation.

If the urinary tract is normal, any stone which can pass through the ureter will immediately be extruded through the urethra, often without the knowledge of the patient. We may say, then, that without an infravesical obstruction there will be no bladder calculi of renal origin. The failure of such a stone to leave the bladder is excellent evidence of the existence of an obstruction. However, a very slight obstruction, giving no urinary symptoms, may be sufficient to cause the retention of a small stone. If the stone is retained, it continues to increase in size in the bladder. If the composition and reaction of the urine are altered from time to time, as by infection, the material deposited on the calculus may vary, as already described. Infection is more apt to occur the longer the stone remains in the bladder, and if this is markedly alkaline in character (usually due to Bacillus proteus) the outer layers of the stone will be phosphatic.

Calculi may *originate* in the bladder either as deposits on foreign substances of various sorts, catheters, sutures, hairs from dermoid cysts, etc., or on the surface of inflammatory lesions. The foreign bodies concerned are of the most varied types. Every kind of foreign body will become encrusted except pure, clean paraffin. They may be introduced by the patient, usually as a means of masturbation, particularly in women where a great variety of objects may be found—hairpins, bonnet pins, needles, etc. In men absolutely extraordinary things which one would think impossible to introduce have been found in the middle of vesical calculi. Filiform bougies and catheters broken off during instrumentation are not uncommon, and shell fragments, bullets, and bits of clothing occasionally form the nuclei of calculi. Blood-clots, masses of coagulated exudate, or pieces of tissue may serve for the laying down of calcareous material, and may become the nuclei of stones. While ulcerated surfaces, from infection or neoplasm, by no means always produce calcareous deposits, they most often do so when the urine is strongly alkaline, and such deposits are usually phosphatic. They are usually seen as sand-like granules scattered over the surface of the lesion, giving rise to the term "encrusted cystitis." These granules may coalesce to form a dense layer, which can sometimes be lifted off the lesion intact, or the individual granules may grow, giving rise to multiple stones. It will be seen that calculi may arise in any of these fashions without infravesical obstruction, but the presence of stasis favors their formation and accelerates their growth. The rate at which these deposits occur is extremely variable, and depends, of course, on the composition and condition of the urine. Calculi 1 cm. in diameter may develop in a week or two, while we have seen a filiform which, after remaining in an infected bladder for five months, had only a few tiny grains of sand-like material adhering to it.

According to their origin, bladder calculi will be single or multiple. In some cases large calculi have been found which were broken into several pieces, the lines of fracture being recent. It has been claimed that this sometimes followed copious water drinking or changes in diet, and suggested that facetted stones may arise in this way. As multiple stones enlarge it is inevitable that their shape will be influenced by mutual pressure, so that such an explanation is not necessary. The occurrence of spontaneous fracture, however, is beyond doubt. We have seen one patient who had just returned from Saratoga Springs where he had drunk large quantities of water from the Congress Spring. On cystoscopy we saw nineteen clean-cut fragments into which a large calculus had broken.

The bladder may become completely filled with one large calculus, or with a number of smaller calculi with flat sides fitted neatly together. In other cases there are large quantities of gravel or sand-like concretions. Single calculi may grow to great size. The largest on record is that of Randall, which weighed 4 pounds (64 ounces). It measured around its greatest circumference 19 inches (48 cm.) and was about 6 inches in diameter. This calculus was removed suprapubically, but the patient died.[1] These enormous stones are now, fortunately, rare. Their size sometimes prevents removal, even at suprapubic operation, without forcible fracture with mallet and chisel. A most remarkable stone is to be seen in the Hunterian Museum, London. Mr. Cline attempted to remove this stone, which was about 5 inches in diameter, through the perineum (without anesthesia!). With a blacksmith's hammer and chisel he succeeded in breaking away a teacupful of fragments, when the patient's fortitude gave out! The patient died in a day or so.

Stone in the bladder irritates the surface, so that there is always a certain degree of reddening and congestion, even in the absence of infection. Hemorrhage is frequently caused, and this is more frequent with rough or spiculated calculi. Direct pressure of larger stones may cause ulceration. Stone favors the development of *infection* and bacterial *cystitis* is then added to the effects of direct trauma. Large single calculi or mutiple smaller ones filling the bladder may occlude the ureters by direct pressure. It is recorded that Sir William Ogilvie could only urinate when he stood on his head. This took the pressure off the ureters, which were so greatly dilated that they acted as bladders, and required only occasional emptying. There may be fibrotic stricture of the ureteral meatus from the inflammation.

Similarly, calculi may occlude the vesical orifice during micturition, either constantly or intermittently. In these cases patients are sometimes able to void by assuming reversed positions which allow the stone to fall into the bas-fond or vertex of the bladder. The results of trauma, inflammation, and infection may produce a fibrotic contracture of the vesical orifice, with obstruction.

In a bladder the seat of obstructive changes, calculi, which have developed in the kidney or elsewhere in the bladder, may drop into cellules or diverticula. In other cases stones originate in diverticula by incrustation of masses of pus or coagulated fibrin or blood when infection is present, or perhaps by the same mechanisms that give rise to kidney stones. Any of these processes is favored by the stasis always present in diverticula. We have seen cases with multiple small diverticula, nearly every one of which contained a calculus (one case had eight, while there was no stone free in the bladder). As a diverticular stone increases in size it may send a process out through the orifice. The process then enlarges at its tip in globular fashion, so that the entire calculus is shaped like a dumb-bell or sheaf of wheat. If the pedicle is small, fracture easily occurs, and the broken end remaining in the diverticulum may be missed, even at cystoscopy or operation. When this occurs, the condition will recur, even if the portion broken off in the bladder be removed by lithotomy or litholapaxy. We have reported 1 case in which seventeen operations for recurrent vesical calculus had been performed. On removing a large stone suprapubically we noticed a small stem, and at once realized that it must have connected with an encysted calculus. A most exhaustive search was necessary to find a small calculus concealed in a diverticulum at the vertex of the bladder. Diverticulectomy put an end to the recurrence of the calculi.[2] In this same paper a case with multiple calculi attached to silk sutures, which had been inserted to close

[1] Randall, A.: Journal of Urology, 1921, v, 119–125.

[2] Young: Transactions Southern Surgical and Gynecological Association, 1911.

a bladder injured in an operation for inguinal hernia, is recorded.   The calculi and sutures were removed with our cystoscopic rongeur, intravesically.   In another case, a calculus was seen at cystoscopy adhering to the anterior wall of the bladder. At operation the most careful search revealed no diverticulum or other explanation of this phenomenon.

Urethra.—Calculi seldom originate in the urethra, and when they do, it is usually when the urethra is much distorted by trauma or the results of inflammation.   Thus calculi occasionally arise in blind passages or diverticula of the urethra.   Those commonly found, however, have originated in the bladder or kidney and are arrested in their passage through the urethra.   This is somewhat more apt to happen in children, where there is not as much disparity in size between the ureter and urethra as in the adult.   In grown persons there will be in most cases an obstruction of some sort, usually an inflammatory stricture.   If this be present, the stone will lodge above it; if not, the usual point of arrest is at the external sphincter, or external layer of the triangular ligament.   Arrest may be at other points, however, as in the penile urethra, or not infrequently at the external meatus.   We had one patient who had been treated at several celebrated clinics, here and abroad, for pyuria, in whom we found a small calculus incarcerated in the fossa navicularis.   There was a urethral discharge, and he had even submitted to the indignity, at the age of sixty-five years, of being treated for "gonorrhea."   Calculi are not infrequently seen which lie both in the urethra and bladder.   The lower portion usually presents a cast of the dilated prostatic urethra (even showing the verumontanum).   The central portion is constricted by the internal sphincter, and the vesical portion is flattened out on the trigone.   In some of these cases it is difficult to say which started first, the vesical or the urethral portion.   We have seen one case in which a round oxalate calculus, nearly 1 inch in diameter, would escape (or be pushed by vesical spasm) into the prostatic urethra, where it would remain, causing the patient violent pain, until he was given morphin.   This would relax the spasm and allow the stone to escape back into the bladder.   This had occurred many times before he came to the hospital.   On one occasion we were able to push it back with a urethral sound.   In individuals with tight phimosis, a stone may be arrested in the preputial cavity.   Many such cases, mostly in children, have been reported from India.   The urethra, above an impacted calculus, may be greatly dilated.

In the presence of *infection* the ulceration due to impacted stone in the urethra may give rise to prostatitis or prostatic abscess, and peri-urethral inflammation or abscess, with or without extravasation or fistula formation.

Prostate and Seminal Vesicles.—Although prostatic and seminal calculi are not urinary calculi, they may well be considered at this point.   They arise by deposition from the secretion present in the ducts just as urinary calculi arise from urine.   The laws of their formation are undoubtedly the same.   They are usually composed of cholesterin.

Prostatic calculi are usually small, round, multiple, and dark colored.   They are generally hard, but may be of such consistence that they can be cut with a knife, suggesting a relation to corpora amylacea.   They usually occur in large numbers, millet seed in size, but they are often seen the size of bird shot, or 3, 4, 5, or even 8 mm. in diameter.   In other cases the stones may be larger and, if multiple, facetted on their adjoining surfaces.   They are often associated with benign prostatic hypertrophy, rarely with cancer, and usually with a chronic inflammatory change with increase of fibrous tissue. The effects of obstruction are usually not obvious, but cystic dilatation of acini may be seen.

Calculi in the seminal vesicles are rather rare. Most common are calcareous deposits in tuberculosis or other chronic inflammations. When true vesicular calculi occur, they are like prostatic calculi, though cases are reported in which compact masses of spermatozoa assumed stone-like hardness (Samensteine).

Stone-like bodies are very rarely found in the ductus epididymis, or in aberrant ducts or cysts at that locality.

SYMPTOMS

Kidney.—In renal calculus the symptoms are predominatingly local, since the disease in a majority of cases is unilateral. Where both sides are involved, where there is a coincident Bright's disease, where one kidney is missing, either congenitally or from previous operation, or where a congenitally atrophic or infantile kidney is present on the opposite side, the general symptoms of renal insufficiency may complicate the picture.

The most important and constant symptom is *pain*. This may be of an aching character, more or less *constant*, or *colicky*. The aching pain has no necessary relation to obstruction. It is oftenest felt in the loin just below the last rib in the region known as the kidney region. It may, however, be more general over the lower back, or radiate like the sharper pain of colic, down into the groin or genitalia, and to the leg. It may be brought on or increased by muscular exertion or sudden and unaccustomed movements. In rare cases it may be most pronounced in the lower abdominal quadrant, or may radiate to the opposite loin, the umbilicus, or the scapular region of the same side. These cases are especially apt to be ascribed to other abdominal diseases, and may be operated upon therefor.

The so-called *renal colic* is more characteristic of kidney conditions. It may have a definite relation to obstruction, but not necessarily so, since it is seen in cases where no obstruction can be demonstrated. In typical cases the attacks come on suddenly with severe pain in the "kidney region" and from there it quickly radiates downward in the abdomen to the groin, scrotum (or vulva), and the anterior surface of the thigh. Sometimes the testicle is retracted and a sickening "gonad pain" is present. Less often the pain also follows the general course of the ureter, and may extend down to the end of the penis in men, or to the vulva in women. Sometimes it shoots down the leg, even as far as the ankle. Rarely it may radiate in atypical directions, as to the opposite kidney, the so-called "renorenal reflex"[1] or to the homolateral scapular region. The pain, while sometimes mild, is usually severe, and in extreme cases appears to be as severe as any that patients are called on to endure. Ordinary doses of morphin are sometimes without effect. The patient often states that the pain "doubled him up," and that he was completely incapacitated by it. Nausea, often with vomiting, is almost the rule. The intestines may become constipated and distended with gas during the attacks. The duration of the attack is usually from four to twelve hours, but it may end in a few minutes, or last several days. While common in cases of stone in the kidney, "renal colic" is by no means confined to this condition. Its cause seems to be anything which irritates the interior of the urinary tract, *e. g.*, a stone, a ureteral

[1] See paper by Johnson: Transactions American Association Genito-urinary Surgeons, 1907, ii, 273–281.

catheter, a strong chemical irritant.   When associated with distention, as in obstruction, it seems to be more severe.   When the pain originates in the ureter it is known as ureteral colic, and shows certain slight clinical differences, as will be taken up in the section on the Ureter.

Renal colic depends upon strong spasmodic constrictions of the smooth muscle of the pelvis and ureter.   The peristaltic sequence is, however, apparently preserved, since, during the contractions, small stones, blood-clots, etc., may move down the ureter.

Statistics show that there is colic at some period in about one-half the cases of kidney stone.   It may be superimposed upon the fixed pain, may alternate with it in any fashion, or may be entirely independent of it.

The second cardinal symptom of stone in the kidney is *hematuria*.   This symptom, of course, does not distinguish it from stone elsewhere in the urinary tract.   Since the hematuria results from traumatism caused by the stone, it will depend on the character and location thereof.   Oxalate stones are most prominent as hemorrhage producers, since they are often rough, and have sharp edges and points.   The hemorrhage is increased, when present, by an attack of renal colic, or if absent before, is often demonstrable for the first time immediately after the colic. Slight or moderate grades of hematuria are often not noticed by patients, especially if the urine is acid and the hemoglobin is converted to the brown acid-hematin before it is voided.   The hematuria may occur at widely separated intervals, at short intervals, or may be continuous.   There may never be more than a few red blood-cells, not detectable macroscopically, or, on the other hand, the bleeding may be enough to form clots.   It is rare, however, for the hemorrhage to be a serious matter in itself, as stones do not erode large vessels—they are obliterated by scar formation before this occurs.

In a series of 184 cases of renal calculus studied at the Brady Urological Institute, renal colic had occurred in 129 cases, or 70.1 per cent.   Definite note of radiation was made in 58 of these cases, but it undoubtedly was present in some of the others. These figures are somewhat higher than those commonly quoted.   Diffused, fixed, or constant pain, in a word, pain definitely not of a colicky nature, was observed in 124 cases, or 67.4 per cent.   It will be seen that in many cases this alternated with attacks of colic.

Hematuria was present at some stage of the process in 107 cases, or 58.1 per cent.

A third symptom, more characteristic, but less frequent than pain or hematuria, is the *passage of sand, gravel,* or *small stones.*   This was noted in 53 cases, or 32.3 per cent.   With the larger ones the extrusion of the stone is usually preceded by an attack of colic, but small fragments may be passed without pain.

Some minute fragments may cause intense pain for a week or more before passing into the bladder.   The history of this occurrence is of special importance in those cases where no stone appears in the x-ray plate.   Such patients manufacture small stones in the kidney, and the circumstances are such that they can be expelled before they grow too large.   The size of stones which can be expelled spontaneously varies greatly and according to the size of the various parts of the tract.   Smooth stones up to $1\frac{1}{2}$ cm. in diameter have been expelled, though it is difficult to say whether any additional growth had taken place in the bladder.   In general, stones passed are not over 8 mm. in diameter.

Symptoms due indirectly to kidney stone occur especially in the intestinal tract and in the lower urinary tract. The *nausea, vomiting,* and *meteorism* associated with renal colic have already been mentioned. There may be vaguer manifestations, such as constipation, belching, anorexia, etc., independent of colic. In the presence of a kidney stone, *bladder symptoms,* including frequency, urgency, and burning not infrequently occur. Pain, burning or tingling, may be referred to the anterior urethra. These symptoms may be due to secondary infection of these parts, but have been observed when the urine was sterile, and no lesion demonstrable in the bladder.

If the stone causes *obstruction* other symptoms occur, and may occupy the foreground. If the obstruction is such as to cause *hydronephrosis,* the symptoms of that condition, already described, and consisting especially of pain and tumor, enter the picture. Stone is a frequent cause of hydronephrosis. Obstruction predisposes to serious *infections.* In obstruction, renal colic is likely to be more severe. When an acute complete obstruction occurs following a change in the position of the stone, a complete *anuria* may occur, the so-called "calculous anuria." This phenomenon has been the subject of much debate, some claiming that it could not occur when the opposite kidney was healthy. Since it has been caused experimentally in healthy animals by clamping one ureter, and since many competent observers have reported its occurrence in cases where the opposite kidney gave every evidence of being sound, we must admit its existence, and call it, for want of a better name, "reflex anuria." This reflex has not been traced. Rovsing reports reflex anuria in a sound kidney during a period in which a clamp was applied to the pedicle of the opposite kidney. When the clamp was removed the anuria disappeared. Apparently it always does disappear, for no case of uremic death due to reflex anuria, where one kidney could be shown to be healthy, has been found by us. When but one kidney is present, sudden blocking is more serious. If there has been no obstruction before, it may occur when the patient is in good health, or even before stone has been suspected. In such an event the symptoms of uremia appear, and immediate action is demanded.

Infection is a serious and frequent complication of nephrolithiasis. Its relation to the genesis and growth of stones has already been discussed. It becomes a factor comparatively late in the disease, as a rule, and is capable of modifying the symptoms extensively. The most characteristic symptomatic evidence of infection is *pyuria.* This may be present in the absence of fever, and when the patient is apparently in good health. It may be the first symptom noted. Small amounts of pus may be present without infection, but even when infection is present the amount may be small. In other cases the quantity is great. The patient may, however, mistake a sediment of phosphate for pus. Pain may be increased by infection. If the infection attacks the parenchyma or is dammed up, fever, leukocytosis, and malaise appear, which, if continued, lead to anemia and cachexia and sometimes to septicemia. When there is obstruction, infection is favored, and if pyonephrosis develops, there may be added to the above symptoms a local tumor. Sudden blocking by stone when only one kidney is affected may lead to an interesting symptom complex. The voided urine, formerly containing pus and bacteria, will become clear, while the patient's general condition will grow worse, with pain, fever, and malaise due to the penning in of the infectious process.

If the *infection spreads outside the kidney* the patient generally becomes quite ill. Abscesses frequently develop which may burrow in various directions, appearing most often in the loin, with redness, swelling, and tenderness, later fluctuation. While deep, they not infrequently give rise to definite tumor. Spreading in other directions they may simulate other abdominal conditions. A full discussion is given in the section on Infections of the Kidney. Sinuses, usually in the upper loin, from previous and unrecognized perinephric abscesses, may sometimes be the principal cause of complaint of patients with renal stone. We know of 1 case in which several operations were done to curet and pack a sinus, which was thought to lead to spinal caries, and which was really due to a kidney practically destroyed by stone. There had been no symptoms whatever referable to the kidney. If the connection with the kidney pelvis remains open, the sinus may discharge varying quantities of urine. If an actual perforation of the kidney occurs fairly suddenly, in the presence of obstruction from stone, urinary extravasation will be added to the symptoms of abscess. These consist of a rapidly spreading tumefaction and the severe prostration accompanying all extravasations. This may be so severe that fever and leukocytosis do not occur, but they are usually present. If the extravasation extends internally, so that it cannot be palpated, the prostration and general symptoms only will be in evidence.

Ureter.—When a stone enters the ureter, the most characteristic and frequent symptom is *colic*. Efforts have been made to distinguish ureteral and renal colic, and it has been said that the pain in ureteral colic may originate at a lower point, that the radiations along the course of the ureter are more severe, and that they more often extend into the genitalia or leg. This refinement is of little value, however, since there is so frequently a ureteral element in colic originating in a kidney lesion, due to the passage through the ureter of blood-clots, etc.

The onset of ureteral colic is sudden, and if diffuse pain has been present before, the distinctive character of the colic is usually recognized at once by the patient. The pain is severe, spasmodic, and radiates to the groin, bladder region, penis, testis, or down the leg. Atypical radiation may be noted, as to the umbilicus, the crest of the ilium, the opposite kidney, or to the shoulder. The pain may begin in the groin and radiate upward, which is spoken of as "reverse radiation." The point of maximum severity of the pain may move downward as the stone advances through the ureter. Stones may pass through the ureter without colic, but when they are spontaneously expelled into the bladder, it is usually during a crisis of colic.

It may be said that colic occurs in practically all cases of ureteral calculus except those where the stone is expelled by normal, painless contractions, and these cases are of minor interest, since they require no treatment.

Diffuse pain may occur at any point along the ureter, due to pressure of the calculus. This pain is often not well localized, and may be referred to other points in the abdomen. Associated with it may be any degree of *tenderness* over the ureter, and sometimes marked *muscle spasm* of the abdominal muscles on the affected side. When combined with a little fever and leukocytosis, which is not infrequently the case, and the usual nausea and vomiting, the picture may easily be mistaken for that of an intra-abdominal lesion, and many appendectomies and other laparotomies have been done on this incorrect diagnosis.

The position of the stone in the ureter will influence the location and character of the pain. After it has passed the pelvic brim there is less likelihood of mistaking it for intra-abdominal pain. When near the bladder, or in the intramural portion of the ureter, pressure may occur on the rectum, seminal vesicle, or bladder, or on all three. We have described cases in which, in addition to the usual symptoms of ureteral colic, painful defecation, pain on ejaculation, and dysuria fixed the location of the calculus at this point.[1] This symptom-complex of Young is pathognomonic of stone at the lower end of ureter, but not always present.

Frequency and dysuria may occur even when the stone is in the upper portion of the ureter, but are the rule when it is in the lower extremity, even if there is no infection.

Hematuria is the second most frequent and characteristic symptom. Even when no hemorrhage has occurred while the stone was in the kidney, the added trauma of the spasmodic contractions of colic will usually cause bleeding after the stone is in the ureter. Hematuria is the most useful finding to distinguish ureteral colic from pain due to intra-abdominal lesions.

Nausea and vomiting occur frequently with ureteral as with renal colic.

Bladder.—The cardinal symptoms of vesical calculus are *frequency, dysuria, hematuria, sudden stoppage of urine,* and *pain* running down to the head of the penis. There is often *difficulty,* which may be affected by changes of position, and, if infection be present, pyuria. A history of renal colic, the cessation of which was followed immediately by increase in frequency and dysuria, is suggestive of a renal origin for the bladder stone. We have recently seen one case in which a renal calculus passed into the bladder ten years before, but had never given any symptom except sudden stoppage during urination. The *passage of sand* or gravel is frequent in encrusted cystitis or other infected cases where small concretions are being formed. As the stone grows larger, its pressure causes constant pain and irritation in the bladder, with *urgency* and *tenesmus.* The difficulty of voiding may become very great, and may be characterized by a sudden stoppage as the stone drops into the vesical orifice. In such cases the patient may void better lying down, or even with the head considerably lower than the hips. In the giant calculus of Sir William Ogilvie he could only void when "standing on his head."

When calculi accompany prostatic obstruction with residual urine, they may cause no additional symptoms. The presence of residual urine may prevent the bladder from contracting upon the stones, and there may be neither pain nor sudden stoppage of urine. On the other hand, calculi may greatly aggravate the symptoms in enlarged prostate, and lead to hematuria, dysuria, and frequency.

In infants pain on urination during which the patient seizes the penis in his hand is characteristic. Sometimes the irritation is so great as to produce very frequent erections and masturbation at a very early age. Sometimes the frequent urination simulates incontinence. Diverticular or encysted calculi usually give no symptoms if they are small in comparison with the pouch in which they lie. If, however, they fill the pouch and particularly if the location is in the base of the bladder adjacent to the trigone, frequent or even constant desire to urinate, with spasm of the bladder and great dysuria, may be present. This is particularly true when a portion of the calculus projects into the bladder.

If, however, the diverticulum is situated in the vertex of the bladder there may be no pain or frequency until the stem breaks and the stone drops to the base of the bladder. In one such case the patient had had no pain until it came on suddenly and violently four weeks before. We found at operation a stone nearly 2 inches in

[1] Young: Transactions of American Association of Genito-urinary Surgeons, 1907, ii, 104–109.

diameter. A slender stem projecting from its surface, showing a recent fracture, pointed to its origin and caused us to search for the encysted "parent" calculus, which we found in a small diverticulum at or near the urachus.

In general, the symptoms of vesical calculus are not very characteristic and it may be confused with various kinds of cystitis, tuberculosis, enlargements of the median prostatic lobe, or vesical neoplasm. Only careful examination can make the diagnosis.

Urethra.—Since calculi do not usually form in the urethra, the entrance into the vesical orifice of a stone large enough to pass with difficulty, or be arrested, is characterized by the sudden onset of great difficulty in voiding, or complete retention. This is especially characteristic in younger patients without previous symptoms pointing to an infravesical obstruction. There may also be hemorrhage. In cases where a stone develops in an irregular urethra or blind pocket, the difficulty will develop more slowly, and no characteristic symptoms be present.

Prostate.—Prostatic calculi may exist without causing symptoms. In other cases the associated chronic prostatitis or benign hypertrophy causes the symptoms associated with either of these two conditions. Pain and dysuria seem sometimes to be accentuated by the presence of stones in the prostate.

Urolithiasis is one of the four important and serious conditions causing *hematuria*, and we again emphasize the gravity of this symptom, and the necessity of always investigating its cause thoroughly.

DIAGNOSIS

Kidney.—The diagnosis of renal calculus has been made a matter of great exactness by the introduction of the x-ray and the wax-tipped ureteral catheter. Other means of investigation should not be neglected, however, since it is incumbent upon us, not only to learn that a stone is present but also to learn how much and what sort of damage has been done.

General physical examination will give little help unless a complication such as hydronephrosis, pyonephrosis, or perirenal abscess, sufficiently large to be palpated, or causing tenderness or muscle spasm, is present. A movable kidney may be disclosed. During renal colic a marked rigidity of the abdominal muscles on the affected side may be present, leading one to suspect an intraperitoneal lesion. There may also be tenderness over the kidney and ureter. These features cause many laparotomies to be done on patients with renal or ureteral calculus with mistaken diagnosis of appendicitis, gall-bladder disease, etc.

The *history* will usually give the first clue to the true nature of the lesion. Renal colic or fixed pain, hematuria, pyuria, or passage of calculous material, or combinations of these symptoms, arouse suspicion of stone. Other fairly common conditions which can give rise to similar syndromes are especially chronic prostatitis, tuberculosis, neoplasm or pyogenic infections of the kidney, and primary hydronephrosis. It is from these conditions, commonly, that kidney stone must be distinguished, and, if the physical examination has given no aid, a careful *examination of the urine* is in order. Besides the usual tests, smears made from centrifugalized second and third glass freshly voided specimens should be examined, both moist and stained. In this manner only can small amounts of blood, pus, or scanty bacteria be discovered. If the findings are positive, the examination must be repeated on specimens obtained by ureteral catheterization to rule out other parts of the urogenital tract as the source of the abnormal elements. The presence of red blood-cells, however, is then of no value, since a few are almost always present resulting from the trauma of the catheterization.

Typical renal colic with blood in the urine and equal in each of the three glasses is strong presumptive evidence of stone and *x-ray* or *wax-tip* examination should be proceeded with at once. It should be stated here that chronic prostatitis may give

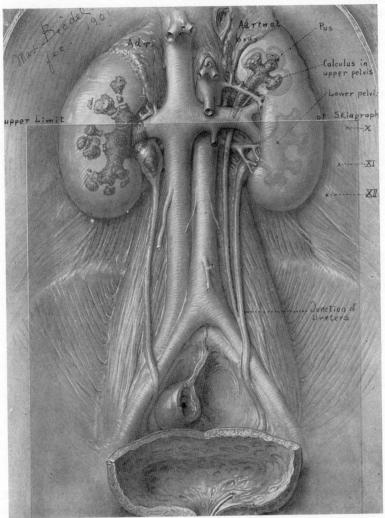

FIG. 193.—Bilateral renal calculi; large branching calculus filling pelvis and calyces of right kidney and also pelvis and calyces of the upper portion of left kidney which is double. The lower portion of the double kidney is normal. *x*-Ray (as indicated) showed a shadow in the right kidney, but none in the left because the plate was placed too low.

rise to pain simulating renal colic, with blood in the urine coming from a congested posterior urethra. This condition can be ruled out by the use of the endoscope, etc. Occasionally an appendicitis or other abdominal inflammation involving the ureter by contiguity may cause hematuria.

Chemical examination of the urine may give an idea of the composition of the stone, as explained in the section on Pathology. The presence of cystinuria and xanthinuria can be determined in this way. Often there is no excess of urates, phosphates, or oxalates to indicate the existence of these stones.

An x-ray photograph should now be made. Care should be taken to see that it is so taken as to include the highest possible location of the kidney. We[1] have observed a case in which the x-ray revealed a large calculus on one side, but failed to show a second one which was in the upper half of a double pelvis on the other side. This stone lay just outside the upper border of the plate (Fig. 193). Exposures should also be made of the lower abdomen and pelvis which might be the seat of a stone in an ectopic kidney.

The Bucky diaphragm adds much to the clearness of these pictures, especially in fat patients. We have seen cases in which stones, long unrecognized, were first disclosed in pictures taken with the Bucky diaphragm. Ordinary x-rays had failed to show them on account of the great thicknesses of fat and muscle present. We now use the Liebel-Florsheim-Young flat diaphragm in the latest model of our cystoscopic x-ray table described elsewhere (Chapter XIII).

Small stones may lie directly in line with a rib and be hard to distinguish. Particles of bismuth remaining in the intestine after gastro-intestinal x-rays some-

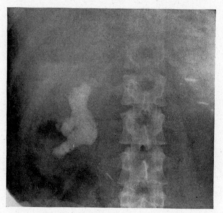

Fig. 194.—Large staghorn or coral calculus of the right kidney making an almost perfect cast of the pelvis and calyces. B. U. I. x-Ray 2631.

times give rise to confusion, as may fecoliths in the appendix or elsewhere. Mark[2] reports an extraordinary case in which the appendix, with two large fecoliths, was adherent to the right ureter. There were renal colic and hematuria. Even after careful urologic examination, the diagnosis of ureteral calculus was made, and the true condition revealed only at operation. Gas in the intestine may prevent a clear view, and it may be said that purgatives often, instead of removing this trouble, increase it. Fecal accumulations must be removed.

Very small stones in large individuals may cast practically no shadows on account of convergence of the rays. Certain stones, as previously mentioned (especially cystin stones), cast no shadows with the x-ray, unless they are very large. In these types of cases especially, the wax-tip catheter lends invaluable assistance.

The importance of the x-ray in the diagnosis of renal calculus is indicated by the fact that in our series of 184 cases roentgenograms disclosed the stone in 154 cases, or 83.7 per cent. of the total. Some typical pictures are shown in Figs. 194 to 201.

[1] Young: Johns Hopkins Hospital Reports, 1906, xiii, 447–454.

[2] Journal of the American Medical Association, 1924, lxxxii, 1689–1691.

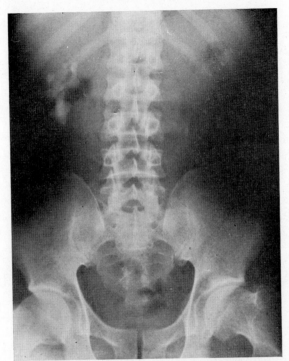

FIG. 195.—x-Ray showing large staghorn calculus in the right kidney; and a long cylindric calculus in the left ureter. B. U. I. x-Ray 5208.

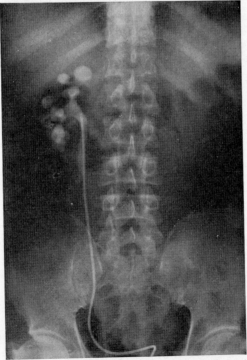

FIG. 196.—Same case as the preceding picture. The cylindric calculus has been removed from the left ureter, but the two small calculi in the kidney substance remain, although they are not well shown in the reproduction. The staghorn calculus is still present in the right side and the pyelogram shows the moderate hydronephrosis which has been caused, remarkably little for such a large calculus. B. U. I. x-Ray 5512.

If the x-ray photograph has shown a stone in the kidney, further measures, including cystoscopy and catheterization of the ureters, should be taken to discover how much damage has been done to the affected kidney. In bilateral stones this is even more important to enable one to form a judicious plan of operative treatment, best fitted to the interests of the patient.

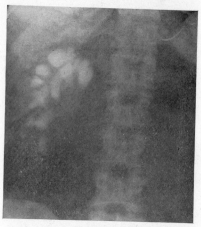

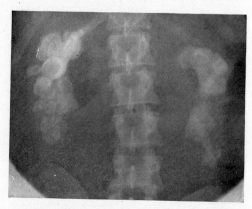

Fig. 197.—Multiple calculi of the right kidney. This kidney was greatly dilated and heavily infected. There were also stones in the lower right ureter with obstruction and several small stones in the left kidney. The ureteral stones alone were removed. The urine cleared up remarkably and the general health improved, showing that it is often wise not to do too much in bilateral stone cases. B. U. I. x-Ray 2561.

Fig. 198.—Very large bilateral renal calculi. History of slight pain in the back for two years. The patient survived nephrolithotomy on one side for a year, but the renal function grew steadily less. Death occurred following attempt to remove the other calculus. B. U. I. x-Ray 2191.

The *cystoscopy* should be preceded by a careful study of the total renal function, including at least a phenolsuphonephthalein test and a determination of the blood urea if the total function is quite low. This gives a valuable guide to the general condition of the patient, and also enables us to estimate, later on, what proportion of the total function is being carried on by each kidney.

Fig. 199.—Stereoscopic x-ray showing catheter coiled about a calculus in the renal pelvis. B. U. I. x-Ray 5804.
These pictures are intended to be used with the ordinary home stereoscope.

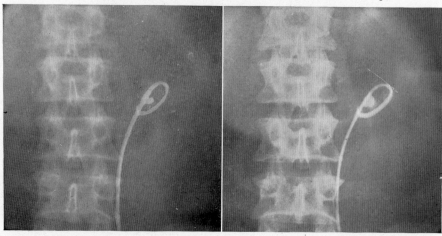

Examination of the bladder should not be neglected. Where stones have passed into the bladder, inflammation of the ureteral meatus, with redness and pouting, may be noticed. If infection has occurred, purulent urine may be seen coming from the affected side. That hematuria is of renal origin may be determined by direct observation. Where it has not been possible to catheterize the ureters the excretion of indigocarmin, as seen by the cystoscope, may give a rough indication of the relative functions.

If other diseases are present, they may be diagnosed at this time, as, for instance, tuberculosis, with vesical ulceration or pulling upward of the ureter, or bladder tumors may be seen. In rare cases a renal neoplasm may have extended down the ureter to the bladder, and appear in the orifice.

After careful inspection of the bladder *ureteral catheters* should be inserted, The general course of the examination then follows the same lines as in the case of hydronephrosis, as given previously. An x-ray photograph with opaque catheters in place shows the relations of the ureter to the stone. Separate specimens of urine are obtained for examination and culture. In this way infection is determined, and lowered specific gravity or urea concentration noted. The pelvic capacities are

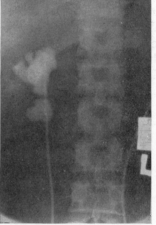

FIG. 201.—Same case as the preceding picture. Right pyelogram in a case of bilateral renal calculi. The catheter has ascended into the upper calyces which alone are filled and which show marked hydronephrotic changes with clubbing of the minor calices. The other calyces were later found to be equally distended. B. U. I. x-Ray 5134.

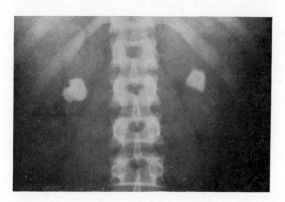

FIG. 200.—Case of bilateral renal calculi. B. U. I. x-Ray 5131.

determined, since one of our principal cares is to determine whether the stone, by obstruction, has caused any hydronephrosis.

Finally, *pyelograms* should be taken. They give further evidence as to the existence of hydronephrosis (Figs. 200, 201), and show any destruction caused by the stone as deformation of the pelvic shadow. One is also enabled to see the relation of the stone to the pelvis, and to judge, somewhat roughly, it is true, the type and extent of operation which will be necessary to remove it. A stone which casts no shadow (*e. g.*, cystin) may appear in the pyelogram as a clear, translucent area in the pelvic shadow. Again, a stone not appearing clearly in the plain x-ray may become more conspicuous, after the pelvis is again emptied, by imbibition of some of the pyelographic medium. Other conditions, especially tuberculosis, neoplasm, and congenital cystic kidney, are frequently disclosed by other types of pelvic deformation.

If the diagnosis of stone is still in doubt at this stage, the *wax-tip catheter* method of Kelly should be used. This procedure has not had the wide use it deserves. Care must be taken, as it is not difficult to produce scratches in the wax from the cystoscope employed. This purely technical objection can, however, easily be overcome by practice.

There are three methods of passing the wax-tip catheter, with any of which satisfactory results may be obtained: (1) The catheter is first passed into the bladder through the urethra. The sheath of a catheter cystoscope with removable sheath is then inserted with the catheter passing through its lumen. Finally, the outer end of the catheter is threaded into the ordinary catheterizing telescope, which is then pushed into the sheath. Certain precautions are, however, necessary. The length of the urethra should be known so that the catheter will not extend more than about 2 inches into the bladder. The bladder should be filled with fluid beforehand, in order that the catheter may not be bent on itself and present its waxed end at the vesical orifice where it may be scratched by the cystoscope as it enters. The catheter should be held in such a manner that it cannot be pushed further into the bladder or pulled partly out while the parts of the cystoscope are being threaded over it. The disadvantage of the method is that the catheter lies alongside the beak of the cystoscope during the insertion of the sheath, which may cause difficulty if there is any narrowing of the urethra.

(2) For this method also a catheterizing cystoscope is employed. The sheath and obturator are inserted in the usual manner, and the bladder irrigated and filled with fluid. A rubber tube is then selected which will just fit in the channel of the sheath, and about 2 inches longer than the cystoscope. Its lumen should readily admit the wax-tip catheter, and should be well lubricated. The inner end is cut off at an angle of about 45 degrees to enable it to ride up over the beak of the cystoscope. When it is in place, the wax-tip catheter is inserted through it until it projects about 2 inches into the bladder. The tubing is then withdrawn, holding the catheter as before, so that it cannot slip in or out. The catheterizing telescope with a rubber nipple is then slipped on over the outer end of the catheter and the insertion into the ureter can be begun at once under guidance of the eye. If an operating cystoscope is used, the rubber tube can be passed in through the large catheter channel.[1]

In both of these methods it is wise to have the patient quiet and with head well depressed, since there is opportunity in both methods for some of the fluid to run out of the bladder. The tip may be inspected through the telescope before insertion, and since, if it is brought close, considerable magnification can be had, any scratches made during the process of entering the bladder can usually be detected. Care should be taken not to pull the catheter back so far during this examination that the wax touches the elevator. Neither of these two methods can be done carelessly, but with a little practice they can easily be mastered, and afford accurate information.

(3) The third method involves the use of the straight open cystoscope, such as the models of Kelly and Luys. The bladder may be distended with air by placing the patient in the knee-chest or extreme Trendelenburg position as shown in Fig. 202. It is possible, however, to dispense with distention by placing the end of the cystoscope directly over the ureteral meatus. This can be accomplished even in

[1] Kirkendall: Journal of the American Medical Association, 1915, lxv, 1253–1255.

the male by elevating the handle of the cystoscope and pressing it slightly to one side. When this is done, it is necessary to have a constant suction drainage at the inner end of the cystoscope, otherwise it continually fills with urine from the ureter. The wax-tip catheter is inserted straight into the ureter under guidance of the eye, the light being furnished either by a small electric bulb at the inner end of the cystoscope, or reflected from a head mirror. The advantages of the method are that there is practically no chance for adventitious scratches, that larger catheters and tips may be used, that stilets may be placed in the catheters giving additional stiffness in ureters difficult to catheterize, and that different size tips may be tried in succession without extra complications.

The disadvantages of the method are, in the male, that distention of the bladder by air is often difficult, and that any abnormalities in the prostate or urethra,

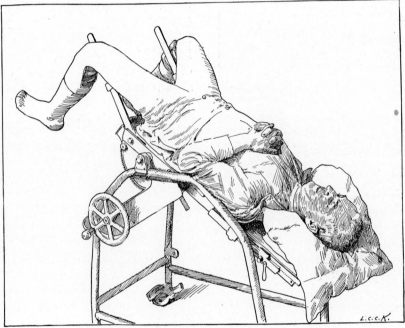

Fig. 202.—Position of patient on a Young cystoscopic table with head lowered to an angle of 60 degrees. Neill.

especially enlargement of the median lobe, make proper exposure of the ureteral meatus difficult or impossible. It certainly is the method of choice for ureteral dilations in women.

The wax-tip should be prepared freshly before use. Kelly recommends a mixture of 2 parts dental wax and 1 part olive oil. Ordinary embedding paraffin may be used. Hunner uses pure beeswax. The end of the catheter is dipped in the melted wax, and the catheter is rotated during the cooling process to secure a smooth, even coating. The end should always be covered. Bands of wax placed at intervals along the catheter sometimes give valuable indications of the location of stones in the ureter, but their use is not practicable when the indirect cystoscope is employed. Solid bougies may be employed as well as catheters. Some urologists prefer to use catheters, being careful not to obstruct the eye with wax, enabling them in this way to conduct the other catheter procedures at the same sitting.

A little experimentation may be necessary to find the size of tip which will ascend into the ureter. When it is found the catheter is pushed home as far as it will go. It is a good plan to impart to the catheter a rotary motion while in its extreme position and during the process of withdrawal. In this manner any stone scratches will be circumferential or spiral, and can be distinguished from any adventitious scratches which may have been made, and which will be longitudinal. Sometimes tiny fragments of stone will be brought out embedded in the wax; this is absolutely diagnostic, and also allows us to determine the composition, at least of the outer layers of the stone. The tip is examined after withdrawal with a hand lens.

The wax-tip is an invaluable aid to diagnosis. Those who have become accustomed to its use find that it not infrequently gives the decision in the presence of equivocal signs and x-ray pictures. It is only in very rare cases of unmixed colloidal soft stones, or of stones embedded in the kidney cortex or in a dense mass of blood-clot that the wax-tip fails to show scratches. The only cause of fail-

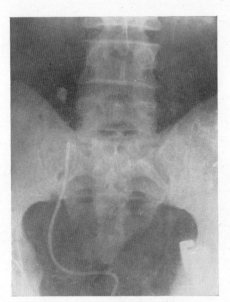

FIG. 203.—Ureteral calculus lodged in the right ureter at the level of the top of the fifth lumbar vertebra. B. U. I. x-Ray 2921.

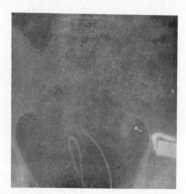

FIG. 204.—The arrow points to a large calculus just below the pelvic brim in the left ureter. Ureteral catheter is coiled in the bladder. B. U. I. x-Ray 2541.

ure which is at all common is inability to insert the catheter in the ureter. We unhesitatingly recommend it as a procedure with which every urologist should be familiar.

A persistent, thorough, and skilful application of these various methods of diagnosis make the elucidation of cases of nephrolithiasis practically certain. In addition we can usually glean from them enough accurate information to plan our operative procedures calmly and confidently before entering the operating room. Exploratory operations for kidney stone have become almost curiosities, if not disgraceful.

Ureter.—The symptoms and signs of ureteral calculus are so like those of certain cases of renal calculus that the distinction cannot usually be made except by the x-ray and wax-tip, unless the stone be arrested at the ureterovesical orifice. The stoppage of ureteral catheters part way up the ureter is no proof of the presence of ureteral calculus, since they may be arrested in so many other ways. On the other hand, a catheter may pass by a stone, even one which is causing obstructive symptoms, without the slightest perceptible hitch. If a calculus does not show in the x-ray plate the wax-tip catheter, armed with multiple bands of wax, may be used to show the location of the stone in the ureter.

From the x-ray, one estimates the size of the stone, whether it is rough or smooth, and the likelihood of its spontaneous passage. Allowance must be made for divergence of the rays (Figs. 203, 204). Further roentgenograms taken at intervals will show whether the stone is moving down the ureter (Figs. 214–220). As long as movement can be detected, we may hope for spontaneous expulsion. If an opaque catheter is placed in the ureter we can distinguish phleboliths, calcified

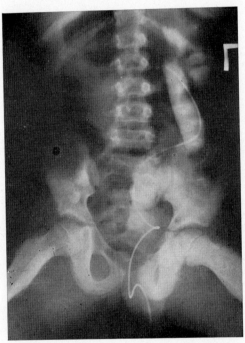

FIG. 205.—Pyelogram and ureterogram showing marked hydronephrosis and hydro-ureter in a child due to three calculi in the lower end of the left ureter. Successfully removed at operation. B. U. I. x-Ray 5519.

glands, etc., which will lie at a distance from the catheter. Stereoscopic pictures aid this distinction. A stone in a dilated ureter may also lie at some distance from the catheter. Errors can be avoided in such cases only by taking a ureterogram, preferably stereoscopic.

By injection of opaque media we can determine the amount of hydronephrosis and hydro-ureter present (Fig. 205). The opaque solution will often pass up by the stone, even when the catheter will not.

Functional studies of the kidneys—as always—are to be made.

If the calculus is at the lower end of the ureter, it may elevate the bladder mucosa over the intramural portion enough so that the swelling can be seen cystoscopically. In other cases the stone itself can be viewed through the ureteral orifice. An inflammatory reaction, with reddening, will be present in such cases.

It will sometimes be possible to feel a grating sensation on rubbing the stone within the ureter with a ureteral catheter or fulgurating wire. This is always advisable, as blood-clots seen through the orifice may simulate stones. Ulcers produced by pressure of such stones can be seen with the cystoscope. Rarely calculi in the lower end of the ureter can be palpated by rectum. In women it is not so rare to feel them through the vagina.

The findings in a series of 180 cases of nephrolithiasis studied at the Brady Institute are given in the following table:

TABLE 47

SUMMARY OF 180 CASES OF NEPHROLITHIASIS, BRADY UROLOGICAL INSTITUTE

46 previously passed stones. (One passed 20, one passed 40.)
20 previous operations with recurrence.
 8 had gravel in urine for years.
   (x-Ray revealed stone in all cases where present as proved by operation, save 2. One of these
     was in ectopic kidney.)
In 75 cases there were multiple stones.
In 105 cases there were single stones.
In 21 cases stones were bilateral (11.7 per cent.).
In 159 cases stones were unilateral.

Urine

Acid	105	No R. B. C. or W. B. C..	42
Alkaline	14	Infected	100 (55.5 per cent.)
Not reported	61	Not infected	80 (44.4 ")
Red blood-cells	70	Sugar	3
White blood-cells	131	T. B. bacilli	1

{ 103 cases had hematuria.
{ 77 cases not reported as to hematuria.

{ 121 had generalized aching over region affected.
{ 59 gave no history of generalized pain.

{ 124 gave history of renal colic.
{ 56 did not give history of renal colic.
   53 cases reported the pain of the colic as radiating.
     11 did not state precisely where.
     17 reported pain as radiating to groin.
      8 reported pain as radiating to testicle.
      2 reported pain as radiating to bladder.
      2 reported testicle retracted.
      4 reported pain as radiating to thigh.
      6 reported pain as radiating to penis.
Bladder symptoms:
     12 cases reported frequency.
      4 cases reported dysuria.
      3 cases reported difficulty.

Bladder.—For the diagnosis of stone in the bladder, we rely upon cystoscopy and the x-ray, with the metal stone searcher as an additional method.

The cystoscope usually discloses the calculi, and enables us to estimate the number and size. It is easy to mistake the size of a stone. Where this knowledge is important, it is best to make sure of the distance of the stone from the lens of the cystoscope by touching it with the tip of a graduated ureteral catheter. The number of centimeters is read off by direct observation, and the size of the stone calculated by noting the degree of magnification at the given distance. It is also possible to measure accurately the diameter of a calculus by pushing the cystoscope

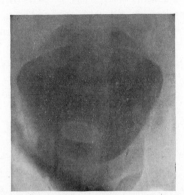

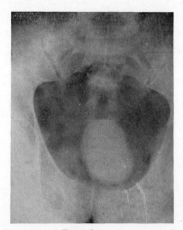

Fig. 206.—x-Ray showing a medium sized vesical calculus. The shadows seen in the left side of the pelvis are due to phleboliths. B. U. I. x-Ray 2432.

Fig. 207.—x-Ray of an enormous vesical calculus. In the original film the laminated structure of the calculus was well made out. B. U. I. x-Ray 2307.

in until the farthest edge is in the center of the field and then withdrawing the cystoscope in a straight line until the other edge of the stone is in the center of the

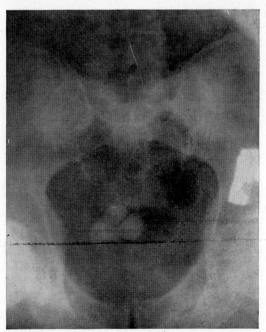

Fig. 208.—x-Ray showing four vesical calculi. B. U. I. x-Ray 2190.

field. An assistant meanwhile measures the excursion of the cystoscope outside, as shown in Fig. 635.

A number of precautions must be noted. Calculi may be concealed behind a hypertrophied trigone, or in diverticula. They may also be hidden by masses of pus or blood, or missed in cloudy media. They may be simulated by blood-clots, tumors, pieces of tissue, etc. In such case one can determine whether the object seen is free or not by rolling the patient from side to side, when a stone will generally move, seeking always the most dependent portion. One may also substitute for a stone searcher the tip of the cystoscope, or a piece of wire introduced through the ureteral catheter channel. A touch with either of these will give the grating sensation if the object is a stone. A coating of firm blood-clot may interfere with this procedure. The calcareous deposits in encrusted cystitis are usually recognizable as small light colored granules. Larger calculi may be adherent to the bladder wall, even in the vertex or in the anterior portion, and simulate tumors. Dumb-bell calculi arising from diverticula give a similar appearance. A touch with a metallic object is usually sufficient to identify them. Bits of tissue remaining in the

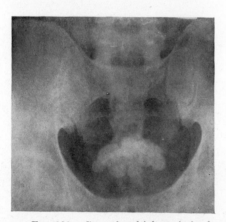

FIG. 209.—Case of multiple vesical calculi. The causative factor in this case was a piece of gauze which had been left in the bladder. The shadow of this piece of gauze encrusted with calcareous material is indistinctly seen below the calculi. B. U. I. x-Ray 3591.

bladder after operation may become encrusted and cause serious symptoms, especially difficulty and pain on voiding. Such cases should always be cystoscoped. Calculi may sometimes lie in parts of the bladder not visible through the cystoscope. The instrument should always be moved about to all possible positions, and sometimes direct vision cystoscopes, like those of Braasch and Bransford Lewis, may be necessary.

The *x-ray* is especially useful to show the size of stones, and to disclose those hidden to cystoscopic examination (Fig. 210). Phleboliths, calcified glands, or tumors, prostatic calculi, and calculi in the lower ureter and the urethra are ruled out by appropriate procedures. Chief of these are the placing of opaque catheters in the ureters and urethra, and the taking of cystograms. The cystogram will show diverticula, if present, and give their relations to the calculi.

In the past, *metal stone searchers*, some with resonating drums or even telephonic tubes to the ear, were in constant use. An evidence of the revolution produced by the cystoscope is the almost complete discarding of these ingenious instruments of our urologic forefathers. A Thompson catheter stone searcher should still be in every cabinet, for it may be of great assistance, especially when the cystoscope and x-ray are not at hand, or great hemorrhage is present, or other conditions (strictures, hypertrophy, cancer, etc.) make cystoscopy unsatisfactory. Small searchers are quite necessary for certain cases in children. The cystoscope should always be used where possible, but one should not forget, however, to try for the grating sensation when in doubt, as it may clear up an otherwise puzzling case. Every effort should be made to count the stones as well as possible before operation, especially if they are in diverticula, to ensure complete removal. Diverticula with large mouths should be cystoscoped if possible, as one occasionally finds stones within them.

PLATE VIII

VESICAL CALCULI

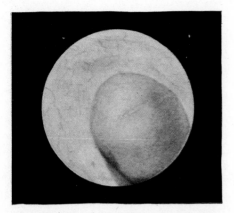

A. Large urate calculus in bladder behind right ureteral orifice. B. U. I. 7325.

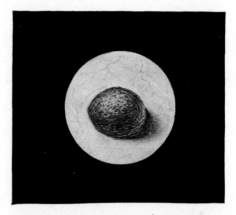

B. Small oxalate calculus. B. U. I. 12,292.

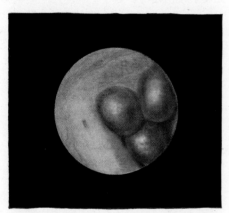

C. Numerous oxalate calculi behind hypertrophied trigone. B. U. I. 8477.

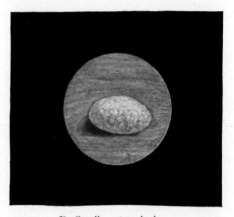

D. Small urate calculus.

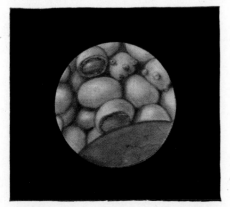

E. Numerous calculi behind hypertrophied lobe. Two calculi spontaneously fractured, outer urate shell absent, disclosing the deep portion of oxalate. B. U. I. 11,514.

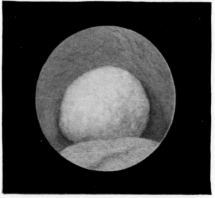

F. Large phosphatic calculus behind hypertrophied lobe. B. U. I. 7769.

x-Rays taken after the removal of opaque media, with or without distention of the bladder with air, may show stones of low density otherwise invisible, if they have adsorbed any of the medium. Large stones of low density may appear in cystograms as clear areas.

Infection, if present, should be discovered by examination of the urine, and studied by culture. Since tuberculosis may coexist with stone an acid-fast stain should be made in suspected cases.

Renal function, of course, must be determined before any operative procedure.

With so many diagnostic measures at command, it is surprising that some vesical calculi escape diagnosis. This, however, is usually in cases where some other condition has held the attention of the examiner, and the study of the bladder has not been as complete as it might have been.

Urethra.—Calculi large enough to lodge in the urethra can usually be *palpated* upon examination of the genitalia or by rectal examination. Additional measures are *urethrograms* and *x-rays*, or they may be seen with the *urethroscope*. Calculi wedged in the urethra at the vesical orifice may prevent instrumental examination, and in such cases the *x*-ray must be relied upon.

After operation for enucleation of the prostate calculi not infrequently form in the greatly dilated or pouch-like prostatic urethra. When small they may lie at a distance from the center of the tract and may not be encountered by a metal instrument passing into the bladder. They may even be difficult to see with the cystoscope.

In 2 of our cases calculi have formed at the line of anastomosis in the radical operation for cancer of the prostate about unabsorbable sutures.

Fig. 210.—Stereoscopic *x*-ray of a case showing (1) a large stone opposite the promontory of the sacrum encysted in a diverticulum, (2) several medium sized stones in the bladder, and (3) numerous small calculi in the substance of the prostate. B. U. I. *x*-Ray 5450. View through stereoscope.

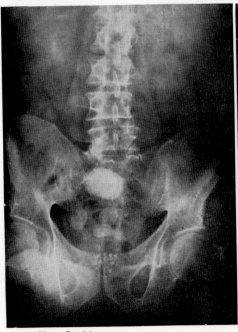 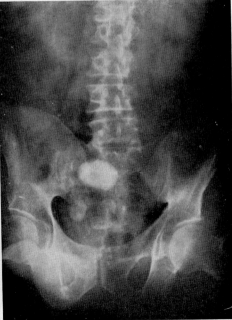

Prostate.—Prostatic calculi, especially those of the millet seed type, may be present in large numbers, and still be unrecognizable on *rectal examination*. This is especially true when accompanied by prostatic hypertrophy. We have not infrequently missed them in both old and young men with prostatitis. Sometimes they cause the prostate to be very *hard* and *nodular*. The picture may resemble exactly that found in prostatic carcinoma, and we must rely on the *x*-ray to show the calculi (Fig. 211). One must not forget that calculi are occasionally found in a carcinomatous prostate, and that there is nothing to prevent the development of cancer in a prostate already the seat of stones. Occasionally a calculus, near the posterior surface of the prostate, can be palpated as a hard, round, smooth nodule in an otherwise fairly normal gland, and in multiple calculi a *crepitus* can sometimes be distinctly felt when pressure is made by the palpating finger.

Seminal Vesicles.—Concretions or calcareous deposits in the seminal vesicle are often closely adherent to the ureter, and give *x-ray* pictures suggesting ure-

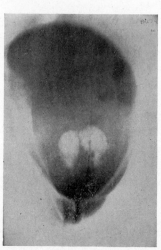

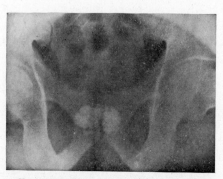

FIG. 211.—Case of prostatic calculi. The calculi here are very numerous and practically outline the prostate which was very hard on rectal examination and indistinguishable except for the *x*-ray from carcinoma. B. U. I. *x*-Ray 4708.

FIG. 212.—Same case as the previous picture. *x*-Ray taken with the tube pointing directly downward through the long axis of the pelvis. Note how much more clearly the shadows of the calculi are seen when not obscured by the symphysis. B. U. I. *x*-Ray 4713.

teral calculus. The diagnosis may be difficult, since the ureter may be strictured at the point where the vesicle is adherent. A thorough study with opaque catheter and ureterogram, preferably stereoscopic, must be depended on to show the extraureteral location of the shadow.

In taking *x*-rays of the prostate and seminal vesicles the tube should be so placed that the rays pass down the strait of the pelvis. In this way the prostatic shadows are thrown well within the bony circle of the pelvis and not behind the symphysis as usual. This is well exemplified in the two *x*-ray plates of the same case—taken in different positions (Figs. 211, 212).

TREATMENT

The *treatment of urolithiasis* may be classified as follows:
1. Preventive and medical treatment.
2. Instrumental.
3. Operative.

Preventive.—The prevention of urolithiasis is based on the avoidance or relief of conditions which have a tendency to cause the formation of calculi. These have been set forth at length in foregoing pages. Briefly stated, the precipitation or deposition of urinary salts should be prevented, and anatomic or pathologic conditions which might lead to stasis or obstruction should be corrected. As most renal and ureteral calculi contain *oxalate of lime* as the principal ingredient it is rational to avoid excess of substances which contain oxalic acid and calcium. The following articles of diet have been found to be rich in oxalic acid: Tomatoes, spinach, beans, rhubarb, strawberries, coffee, tea, pepper, and milk. Calcium is found to excess in cereals, milk, eggs, and fresh vegetables as well as limestone waters. Theoretically all these food-stuffs should be avoided more or less strictly by individuals who have once had an oxalate calculus, or are subject to oxaluria. Persons wishing to avoid having a "stone" might also take similar precautions. As a matter of fact, however, it is practically impossible to exclude even for a short time the multitude of valuable food-stuffs which might contribute to the formation of an oxalate calculus. The use of *water* in large amounts is probably the most valuable prophylactic treatment which can actually be put into practice, but the use of urine acidifiers, such as acid sodium phosphate (gr. xx t. i. d. p. c.), may well be tried for a time.

When the oxaluria is prolonged, and especially if accompanied by annoying symptoms, a careful dietary regimen, with mineral waters rich in sodium and magnesium phosphate, is recommended. Certain mineral springs in Europe and also in America are of high repute in the treatment of gravel, and undoubtedly many calculi are passed after great imbibition of such waters. In certain cases definite fracture of calculi and passage of the fragments occur.

The use of turpentine internally is found in the very early literature, and is referred to by Samuel Pepys in his celebrated diary. Watson has, in recent years, reiterated his faith in turpentine, which he says should be given in 10-minim doses in gelatin capsules thrice daily—but not for longer than a week.

Phosphaturia and phosphatic calculi may be combated by a diet poor in calcium salts, meat in place of milk, and acid sodium phosphate or nitrohydrochloric acid. The most important thing is to remove the alkaline infection and allow the urine to become acid.

Uric acid in excess and urate calculi call for a treatment directed toward reduction of the uric acid in the urine, viz., by improving the metabolism of nitrogenous foods, reducing the excess of uric acid derivable from foods, and preventing the uric acid from crystallizing in the urine. That these desiderata are often unobtainable, or too obnoxious to be worth while, is a fact, but much can be gained by avoidance of overeating, careful regulation of the bowels, reduction in nitrogenous foods, especially those rich in purin bodies (limiting but not excluding meat) and the abundant use of waters containing antacids. Soda bicarbonate and citrate of potash are valuable adjuncts. But here again good pure water in abundance is about the best treatment to employ and may be continued indefinitely without disgust. Dozens of uric acid solvents have been promulgated—of which piperazin (gr. 6 to 15), hexamethylenamin (gr. 10 to 20 t. i. d. p. c.), and turpentine are the best known—but of uncertain value.

Instrumental.—The present indications for treatment of *renal* and *ureteral* *calculi* by *cystoscopic manipulation* may now be set down briefly as follows: Careful study of the case by x-ray, cystoscopy, ureter catheterization, cultures, functional tests, pyelograms, and wax-tip catheter to determine accurately the position, shape, size, and character of the stone, the condition of the kidneys, and the possibility of a non-operative treatment succeeding, should have been done.

If a calculus is found projecting from the lower end of the ureter, an attempt should be made to dislodge it with ureteral catheter, bougie, or forceps, or by the cystoscopic rongeur. Failing in these, the ureteral orifice may be enlarged by fulguration—burning through the mucous membrane upon the impacted calculus along the line of the ureter, or by slitting up the ureter with cystoscopic scissors or knife.

The following case, which we reported in 1902, is apparently the first case in which a calculus has been removed from the lower end of the ureter by cystoscopic manipulation. The patient, a male, aged thirty-one years, had suffered with constant pain in bladder and penis. The cysto-

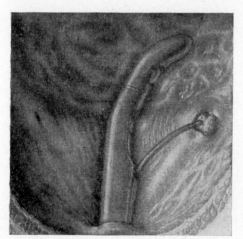

scope showed a calculus projecting from the orifice of the left ureter (Fig. 213). With Casper's catheterizing cystoscope we were able to dislodge the stone—prying it out of the ureter. It rolled down the trigone, leaving a large open ureteral orifice.[1]

If the calculus is located in the ureter above its vesical orifice, passage of instruments (ureteral catheters, bougies, dilators, stone extractors, etc.) may be employed in increasingly larger sizes so as to dilate the ureter and facilitate the passage of the stone. Cocainization of the ureter, and the injection of papaverin below or glycerin above the site of the stone in the ureter are highly recom-

FIG. 213.—First extraction of calculus caught in lower end of ureter by means of a catheterizing cystoscope.

mended. Hydrotherapy and large doses of glycerin internally (200 c.c., H. Casper) have also been advocated. By these methods great numbers of calculi, some amazingly large, have been induced to pass, though repeated catheterizations and employment of two or three large bougies (2 of 11 and one 6 F., Crowell) may be necessary to secure sufficient dilation. It may even be desirable to leave the bougies in place twelve hours or more. Stones may pass slowly, as in one of our cases where one took seven weeks to traverse the ureter. Operation was contemplated several times, but each successive x-ray showed that the calculus had progressed, and the patient's condition was excellent (Figs. 214–220).

Failures should not discourage one, as numerous repetitions of ureteral instrumentation may be necessary to induce the passage of a calculus.

The non-operative methods make a particular appeal in cases of bilateral calculi, multiple calculi, recurrent calculi, and in patients who are not good operative risks. With the earlier recognition of stones—while still small—it seems probable that the future will see nearly all ureteral stones removed by cystoscopic instrumentation.

There are, however, very definite and serious dangers associated with the

[1] Young: American Medicine, 1902, iv, 209–217.

manipulative treatment of ureteral calculi, consisting of infection, and injury to the ureter. If unsuccessful instrumentation is followed by an infection above the stone, the obstruction, which of course has not been removed, favors the rapid

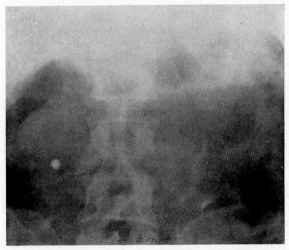

Fig. 214.—Case of spontaneous expulsion of ureteral calculus (1): Stone as first seen. At this time patient had fever, severe pain, leukocytosis, rigidity of right abdomen, and slight hematuria (May 15, 1922). B. U. I. x-Ray 3676.

progress of this infection. We have described elsewhere a case in which this complication occurred in a patient with but one kidney and led to a fatal ending.

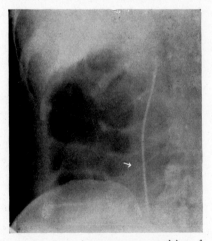

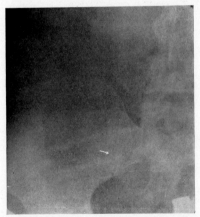

Fig. 215.—Case of spontaneous expulsion of ureteral calculus (2): The arrow points to the calculus which has moved a little ways down the ureter and which lies about ¾ cm. away from the catheter (May 16, 1922). B. U. I. x-Ray 3680.

Fig. 216.—Case of spontaneous expulsion of ureteral calculus (3): The arrow points to the calculus which has moved down opposite the sacro-iliac synchondrosis. At the time this film was taken we were not sure that this shadow represented the calculus (May 17, 1922). B. U. I. x-Ray 3682.

It is incumbent upon all who treat ureteral stones in this fashion to develop their technic to the highest point so that infection will not occur, and to reinforce their care by the injection of efficient antiseptic drugs at the conclusion of the manip-

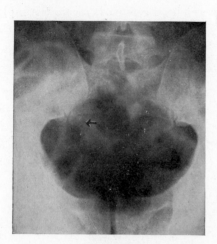

FIG. 217.—Case of spontaneous expulsion of ureteral calculus (4): Further movement of the calculus which now appears just below the pelvic brim. Arrow indicates calculus (May 24, 1922). B. U. I. x-Ray 3689.

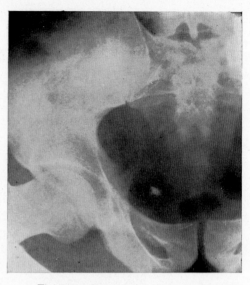

FIG. 218.—Case of spontaneous expulsion of ureteral calculus (5): Calculus has now moved down to a position near the bladder. No symptoms (June 29, 1922). B. U. I. x-Ray 3768.

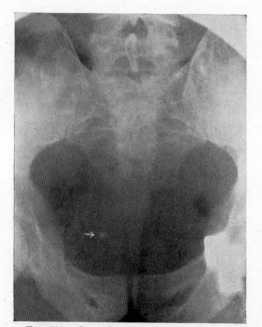

FIG. 219.—Case of spontaneous expulsion of ureteral calculus (6): This picture shows the calculus after it has descended to the lowermost part of the ureter (July 8, 1922). B. U. I. x-Ray 3776.

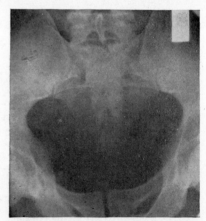

FIG. 220.—Case of spontaneous expulsion of ureteral calculus (7): Final x-ray after the passage of the calculus (July 15, 1922). B. U. I. x-Ray 3814.

ulation. It is desirable to have the patient at all times under close observation, so that the first signs of beginning infection can be detected and the proper measures taken. Even so, there is a certain risk, just as in operative treatment, since

PLATE IX

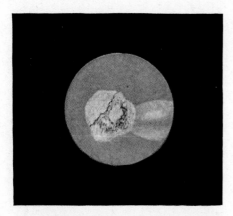

A. Floating calculus next to air bubble on anterior wall of bladder. (Ball of paraffin covered with a thin layer of urinary salts.) B. U. I. 12,787.

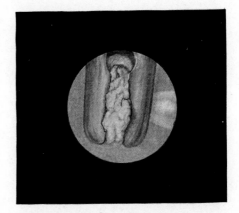

B. Removal of paraffin calculus with cystoscopic rongeur. Calculus grasped by blades of rongeur.

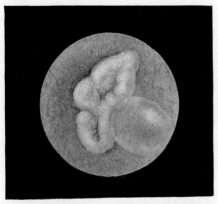

C. Irregular mass of paraffin floating in urine next to air bubble on anterior wall. B. U. I. 10,419.

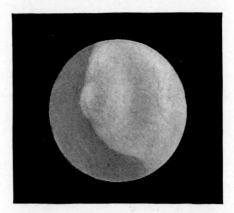

D. Intravesical hernia, abdominal contents pushing mucous membrane into bladder through hole in muscular wall. B. U. I. 7258.

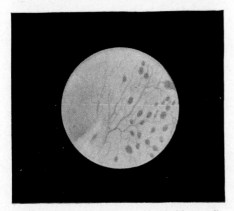

E. Small hemorrhages in bladder wall along course of terminal arteries. B. U. I. 8573.

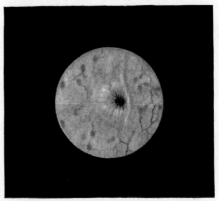

F. Cellule of bladder produced by great intravesical pressure. Terminal hemorrhages in bladder wall.

infections beginning in this manner may occasionally develop with such rapidity that even immediate operation does not cut short their course. It is also essential to use great care not to injure the ureter, and we unhesitatingly condemn instruments which are too stiff or which make use of sharp or angular projections of any sort designed to pull the stone along the ureter by brute force.

If no movement of the stone can be detected as a result of manipulation, it is better not to wait more than a few days before operating, although, of course, the size of the stone will have an influence on this decision. If it is very small, one may be inclined to wait a little longer. If, on the other hand, progressive movement down the ureter can be demonstrated on successive occasions, if the patient is not too uncomfortable, and if no signs of infection develop, operation may be deferred for a much longer time, and we may even see the stone pass spontaneously at the end of several weeks, as in the case illustrated in Figs. 214–220.

Vesical calculi, if small, are often voided with the urine. It is remarkable how large a calculus may pass through the urethra without difficulty. Sometimes they cause lancinating pain and occasionally hemorrhage. Where a prostatic obstruction, bar, or hypertrophied lobe is present, there is much less chance of a calculus, even if small, passing out of the bladder. Sometimes, after having left the bladder, they may be arrested in the urethra, generally the prostatic, but sometimes in the pendulous urethra, especially behind a congenitally narrowed meatus.

Small vesical calculi may be removed by our cystoscopic rongeur, even when found at the bottom of large diverticula (2 cases). The rongeur may also be used to pull out an intravesically projecting ureteral calculus. If the stone is covered by mucous membrane it will be removed by rongeur in such cases. We usually prefer to split open the ureteral pouch covering the stone with a linear application of the high-frequency current,[1] after which the stone has always passed into the bladder.

Small stones may be picked up by a cystoscopic lithotrite or the ordinary lithotrite may be used, followed by evacuation of the fragments as described elsewhere.

Where the stone is not too large and no obstruction of the prostate, no residual urine or trabeculation, no cellules nor diverticula are present, litholapaxy is generally the method of choice.

But when prostatic disease with the above-mentioned complications is found, the stone can generally be removed simultaneously with the prostatic enlargement (by perineal or suprapubic prostatectomy). Incarcerated or encysted vesical calculi generally require suprapubic lithotomy. The technic of these various procedures is described in Chapter XVI.

Continuation of obstruction, vesical pouches, and incomplete removal of fragments is the frequent cause of recurrence of vesical calculi. Great care should, therefore, be taken to suit the operative procedure to the case and to remove thoroughly every fragment, as well as to relieve the obstruction by prostatectomy, punch, urethral dilation, etc., as indicated.

The old median and lateral lithotomy, so famous in the early days of surgery, are discarded now.

Urethral calculi usually come from the bladder, and generally pass out spontaneously, but sometimes require meatotomy. In rare instances they may lodge

[1] Young: Journal of Urology, 1918, ii, 35–38.

in the urethra and may be removed with forceps, sometimes with the aid of an endoscope.

If irregular or furrowed, the patient may be able to pass urine (with difficulty), but a urethritis usually comes on and its cause may not be recognized. We once saw a dignified old gentleman who had patiently suffered himself to be treated for chronic urethritis in Europe and America, when the discharge was produced by an incarcerated calculus near the meatus, which was quickly removed, thus curing the "gleet."

Stones which lodge or develop in the deep urethra may sometimes be pushed back with a sound into the bladder where they may be crushed.

In some cases a perineal operation—prostatotomy or urethrotomy—may be required to remove the stone. In one of our cases a stone, nearly an inch in diameter, had been present in the membranous region of the urethra for years, causing little discomfort. The symptoms were those of urethral stricture.

Prostatic calculi are usually associated with prostatic hypertrophy, and may be removed during prostatectomy. Occasionally these small calculi occur in an otherwise normal prostate (often in young men). If producing symptoms, they may be removed by perineal prostatotomy. Where the stone is larger and projects into the urethra, perineal section back of the sphincter and triangular ligament may be the operation of choice.[1]

Stones in the seminal vesicle seldom require treatment, but may, on occasion, be removed through the perineum.

Operative.—In accordance with the preceding paragraphs, it will be supposed that before operation is considered the patient has been carefully studied with the idea of trying a non-operative course of treatment if possible. As stated above, not infrequently, after repeated passage of catheters and bougies of increasing size into the ureter, the calculus may be induced to pass. Such treatment has to be done with caution and very careful study of the urine to determine that no infection has occurred, and that the kidney is not being impaired either by the continued presence of the stone or the traumatism of the treatment. We have seen one sad case in which, with a single kidney, efforts to induce a ureteral calculus to pass suddenly ended in an acute infection and death. It is, therefore, advisable to use great care in carrying out the non-operative treatment and to realize that serious damage may result. In most cases the removal of a calculus of the ureter or pelvis of the kidney is such a simple affair that one is not justified in taking grave risks by non-operative measures.

The operation to be done will depend on many factors. The location, size, shape, multiplicity, and character of the calculi; the anatomic and pathologic characteristics of the kidney, and the situation in which the calculus is found; the presence or absence of infection and destructive changes in the kidney, the condition of the second kidney, the condition of the patient and the previous stone history.

In deciding upon the operation to be performed one is influenced by the fact, as shown by Hinman, that a kidney damaged by a stone and by the operation necessary to remove it will resume its function if the other kidney is insufficient for any reason, but if the other kidney is perfectly normal and healthy, the damaged kidney will not regain its function after operation.

It seems best to us to divide the question into the following categories:

[1] Young: Johns Hopkins Hospital Reports, 1906, xiii, 385–400.

1. *A Small Stone in Pelvis or Ureter.*—Here if the calculus is in the ureter or at the ureteropelvic juncture and efforts to get it to pass have failed completely, the stone should generally be removed by ureterotomy or pyelotomy in case there are no serious contraindications. If there is a stricture below the stone the longitudinal incision in the ureter or at the ureteropelvic juncture may be closed in a transverse line, thus enlarging the lumen. Before closure very careful determination that the ureter is patent to the bladder and up to the kidney should be made. For this purpose a flexible spiral ureteral bougie is of great value. Catheters and bougies of other types may also be used. In pyelotomy cases very careful investigation of the entire pelvis and its branches, and, as far as possible, the calices, should be made to be sure that no fragments remain. For this purpose to and fro suction lavage is valuable. In this way not only small fragments of stone may be evacuated, but also mucus etc., which might lead to the formation of a calculus. It is very important to make use of the *x*-ray, either by fluoroscopy of the kidney drawn out at operation, or with a radiographic film which is immediately developed, to determine whether the removal has been complete. Where the pelvis is infected, one may consider the advisability of inserting a small ureter catheter into the pelvis, either through the pyelotomy wound or through a puncture, so that continuous irrigation with some mild antiseptic may be carried out, but we have rarely been successful in securing sterilization by this means.

2. *A Large Stone in Pelvis or Ureter.*—It is presumed that the case is such that the possibility of its passage is too remote to be considered. Keyes states that a stone 1 cm. in diameter may pass down the ureter into the bladder, and Crowell has published some cases in which very large stones passed after instrumental dilation. Where the stone is completely obstructing the passage of urine, operation should be carried out as soon as possible to avoid serious injury of the kidney. Not infrequently, however, the stone is tunneled or furrowed and its position is such that it does not obstruct the urine, and in fact causes no pain or discomfort. If the urine from this side is sterile, and the age and general condition of the patient is such as to make conservatism desirable, such calculi may occasionally be left *in situ*. We have seen one case in which a calculus, the length and diameter of a small cigar, caused no obstruction or pain in the ureter, and had been present probably fourteen years.

As a rule these stones should be removed, and the sooner the better. Pyelotomy is greatly to be preferred to opening the kidney, and if the stone is confined to the pelvis or has very short branches extending toward the calices, unless the pelvis is an intrarenal one, no difficulty is usually encountered in removing the stone through the pyelotomy incision. Where the pelvis is largely intrarenal, and the portion exposed at operation is so small and so surrounded by renal tissue that it is impossible to remove a large pelvic stone through the pyelotomy wound, it may be necessary to do nephrolithotomy.

3. *Stone in Calyx.*—If it is possible to remove such stones through the pyelotomy incision, this should be done, as the operation is simpler, safer, and far less destructive to the kidney substance than nephrotomy. Where the calyx is short, and the passage-way connecting it with the pelvis is sufficiently wide, as shown by the pyelogram, one may often succeed in the removal of a calculus from such a calyx through a pyelotomy wound. If difficulty is experienced in entering the calyx and finding the calculus, needling directed by accurate measurements from

the cortex, as suggested by Burns,[1] may be of assistance (Fig. 221).   Care should
be taken not to fracture the calculus, and to be sure that everything shown by the
x-ray has been removed, careful exploration of the other calices being done as far
as possible.   Where the stone is larger than the exit from the calyx or where the
exit itself is very long and narrow, chances of removing calculi completely may be
remote, particularly if there are several present.   In such cases nephrotomy directly upon the calculus is the accepted method.   The incision should usually be

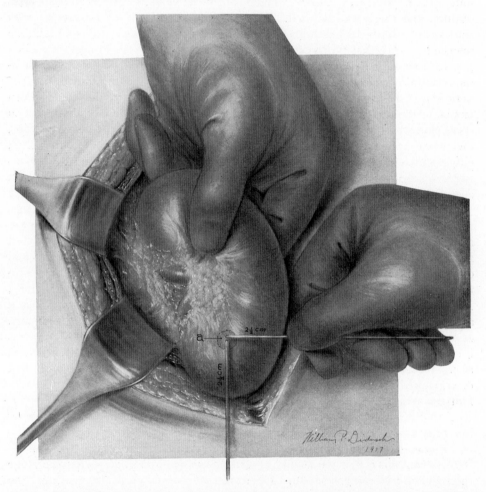

FIG. 221.—Method of locating calculus within kidney.   Its location in relation to the kidney
outline is measured from the x-ray.   By measuring on the kidney in the same manner after it is exposed
one can locate the stone with accuracy.   a, Stone.

parallel with the main vascular trunks so as to divide as few vessels as possible.
The calyx should be well exposed so that a complete operation is carried out and no
fragments or other calculi left behind.   Careful search of the rest of the calices
and remainder of the pelvis should be carried out and the kidney carefully palpated
for other areas which might mean stone.   In cases of multiple calculi the stones
removed, when placed together, should conform to the x-ray shadow.   If possible,

[1] Journal of Urology, 1917, i, 559–570.

the ureter should be probed through to the bladder, and examination of the uretero-pelvic juncture be made for strictures and congenital abnormalities. When the calyx is situated so that it drains up hill through a small connection with the pelvis, and particularly if there is a dilatation of the pelvis and other pathologic changes which indicate that a recurrence of the calculus will probably take place, it is our opinion that resection of this dependent portion of the kidney, thus radically excising the stone-bearing area and the dependent pouch-like calyx, should be carried out. In the discussion of operative technic we have given the details of this procedure, and the cases upon which it has been performed. The results obtained justify, we believe, the opinion that this procedure should become the method of choice in such cases (which are limited in number).

4. *Stones in Pelvis and Calyx.*—Here again, if possible, the operation of choice is pyelotomy, and as mentioned in previous paragraphs, much will depend on the size, shape, multiplicity, and character of the calculi and the anatomic configuration of the calyx and its connection with the pelvis. Where it is manifestly impossible to do a radical operation through the pelvis, the kidney should be opened. Where several calyces are involved it may still be possible to empty them completely through the pelvis, but if not, either multiple small incisions or a single large wound may be necessary, but this should be done with the realization that the procedure is much more serious and destructive of kidney function than pyelotomy or small nephrotomies.

5. *Large Stone in Pelvis with One or More Branches in Calyces.*—In some cases such a stone may be satisfactorily removed through a pyelotomy, as above described, but in other cases, particularly where the branches are multiple or clubbed at their ends, a wide nephrotomy may be necessary for complete removal. These cases are very often associated with serious impairment of the kidney and with chronic infection often characterized by accumulation of pus above the stone or focal areas in the kidney. In such cases nephrectomy is preferable to extensive nephrolithotomy in an effort to save the kidney, which is necessarily badly injured by the incision and the sutures required to stop the hemorrhage. One should determine before operation just what the kidney function is, whether infection is present, and its extent. Forearmed in this way one can usually determine as soon as the kidney is exposed whether nephrectomy, nephrolithotomy, or pyelotomy should be chosen, the desideratum being to cure the patient and eliminate the possibility of recurrence of the calculus or a continuation of a chronically infected kidney.

Unfortunately the recuperative power of kidneys which have been badly injured by the long presence of large stones, particularly when infection is present, is very poor, so that in many cases nephrectomy is the method of choice. It is in these cases that an exact foreknowledge of the condition of the other kidney is so important.

Stone in Kidney Substance.—Statistics show that cortical stones occur in about 20 per cent. of the cases. As they do not usually communicate with the pelvis or calyces they are best removed through small incisions through the substance of the kidney, so made as to injure as little as possible of the blood-supply. The opening should be sufficiently large for thorough exploration of the other calyces or pelvis so as to insure against calculi being left behind. If the stone-bearing area is small and suppurative, it may be packed, otherwise several sutures to close the area and arrest hemorrhage should be provided.

Small "silent" calculi embedded in the substance of the kidney may often be causing so little harm that they may be safely left without operation, especially if the patient is old or his general condition such that conservatism is desirable. One should ascertain with certainty that the kidney function is good and infection not present before advising a non-operative course in these cases unless the disease is bilateral, which completely alters the problem. "Silent" stones in calyces may also be treated according to the same principles. In all these cases the patient should be seen occasionally to determine that no harm is resulting. Not infrequently, especially if the patient becomes neurasthenic, removal of the calculus from the cortex or pelvis, even though "silent" and producing no symptoms, is the better procedure.

7. *Bifid Pelvis, Stone in One Portion.*—The frequency of this form of abnormality is so great that it is remarkable that calculi do not form more often in these cases. We have called attention to the importance of this condition in previous papers, and have advised that where a calculus has led to more or less complete destruction of the kidney surrounding the pelvis which it occupies, resection or heminephrectomy should be carried out.

Our attention was drawn to the importance of this condition by a case in which the ureter catheter on the left side passed into the normal lower half of the kidney, thus failing to detect the suppurative condition in the upper half of the kidney.[1] With the further development of the x-ray and pyelogram, such cases are now recognized with the greatest ease, and we believe resection or heminephrectomy is the method of choice. In taking pyelograms it is important to withdraw the catheter to the lower half of the ureter in order to detect cases of bifid ureter and pelvis. The advantage of resection is that it leaves a healthy remaining kidney half which probably hypertrophies with time. Where the stone in half of a bifid pelvis is small or associated with little or no renal destruction and particularly if infection is absent, and the phthalein test or careful examination at operation shows that this portion of the kidney is of functional value, conservative pyelotomy or nephrotomy may be the method of choice.

8. *Stone in Kidney and Ureter Simultaneously (Unilateral).*—If possible, the ureteral calculus should be induced to pass by physical or non-operative methods so that the operator will only have the renal stone to deal with. Where the ureteral stone fails to pass and its location is near the kidney both may be successfully attacked through the usual kidney incision. If one stone is in the pelvis the ureteral stone may sometimes be pushed or "milked" upward into the pelvis and both removed through a single pyelotomy, or after pyelotomy a delicate forceps may be passed down the ureter to withdraw the ureteral stone through the pelvis. Otherwise both will have to be removed through separate incisions, ureteral, pelvic, or renal, as the case may be. If the ureter is blocked by the calculus within it and grave symptoms are present as a result of back-pressure, it may be advisable only to remove the ureteral calculus, particularly if the renal stone is where it may do little harm. Complete removal of both stones, however, is usually desirable.

9. *Stone in Both Kidneys or Ureters (Bilateral Nephrolithiasis).*—The problem is immensely aggravated by the presence of a calculus in the opposite side, and many of the rules which apply in unilateral calculus have to be discarded. In the first place, it is very desirable to do as little traumatism and permanent injury as

[1] Young: Johns Hopkins Hospital Reports, 1906, xiii, 447–454.

possible.   The kidney function on both sides should be preserved or as little injured as possible.   One does not dare to do a nephrectomy unless almost compelled to do so, and stones which would be removed immediately without hesitation (often along with the kidney) in the unilateral cases may best be left behind when bilateral nephrolithiasis is present.   The problem is so varied that it is extremely difficult to lay down any fixed rules.   Perhaps it may be discussed as follows:

(*a*) *When both kidneys are in good condition and uninfected.*   In such cases one may go in and remove a calculus from the ureter, pelvis, or kidney with as little traumatism as possible.   Operations through the renal cortex should be avoided at all costs, if possible, and the sterility and function of the kidney preserved.   At a subsequent operation the other side may be likewise operated on if the stone is producing symptoms, pain, hemorrhage, pyuria, and particularly if associated with infection.   Here again the procedure should be as conservative as possible.   Bilateral cases of this type are constantly operated upon with impunity.

(*b*) *Bilateral nephrolithiasis with marked impairment of the kidneys.*   Here the problem is a grave one.   The presence of renal impairment, especially if progressive, may demand operative relief, and a most careful study should be made to determine the comparative value of the two kidneys and to weigh most carefully operative procedures for extraction of the calculus from either side.   Here again the conservative pyelotomy should be preferred to nephrotomy.   As a rule, it is better to operate upon the worst kidney so as to have the better renal function to carry the patient through the convalescence.

With bilateral nephrolithiasis and one kidney greatly impaired or destroyed, no operation is indicated unless pain, infection, toxemia, etc., call for relief, in which case, if the renal function on the other side is good, and the stone located in a position where it does not obstruct, nephrectomy upon the badly injured kidney may be carried out.

(*d*) *Large "silent" stones* associated with calculi in the opposite kidney or ureter should generally be left alone.   By "silent" stones it is understood to mean cases in which pain is absent and the infection and general symptoms are such as to warrant the conservative treatment.   When the stone is of the "stag-horn" type, the kidney may often be of fair function, and not infrequently bilateral stag-horn calculi are seen with remarkably few symptoms and fairly good renal function.   Geraghty[1] has discussed cases from this clinic and mentions one case in which a kidney containing a very large stag-horn calculus continued to have good phthalein output during eight years.   He notes that such calculi are only exceptionally the cause of hydronephrosis or pyonephrosis.   Removal of these calculi always necessitates a complete nephrotomy, and the renal impairment resulting will usually be greater, according to Geraghty, than that produced by the stone.   He thinks these kidneys should rarely be operated on, and that if operation is necessary, nephrectomy should usually be done.

In cases of bilateral nephrolithiasis when the development of an acute pyonephrosis or a ureteral block requires immediate operative interference, drainage of the renal cortex, pelvis, or ureter may be sufficient to relieve the crisis or, in fact, restore the patient to comparative health.   The problem is one requiring the greatest care, and about which there is much discussion and uncertainty.   Undoubtedly where calculi are present on both sides and can be safely removed

[1] Journal of the American Medical Association, lxx, 901–903.

without injury of the renal tissue, this should usually be done. Where the patient's life would be endangered conservative measures should be adopted. Pain, infection, fever, and progressively diminishing renal function and increasng evidence of uremia may force the surgeon to operate even in desperate cases.

10. *Stone in Single Kidney or Ureter.*—Here again conservatism is forced upon the surgeon by the nature of the case, and many of the principles laid down in the preceding paragraph are directly applicable here. Conservative operations must be chosen. If the stone can be induced to pass by physical, instrumental, or ureteral methods, these should be employed. Where the stone is "silent" or producing little or no trouble, and the kidney function is well maintained, it may often be left alone. Such is the case when the stone in the ureter allows the urine to pass through grooves upon its surface. The greatest care should be employed in watching these cases from year to year, operation being carried out when the picture changes, and the patient's life is in danger. Pain, infection, decreasing phthalein, and increasing uremic symptoms force intervention, and sudden complete blockage, of course, demands immediate attention. In such cases the passage of a ureter catheter past the calculus and drainage through it for a day or more may give complete relief, and even lead to the passage of the stone. In others this procedure may be repeated a few times as long as no infection is present, but if infection occurs or the condition of the patient becomes aggravated regardless of the relief afforded by ureter catheterization, operation should be undertaken for the removal of the stone and the cure of the blockage. It is very important not to persist in conservative methods too long, as shown in the following case (B. U. I. 6364): A man with the left kidney removed came in with a calculus in the right ureter and complete anuria. The x-ray showed a calculus about 3 inches above the bladder. No difficulty was experienced in passing a catheter and relieving the block. The patient rapidly improved and during successive days other catheters and bougies were inserted in the hope that the stone would be passed, but it did not move. For a time the urine would pass by the calculus, then blockage would suddenly occur, and hasty ureter catheterization would become necessary. Finally infection occurred and spread rapidly. The stone was removed through an extraperitoneal low abdominal incision, but the patient died of uremia and sepsis, and autopsy showed an acute pyelonephritis. Unquestionably in this case operation should have been carried out much earlier.

11. *Stone in horseshoe or ectopic kidney* may present serious problems. A most careful study, by means of pyelograms, of the relation between the kidney and the surrounding structures, and particularly the great vessels, should be made. If possible the mobility of the kidney, as shown by x-rays, taken in both vertical and horizontal positions, should be determined. The relation of the stone to the ureters and pelves must be accurately determined. The operation to be carried out will depend upon the character of the anomaly and the complicating conditions. (See description elsewhere.)

12. *Stones in kidneys subject to tuberculosis, tumor, or polycystic disease,* etc., occasionally require relief. The principles guiding the treatment of the major pathologic conditions will determine largely the operative attack for the removal of the calculus. In tuberculous kidneys, when the kidney is completely destroyed by "autonephrectomy," and the stone is simply a concretion in a caseous kidney which is doing no harm, a non-operative treatment is usually the safest course to

TABLE 48

116 Cases Were Treated Operatively

Pyelolithotomy

31 cases.

9 well, 5 improved, 1 unimproved, 16 no reply, 3 dead (recurrence of stone).

Well, 1—eleven years, 3—ten years, 3—four years, 2—three years.

Improved, 1—ten years, 1—two and a half years, 3—two years.

Unimproved, 1—five years.·

Nephrotomy

24 cases.

7 well, 2 improved, 4 unimproved, 1 (bilateral), no reply, 11 no reply, 1 dead (recurrence, bilateral stone and shock), 3 dead other causes.

Well, 1—six years, 1—four years, 2—three years, 1—two years, 2—one year.

Improved, 1—five years, 1—three years.

Unimproved, 2—six years, 1—three years, 1—two years.

Ureterolithotomy

6 cases.

3 well, 1 improved, 1 dead, 2 no reply.

Well, 1—eight years, 1—four years, 1—two years.

Improved, 1—seven years.

Nephrectomy

43 cases.

15 well (1 nephrectomy and nephrotomy well), 2 improved (1 recurrence in other kidney), 26 no replies, 2 dead (shock), 4 dead other causes.

Nephrectomy and Operation on Other Side

4 cases.

1 well, 1 no reply, 2 dead.

Pyelotomy and Ureterotomy

2 cases.

1 dead, 1 not improved

Nephrotomy and Ureterotomy

2 cases.

1 well, 1 no reply.

Well, 1—seven years.

Passed Stones

24 cases.

6 are well—no recurrence.

1 operated upon later—well.

2 operated upon later—unimproved.

3 dead.

12 not heard from.

40 Cases Not Operated Upon at the Brady Institute

Not Treated at All

16 cases.

Well, 1—five years, 1—four years, 1—three years, 2—? years.

Improved, 1—nine years, 1—five years.

Unimproved, 1—five years, 1—four years.

Dead, 7 cases.

Not heard from, 2 cases.

Operated Upon Elsewhere

12 cases.

Well, 1—ten years, 1—five years, 1—four years, 1—three years, 1—one and a half years, 1—one year, 2—? years.

Improved, 1—ten years.

Unimproved, 1—ten years, 1—four years, 1—? years.

pursue. In such cases there are often lesions elsewhere (lung, glands, pleura, or genito-urinary tract) which may give trouble if nephrectomy is attempted. Therefore, conservatism is the better course. In one of our recent cases of double polycystic kidney a stone which was giving pain was removed and at the same time the cysts, superficial and deep, were incised as completely as possible, with very good result.

13. *Stones accompanied by great destruction of the kidney* and with a healthy kidney on the other side should be treated by nephrectomy, other conditions being favorable. Where the kidney is completely or largely destroyed by pyonephrosis, or where the stone is such that only by a very extensive nephrotomy can it be removed, nephrectomy is the better procedure. It must, of course, be determined beforehand that the opposite kidney has hypertrophied, and is well able to carry on the work of the two. Nephrectomy is quicker, less bloody, and a much safer operation than wide nephrolithotomy. The great destruction of the kidney substance which follows the incision and sutures necessary for hemostasis in nephrotomy make nephrectomy the method of choice in such cases.

Results of Treatment.—The results of treatment in our series of 180 cases of nephrolithiasis is shown in Table 48 on page 415.

Vesical Calculi.—The operative treatment for vesical calculi has already been considered (page 407).

CHAPTER VII

BENIGN HYPERTROPHY OF THE PROSTATE

PATHOLOGY

The pathologic nature of hypertrophy of the prostate has been the subject of endless dispute, not only as to its point of origin, but as to whether it is a hyperplastic process or a true neoplasm. The latter question is academic, and we prefer to let it rest with the statement of our belief that the process is a hyperplastic one. On this basis we are discussing the lesion as a separate subject. Further comment on "adenoma of the prostate" will be found in the section on Carcinoma of the Prostate.

Benign hypertrophy of the prostate is associated with senescence. It occurs in dogs, and Goodpasture[1] has shown that the process here is entirely analogous to that in the human. It is not known what initiates the hyperplasia. Castration produces an atrophy of the normal prostate, but has no effect on a hypertrophy when already established. We have noted that most of our patients have been married men, and that none have come from the celibate priesthood. It has also been suggested that hypertrophy follows sexual repression where desire is present. These hypotheses, while interesting, cannot be said to be proved. Equally, it has not been possible to lay the blame upon pre-existing gonorrheal or other infections. It is now believed that prostatic hypertrophy is confined largely to the small suburethral glands, and it has been suggested that this may occur as a compensatory phenomenon when the remainder of the prostate undergoes the usual senile atrophy. Since in all cases of hypertrophy the atrophy of the uninvolved portions of the gland can equally well be ascribed to pressure, it has not been possible to prove this hypothesis.

In the majority of men the prostate undergoes atrophy in old age, comparable and parallel with the atrophy of other organs. Thompson found the prostate hypertrophied in 34 per cent. of cases over sixty years old, but in only half of these had any obstructive symptoms been caused. In most of the remainder the prostate was smaller than normal. This atrophy causes no symptoms.

Prostatic hypertrophy tends to increase constantly in size. In occasional cases this growth is rapid, but is usually very slow, and there may apparently be remissions in the growth. In an occasional case increase will stop entirely at a certain point. Since there is no tendency to necrosis, ulceration, or metastasis, and the growth is painless, prostatic hypertrophy causes no symptoms whatever except as it presses upon and obstructs the urethra or occasionally the rectum. Exception is also made for a few cases where hemorrhage occurs. This disease is, therefore, important as one of the chief causes of the obstructive uropathy.

---

[1] Journal of Medical Research, 1918, xxxviii, 127–190. (See also Smith: Journal of Medical Research, 1919, xl, 31–49.)

We will recall a few salient anatomic facts (see Fig. 222). Lowsley[1] has shown that the prostatic glands arise in five groups—median posterior, two lateral, and anterior or ventral. According to him, those of the lateral groups grow in length and complexity until they make up most of the substance of the normal gland, and the dual origin is suggested by the shallow median furrow felt per rectum. The posterior group develops to a lesser extent, and as a somewhat flattened layer. The median group shows a still smaller development, while those of the anterior group usually remain short and simple. On the posterior or dorsal aspect of the urethra, between the verumontanum and the vesical orifice, are found other glands, which also remain short and simple. These are known as the suburethral glands, and were first described by Jores.[2] They lie between the median group of prostatic tubules and the urethral lumen. Homologues of these glands are also found, but not in all cases, beneath the epithelium of the vesical orifice, of the trigone (sub-trigonal glands), and even back of the interureteric bar in the lower half of the bladder.

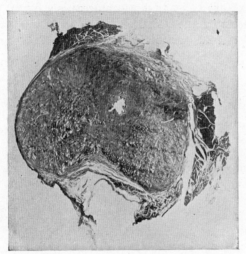

FIG. 222.—Low-power magnification of a cross-section of the entire prostate of a young adult, aged twenty-one. From Mr. Henry Wade.

Loeschke[3] and Adrion[4] restudied the anatomy of the adult prostate, and they concluded that it differed markedly from that of the hypertrophied prostate. They divided the glands into three categories, according to their length. First, the very short and simple "mucosal glands" which arise principally on the lateral and anterior walls of the urethra at the level of the verumontanum, but which are also found on the posterior wall in the region of the sphincter, and indeed are more numerous posteriorly at this point. They may also extend up on the trigone for varying distances. Second, there are somewhat longer and more branched glands, called "submucosal glands," which run principally in an anteroposterior direction, on each side of the urethra, and curve around posteriorly to empty into the posterolateral sulci of the urethra, at either side of the verumontanum. Third, the principal mass of the prostate is made up of the prostatic glands proper, which are long and show much branching and which lie outside the two above-mentioned gland groups, and curve around to enter the posterolateral sulci. These relations are represented graphically in the diagram (Fig. 224). These authors state that there is a definite fibrous capsule in the position indicated by the dotted line, separating the mucosal and submucosal glands, which they speak of collectively as the "inner glands," from the prostatic glands proper, or "outer glands" (Fig. 223).

[1] American Journal of Anatomy, 1912, xiii, 299–346.

[2] Virchow's Archiv, 1894, cxxxv, 224–247.

[3] Münchener Medizinische Wochenschrift, 1920, lxvii, 302.

[4] Ziegler's Beiträge zur pathologischen Anatomie und Allgemeinen Pathologie, 1922, lxx, 179–202 (Lit.).

Jacoby,[1] in an excellent article based on the study of some 200 autopsy specimens of prostates of all ages, confirms these findings, except that he states that the capsule separating the inner from the outer glands is by no means constant.

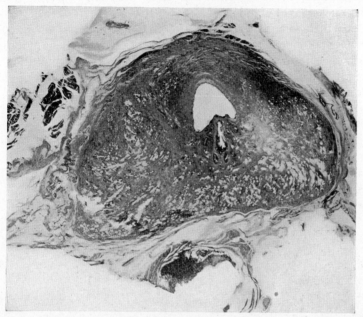

Fig. 223.—Low-power magnification of a cross-section of the entire prostate of a normal individual, aged forty-one. Note how close the fibrous layer marking the anterior boundary of the posterior lamella comes to the urethra. This indicates that the urethral glands are not hypertrophied. The ejaculatory ducts and utricle are well shown. From Mr. Henry Wade.

These inner, mucosal, suburethral, central, or peri-urethral glands, although known since 1894, first took on importance when Albarran and Motz[2] in 1902 dis-

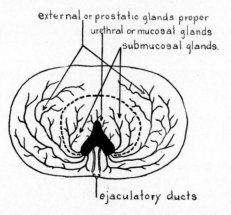

external or prostatic glands proper
urethral or mucosal glands
submucosal glands.

ejaculatory ducts

Fig. 224.—Diagram showing the anatomy of the normal prostate gland, according to Loeschke and Adrion.

covered that the hypertrophied median lobe was derived from those located at the

[1] Zeitschrift für Urologische Chirurgie, 1923, xiv, 6–37 (Lit.).
[2] Annales des Maladies des Organes Génito-Urinaires, 1902, xx, 769–817.

posterior aspect of the vesical orifice. The mucosal glands in this locality have since been known as "Albarran's glands."

To Motz and Perearneau,[1] however, goes the credit for perceiving that all hypertrophies of the prostate arise from these mucosal or suburethral glands. Tandler and Zuckerkandl,[2] Papin and Verliac,[3] Ribbert,[4] and others have confirmed this work, and there is no longer any reason to doubt its essential truth. Jacoby shows splendid photomicrographs of very small and early spheroids of hypertrophy, just beneath the urethral mucosa, and with ducts still communicating with the urethra (Fig. 225). This seems to dispose of the contention that the growth is a true neoplasm, or adenoma.

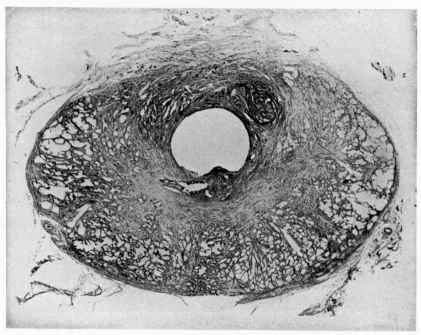

FIG. 225.—Cross-section of the entire prostate of a man sixty-two years old, showing a very early stage of beginning prostatic hypertrophy. Note that the two small spheroids are both very closely applied to the mucosa while the rest of the prostate is normal. The acini of the lower spheroid are connected by ducts which join and open into the urethra by a single channel, indicating that the process is not a true adenoma. From Jacoby, Zeitschrift für Urologische Chirurgie, 1923, xiv, 6–37.

The conception of Motz and Perearneau explains perfectly the findings in hypertrophy of the prostate. Since the enlargement always begins in the "inner" or mucosal glands, it is always central, in close relationship with the urethra, and surrounded by a layer of prostatic tissue, normal except for the results of compression. Since these prostatic glands proper all empty into the posterior aspect of the urethra (Fig. 226), they tend to be spread out over the posterior and lateral surfaces of the hypertrophied masses, forming the "posterior lamella" as seen at operation or autopsy. Thus the posterior lamella, with the ejaculatory ducts within it, does

[1] Annales des Maladies des Organes Génito-Urinaires, 1905, xxiii, 1521–1548.

[2] Studien zur Anatomie und Klinik der Prostatahypertrophie, Berlin, 1922.

[3] Archives Urologiques de la Clinique de Necker, 1919, ii, 425–567.

[4] Zeigler's Beiträge zur pathologischen Anatomie und Allgemeinen Pathologie, 1916, lxi, 149–168.

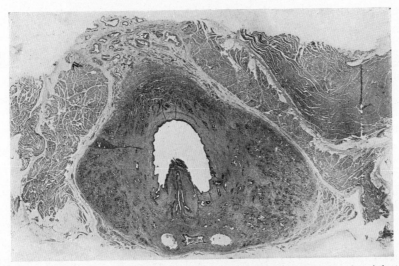

Fig. 226.—Low-power magnification of a cross-section of the entire prostate of an infant of four months. The fascia surrounding the prostate and separating it from the levator ani muscles is well shown, also the preprostatic venous plexus. The prostatic ducts curving around and entering the lateral sulci at either side of the verumontanum are seen. In the posterior lamella appear the two large ejaculatory ducts and, between them, the prostatic utricle. From Mr. Henry Wade.

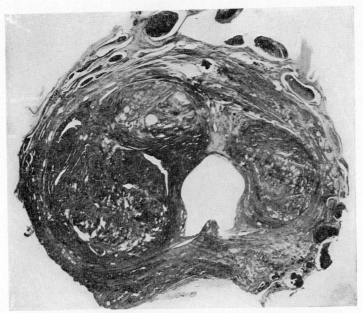

Fig. 227.—Low-power magnification of a cross-section of the entire prostate which is the site of benign prostatic hypertrophy. Note how the fibrous band marking the anterior boundary of the posterior lamella is pushed outward and backward by the masses of hypertrophied tissue which have developed adjacent to the urethra. One "lateral lobe" is much larger than the other. From Mr. Henry Wade.

not represent a "posterior lobe" of the normal prostate, but rather the entire normal prostate, distended and thinned out by the growth of the hypertrophied masses within it (Fig. 227).

The mucosal glands which undergo hypertrophy are always above the verumontanum—that is, between it and the bladder. We have observed no exception to this rule, nor have Tandler and Zuckerkandl in their great experience. Consequently, the verumontanum will always be found, no matter how large the prostate, at a point very near the apex and membranous urethra, and can be avoided in a properly conducted operation. The ejaculatory ducts, running in the posterior lamella, are never included in the hypertrophied masses.

It should be mentioned that, while the hypertrophic process very seldom begins in the prostatic glands proper, or outer glands, it may rarely do so, and occasionally one sees an isolated spheroid of hypertrophy within the substance of the posterior lamella (Fig. 228). This circumstance accounts for certain cases in which there is recurrence of the hypertrophy even after complete and thorough operation, and also for certain cases in which spheroids are seen projecting as nodules on the posterior surface of the prostate.

As the hypertrophied masses enlarge, their development varies greatly according to the point at which the initial enlargement occurs. If the process begins in the region of the vesical orifice (Fig. 229), the line of least resistance must be upward through the sphincter, and as the mass increases in size it pushes into the cavity of the bladder (Fig. 230). In its growth it is influenced by the sphincteric and trigonal muscles which, as we have shown, hypertrophy as a result of the increased work put upon them in opening the vesical orifice by the increasing growth of the prostatic obstruction. The frequent contractions of the sphincter cause a groove to appear in the mass as it enlarges so that, eventually, as the intravesical portion increases in diameter, the whole will have a pedunculated appearance. If the growth gets very large, the sphincter may be so widely dilated that it atrophies and eventually practically disappears. If the growth pushes up exactly in the midline, it is probable that the trigonal muscles (muscles of Bell), passing over or around it, play an important part in determining its shape, and account for the bilobed and trilobed appearances sometimes seen.

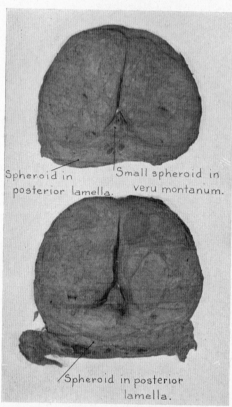

Fig. 228.—Cross-sections of the entire prostate removed at autopsy from a case of benign prostatic hypertrophy. Note that the enlargement is mostly in the "lateral lobes," but that a few small spheroids are to be seen in the posterior lamella and verumontanum. This is an unusual finding and in such a case obstruction may recur after removal of the lateral masses by the ordinary technic of prostatectomy.

The intravesical mass is usually posterior, but occasionally may arise anteriorly (Fig. 231), apparently from the ventral group of glands, which are short and belong

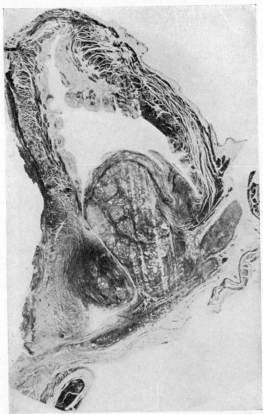

FIG. 229.—Low-power magnification of a median sagittal section showing the bladder, prostate, seminal vesicles, and membranous urethra. The bladder is hypertrophied, contracted, and the mucosa is edematous. The prostate is hypertrophied. A large middle lobe is shown extending up into the bladder. One lateral lobe is evidently enlarged more than the other since it pushes across the midline and a section of it appears below and in front of the median lobe. Note how the median lobe pushes up the trigone and obstructs the orifice. From Mr. Henry Wade.

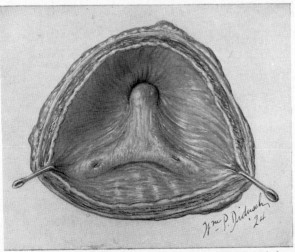

FIG. 230.—Autopsy specimen showing small median prostatic lobe, with hypertrophy of trigone and ureteral ridges and pouch behind them. This hypertrophy of trigone is undoubtedly due to increased exercise required to pull down obstructive median lobe during micturition.

to the same type as the suburethral ones.   In still other cases the growth may extend almost or quite around the entire urethra, so that a structure shaped like the uterine cervix pushes up into the bladder.   When mucosal glands are present on the trigone, or even beyond the interureteric bar, they also may hypertrophy, causing true intravesical masses.   Sometimes this occurs in younger individuals, the resulting "cystic adenoma" markedly resembling prostatic hypertrophy under the microscope.   (See Neoplasms of the Bladder.)

This intravesical type of growth is the most apt to produce obstruction as it pushes up through the sphincter.   If the mass develops from gland groups at or above the sphincter, as it becomes pedunculated it may fall into the orifice during micturition, and produce obstruction in the manner of a ball-valve while still very small (Fig. 230).

If, however, the growth begins further down the urethra, it increases laterally, and shows no tendency to push through the sphincter, presumably because it becomes too wide before its upper margin reaches the sphincteric region.   This form of growth is much more apt to extend around the urethra, but is usually seen as two masses, lateral to the urethra (Fig. 228).   This suggests origin from two different foci.   The two masses may be equal in size, one may be larger than the other, or, rarely, the growth may be confined to one side.   Posteriorly, the masses are separated by the posterior lamella.   They press upon the urethra, converting it into a narrow slit, with its long diameter extending anteroposteriorly.   This slit may extend as far anteriorly as do the lateral masses, or they may come in contact with each other in front of it.   If the ventral group of glands take part in the growth, there may be a layer of hyperplastic tissue

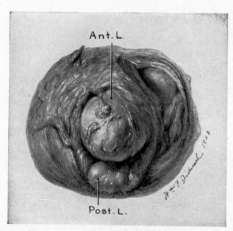

Fig. 231.—Perineal prostatectomy, prostate removed in one piece showing unusually great hypertrophy of the ventral group of glands (anterior lobe).   The posterior group (median lobe) is also hypertrophied, but to a less degree.   B. U. I. 11220.

running across in front, but more usually this does not occur, and the lateral masses are united, anteriorly to the urethra, only by a thin sheath of fibrous tissue. It is through this sheath that the finger breaks in the first stage of a suprapubic prostatectomy.

Sometimes the lateral masses in their upward extension expand within the internal sphincter so that intravesical masses may appear lying to the side of the urethra.

This infravesical growth is less apt to cause obstruction.   Often the urine flows freely through the slit-like urethra until the lateral pressure becomes very great.

It is infrequent for the infravesical or intravesical form to exist alone, but usually there is a combination of the two, with one or the other predominating.   Whatever the form, however, the growth always originates above the verumontanum, since while the distance from the veru to the apex of the prostate remains practically unchanged, the veru may be pushed very far away from the vesical orifice by the growth. This lengthening of the prostatic urethra, which may reach 4 inches or more, is a characteristic feature.

As the hyperplastic masses grow, the unaffected portions of the prostate, which now form a sheath or capsule about the growth, undergo a certain amount of fibrosis, like the thin sheet of renal tissue about a hydronephrosis. On account of this increased firmness, the masses can be easily distinguished at operation, by touch or vision, from the sheath, and separation along this "line of cleavage" is easily accomplished by blunt dissection. There is no such line of cleavage in a normal prostate.

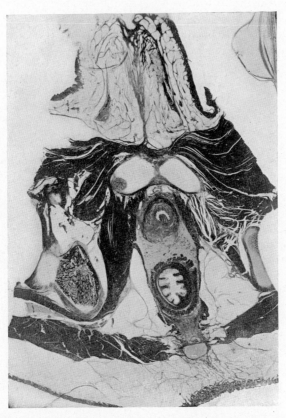

Fig. 232.—Low-power magnification of a cross-section of the entire pelvis of a term fetus. Note the fascial planes at either side of the rectum going forward to surround the prostate and walling off the ischiorectal fossæ. The section passes through the prostate at the level of the verumontanum showing the ejaculatory ducts. The external sphincter is shown forming a layer on the anterior surface of the prostate. The recto-urethralis muscle is not shown, section passing above it. From Mr. Henry Wade.

It is owing to the fact that there are prostatic glands in this sheath or "capsule" that the prostate may return practically to normal after enucleation of hypertrophied masses, and normal prostatic secretion be obtained. Figure 232 shows the gross relations of the prostate with the surrounding structures.

The cut surface of a hyperplastic prostatic mass is usually light colored, and of moderately soft, elastic consistence. There may be seen definite, rounded areas known as "spheroids," which represent portions of the tumor arising from subsidiary centers of growth. Sometimes the contents project in convex form after section, indicating the existence of internal pressure in the spheroids. Occasionally individual spheroids project beyond the general surface of the mass, causing nodules which may even be felt per rectum.   The fibrous stroma may be seen as grayish, translucent strands, generally more abundant between the spheroids.   The epithelial portion has a more yellowish cast, and is opaque, though less so than carcinoma. Cystic dilatation of acini may give the mass a sponge-like appearance.   A milky secretion, similar to normal prostatic secretion, flows from the cut surface.   It is more abundant in cystic cases.

Microscopically, one sees the epithelial hyperplasia represented by folds and villous formations within the acini, the normal architecture of the epithelial layer itself being preserved (Fig. 233).   That the growth is slow and ordered is indicated by the absence of mitoses, by the failure of fusion between the tips of villi which come in contact, and by the presence of connective-tissue stalks, with capillaries,

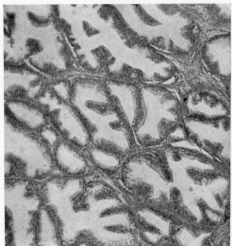
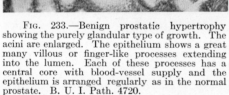
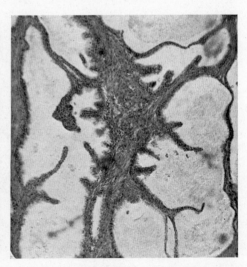

FIG. 233.—Benign prostatic hypertrophy showing the purely glandular type of growth. The acini are enlarged.   The epithelium shows a great many villous or finger-like processes extending into the lumen.   Each of these processes has a central core with blood-vessel supply and the epithelium is arranged regularly as in the normal prostate. B. U. I. Path. 4720.

FIG. 234.—Benign prostatic hypertrophy showing cystic dilatation of the hypertrophied acini.   This picture is often associated with chronic inflammatory changes and is thought to represent the result of occlusion of ducts with subsequent retention of secretion. B. U. I. Path. 4716.

in all the new-formed processes.   The tubules undoubtedly increase in length and complexity, and it would seem that the enormous masses sometimes occurring could not be produced without multiplication of acini.   Frequently the acini undergo cystic dilatation (Fig. 234), and become filled with secretion and desquamated epithelium.   The cast-off cells, like those of the normal prostate, undergo fatty degeneration, showing many droplets of lipoid material in the cytoplasm. Later the nuclei may disappear, and the droplets fuse into large globules of fatty matter.   The epithelium is stretched out into a single layer, and often flattened until it is as thin as a serous coat.   The thinning is most marked on those aspects of the cyst which are freest to bulge outward.   The partitions between adjacent cysts become very thin, and may be absorbed in part or whole, giving complex multilocular cysts.   The cysts sometimes at least remain in communication with tubules, for on massage the partial obstruction may be overcome and the cysts emptied into the urethra. Such cases are the ones which show temporary diminu-tion in size, and improvement in symptoms of obstruction, after massage. The posterior lamella may be the seat of a cystic change, without evidence of epithelial hyperplasia. This is probably due to obstruction of its ducts by the hypertrophied masses between it and the urethra.

In uninfected cases the stroma undergoes no more overgrowth than is necessary to form a framework for the epithelium. If chronic infection is present, fibrous tissue is laid down in varying amounts, sometimes distorting the architecture greatly. This process is, no doubt, responsible for much of the cyst formation (Fig. 235).

When only portions of specimens are studied microscopically, one may be de-ceived into thinking that the growth is largely fibromuscular if the section happens to pass through portions of the internal sphincter removed at the operation. This may easily happen since, in the normal, a considerable part of the prostatic mass lying in front of the urethra consists of the large outer loop of the internal sphincter (external arcuate muscle) which passes around the urethra at this point. Some observers, however, who have sectioned the whole gland have found cases in which large portions of the mass were com-posed of fibrous tissue and smooth muscle (Figs. 236, 237). Ribbert,[1] Simmonds,[2] Niemeyer,[3] Horn and Orator,[4] Jacoby,[5] and others believe that these cases rep-resent a true myomatous hyperplasia. Jacoby, however, observes that a pure my-oma of the prostate apparently never oc-curs, epithelial hyperplasia also being in-variably present at some point in the gland. Others, as Ciechanowski,[6] Loeschke,[7] Ad-rion,[8] and Tandler and Zuckerkandl[9] feel that myoma does not occur, and that the pictures described above are to be ex-

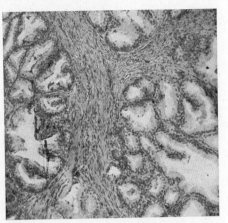

Fig. 235.—Benign prostatic hypertrophy. Similar to Fig. 233, but showing the connective-tissue trabeculæ separating the small groups or spheroids of the glandular growth. B. U. I. Path. 2051.

plained as scars from infectious processes, or the result of arteriosclerosis, with occlusion of the vessels and consequent degeneration of the originally epithelial mass.

Infection is rarely absent, since most cases coming to operation have been instrumented, and urinary infection may occur even without instrumentation.

[1] Zeigler's Beiträge zur pathologischen Anatomie und Allgemeinen Pathologie, 1916, lxi, 149-168.

[2] Aschoff's Lehrbuch der Pathologischen Anatomie, 5th ed., 1921, ii, 561–568.

[3] Deutsches Archiv für Chirurgie, 1921, clxvii, 65–80.

[4] Frankfurter Zeitschrift für Pathologie, 1922, xxviii, 340–358.

[5] Zeitschrift für Urologische Chirurgie, 1923, xiv, 6–37.

[6] Mitteilungen aus der Grenzgebiete der Medizin und Chirurgie, 1901, vii, 184–301.

[7] Münchener Medizinische Wochenschrift, 1920, lxvii, 302.

[8] Ziegler's Beiträge zur Pathologischen Anatomie und Allgemeinen Pathologie, 1922, lxx, 179–202.

[9] Studien zur Anatomie und Klinik der Prostatahypertrophie, Berlin, 1922.

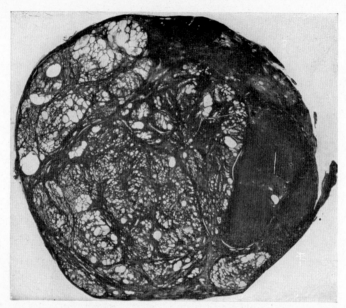

Fig. 236.—Low-power magnification of a section of a prostatic "lobe" removed at operation showing benign hypertrophy and a good sized area composed entirely of fibromuscular tissue. From Mr. Henry Wade.

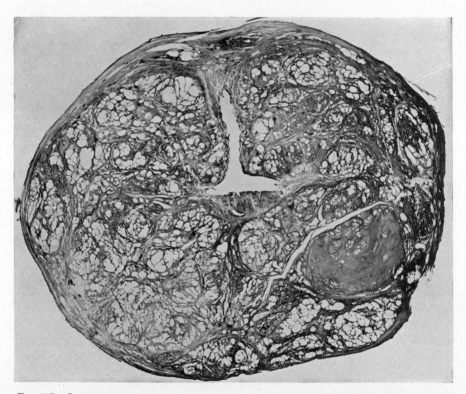

Fig. 237.—Low-power magnification of a section of a prostatic specimen removed at operation in one piece showing benign hypertrophy everywhere excepting the nodule in the right lower corner, which is composed of fibromuscular tissue. From Mr. Henry Wade.

The results are a cellular infiltration, round-celled in chronic cases, polymorphonuclear in acute, and at the beginning more pronounced in the region of the urethra. Later it spreads along the ducts, and eventually may involve the entire mass. As it continues, more and more fibrous tissue is laid down. The process may involve the outer "capsular" layers, in which case adhesions, palpable per rectum, bind the prostate to the surrounding tissues. Abscesses may occur at any point. In a prostate the seat of an old diffuse infection, with scarring and contraction, a very small amount of hypertrophy may cause obstruction (Fig. 238). This is sometimes called "small fibrous prostate."

Prostatic calculi may occur in hypertrophy, but are rare, and apt to be associated with chronic infection. They are usually at or near the line of cleavage between the hypertrophied lobes and the posterior lamella.

Necrosis and ulceration do not occur, except in connection with abscesses. The blood-vessels in the stroma of the largest masses are always large enough to nourish the tissue.

Occasionally, in connection with acute cystitis, and especially with pedunculated intravesical masses, vascular congestion will occur, and ulceration and hemorrhages into the bladder may take place. In such cases the cystoscopic picture and history may simulate carcinoma of the bladder or prostate.

A few isolated but well-studied cases seem to show definitely that malignant changes may begin in hypertrophied portions of the prostate.[1] In many cases benign hypertrophy complicates carcinoma arising in the posterior lamella.

Instrumental injuries to enlarged prostates are common, and result from the

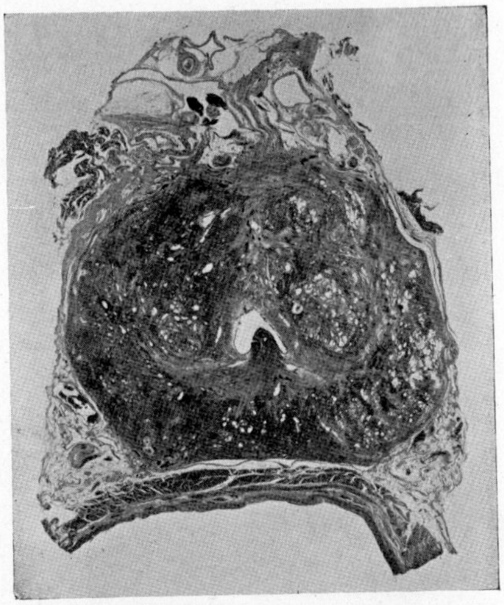

FIG. 238.—Low-power magnification of a cross-section of the entire prostate from a man of seventy-three. There is a very slight hypertrophy of the "lateral lobes." The line of demarcation between these and the posterior lamella is well shown. There is also chronic inflammatory change. In spite of small size of this prostate the patient suffered from urinary obstruction. From Mr. Henry Wade.

distortion of the urethra. They may lead to false passages, tunneling of median enlargements, abscesses, extravasations, etc. If the false passage goes anteriorly, it may penetrate the capsule, and lead into the prevesical space.

The pathology of the obstructive changes caused by prostatic hypertrophy is fully considered in the section on Obstructive Uropathy. There are, however, a few special points in connection with this disease. The trigonal muscle, taking origin from the ureteral orifices, and being of the same origin, developmentally, as the ureteral musculature, runs down, converging as it goes, to the vesical orifice. Here it passes down over the edge, continuing along the posterior wall of the urethra to and beyond the verumontanum. Its course, therefore, makes an angle at the vesical orifice, so that as it contracts it tends to straighten and, therefore, to pull open the orifice, overcoming the tone of the sphincter and aiding in the act of voiding. Especially in median enlargements, which obstruct the orifice and push

[1] Shaw: Journal of Urology, 1924, xi, 63–74.

up and distort the trigonal muscle (Bell's muscles) this action is hindered, and as the muscle contracts more strongly in efforts to pull down the bar and open the sphincter and empty the bladder it hypertrophies. In some cases this hypertrophy becomes very great. The trigone becomes a firm, projecting mass of muscle, and the bladder wall, just behind the interureteric bar may, if it dilates, push down under the trigone and gradually undermine it. A large pocket, like a diverticulum, and reaching even as far as the level of the vesical orifice, may be produced at this point. When this occurs, the projecting trigone may be allowed to push forward against the orifice, and act as an obstruction itself, which will continue even after the prostatic enlargement, the original cause of the trouble, has been removed.

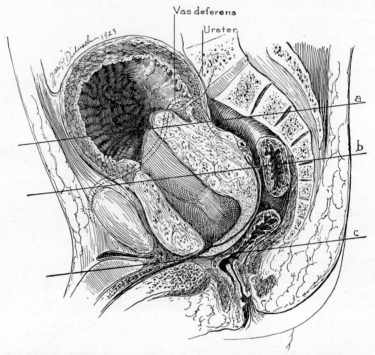

Fig. 239.—Cross-section of an enormous prostatic hypertrophy which is mostly extravesical. As the prostate has enlarged the ejaculatory ducts have failed to elongate concurrently, and the seminal vesicles, therefore, occupy a position on the posterior surface of the prostate instead of above it. Note how the sphincter is dilated and also the wide slit-like urethra. Line *b* shows the level of the intervesicular notch which is almost half-way between line *a*, the upper border of the prostate, and line *c* the level of the apex. Redrawn from Die Prostatahypertrophie, Tandler and Zuckerkandl.

This is undoubtedly the condition sometimes spoken of as "myoma of the vesical orifice." In treating this condition, it is better not to remove or destroy the entire trigone, as absence of Bell's muscles may make voiding difficult. In those cases requiring operation we have simply divided the trigone in the median line. (See section on Physiology and Pathology of Micturition.)

During the growth of prostatic hypertrophy, if it is of the extravesical type, the bladder is pushed upward, sometimes 3 or 4 inches. At the same time, since the verumontanum does not rise, the ejaculatory ducts will be pulled upon and lengthened. The vesicles may not always ride upward on the prostate, but come to lie on the posterior surface of the tumor; doubtless due in part to the pull downward of the ejaculatory ducts. When this happens the vasa deferentia will be pulled upon, even to the extent of compressing the ureters where they hook around them, as in a case illustrated by Tandler and Zuckerkandl (Figs. 239, 240), at the same time the lateral growth of the tumor tends to spread the vesicles apart and widen the angle between their lower ends. In such cases the tumor may be felt in the widened intervesicular space, and would have to be distinguished from a plateau of inflammatory tissue.

Other forms of prostatic obstruction, grouped under the general head of "contracture of the vesical orifice," are considered under Inflammations of the Urogenital Tract. These inflammatory contractures may be combined with various degrees of glandular hypertrophy, which has given rise to some confine confusion concerning their origin. When, for instance, a mass of fibrosis, confined largely to the posterior aspect of the orifice, and forming, therefore, a "median bar," has in its interior some groups of glands showing epithelial hyperplasia, it represents two distinct pathologic processes—inflammatory fibrosis and glandular hypertrophy. In the same way, an inflammatory contracture may exist at the orifice above an infravesical hypertrophy, and demand separate treatment.

SYMPTOMS

The symptoms of prostatic hypertrophy in the early stages result from the pathologic changes at the vesical orifice, and the consequent interference with the normal physiologic function of micturition.

The amount of obstruction produced by a gradually growing "spheroid," or group of spheroids, depends much on their location, and the ability of the muscles, which take part in the act of micturition, to open the prostatic orifice, and expel the urine from the bladder.

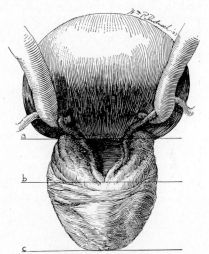

Fig. 240.—Posterior view of the same specimen shown in the preceding diagram. The manner in which the seminal vesicles lie on the posterior surface of the prostate is shown and also how it is possible to palpate prostate between the vesicles. It is no doubt in such cases that observers report the palpation of the median lobe. Note the dilatation of the ureters above the points at which they are crossed by the vasa deferentia. Redrawn from Die Prostatahypertrophie, Tandler and Zuckerkandl. (The lines *a*, *b*, *c* are the same as in the preceding diagram.)

A small middle lobe, for example, may be pulled down by the contraction of the trigone, so as to enable the bladder to empty itself completely. Not infrequently there is some delay or hesitation before the way is cleared and urination begun, and the increased effort put upon the trigone may cause it to tire, and relax before the urinary act is complete. Micturition in two or more stages therefore results. This increased effort causes the trigone to hypertrophy, and become congested. The bladder also becomes thicker, and reduced in capacity, so that increased frequency of urination is usually due to a smaller bladder in the early stages of prostatic obstruction.

In most cases the bladder soon becomes unable to empty completely, and "residual urine" remains after the patient has apparently completed urination. This residuum gradually increases in most cases, thus reducing the working capacity of the bladder and increasing the frequency of urination.

In some instances, however, as the residual urine increases, the bladder dilates so that the working capacity of the bladder remains nearly normal.

The varying conditions present may be expressed thus:

$F = \dfrac{TU}{WC}$. Where F = frequency, TU = total urine in twenty-four hours, and WC = working capacity of the bladder.

Thus in normal cases:

$$F = \frac{TU}{WC} = \frac{1600 \text{ c.c.}}{400 \text{ c.c.}} = 4.$$

This figure is, of course, not absolute, varying with the amount of water drunk, and the habit of the individual. In diabetes great increase in production of urine (TU) similarly increases the frequency. If the capacity of the bladder is reduced by irritation or a habit of the individual of voiding frequently, F is correspondingly increased.

In cases of prostatic hypertrophy, the working capacity of the bladder is reduced by the amount of residual urine present. If the bladder capacity is expressed by BC, and the residual urine by RU, the working capacity will be the difference between them, or BC — RU = WC.

If, as RU increases, BC increases correspondingly, the frequency of urination may remain normal. For example, we may cite a case where urination was normal in frequency, although RU was 2100 c.c. In this case the BC was 2600 c.c. and the working capacity was normal. (2600 c.c. — 2100 c.c. = 500 c.c.)

The presence of inflammation, calculi, ulcers, diverticula, etc., may lead to irritation and increased desire to urinate, incommensurate with the actual working capacity (WC).

Difficulty of urination usually increases gradually, being accompanied with more hesitation, more straining, a smaller stream, and greater frequency, and sometimes with pain and bleeding. Here again cases vary greatly.

The increased frequency and difficulty of urination may be borne by the patient for years, or he may decide to demand relief while still voiding fairly well.

In other cases the patient may gradually or suddenly become unable to urinate. A condition known as complete retention (RC) has set in and relief is demanded.

In many cases when the patient has once been catheterized, he is thereafter unable to urinate and a catheter life is begun. In others, after one or more catheterizations, ability to void returns, but, as a rule, attacks of complete retention requiring catheterization come on from time to time until permanent complete retention supervenes. The patient, therefore, never knows when or where he may urgently require relief and, as the operation of catheterization is one requiring, at times, a varied assortment of instruments and great skill in using them, the situation is often fraught with considerable danger.

The use of a catheter may also lead to complications; traumatism, false passage, hemorrhage, infection, etc., any of which may change the subsequent course of the case, and even make further catheterization very painful, difficult, or impossible.

More serious still are the functional changes which may occur in the kidneys, as a result of catheterization. As mentioned elsewhere, suppression of urine, partial or complete, accompanied by uremia, may follow immediately after emptying the bladder with a catheter. This is particularly apt to occur if the amount of residual urine is large and the renal function markedly impaired by back pressure.

A chronic uremia may gradually develop in cases that have not been catheter-ized, the symptoms often being a gradual loss of appetite, nausea, or even vomiting, headache, dizziness, drowsiness, impairment of mental alertness, and sometimes of vision. These symptoms vary greatly. Sometimes there is only a foul breath, and loss of vigor on the part of the patient.

As remarked before, the symptoms vary greatly, there being very little definite relationship between the size of the prostate, and the resultant conditions in the bladder and kidney or the accompanying symptoms. We frequently see very slightly enlarged prostates causing severe changes and marked symptoms, and again very great hypertrophies of the median or lateral lobes may cause so little obstruction, or be so thoroughly compensated as to produce few symptoms.

One of the greatest dangers lies in the insidious development of grave renal changes with few symptoms of either marked frequency or difficulty of urination, or of chronic uremia, to warn patient or physician of the seriousness of the situation. It is such cases that should bring home to the medical profession the urgent necessity of periodic examinations, including the prostate, as shown by rectal examination. Two recent cases in which early carcinoma of the prostate was discovered in patients who gave absolutely no symptoms referable to the prostate or bladder may be cited.

Hemorrhage may be a prominent symptom, even in cases where no instrumenta-tion has been done. It is more common in hypertrophy than in cancer of the prostate according to our clinical studies.

Pain, irritation, and local discomfort vary greatly. At times there is simply a burning in the deep urethra or during urination. Sometimes there is sexual irrita-tion, or painful ejaculation—but more often a suppression of the sexual powers, and even disappearance of erections, libido, and a condition of impotence.

Not infrequently the distress of the patient becomes very great, urination being very painful, difficult, and frequent. The patient's rest may be so disturbed, and his general health so greatly impaired that the condition presented on entrance to the hospital is grave in the extreme. In such cases, and particularly those associ-ated with large residuals, much renal back pressure, and severe impairment of the kidneys, only by the most careful preparatory treatment can the patient's life be saved by operation.

When infection supervenes, and especially if the kidneys become involved (as often happens) the dangers are aggravated.

Some form of cardiovascular disease has been present in 50 per cent. of our cases, viz., arteriosclerosis, hypertension, myocarditis, and valvular lesions.

Cerebral symptoms produced by arteriosclerosis are not infrequent, particularly in the very aged. In some cases the patient has a severe psychosis which may amount to acute insanity. The relation between this and the prostatic condition has never been satisfactorily explained.

To recapitulate: A typical case of moderately large hypertrophy of the prostate often gives a history such as this: Several years ago he first had to get up twice at night to urinate and about the same time noted that the outflow of urine was not quite normal. At times two or three attempts were necessary to start the flow of urine, and also to complete the act. Micturition gradually became more frequent and difficult, until he was voiding urine every hour. Finally, one day he was un-able to urinate, and catheterization became necessary. After that complete reten-tion of urine persisted, and a catheter life began and has persisted to date. Shortly after being catheterized he had a chill followed by fever, and soon noticed that the urine was cloudy. Pain, which had been absent, now gave him increasing discomfort. Catheterization was usually easy, but often required a prostatic catheter (gum coudé or a rubber catheter armed with a stilet with a long prostatic curve). At times it was extremely difficult to pass a catheter, and occasionally considerable bleeding occurred, followed by a urethral chill and fever. During recent months he has been able to urinate, although with difficulty, and catheterization has been done only at irregular intervals. He has been bothered with lack of appetite, and occasional nausea and vomiting, headaches, dizziness, and gradual loss of vigor and mental alertness. At present he urinates four or five times at night, every hour during the day, with straining and pain. On examination a moderately enlarged prostate with 300 c.c. of residual urine, and a bladder capacity of 400 c.c. was found (WC = 100 c.c.). The urine was of low specific gravity, contained pus-cells and bacilli in large numbers, and the phthalein test showed considerable impairment of renal function (appearance time fourteen minutes, elimination 20 per cent. in two hours). The blood urea was 0.60 gm. per liter, thus confirming the damage to the kidneys and explaining the symptoms of slight uremia.

In our thousand cases[1] the onset was gradual in 93 per cent., and the mean duration of symptoms was 7.4 years before the patient entered the hospital. Prostatectomy was done on 41 patients under forty-five years of age, in nearly all of whom the prostate was small and the obstruction due to a fibrous bar or contracture of the vesical orifice. These cases would now be successfully cured by the punch operation. The following table shows the age at onset of prostatic symptoms in patients forty-five years of age and over.

TABLE 49

AGE AT ONSET

45–49 years	67
50–54	132
55–59	219
60–64	197
65–69	143
70–74	103
75–79	31
80–84	5
85–89	1

It is seen here that only 7.5 per cent. are under fifty years of age; 40 per cent. between fifty and sixty years; and 60 per cent. in the fifteen years between fifty and sixty-five years of age.

TABLE 50

SYMPTOMS WHICH PATIENT HAD HAD

	Per cent.
Difficulty of urination	77
Frequency of urination	99
Hesitancy of urination	85
Urgency of urination	30
Hematuria	24
Weak urinary stream	86
Passage of calculi	4
Pain	79
Incontinence	10

[1] Prepared by Miss Mary Gover.

It has been interesting to analyze the location and severity of the *pain:*

TABLE 51

PAIN—LOCATION AND INTENSITY

Total number of cases studied....................................... 983
No information....................................... 122
No pain....................................... 182—21 per cent.
Slight pain....................................... 861—40 "
Considerable pain....................................... 338—39 "

Location of pain.	Slight.	Per cent.	Much.	Per cent.
Neck of bladder...........................	258	76	280	83
Perineum...........................	26	8	50	15
End of penis...........................	70	20	97	29
Rectum...........................	17	5	40	12
Back...........................	37	11	78	23
Thighs...........................	19	6	37	11
Legs...........................	7	2	23	7
Kidney...........................	7	2	28	8
All others...........................	4	1	12	4

It is thus seen that pain plays an important rôle in the symptomatology of benign prostatic hypertrophy, being present in 79 per cent. of the cases, and in 39 per cent. severe. It is not so frequent or severe as in cancer, but the distribution and radiation are much the same.

Hematuria was present in 24 per cent. of the cases. Of these 223 cases, 49 had stones removed at operation (22.5 per cent.). It is, therefore, shown that in nearly 80 per cent. of the cases in which hematuria has been present it is not caused by calculi.

Hematuria and pain, which have been supposed to be so diagnostic of cancer, are thus shown to be present in 80 per cent. of the cases of hypertrophy.

Of the 168 cases with hematuria, 36 patients had not used a catheter. In about three-fourths of the cases, therefore, a catheter had been employed either occasionally or frequently, and traumatism probably contributed to the bleeding.

Incontinence of urine was present on admission in 96 cases (nearly 10 per cent.). In 14 of these cases the residual was over 1000 c.c., and in 3, over 2000 c.c. In 18 cases it was between 400 and 1000 c.c., but in 38 cases it was less than 400 c.c., in 3 only 10 c.c., and in 2 cases no residual was present.

While it is evident that high residuals are more common in these cases of incontinence, these statistics show that low residuals are not uncommon, 20 per cent. being below 100 c.c. They cannot, therefore, be explained as typical paradoxic incontinence—simple overflow from a greatly distended bladder. The urine probably leaks out through apertures between the hypertrophied lobes; this may occur with any degree of residual and vesical distention. As a rule, the history of incontinence should be viewed with alarm and the bladder carefully palpated and percussed to determine its size. If found to be distended well above the symphysis, the patient should be put on a decompression apparatus and blood urea carefully estimated. Cystoscopy should be delayed several days until the pressure has been reduced to normal and the bladder should not be emptied at the first catheterization.

Sexual Powers.—In 665 histories satisfactory notes as to the sexual powers of the patient are at hand and show that erections were normal in only 34 per cent. of the cases, and completely lost in 28 per cent. of the cases. Gonorrhea had been present in 33 per cent. of the cases. In 978 cases only 51 patients had not been married (5.2 per cent.). There were very many Protestant ministers and not one Catholic priest in this series of 1000 cases.

Symptoms accompanying large *residual urine:* There were 96 cases in which R. U. 400 c.c. or more was present. Of these, 37 per cent. had incontinence, 14 per cent. hematuria, and 25 per cent. uremia. It is noteworthy that 12 of these patients had no difficulty of urination and 8 said the stream was normal. One patient with 2100 c.c. residual urine had normal urination at intervals of five or six hours; his only complaint was enlargement of the lower abdomen.

Complete *retention of urine* was present on admission in 17 cases. The onset had been gradual in 86 per cent.; 7 per cent. had had incontinence; 24 per cent. hematuria, and 16 per cent. uremia. The condition was distinctly better than patients with high residuals who had not been using a catheter.

Catheter Life.—Among 711 cases with incomplete retention of urine, 272 patients had never used a catheter; 252 used it occasionally; 27 from one to six times a week, 96 once or twice a day, 47 three or four times, and 17 five times or over.

Among 730 cases there were 209 patients who had not used a catheter, but in 150 the urine was infected (73 per cent.).

In 229 who had used a catheter occasionally 84 per cent. were infected, and in 297 who had used a catheter frequently 269, or 90 per cent., were infected. It is evident that residual urine is apt to become infected even though a catheter is not used.

Diverticula were present in 121, or 16 per cent., of the cases noted. Of these, 15 per cent. had incontinence, 78 per cent. difficulty, 96 per cent. frequency, and 89 per cent. a small urinary stream. The symptoms were in no way characteristic or diagnostic.

The location of the diverticula was as follows: On the lateral walls in 33 per cent., at the corner of the trigone 33 per cent. (containing the ureter in one-fifth of these, or 6 per cent.), on the posterior wall 3 per cent., on the anterior wall 3 per cent., and at the vertex 1 case.

Among the 1000 prostatectomy cases (a few being suprapubic) analyzed by Miss Gover the following operations had been performed before admission to the Brady Clinic:

Suprapubic for drainage, 30; for hemorrhage, 1; for bladder calculus, 17; for tumor, 1; punch, 8; perineal prostatectomy, 4; suprapubic prostatectomy, 4; cancer of prostate, 1; Bottini, 8; prostatitis, 1; vesiculitis, 1; seminal vesicle stones, 3; epididymitis, 4; tuberculosis of epididymis, 1; castration, 4; hydrocele, 12; urethral stricture, 15; stones in kidney and ureter, 1; pyonephrosis, 1.

There were 34 cases in which the cystoscope showed an anterior lobe.

The findings, as to size, on *rectal examination* cannot be considered absolutely dependable as shown by the fact that in 254 cases in which the enlargement of the prostate was called "small" or not at all enlarged, the operative findings were: "small" 100, "medium" 152, and "large" 2. This simply means that one or more lobes of the prostate which were moderately enlarged either projected into the bladder or anteriorly toward the prevesical space, and did not present rectally.

The cystoscope generally corrected the mistaken impression given by the rectal examination which was correct in only 39 per cent. of the cases.   Among 254 cases "rectally small," the cystoscope showed 190 with moderate intravesical hypertrophy, thus showing the great value of the cystoscope.   In other words, in 61 per cent. of the cases, where rectal examination showed a slight enlargement, operation proved it wrong.   Among these "rectally small" prostates the weight of the operative specimen is shown in the following table in which the amount of R. U. found in each class is also given:

TABLE 52

SMALL PROSTATE ON RECTAL EXAMINATION: RESIDUAL URINE AND WEIGHT OF PROSTATE
AT OPERATION

Residual urine in cubic centimeters.	Weight of prostate in grams.									
	No information.	0–9.	10–19.	20–29.	30–39.	40–49.	50–59.	60–69.	70–79.	Total.
No information....	10	2	3	1	..	..	..	..	..	16
Complete retention.	24	5	7	6	2	1	1	..	1	47
0–199 c.c..........	74	16	25	20	6	5	3	..	..	149
200–399..........	20	6	6	2	1	2	..	..	..	37
400–599..........	4	2	1	..	..	..	..	..	..	7
600–799..........	2	1	..	1	1	..	..	..	..	5
800–999..........	...	..	1	..	..	..	..	..	..	1
1000 and over......	4	..	1	2	1	..	..	..	..	8
Total..........	138	32	44	32	11	8	4	..	1	270

TABLE 53

"SMALL PROSTATES."   RELATION BETWEEN WEIGHT AND RESIDUAL

Grams.	Total.	Residual urine under 400 c.c.	Residual urine 400 c.c. or over (including complete retention).
0– 9.............	30	22	8
10–19............	41	31	10
20–29............	31	22	9
30–39............	11	7	4
40–49............	8	7	1
50–59............	4	3	1
60–69.............			
70–79............	1	..	1
Total.................	126	92	34
Weight, mean..........	20.48 gm.	Mean 20.11	Mean 21.47

Including cases where exact weights were not taken, we have among the 254 "rectally small" prostates 186 in which the residual urine was under 400 c.c. and 68 over 400 c.c., or 26.8 per cent.   As a residual of 400 c.c. or over is almost always associated with renal impairment, the danger of relying on a rectal examination alone to determine the enlargement of the prostate is evident.   Or, stated otherwise, finding a "small prostate" by rectum is no sure indication that considerable obstruction and large residual may not be present.

TABLE 54

HEMATURIA AND STONE IN BLADDER

Cases that had hematuria: 223   Number.
    Stone in bladder at operation.. 49
                (or 22.5 per cent. of hematuria cases had stone)
    No stone in bladder at operation....................................... 168
    No information... 6
        Total.. 223

Those that had no stone in bladder:
    Use of catheter: Number.
    None... 36
    Occasionally... 65
    One to six times a week.. 5
    One to two times a day... 24
    Three to four times a day.. 15
    Five and over times a day.. 10
    Suprapubic drainage.. 2
    Retention catheter... 4
    Complete retention(?). No information.................................. 4
    No information... 3
        Total.. 168

Those that had no stone in bladder at operation:
    Stone in bladder in past history....................................... 4
    No stone in bladder in past history.................................... 164
    No information... 0
        Total.. 168
        (Only 4 had history of stone before.)

TABLE 55

INCONTINENCE: HAD INCONTINENCE ON ADMISSION: 96 CASES

B. U. I. No.	Use of catheter Code No.	R. U.* in c.c.	Bladder capacity.	B. U. I. No.	Use of catheter Code No.	R. U. in c.c.	Bladder capacity.	B. U. I. No.	Use of catheter Code No.	R. U. in c.c.	Bladder capacity.
1313	1	10	190	3123	1	50	70	5154	0	750	N. I.‡
1414	4	C. R.†	500	3273	N. I. C. R.	C. R.	N. I.	5155	1	100	500
1428	4	C. R.	N. I.	3297	0	10	100	5269	3	C. R.	N. I.
1554	0	470	N. I.	3329	1	400	460	5290	0	200	400
1598	3	260	520	3332	4	450	470	5352	0	10	170
1619	3	150	400	3366	1	N. I.	N. I.	5367	1	30	150
1768	0	1000	1500	3383	0	540	Large	5371	3	250	300
1780	4	370	400	3412	0	N. I.	N. I.	5376	0	750	N. I.
1808	0	800	N. I.	3421	3	130	420	5378	1	130	550
1820	1	2500	N. I.	3495	1	N. I.	320	5592	0	60	250
1931	2	740	N. I.	3531	2	180	480	5441	4	170	N. I.
1933	1	None	340	3539	3	30	360	5503	1	20	80
1971	0	400	N. I.	3557	3	100	420	5557	0	2100	N. I.
2010	2	540	N. I.	3595	1	10	180	5604	0	170	170
2020	0	180	200	3648	0	830	N. I.	5648	0	830	N. I.
2067	0	1000	1100	3673	0	700	N. I.	5706	1	60	60
2100	0	N. I.	360	3717	0	500	660	5843	0	1400	N. I.
2174	3	C. R.	N. I.	3795	0	20	310	5899	0	2100	N. I.
2195	0	200	220	3866	0	320	320	5908	1	500	550
2253	1	650	800	4034	0	1300	N. I.	5961	5	C. R.	N. I.
2276	3	1040	1300	4131	2	720	950	5997	6	C. R.	N. I.
2279	4	1200	N. I.	4177	1	160	560	6509	1	N. I.	N. I.
2311	0	380	380	4249	0	60	250	7452	0	500	N. I.
2367	1	None	500	4278	0	250	330	7797	0	300	N. I.
2380	0	1400	N. I.	4386	0	Large	N. I.	8547	0	250	600
2394	2	1180	250	4388	0	40	200	8703	0	70	250
2420	1	200	240	4580	0	C. R.	N. I.	9030	1	C. R.	1200
2446	0	1550	N. I.	4597	0	40	150	9034	1	N. I.	N. I.
2475	4	690	N. I.	4626	0	1120	N. I.	10,136	N. I.	1800	N. I.
2515	0	60	60	4654	3	C. R.	270	10,179	4	C. R.	N. I.
2518	3	N. I.	450	4664	0	1230	N. I.				
2611	5	C. R.	N. I.	4738	1	N. I.	N. I.				
2683	0	...	...	4876	0	1150	N. I.				

*R. U. = residual urine
† C. R. = complete retention
‡N. I. = no information

CODE:
0 = none
1 = cath. used occasionally
2 = 1 to 6 weekly
3 = 1 to 2 daily
4 = 3 to 4 daily
5 = 5 or more daily
6 = suprapubic drain
7 = retained catheter

TABLE 56
Symptoms: On Admission

	Number.	Per cent.
Gradual onset	877	92.71
Sudden onset	69	7.29
Total	946	
No incontinence	842	89.77
Has incontinence	96	10.23
Total	938	
No difficulty of urination	186	22.85
Has difficulty of urination	628	77.15
Total	814	
No abnormal frequency	11	1.18
Has abnormal frequency	923	98.82
Total	934	
No hesitancy at urination	113	14.75
Has hesitancy at urination	653	85.25
Total	766	
No urgency	653	69.99
Has urgency	280	30.01
Total	933	
Stream good force	99	13.62
Stream weak force	628	86.38
Total	727	
Has not had hematuria	718	76.22
Has had hematuria	224	23.78
Total	942	
Has not passed any calculi	903	96.06
Has passed calculi	37	3.94
Total	940	

TABLE 57
Features in History

Sexual Powers at Operation:	Number.	Per cent.
Erections, normal	227	34.14
Erections, impaired	255	38.35
Erections, lost	183	27.52
Total	665	

Venereal History:	Number.	Per cent.
No venereal disease	596	64.71
Gonorrhea only	254	27.58
Gonorrhea and some other venereal	47	5.10
Some other venereal	24	2.61
Total	921	

Social Status:

Single.................. 51
Married................ 764
Widowed............... 159 } Including only those who were forty-five and over at operation
Divorced.............. 4
Total................ 978

Expected number of single men (forty-five years or over) on the basis of the 1910 census = 90.43. There were actually 51 single men in this group.

Or, there is a difference of 39.43 men between the actual and expected number of single persons. The chance of getting a difference as large as this due to errors in sampling is only 7 in 1,000,-000. Therefore, the number of single men in the prostatic hypertrophy group is significantly smaller than the expected number, based on the 1910 census.

TABLE 58

TIME ELAPSING FROM ONSET OF SYMPTOMS TO ADMISSION

Years.	Number.
0– 1	144
2– 3	213
4– 5	183
6– 7	94
8– 9	50
10–14	153
15–19	51
20–24	37
25–29	10
30–34	6
35–39	1
40–44	
45–49	
50–54	1
Total	943

Mean duration of symptoms before operation = 7.427 ± 0.142 years.

TABLE 59

AGE AT ONSET OF SYMPTOMS

Years.	Number.
15–19	2
20–24	2
25–29	2
30–34	7
35–39	9
40–44	19
45–49	67
50–54	132
55–59	219
60–64	197
65–69	143
70–74	103
75–79	31
80–84	5
85–89	1
Total	939

Mean age at onset of symptoms = 60.221 ± 0.203 years.

TABLE 60

PHTHALEIN ON ADMISSION

Two-hour percentage.	Number.
0– 4	8
5– 9	5
10–14	15
15–19	9
20–24	21
25–29	20
30–34	32
35–39	52
40–44	55
45–49	80
50–54	93
55–59	91
60–64	92
65–69	61
70–74	13
75–79	8
80–84	3
85–89	3
90–94	3
Total	664

Mean = 46.525,600 per cent.

TABLE 61

SYSTOLIC BLOOD-PRESSURE ON ADMISSION

Mm. Hg.	Number.
90– 99	2
100–109	14
110–119	28
120–129	64
130–139	71
140–149	106
150–159	79
160–169	56
170–179	38
180–189	26
190–199	24
200–209	16
210–219	16
220–229	1
240–249	3
290–299	1
Total	545

Mean B. P. = 153.092.

TABLE 62

LARGE RESIDUAL: SYMPTOMS ON ADMISSION

(Residual urine = 400 c.c. or more on admission. 96 cases)

	Number.	Per cent.
Onset: Gradual	89	
Sudden	3	$\dfrac{89}{92} = 96.7$
N. I.[1]	4	
Total	96	
Incontinence: None	58	
Had	34	$\dfrac{34}{92} = 37.0$
N. I.	4	
Total	96	
Difficulty: None	12	
Had	66	$\dfrac{66}{78} = 84.6$
N. I.	18	
Total	96	
Frequency: None	1	
Had	90	$\dfrac{90}{91} = 98.9$
N. I.	5	
Total	96	
Hesitancy: None	7	
Had	70	$\dfrac{70}{77} = 90.9$
N. I.	19	
Total	96	
Urgency: None	61	
Had	31	$\dfrac{31}{92} = 33.7$
N. I.	4	
Total	96	
Stream: Good force	8	
Weak force	67	$\dfrac{67}{75} = 89.3$
N. I.	21	
Total	96	
Hematuria: None	79	
Had	13	$\dfrac{13}{92} = 14.1$
N. I.	4	
Total	96	
Passed calculi: None	91	
Had	1	$\dfrac{1}{92} = 1.1$
N. I.	4	
Total	96	
Kidney colic: None	92	
Had	0	$\dfrac{0}{92} = 0$
N. I.	4	
Total	96	
Uremia: None	70	
Had[2]	23	$\dfrac{23}{93} = 24.7$
N. I.	3	
Total	96	

[1] N. I. = no information.

[2] Including: blood urea = 0.3 and over.

TABLE 63

DIVERTICULA: SYMPTOMS ON ADMISSION. 121 CASES

		Number.	Per cent.
Onset:	Gradual	109	
	Sudden	8	$\dfrac{109}{117} = 93.2$
	N. I.	4	
	Total	121	
Incontinence:	None	99	
	Had	18	$\dfrac{18}{117} = 15.4$
	N. I.	4	
	Total	121	
Difficulty:	None	22	
	Had	78	$\dfrac{78}{100} = 78.0$
	N. I.	21	
	Total	121	
Frequency:	None	4	
	Had	114	$\dfrac{114}{118} = 96.6$
	N. I.	3	
	Total	121	
Hesitancy:	None	14	
	Had	85	$\dfrac{85}{99} = 85.9$
	N. I.	22	
	Total	121	
Urgency:	None	75	
	Had	41	$\dfrac{41}{116} = 35.3$
	N. I.	5	
	Total	121	
Stream:	Good force	9	
	Weak force	75	$\dfrac{75}{84} = 89.3$
	N. I.	37	
	Total	121	
Hematuria:	None	87	
	Had	31	$\dfrac{31}{118} = 26.3$
	N. I.	3	
	Total	121	
Passed calculi:	None	109	
	Had	7	$\dfrac{7}{116} = 6.0$
	N. I.	5	
	Total	121	
Kidney colic:	None	112	
	Had	4	$\dfrac{4}{116} = 3.4$
	N. I.	5	
	Total	121	

TABLE 64

DIVERTICULA

		Number.
N. I.: Probably no diverticula		225
No diverticula		625
Doubtful cases (not included in later tabulation)		12
Diverticula: Unlocated		11
(Code No.)		
"	1	1
"	1, 3	3
"	3	31
"	3, 5	2
"	3, 5, 7	1
"	3, 7	2
"	3, 7, 9	1
"	3, 9	4
"	5	13
"	7	10
"	7, 9	2
"	9	32
"	9, 19	1
"	19	7
Diverticula: Subtotal		121
Total		983

No diverticula = 625
Had diverticula = 121
$$\overline{746}$$

Percentage had diverticula $= \dfrac{121}{746} = 16.2$

Code to above tabulation.

  1 = diverticula at vertex.

  3 = diverticula on lateral wall.

  5 = diverticula on anterior wall.

  7 = diverticula on posterior wall.

  9 = diverticula near trigone and not containing the ureteral orifice

19 = diverticula near trigone and containing the ureteral orifice.

TABLE 65

COMPLETE RETENTION: SYMPTOMS ON ADMISSION AND JUST PREVIOUSLY
197 cases of complete retention on admission: No record of residual urine.

	Number.	Per cent.
Onset: Gradual	163	
Sudden	26	$\dfrac{163}{189} = 86.2$
N. I.	8	
Total	197	
Incontinence: None	172	
Had	13	$\dfrac{13}{185} = 7.0$
N. I.	12	
Total	197	
Difficulty: None	36	
Had	118	$\dfrac{118}{154} = 76.6$
N. I.	43	
Total	197	
Frequency: None	11	
Had	176	$\dfrac{176}{187} = 94.1$
N. I.	10	
Total	197	
Hesitancy: None	23	
Had	124	$\dfrac{124}{147} = 84.4$
N. I.	50	
Total	197	
Urgency: None	142	
Had	40	$\dfrac{40}{182} = 22.0$
N. I.	15	
Total	197	
Stream: Good force	15	
Weak force	120	$\dfrac{120}{135} = 88.9$
N. I.	62	
Total	197	
Hematuria: None	140	
Had	45	$\dfrac{45}{185} = 24.3$
N. I.	12	
Total	197	
Calculi passed: None	174	
Had	11	$\dfrac{11}{185} = 5.9$
N. I.	12	
Total	197	
Kidney colic: None	180	
Had	4	$\dfrac{4}{184} = 2.2$
N. I.	13	
Total	197	
Uremia: None	166	
Had[1]	31	$\dfrac{31}{197} = 15.7$
N. I.	0	
Total	197	

[1] Including: Blood urea = 0.3 and over.

The cases where a catheter has been used have been distributed between the occasional users and the more or less constant users, chiefly to the latter.

Those who said they did not use a catheter on admission, but had a record of having had complete retention at some time were put into the occasional group.

TABLE 66

USE OF CATHETER

Condition of urine.	N. I.	No catheter.	Occasional use of catheter.	Frequent use of catheter.	Total.
N. I.	14	49	64	107	234
Not infected	6	59	43	28	136
Infected	13	150	181	269	613
Total	33	258	288	404	983

	Uninfected urine.	Total.	Uninfected urine, per cent.
No catheter	59	209	28.2 (or 77.2 per cent. of those who had not used a catheter before operation had infected urine on admission).
Occasional use of catheter	43	224	19.2
Frequent use of catheter	28	297	9.4

The relation between the blood urea and the phthalein test made at approximately the same time are shown in Table 67 on page 447 for 88 cases of urinary obstruction due to prostatic hypertrophy.

It will be seen from Table 67 that there is a distinct parallelism between high phthalein and low blood urea. While a fair number of cases (upper left corner) show low blood urea with low phthalein, yet in only 1 case is a very low phthalein associated with a blood urea of normal or below. On the other hand, a high phthalein exists with a high blood urea (lower right corner) in only 3 cases. These may represent errors in technic, or the phthaleins may have been made shortly *after* the blood urea tests at a period when the renal function was improving rapidly.

The relation between the total phthalein and the appearance time is shown in Table 68 on page 448 for 625 cases of urinary obstruction due to prostatic hypertrophy.

There is a broad general parallelism between short appearance time and high phthalein, with rather wide limits. Thus while a good phthalein may be associated with an appearance time as great as thirty minutes, there is no case of a good phthalein with appearance time over fifty minutes. The great majority of good phthaleins appear in fifteen minutes or less. There are a few cases of poor phthalein with short appearance time. In these we may assume that although there is considerable destruction of renal tissue, that which remains is functioning under fairly good conditions.

TABLE 67

RELATION, OF BLOOD UREA TO PHTHALEIN

Phthalein, total for two hours after appearance.

Blood urea.	0–4%	5–9	10–14	15–19	20–24	25–29	30–34	35–39	40–44	45–49	50–54	55–59	60–64	65–69	70–74	75–79	80–84	Total
0– .09								1		1		1						3
.10– .14																		
.15– .19						1		1	1							1		4
.20– .24			1		1		2	1	1	1	1	1	1	1				11
.25– .29													1	2	1			4
.30– .34			1			1	1	1	2	1	1		1	1				10
.35– .39	1		1		1													3
.40– .44					1			1				2	1					5
.45– .49					1			2			2							5
.50– .54			1		2		1				1						1	6
.55– .59	1										1							2
.60– .64								1					1					2
.65– .69				1					1		1							4
.70– .74		1	1		1			1		1								5
.75– .79		1		1	1													3
.80– .89	1			2		3	1	1										8
.90– .99	1			1	1		1											4
1.00–1.09			1					1										2
1.1 –1.19																		
1.2 –1.29	1									1								2
1.3 –1.39					2													2
1.4 –1.49	2			1														3
1.5 –																		
Total	7	2	6	6	11	5	7	11	5	5	7	4	5	4	1	1	1	88

TABLE 68

Relation Between the Appearance Time and the Total Phthalein Eliminated in Two Hours

Appearance time, minutes.	Phthalein percentage.																			Total.
	0–4.	5–9.	10–14.	15–19.	20–24.	25–29.	30–34.	35–39.	40–44.	45–49.	50–54.	55–59.	60–64.	65–69.	70–74.	75–79.	80–84.	85–89.	90–94.	
0– 9	...	...	...	...	1	3	2	9	9	14	26	27	25	23	5	2	1	2		
10– 14	4	...	5	1	5	7	17	24	30	42	45	50	54	27	8	3	2	1	3	
15– 19	...	1	2	...	6	6	7	8	11	12	8	8	7	4	...	2				
20– 29	2	2	4	3	1	1	2	5	3	7	7	1	1	3						
30– 39	2	1	2	1	2	1	...	1	...	3	1	...	1							
40– 49	...	1	...	2	1	...	...	1	...	...	2									
50– 59																				
60– 69																				
70– 79																				
80– 89	...	...	...	...	...	1									...					
90– 99	...	...	...	...																
100–109	...		1																	
Total	8	5	14	7	16	19	28	48	53	78	89	86	88	57	13	7	3	3	3	625

DIAGNOSIS

In simple cases the diagnosis of prostatic hypertrophy is easy. With a history of frequency and difficulty of urination, rectal examination shows to the palpating finger a uniform enlargement which is smooth, elastic, and confined to the prostate; the catheter finds residual urine or a contracted bladder, and the cystoscope, enlarged lobes at the prostatic orifice and trabeculation of the bladder.

There may be, however, great variations in the findings, *e. g.:*

Size.—Not infrequently the prostate is no larger than normal on rectal palpation. This may be due either to the fact that the spheroids are small or that they lie anteriorly or project into the bladder and are not perceptible on rectal examination. The use of the finger in rectum and cystoscope in urethra will generally show the presence of the enlargement which was previously unrecognized. When the prostate is very small, one must make a diagnosis between hypertrophy, *prostatic bar*, or *contracture* at the vesical orifice. Here again cystoscopy, and the examination with finger against cystoscope, as above mentioned, is of very great value. Sometimes it is impossible to say that a small enlargement, especially if it is confined to the median portion of the prostate, is not a small adenoma, but it is important to make a positive diagnosis, because a punch operation, which is adequate for contractures and bars, is unsuited in hypertrophy if not localized to the median portion of the prostate.

If the prostate becomes very large and soft, one must consider *sarcoma*, and sometimes diagnosis is quite difficult. As a rule, however, sarcoma does not involve the whole prostate and may only involve the upper portion and the tissues of the retrovesical region, so that the prostate really lies upon and embedded in the surface of the huge sarcoma. Cystoscopy will show a greatly elevated prostatic orifice and bladder base, and with finger in rectum it is impossible to feel the instrument at all. A cystogram will show a bladder greatly compressed from behind and below. Where the enlargement of the prostate is almost entirely intravesical, the presence of a bladder tumor may be suspected. Even with the cystoscope and in the presence of hemorrhage, diagnosis may be quite difficult, particularly if the surface of the prostate is covered with edematous polyps.

Consistence and Contour.—This may vary between soft and considerable induration. Even in benign hypertrophy, induration may be either localized or general, smooth or nodular. Where it is very extensive, of almost stony hardness (or third degree induration) cancer must be suspected and ruled out by very careful study. The frequent presence of both hypertrophy and carcinoma within the same prostate makes it very important to make a diagnosis before operation if possible. The carcinomatous induration is usually in the posterior part of the prostate and most extensive between cystoscope and finger in rectum in the majority of cases. A localized area of carcinoma may exist in the lateral lobes covered by an area of elastic prostatic tissue and may not be recognized as cancer. Where hypertrophy is associated with chronic inflammation, and if the prostate is still small, it may be extremely difficult to rule out a chronic prostatitis. Presence of hypertrophied lobules as seen with cystoscope or urethroscope and as felt on each side of the urethra by palpation with the rectal finger is usually diagnostic. The consistence of the seminal vesicles is also important. Not infrequently a chronic seminal vesiculitis will give indurated, enlarged vesicles or even a broad plateau of induration above the prostate, which may simulate tuberculosis, or suggest merely a chronic prostatitis with vesiculitis. Here again the cystoscope, urethroscope, combined digital palpation, and study of the prostatic secretion microscopically and bacteriologically will usually clear up the diagnosis. Areas of nodulation or induration may be produced by calculi in the substance of the prostate cr in the urethra. In some cases only the x-ray will make a diagnosis plain and rule out carcinoma.

Hemorrhage.—As this occurs quite frequently in benign hypertrophy, it may obscure the diagnosis considerably and suggest vesical tumor or ulcer, or carcinoma of the prostate. If sufficient to render cystoscopy difficult and unsatisfactory, diagnosis may be impossible. Here again, the configuration of the prostatic orifice, the presence of lobes or median bar, the increase in the median portion as felt with finger in rectum and cystoscope in urethra, and the absence of stony induration, will make the diagnosis of hypertrophy clear. Hemorrhage from the bladder is apt to be well mixed with all of the urine, whereas hemorrhage from the prostate is more apt to be in the first and third glasses of urine voided.

Residual Urine.—This may be absent, and in the presence of a bladder of normal capacity (400–500 c.c.) prostatic obstruction can usually be ruled out, although definite enlargement of the prostate may be present. In many cases with marked symptoms the residual is small, but these are usually associated with contractures of the bladder and the diagnosis of obstructive prostatic hypertrophy is still justified, and operation may be indicated. Occasionally one sees no residual and very small bladder capacity, and here it may be difficult to determine whether an obstructing prostate or chronic cystitis with contracture of the bladder is responsible for the condition. In such cases treatment by forced distention to see what can be accomplished in enlarging the bladder may be necessary. The examination with finger in rectum and cystoscope in urethra is generally of great help in recognizing a bar or collar. In the same way the presence of diverticula may so complicate the picture as to render diagnosis difficult, particularly when infection is present. Cystitis, general or localized, with or without ulcer, or with interstitial cystitis, may alone be responsible for the symptoms present or complicate the prostatic obstruction. Here again most careful study and perhaps a preliminary course of treatment may be necessary.

Differential Diagnosis.—Speaking specifically, the following are the most important diseases or conditions which require diagnostic consideration.

Polyuria, in form of either diabetes insipidus or mellitus or accompanying true nephritis, may produce such a marked frequency of urination as to suggest prostatic hypertrophy. These conditions can generally be excluded by careful urine charts, showing that the amount of urine voided is large, and by urinalysis. If the prostate is found to be enlarged, cystoscopy with determination of the residual urine and bladder capacity, inspection of the prostatic orifice for hypertrophied lobes and the bladder for trabeculation and cellules is indicated.

Vesical and *urethral irritability* may produce such frequency of urination, pain, and even strangury as to suggest prostatic hypertrophy. Often the urine is clear and normal, chemically and microscopically, and very careful examination may be necessary to exclude prostatic obstruction. In such cases the urethroscope may show pathologic changes in the posterior urethra, particularly in the verumontanum—granulations, polyps, hypertrophy, ulcers, etc. In other cases the trigone and median portion of the prostate may show marked congestion, granulation, edema, cysts, and polyps, the cure of which will often restore normal urination.

Infections of the urethra, prostate, and bladder may produce irritation, frequency, and difficulty of urination, pain, hemorrhage, and many of the classical symptoms of prostatic hypertrophy. The history of the case (generally acute), bacteriologic study of the urine, rectal examination, and cystoscopy may be necessary to show the absence of prostatic hypertrophy.

Chronic prostatitis may be accompanied by irritability, frequency, and closely simulate the symptoms of hypertrophy.

Contractures and Bars at the Vesical Orifice.—These may produce exactly the same symptoms and complications as prostatic hypertrophy and most careful study is often necessary for an accurate diagnosis. They frequently occur at a much younger age (under forty-five years). The prostate is usually little if at all enlarged and is apt to be quite indurated. On deep palpation in the median line, the finger does not sink in between lateral hypertrophied lobes as it usually does in hypertrophy.

The urethroscope does not show the prostatic urethra in the form of a vertical slit compressed between two lateral hypertrophies and the cystoscope does not show intravesically hypertrophied lobes, but an irregularly contracted orifice. The cystoscope is often grasped tightly (as if by a stricture). In many cases only a small bar is seen posteriorly. Sometimes the bar is anterior to the cystoscope and occasionally one sees both an anterior and posterior bar, the latter obscuring the anterior part of the trigone and with a pouch behind it. With finger in rectum and cystoscope in urethra, a thick bar is felt, but the lateral lobes are not found to be enlarged and at most form only a collar of small dimensions (along with the median bar) around the shaft of the instrument. In some cases it is difficult to decide whether a case is one of inflammatory contracture or bar or an early hypertrophy at the vesical orifice associated with chronic prostatitis. Occasionally both conditions occur at the same time. If there is much doubt, prostatectomy is a surer procedure, although the punch operation is eminently satisfactory for simple contractures and bars.

Cancer.—"Stony" is the one characteristic of cancer which should make its presence always suspicious. The induration in cancer may be localized to a small part of the prostate, generally in the posterior lobe, but sometimes in the median or lateral lobes. In most cases the induration is general and the entire posterior surface of the prostate is extremely hard, fixed, and sometimes nodular. The induration may extend up into the region of one or both vesicles, ultimately forming a broad plateau of induration from one side of the pelvis to the other. When the latter is present there is no difficulty in making a diagnosis, but when induration is localized to the prostate or especially to a small part of it, diagnosis may be difficult, especially as it is not infrequently accompanied by hypertrophy of the lateral and median lobes, anterior to the layer of cancer. This condition has been present in several cases. There is considerable increase in the suburethral portion of the prostate up to the very apex, and with finger in rectum and cystoscope in urethra the subcervical and suburethral tissues are found to be very hard. This is rarely found in prostatic hypertrophy and may be considered almost diagnostic. A hard nodule or area in one or more lobes may be due to a very chronic localized prostatitis or to a calculus in the prostatic substance, but, as a rule, carcinoma is to be suspected, and if it is impossible to make a diagnosis early, perineal operation should be carried out so that a diagnosis can be made on the operating table, either by palpation, inspection of the prostate, or by excision of prostatic tissue for micro-scopic study. It is only by great vigilance and being suspicious of areas of marked induration that early diagnosis of carcinoma can be made and radical cure by operation obtained. The fact that 20 per cent. of obstructive prostates are carcinomatous and that fully 50 per cent. of these are hypertrophies associated with carcinoma shows the great care that is necessary to avoid serious mistakes.

Tuberculosis.—This disease of the prostate has been shown in recent years to be much more common than previously supposed, and not infrequently must be seriously considered in the diagnosis of supposed hypertrophy of the prostate. Like carcinoma, it may occasionally be seen associated with hypertrophy. In one of our recent cases, a few months after removal of tuberculous seminal vesicles and posterior portion of the lateral lobes of the prostate, it was necessary to remove obstructive hypertrophied lateral lobes by suprapubic prostatectomy.

In most cases of tuberculosis of the prostate there is a concomitant tuberculosis of the seminal vesicles which is easily recognized. In one of our cases there was a localized area of great induration of the right lobe of the prostate which after careful study was diagnosed carcinoma, but at operation tuberculosis alone was found present. We do not see at present how correct diagnosis could have been made in this case, in view of the fact that carcinoma is so common and localized tuberculosis of the prostate so rare, but it is possible that by more careful study of the prostatic secretion for tubercle bacilli such diagnostic errors can be avoided. Where the tuberculosis is extensive the prostate is generally more irregular in contour and variable in consistence than in either cancer or hypertrophy, areas of nodulation and induration intervening between elastic and soft areas. Tuberculous epididymitis, vasitis, and seminal vesiculitis are frequently present, making the diagnosis easier.

Calculi of bladder, urethra, and prostate may give symptoms suggesting prostatic hypertrophy. A large urethral calculus may be palpated by rectum and if surrounded by sufficient elastic prostatic tissue may simulate an enlargement without marked induration. The passage of a metal instrument will give the characteristic crepitus or meet with obstruction and make the diagnosis clear. Where the calculi are not in the posterior urethra, but are in the substance of the prostate, they may not be recognized even on rectal examination or cystoscopy. They may be very minute, present no palpable nodules, and the prostate may be only moderately indurated. Sometimes their character can be made out by rectal examination and occasionally crepitus can be felt, especially with finger in rectum and cystoscope in urethra. The symptoms may be frequency, obstruction, and irritation, quite similar to that of prostatic hypertrophy which will generally be ruled out by cystoscopy and simultaneous palpation with finger in rectum. Not infrequently the calculi are only discovered in x ray plates, which should be made routinely when suspicious areas of induration are present in the prostate or the symptoms cannot be explained by the usual diagnostic methods. Calculi in the bladder may lead to obstruction, frequency, irritation, pain, hemorrhage, and other classical symptoms of hypertrophy of the prostate. They are frequently associated with prostatic bars or contractures and can only be ruled out by cystoscopy, sounding with metal instruments, or the x-ray.

Vesical diseases of various types may give symptoms strongly suggesting the obstructive prostate, viz.:

Submucous cystitis is shown cystoscopically by the presence of the peculiar linear, red areas associated with localized contracture of the bladder wall, and hemorrhage from the mucous membrane when the bladder is distended.

Ulcers and *tumors* are also revealed by the cystoscope.

The same is true for *tuberculosis of the bladder*, which is apt to be more pronounced around a ureteral orifice if a kidney is involved, or in the base of the bladder or trigone if the seminal vesicles are involved.

Diverticula, by encroaching upon the bladder or elevating the floor of the bladder and trigone, may lead to frequency and even difficulty of urination. Sometimes their orifices are so small that they can hardly be seen with the cystoscope, but they can be probed with a ureteral catheter and filled through it with a shadow-graphic medium. They may be demonstrated by a simple cystogram.

In most cases, however, they are associated with obstruction of some sort, either hypertrophy, contracted bar, or prostatic valve.

Trigonal diseases have been recently shown[1] to play a much more important part in obstruction to urination than heretofore supposed. Trigonitis may be associated with marked frequency of urination and pain, but the absence of residual urine, prostatic enlargement, etc., rules out hypertrophy, and cystoscopy demonstrates the congested, irritable trigonal mucosa. Hypertrophies of the trigone are usually associated with contractures or bars or hypertrophy of the prostate. They may become so pronounced as to dominate the picture and cause most of the obstruction, rising as great transverse enlargements close behind the prostatic orifice. In one case we made a diagnosis of bladder tumor, but at suprapubic operation found a trigone 3 inches high and nearly an inch thick immediately behind the prostatic orifice. When they occur with prostatic obstruction, operative cure of the obstruction generally leads to atrophy of the trigone as heretofore described. Only in rare instances is surgical attack upon the trigone necessary.

Hour-glass bladder may produce obstructive symptoms and simulate prostatic hypertrophy. The findings are quite similar to those of hypertrophied trigone, except that they extend around the entire bladder. Rectal examination and cystoscopy will usually eliminate prostatic hypertrophy, although the two are often concomitant.

Bladder paralysis due to spinal cord disease is often the source of diagnostic errors. The pupillary reflexes and those of the extremities should be tested as a routine in all cases with symptoms of urinary obstruction, and a Wassermann test is a wise precaution. The failure of an atonic bladder to regain its tone promptly after drainage is established should always arouse suspicion. If prostatic hypertrophy is actually present in addition to the paralyzed bladder, the difficulties are multiplied, and the nervous disease more apt to be overlooked until after the operation, when it is found that the symptoms persist. Careful study of the bladder tone during the period of catheter drainage, thorough physical examination, and the constant keeping in mind of this by no means uncommon complication will serve to prevent mistakes.

UROLOGIC EXAMINATION IN CASES OF PROSTATIC HYPERTROPHY

Before beginning the examination an adequate history of the patient should be obtained, which, as remarked before, should bring out in detail the symptoms at onset and the subsequent progress of the disease. An effort should be made to

[1] Young and Wesson: Archives of Surgery, 1921, iii, 1–37.

obtain evidence of gradually increasing obstruction and whether any changes in renal function have occurred. Symptoms of uremia should be carefully noted and finally the status præsens, in which the urinary, gastro-intestinal, cardiovascular, sexual, and general symptoms should be recorded.

As the patient is generally seen at the office, the general physical examination is usually postponed. As a preliminary to the urologic examination the patient should be asked to urinate in three glasses and much can often be learned by watching the act of micturition. The size, force, character, and curve of the urinary stream often indicate the amount of obstruction that is present. When micturition is intermittent and completed only after several efforts, prostatic obstruction is usually present. Terminal pain and dribbling are also of diagnostic value as well as hematuria. The character of the urine voided in the three glasses should be noted, and if cloudy, acetic acid may be added to eliminate phosphaturia. Specimens are then sent to the laboratory for examination. If cultures are desired the technic previously described should be followed.

Genitalia.—The condition at the meatus should be carefully noted. The epididymes should be examined for nodules or evidence of epididymitis. The perineum should be studied for scars, and the anus for fissures, fistulæ, and hemorrhoids.

Rectal.—When the finger is inserted into the rectum, the character of the anal sphincter should be noted, and its tonus described. Strictures or other important pathologic conditions of the rectum should be noted. The description of the prostate should be complete and systematic. The size, shape, prominence, and effect upon the rectal lumen are first noted. The median notch and furrow are then examined and the consistence of the tissue in the median line recorded. Making pressure in the median line, one is usually able to detect lateral hypertrophy. Where the median furrow and notch are replaced by a very indurated plateau, carcinoma may often be suspected. A middle lobe generally obliterates the notch at the upper end and can sometimes be felt by rectum as it projects upward into the bladder. Each lateral lobe should be studied and noted separately, and its size, enlargement, contour, surface, consistence, tenderness, and adhesions should be carefully recorded on a chart, as shown in Fig. 241. On these charts the consistence is graded in four degrees—unlined for normal, parallel lines in one direction for slight induration, in two directions for moderate, and in three directions for great induration—as shown in Fig. 242. The third degree induration is usually present in carcinoma, although areas of third degree induration are sometimes seen in prostatic hypertrophy associated with chronic inflammation. Other conditions producing extreme induration are tuberculosis and calculus. Adhesions are indicated along the lateral margins of the prostate and seminal vesicles as shown in Fig. 242, A. The opposite lobe is then studied and recorded in the same way. The examiner then studies the seminal vesicles, recording their size, contour, surface, consistence, tenderness, and adhesions. The relation between the rectum and the prostate and seminal vesicles should be noted. In carcinoma the muscular coat of the rectum is occasionally invaded and the rectal wall fixed to the enlarged prostate. The mucous membrane is but rarely involved or an intrarectal ulceration present. In simple hypertrophy with marked inflammation the rectum is occasionally adherent and at times areas of contracture or septum formation in the rectal wall are found. Not infrequently one finds in chronic seminal infections a marked plateau of induration which restricts the anterior wall of the rectum. The importance of infections of the seminal vesicles in conjunction with prostatic hypertrophy has been stressed of late.[1] Adhesions are of importance and often explain referred pains, particularly those located in the back. By rectal examination one can generally determine whether adenomatous hypertrophy of the prostate is present, but occasionally the growth is entirely toward the bladder and the rectal surface is normal. The spheroidal masses along the urethra, while sufficient to produce obstruction, may not be large enough to be felt per rectum. The great importance of cystoscopy and urethroscopy is, therefore, evident. The secretion of the prostate and seminal vesicles should be obtained by massage and studies of the cells and stained smears for bacteria made. This is of importance as placing the operator on his guard against infections after instrumentation or inlying catheters, and if considerable, may warrant treatment by massage and instillations of the deep urethra before carrying out prostatectomy. We have known one patient with pronounced suppurative prostatitis to

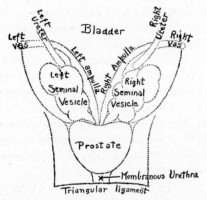

FIG. 241.—Diagram representing the rubber stamp which is used to indicate the normal outline of the structures felt upon rectal examination. The sketches showing the pathologic changes present are superimposed upon this outline. (Reduced one half.)

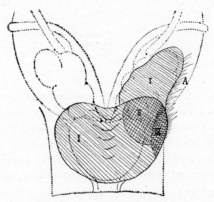

FIG. 242.—Diagram indicating manner of showing pathologic changes in prostate and seminal vesicles. The outline of the prostate indicates that it was enlarged and smooth. The single cross-hatching (I) indicates a very slight degree of induration. The addition of a second series of lines (II) indicates more marked induration, while triple (III) indicates extreme or stony induration. Adhesions are indicated by shading as at A.

develop septicemia immediately after prostatectomy, evidently due to infection of the wound from the pus present in the prostate around the hypertrophied lobes.

Cystoscopy.—An evacuating cystoscope with a right-angled telescope is the instrument of choice in examinations of the bladder and prostate. The lens system may give either a corrected or uncorrected image. Either is satisfactory. The cystoscope with uncorrected image gives more continuous prostatic pictures, but the corrected image is better for the study of the bladder. The posterior cysto-urethroscope is very satisfactory in prostatic examinations because it is possible also to study the posterior urethra with this instrument.

Before mounting the cystoscopic table the patient is instructed to empty the bladder as completely as possible. After the usual preparatory cleansing and sterilizing of the genitalia and urethra, 4 per cent. novocain is injected with a bulb syringe into the anterior urethra and forced through the external sphincter into the

[1] Boyd, M. L.: Journal of Urology, 1923, x, 387–392.

posterior urethra and bladder with a second injection. After five minutes the cystoscope, lubricated with liquid paraffin, is introduced slowly into the bladder. When approaching the median lobe care should be taken to depress the suspensory ligament sufficiently to pass the prostatic enlargement without traumatism. It

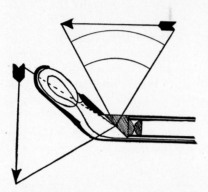

Fig. 243.—The cystoscope: Schematic longitudinal section showing right-angle view obtained with simple prism and lens system. The object is inverted.

may be necessary to turn the instrument slowly to one side or the other, by rotation of the shaft, in order to enter the bladder. Often the cleft on one side of a median lobe is deeper than on the other, and this should be carefully sought for in introducing the cystoscope. After the sheath of the cystoscope enters the bladder the obturator is withdrawn and the residual urine carefully determined, the bladder tonicity being noted as the urine is expelled. The bladder is then slowly filled with a weak antiseptic solution and the vesical capacity obtained. The irrigation is then continued until the fluid is clear enough to make a satisfactory examination. After a cursory view of the bladder with special attention to the base, trigone, and ureteral orifices, noting the presence or absence of stone, diverticula, etc., a systematic study of the prostatic orifice is made.

Cystoscopy in the Hypertrophied Prostate.—The oft-repeated assertion of certain surgeons and even of some cystoscopists that the cystoscope is of little or no value in cases of prostatic hypertrophy comes, we believe, from the difficulty in interpreting what is seen, and has led us to make a detailed study of the subject.[1]

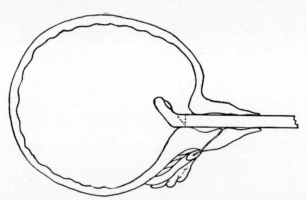

Fig. 244.—Study of prostatic orifice with cystoscope. As shown here it is necessary to draw the instrument out until the prism is within the orifice, only a small part of which is seen with each view.

As shown in Fig. 243, in the plain cystoscope the rays of light are deflected 90 degrees by the rectangular prism, and the line of vision is, therefore, at right angles to the shaft of the instrument. The base and lateral walls of the bladder, being more or less parallel to the shaft of the cystoscope, are easily viewed by the simple cystoscope. The anterior wall of the bladder can only be seen by considerably depressing

[1] Young: Johns Hopkins Hospital Bulletin, 1904, xv, 348–359.

the handle of the cystoscope, but in order to see the margins of the prostatic orifice it is necessary to withdraw the cystocope until the prism enters the prostatic orifice (Fig. 244), when, for the first time, the margin comes into the field of view. But then, owing to the close proximity of the prism to the object viewed, considerable magnification is produced. The picture thus obtained is as represented in Fig. 245, a segment constituting about one-sixth of the margin of the orifice. It is necessary, therefore, to make at least six successive views in order to see the entire circumference of the prostatic orifice. Owing to the spherical aberration, which is more or less pronounced near the periphery of the field of the cystoscope, it is better to take eight successive views.

We thus see that the study of the normal orifice is beset with difficulties, but when we come to deal with the multitudinous forms of irregular and abnormal orifices produced by hypertrophied prostatic lobes, the chances of error and difficulties of interpretation are greatly increased.

This led us to have constructed by Hirschmann in Berlin in July, 1900, a cystoscope with which we could look almost directly backward so as to view the prostatic orifice and its surrounding structures (Fig. 246). This cystoscope differed greatly in construction from the cystoscope No. 3 of Nitze, which was intended to view the

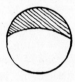
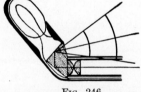

FIG. 245.   FIG. 246. 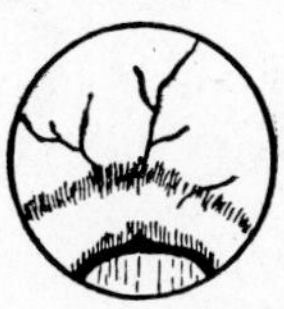   FIG. 247.

FIG. 245.—Anterior margin of prostate as seen looking forward with corrected view lens system.
FIG. 246.—Young's retrograde cystoscope, showing compound prism looking almost directly backward.
FIG. 247.—View of anterior wall of bladder, prostatic margin and shaft of cystoscope below, as seen with Young's retrograde cystoscope.

anterior wall of the bladder and gave no view of the prostatic orifice, and which, we understand, was never a mechanical success, owing to the fact that a mirror was used to produce the reflection.

The design of our cystoscope is shown in Fig. 246. As seen here, the prism with two reflecting surfaces was employed to enable the operator to see almost directly backward; the field of vision, as shown in Fig. 247, included the shaft of the instrument, one-half of the margin of the prostatic orifice, and the adjacent vesical mucosa. It was thus possible with three or four successive views to examine the surface circumjacent to the prostatic orifice, and to see it without magnification or aberration.

This instrument was demonstrated in 1900 to Professors Nitze and Casper in Berlin, and presented to the meeting of the American Association of Genito-Urinary Surgeons, May 12, 1903.

Very soon after our publication there appeared a description of a retrograde cystoscope devised by Schlägintweit,[1] in which he made use of a different system of prisms and lenses to accomplish the same object, as shown in Fig. 248.

Since then Nitze has constructed a retrograde cystoscope (Fig. 249), which is

[1] Centralblatt für die Krankheiten der Harn- und Sexual-Organen, 1903, xiv, 202–207.

similar to ours, except that the prism is split into two and a lens placed between them as was done by Schlagintweit.

After using all these instruments we have, however, reverted to the use of a simple cystoscope with either a corrected or uncorrected view.

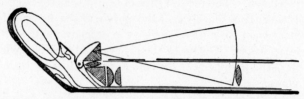

FIG. 248.—Schlagintweit's retrograde cystoscope. The upper prism is hinged to the telescope and can be drawn into the sheath.

The Mechanics of Cystoscopy.—Before discussing the cystoscopic findings we shall consider the changes which occur at the prostatic orifice as a result of hypertrophied lobes. We need hardly refer to the multiplicity of forms in which prosstatic enlargements may be present. The prostate may be larger than an orange or not appreciably enlarged at all. It may present little or no change within the

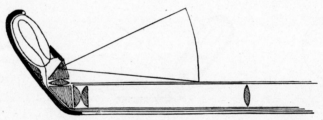

FIG. 249.—Nitze's retrograde cystoscope.

bladder or it may almost fill the cavity. One or all of the respective portions of the prostate may be involved, thus presenting many varieties and forms.

As a rule, the median portion of the posterior commissure (the so-called median lobe), and the lateral lobes are the principal seats of change, but in rare instances the anterior commissure may furnish definite or even great enlargement. The

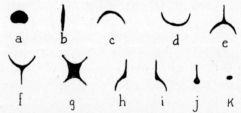

FIG. 250.—The normal orifice (*a*) and changes made in it by lobes arising from different quadrants of the prostate.

shape of the prostatic orifice depends on the pressure which is brought to bear upon it by single or multiple enlargements of the prostate.

This is best shown diagrammatically, as in Fig. 250.

As shown here, *a* represents the normal; *b*, the orifice compressed by the two enlarged lateral lobes; *c*, the orifice elevated by a median posterior lobe; *d*, the orifice depressed by a rounded anterior lobe; *e*, the orifice changed by compression of two lateral and one posterior lobe; *f*, the compression of an anterior and two lateral lobes; *g*, four lobes present at the same time; *h*, the left lateral and median lobes confluent, the right lateral lobe separated from the median by an intervening cleft; *i*, median lobe confluent with the right with sulci between them and the enlarged left lateral; *j*, the median and both laterals confluent with only a cleft in front; and *k*, an enlargement entirely around the orifice leading to circular contracture without sulci.

The normal orifice (*a*) as seen with the right-angled telescope with corrected vision is shown in Fig. 251. The same seen with the uncorrected or inverted image is

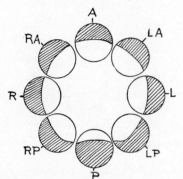

Fig. 251.—The normal prostatic orifice as seen with the corrected cystoscope (non-inverted).

Fig. 252.—Normal orifice, inverted views, as seen with uncorrected lens system.

shown in Fig. 252. In these charts the direction of the cystoscope is shown by the arrows, and the separate views are marked A, anterior; P, posterior; R, right; L, left; RA, right anterior; RP, right posterior, etc. The pictures shown by the cystoscope in various types of prostatic hypertrophy are as follows: Figure 253 shows a series of pictures taken in a case of bilateral hypertrophy (*b*). The orifice is

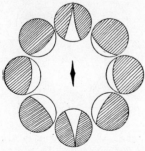
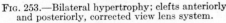

Fig. 253.—Bilateral hypertrophy; clefts anteriorly and posteriorly, corrected view lens system.

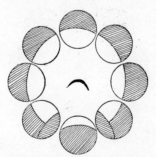

Fig. 254.—Median lobe hypertrophy. Clefts in LP and RP. Lateral and anterior views of margin normal.

shown diagrammatically in the center of the picture. Figure 254 shows the urethral orifice in the case of a small median lobe with no lateral hypertrophy (*c*). As shown here, it is in the form of an inverted crescent with sulci on each side of the median lobe.

As seen here there is no change from the normal when looking upward (A) or to either side (R, RA, L, and LA), but the three inferior views are greatly changed, P showing a rounded intravesical outgrowth, and RP and LP the sulci which lie on each side of it (the ends of the crescent).   Sometimes the median lobe is greatly depressed by the cystoscope (which lies against its anterior surface) and the sulci are then seen in R and L, as shown in Fig. 255.

Care must be taken not to be deceived as to the size of the lobe.   Owing to the immediate juxtaposition of the prism of the cystoscope, such a lobe is always greatly magnified, and the fact that it is seen in five fields (R, RP, P, LP, and L) should not be taken to mean that it is large; the cystoscope may lie in a depression on its surface.

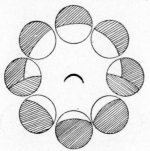

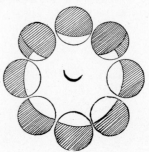

FIG. 255.—Median lobe hypertrophy, sulci appearing higher (in R and L).

FIG. 256.—Anterior lobe hypertrophy. Lateral and posterior margins normal. Sulci in RA and LA.

(d) *Anterior Lobe Hypertrophy.*—The cystoscopic pictures obtained in such a case are seen in Fig. 256.   The three anterior pictures show the changes which correspond to the crescent-shaped orifice, a rounded mass in A, and a sulcus to each side of it, in RA and LA.

(e) *Median and Both Lateral Lobes Enlarged.*—The orifice in this case is in the shape of an inverted Y (Fig. 257), which is a combination of Figs. 253 and 254.   The cystoscopic pictures shown in Fig. 257 show sulci in A, RP, and LP.   The middle

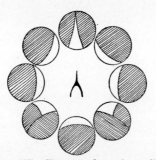

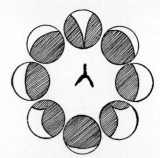

FIG. 257.—Hypertrophy of median and both lateral lobes. Sulci in A, RP, and LP. Corrected view lens.

FIG. 258.—Median and both lateral lobes enlarged. Views obtained by uncorrected lens system. Inverted.

lobe is shown in P and partly in RP and LP.   The right lateral lobe is in RP, R, and RA, and partly in A.   Left lateral lobe is in LP, L, LA, and A.   Figure 258 shows views obtained with the uncorrected lens system cystoscope in a case of median and lateral hypertrophy.

(f) *An anterior and two lateral lobes* are shown in Fig. 259.   They are the opposite of the last pictures.

(g) *Both Lateral, Median, and Anterior Lobe Hypertrophy.*—As stated before, the urethra is here compressed from all four directions and the shape of the orifice is shown in the center of Fig. 260. The location of the clefts and lobes is self-evident.

Most confusing sometimes is it when one finds a lateral and a median confluent on one or both sides. The following pictures show the variations.

(h) *Median Lobe Confluent with Left Lateral Lobe.*—In such cases the three lobes are enlarged, but there is no intervening sulcus between the median and the left lateral lobes. The orifice is shown in the center, and the clefts appear in A and RP

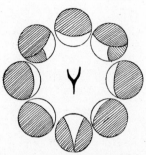 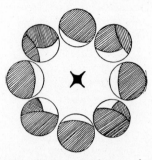

Fig. 259.—Anterior and two lateral lobes. Sulci at P, RA, and LA. Lobes between.

Fig. 260.—Cystoscopic pictures of prostatic orifice with enlarged lobe on each side, posteriorly, and anteriorly, with clefts between.

(Fig. 261). LP shows the confluence of the median and left lateral lobes without intervening sulcus.

(i) *Median Lobe Confluent with Right Lateral Lobe.*—As shown in Fig. 262 these are the counterpart of Fig. 261.

(j) *Median Bar Confluent with Both Lateral Lobes.*—In such a case we have only one cleft and that in A, the median bar or lobe being continuous with the left lateral

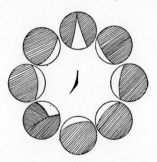 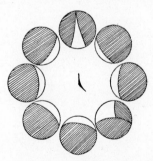

Fig. 261.—Cystoscopic chart in case in which hypertrophied median and left lateral lobes are confluent. Right lobe hypertrophied, clefts in A and RP.

Fig. 262.—Hypertrophied median lobe confluent with right lateral lobe. Both lateral lobes hypertrophied. Sulcus in A and LP.

lobe without intervening clefts as shown in Fig. 263. This is the horseshoe type of intravesical hypertrophy.

(k) *All Portions Being Enlarged and Continuous Without Intervening Clefts.*—In these cases the enlarged prostate projects into the bladder in the shape of a ring of hypertrophied tissue, the anterior, lateral, and posterior portions being confluent without intervening sulci. In such cases the cystoscopic pictures show continuous enlargement, which obscures the anterior part of the trigone below and the adjacent portions of the bladder elsewhere, as shown in Fig. 264.

Large Median Lobes.—In Fig. 257 we saw the inverted crescent-shaped orifice produced by the median lobe, the urethra being divided in the form of a Y, with sulci on each side of the median lobe. If the lobe is small or flat and the sulci on each side shallow, the cystoscope will generally rest on the summit of the lobe.

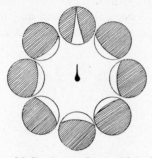

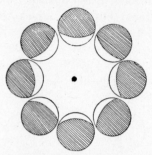

FIG. 263.—Median bar confluent with both lateral lobes. Sulcus only in A.

FIG. 264.—All portions of prostate enlarged and continuous without intervening sulci.

Cystoscopic pictures are then such as shown in Fig. 257, 258. If one or both of the sulci are deep and a median lobe prominent, the cystoscope will generally either pass into the bladder along one of the branches of the urethral Y (Fig. 265), or will slip into the sulcus after introduction. It is an easy matter, as a rule, to carry the cystoscope into the opposite sulcus by successively depressing the outer end of the instrument, pushing it in the opposite direction, and then elevating it. This maneuver will generally cause the vesical end of the cystoscope to traverse the front of the middle lobe from one

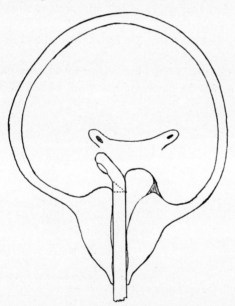

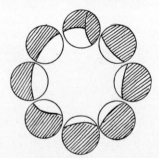

FIG. 265.—Middle lobe, crescentic orifice, Y-shaped urethra. Cystoscope in right branch of Y on right side of middle lobe.

FIG. 266.—Prostatic orifice in large median lobe hypertrophy, cystoscope in sulcus to right of lobe.

sulcus to the other. If the middle lobe is quite high it is advisable to hug the anterior vesical wall with the beak of the cystoscope while rotating the shaft so as to keep the beak continually directed away from the middle lobe and to facilitate its passage into the sulcus on the opposite side of the middle lobe. These maneuvers were used by us in performing the Bottini operation in middle lobe cases.[1]

[1] Young: Monatsberichte für Urologie, 1901, vi, 1–13.

If, in a case of marked median lobe hypertrophy, the cystoscope lies in the sulcus to the right of the lobe, when looking to the left, one will see not the left lateral lobe, but the right side of the median lobe (Fig. 266). As seen here R, RA, and RP show that the right lateral lobe is not at all intravesically enlarged. There is no sulcus or cleft in RP, because the cystoscope lies at the bottom of the cleft, separating it. Rotating the instrument to the left we see the increasing prominence of the median lobe in P, LP, and L. In LA the summit appears and in A we see the cleft which separates it from the anterior border of the prostate. We notice that the mucous membrane is not continuous as is the case with sulci which separate the median and lateral lobes because the middle lobe is separated from the anterior border of the prostatic orifice by the crescentic urethra.

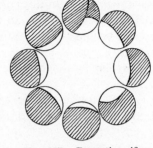

FIG. 267.—Prostatic orifice in large median lobe hypertrophy, cystoscope in sulcus to left of lobe.

After preparing these pictures we place the cystoscope in the bottom of the sulcus on the left side of the middle lobe by the maneuver described above, and obtain the pictures shown in Fig. 267, which are the counterpart of those taken in the opposite sulcus (Fig. 266).

In many cases it is possible to get three sets of pictures from a middle lobe case. One from the top of the middle lobe (Fig. 257), and one from each lateral sulcus (Figs. 266, 267).

In certain cases with a very large anteriorly projecting lateral lobe on one side, and with little enlargement of the other lateral lobe,

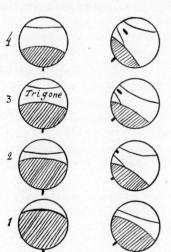

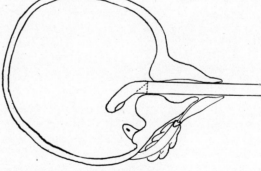

FIG. 268. FIG. 269. FIG. 270.

FIG. 268.—"Motion pictures" showing how trigone, obscured behind median lobe (1), becomes more and more visible on gradually elevating handle of cystoscope (2, 3, 4).

FIG. 269.—"Motion pictures" showing how right ureter, obscured behind hypertrophied lobe, becomes visible by gradually elevating the handle of cystoscope.

FIG. 270.—Schematic longitudinal section. Cystoscope on top of large median lobe showing difficulty in seeing trigone and ureters in such cases.

pictures very similar to those given in Fig. 266 or Fig. 267 for a large median lobe may be obtained. The diagnosis is made by the demonstration of the continuity of the two lateral lobes in front and the inability to obtain two sets of pictures, as shown above in median lobe cases.

In a normal prostate, if the handle of the cystoscope is greatly depressed with the beak looking backward, the interureteral bar may be obscured behind the median portion of the prostate, as shown in 1 (Fig. 268). If the handle is gradually elevated, the distance between the two will be correspondingly increased, as shown in 2,3, and 4, the latter being the position in which the handle is most elevated above the horizontal. In this position the entire trigone is seen up to the prostatic orifice and none is obscured. In the same way the ureteral orifices may be made to disappear behind the prostatic orifice by depression of the handle of the cystoscope, as in 1 (Fig. 269), in which the beak is directed toward the right ureter. By elevating the handle the distance between the two is progressively increased, as shown in 2, 3, and 4.

Such a series of observations is of great value in determining the height of a median bar or lobe (Fig. 270). If one is unable, even with considerable elevation of the handle of the cystoscope, to see the ureteral orifices or the ligamentum interuretericum, one knows at once that the ureters lie beneath a fairly large median bar. If, however, they are brought into plain view, well above the median portion of the prostate, and almost all of the trigone is visible when the handle of the cystoscope is elevated (Fig. 268, 4 and 269, 4), we know the median bar is small. The same rule holds for median lobes when the cystoscope remains on top of the enlargement. If it slips to one side, the orifices and trigone may be easily visible even though the lobe is large.

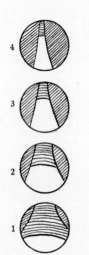

FIG. 271.—Motion pictures of the prostate. Looking anteriorly between two hypertrophied lobes. In upper figure, handle is greatly elevated. It is then gradually depressed, inner end rises and pushes lobes apart until finally they are almost obscured by anterior margin.

Likewise the picture presented by a cleft between two lobes varies greatly according to the position of the cystoscope, as shown in Fig. 271, in which the beak is directed anteriorly between two enlarged lateral lobes. When the handle of the instrument is greatly depressed the inner end of the shaft is pressed up into the upper limit of the sulcus. The lobes are widely separated and the cleft is flattened out. The prism of the instrument then shows only the tautly stretched transverse fold of mucous membrane which runs across from one lobe to the other, as seen in 1. As the handle of the cystoscope is gradually elevated the prismatic end descends and the lateral lobes begin to appear on each side (2 and 3), the transverse fold of mucous membrane disappears from view (4), and finally we see only the narrow chink which separates the lobes. We call these "motion pictures."

This series of pictures is of great value in showing the extent of the hypertrophy, and the depth of the urethral cleft between the lateral lobes. In cases where lateral lobes are smaller and less pronounced, the cleft is shallower and does not appear as a slit.

We have thus given in detail the many changes of view which may be obtained in cases of prostatic hypertrophy, with the feeling that when the mechanics is understood the interpretation will be easy.

In routine practice we employ a chart with circles 2 cm. in diameter, as shown in Fig. 272 (reduced $\frac{1}{4}$). As seen here, the central set of 8 circles is present and around it a square of 16 circles, which may be used for other interesting views which are obtained. Those on each side are used for the "motion pictures" of the anterior or posterior portions of the prostate. As seen in the two accompanying charts taken from clinical cases these "motion pictures" are very valuable in showing the different sets of views obtained in these cases, and the extent of the cleft when the cystoscope is moved by elevating or lowering the shaft of the instrument (Figs. 272, 273, 274).

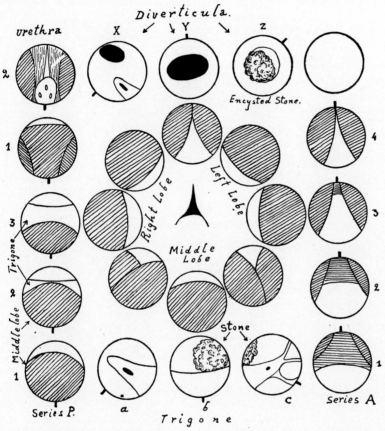

Fig. 272.—Case of bilateral and median hypertrophy of prostate with hypertrophied trigone, trabeculated bladder (c), diverticula (XY), and encysted calculus (Z). Series A shows the anterior margin in 1. As the handle of the cystoscope is elevated the lateral lobes come closer together and the anterior margin disappears in 4. Series P shows appearance of trigone as handle is gradually elevated (2 and 3). Urethra is shown by drawing out the cystoscope; the verumontanum, ducts, and hypertrophied lateral lobes are visible (2). Stone free in bladder (b, c).

The "motion pictures" of the posterior view are most important in demonstrating the size and extent of median bars. We have had many cases in which on rectal examination the prostate was normal in size and the cystoscopic picture was normal in every respect, except that the anterior part of the trigone was obscured behind an elevated median bar. This was only brought out by the "motion pictures," series P, as shown in Fig. 268. As seen here in series P, No. 1 with the handle greatly depressed, the median bar almost completely obscures the trigone and ureters. As the handle of the cystoscope is gradually elevated (2 and 3), more of the trigone is seen and the distance between the ligamentum interuretericum and

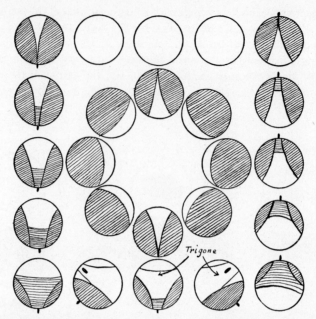

FIG. 273.—Cystoscopic chart in case of hypertrophy of both lateral lobes, median lobe not enlarged. Motion pictures on each side only reveal the anterior and posterior margins when the lateral lobes are pushed aside by depressing or elevating (respectively) the handle of cystoscope.

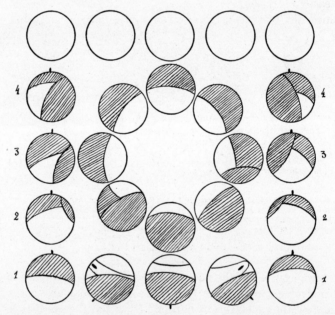

FIG. 274.—Cystoscopic pictures in a case of fairly large median lobe hypertrophy without lateral or anterior lobes. The trigone is largely obscured. By carrying handle of instrument forcibly to either side shaft of the instrument drops into sulcus on opposite side of middle lobe. When handle is depressed in that position (No. 1) the anterior margin alone is seen. As it is gradually elevated (2 and 3) it passes to one side of median lobe which finally obscures portion of anterior margin (4).

the top of the median bar is recorded as farther apart, but when the handle of the cystoscope is greatly elevated, as in 4, there is still a portion of the trigone obscured behind the bar.   The gloved finger is then inserted into the rectum, and the diagnosis may be confirmed by finding increased thickness in the median portion of the prostate beneath the vesical neck and, as a rule, induration of the tissues.   Usually the

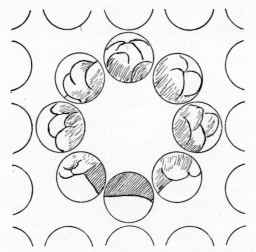

FIG. 275.—Hypertrophied lateral and anterior lobes covered with bullous edema.   Median portion normal.   Inverted view.   B. U. I. 11,352.

beak can be easily felt through the trigone above the median bar.   If the trigone is hypertrophied and thickened, it may be difficult to feel.   This method of accu-

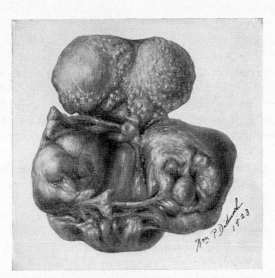

FIG. 276.—Specimen removed by perineal prostatectomy.   History of hematuria at the beginning of urination.   No nycturia, no increased frequency of urination.   Prostate moderately enlarged, elastic.   Residual urine, 40 c.c.   Cystoscope shows enlarged lateral and median lobes covered with large translucent cysts (Fig. 275).   At operation entire adenomatous prostate removed in one piece, some of cysts broken, numerous small cysts remained as shown.   B. U. I. 11,352.

rately determining the presence of median bars was first pointed out by us in 1904,[1]

[1] Young: Johns Hopkins Hospital Bulletin, 1904, xv, 348–359; see also Transactions of the American Association of Genito-urinary Surgeons, 1909, iv, 229–247.

and has since been employed with great success in determining when the punch operation was necessary or advisable in such cases. It is often the only method by which this can be accurately determined.

The appearance of intravesical lobes may be so altered by congestion, edema, polyps, cysts, or ulceration that a question of neoplasm or other disease arises. Figures 275 and 276 depict such a case, where the median lobe was covered by a multitude of small cysts. A few days' antiseptic treatment of the bladder will usually change the picture sufficiently to allow a positive diagnosis.

TREATMENT

Before the question of treatment can be considered certain facts should, if possible, be known in regard to the case, viz.:

The size, character, and induration of the prostate and seminal vesicles as shown on rectal examination. The amount of residual urine and the bladder capacity as shown with a catheter or cystoscope. The condition of the bladder (trabeculation, cellules, diverticula, stone, inflammation, etc.), as shown with the cystoscope. The character of urine, specific gravity, albumin, presence of infection or not. Two-hour phthalein test to determine kidney function, and if low, the blood urea. The condition of the heart, arteries, blood, etc. Treatment may be divided into the non-operative or hygienic, the preoperative, and the operative.

Non-operative.—This is applicable only to early cases or those in which operation is contraindicated. In early cases, where the symptoms are not aggravated—the urine sterile, the residual urine small (less than 100 c.c.) vesical capacity fairly good (say 300 c.c.) and the bladder wall showing no great trabeculation, cellule or diverticulum formation, the kidney function good and no evidence of cardiorenal disease—such patients may often be safely told that they may wait. It should always be made clear that an operation may at any moment become imperative and that careful hygiene must be observed. These patients should avoid exposure to cold or chilling, particularly of the pelvic region. The bowels should not be allowed to become very constipated, urination should be carried out at fairly normal intervals, and the bladder not allowed to become overdistended before urinating. If the urine is very acid and irritating, alkalines in the form of drugs or drinks may be indicated.

Occasionally, prostatic massage carried out at intervals of three to four days or rectal douches of ice-water may be of benefit in reducing prostatic congestion and irritation, particularly if associated with chronic prostatitis. If the latter is present to a marked degree, regular treatment, consisting of posterior urethral injections of 1 per cent. mercurochrome following prostatic massage, and occasionally instillation of nitrate of silver into the posterior urethra or application of nitrate of silver to an enlarged, congested verumontanum may be desirable.

It must be remembered, however, that violent treatment or instrumentation may at any time bring on complete retention of urine. In a few cases we have tried radium in the hope of reducing the prostatic enlargement and doing away with obstruction. In one case, in which there was serious heart disease, contraindicating major operation, the systematic use of radium by rectum, urethra, and perineum, and also through the suprapubic region, in massive doses, led to a great reduction in the hypertrophied prostate, but obstruction and complete retention of urine persisted until relieved by a punch operation under local anesthesia.[1] As a whole, however, the experiences here and elsewhere with radium and x-ray in the treatment of prostatic hypertrophy have been very disappointing. Drugs are likewise of little or no value in the treatment of prostatic hypertrophy, other than to relieve irritation, inflammation, pain, hemorrhage, etc.

If, owing to the incipiency of the disease or the slightness of the symptoms, operation is postponed, the patient should be asked to appear occasionally for a thorough medical examination, at which it should be carefully determined that the renal function is not becoming impaired, that cardiorenal disease is not developing or the general condition of the patient becoming weakened. If the condition remains about the same and the symptoms are slight, operation may be further withheld, but if there is a gradual increase in the difficulty, frequency, pain or discomfort and the patient is losing sleep and generally becoming weaker physically, he should be told that surgery offers the safest course.

The second class of cases in which a non-operative treatment may be advised are those in which immediate operation would be dangerous. In some of these cases a careful preparatory treatment will eventually make a radical operation safe. The handling of these cases will be described at length later on. There are other cases (rare) which will probably never be got into sufficiently good condition for operation to be safe, and for these a method of treatment must be advised, which will make them as comfortable as possible and improve their condition. As previously stated, such cases are those of greatly weakened physical condition, with grave maladies which would not be benefited by careful preparatory treatment, and in the presence of which operation would never be at all safe. Here, treatment to relieve the difficulty and frequency of urination, pain, hemorrhage, etc., must be provided. For such cases, if the symptoms are severe, a catheter life may be necessary. A careful study of the condition should be made and proper catheters selected. The physician, family, or patient should be instructed in the technic of careful catheterization, stress being laid on asepsis of catheter, hands, and urethra, and antiseptic treatment of the bladder to prevent infection. This is particularly important in the early stages. It is impossible here to lay down full rules for the conduct of such cases for the succeeding months or years. Whereas the gum coudé or prostatic catheter enters more easily, most patients prefer a rubber catheter and in many cases a No. 16, 18, or 20 catheter passes without difficulty and with little or no traumatism. A coudé rubber catheter may now be obtained. The outside of the penis is cleansed with soap and water and preferably with a small alcohol sponge, but it is too much to expect patients leading a catheter life to carry out perfect asepsis. If the catheter is carefully cleaned after use in soap and water, boiled, and placed in a clean towel or immersed in some efficient antiseptic solution, its use will be sufficiently safe if the patient is careful to wash and sterilize his hands and not to touch that portion of the catheter which reaches the bladder.

A soft-rubber catheter will occasionally meet with an impassable obstruction and a coudé gum catheter, 16 to 18 F., should always be on hand for such emergencies. The coudé rubber catheter is also a valuable instrument; both can be boiled and are safer than the silver or metal catheter. A stilet of wire with a prostatic curve is often necessary to give a rubber catheter the proper curve, and patient and physician should always be able to procure one of these for such an emergency. If a

[1] Young: Annals of Surgery, 1917, lxv, 633–641.

silver catheter is used and meets with an obstruction, the physician can simply bend it into a wide prostatic curve with the fingers and thus catheterize cases which are otherwise impassable.

When retention of urine is complete and catheterization impossible, aspiration of the bladder, suprapubically, may be carried out. It is preferable to use a needle of moderate size (the usual subcutaneous infusion needle, 5 inches long, is satisfactory). Often after a single-suprapubic aspiration, voluntary urination may be restored or urethral catheterization can be successfully carried out. In some cases suprapubic drainage may be required, other methods failing.

In the majority of cases in which catheter life is begun, the patient may be able to void urine in small amounts and the catheter only be necessary sufficiently often to keep the patient fairly comfortable and to avoid frequent disturbance at night. The physician should be guided by circumstances, there being no hard-and-fast rules to follow. The obstruction of urination, residual urine, and back pressure should not become so great as to cause progressive impairment of the kidneys, and the patient should, if possible, show a steady improvement under the treatment. While many patients follow a catheter life for years, sometimes with little or no trouble, many have "stormy periods" in which catheterization is difficult or required very often, or crises of infection, chills, fever, etc., occur. Statistics show that the catheter life has far more fatalities than operation. Patients who oppose the latter should be made to face the facts, so that they will at least take proper precautions in following the catheter life. The use of internal antiseptics and urethral and bladder irrigations to prevent or minimize infection of the urinary tract is discussed elsewhere.

Suprapubic drainage may be classed under palliative treatment and is often necessary where a catheter life is unsuccessful; a large group of surgeons employ it as the first stage of a "two-stage prostatectomy," but we wish to refer here to its use in cases where radical operation is out of the question, and relief is necessary on account of the inability to follow successfully a catheter life. In such cases the bladder should be opened through a very small incision and a rubber tube fastened into the bladder in proper position to form a good fistula for permanent drainage. The de Pezzer mushroom catheter or some other form of self-retaining catheter is of great value in this procedure. If the bladder is greatly distended, the urine should not be completely evacuated at once, but some form of pressure apparatus applied to prevent too rapid evacuation and consequent uremia or suppression. With the formation of a good fistula, the suprapubic drainage can be worn indefinitely with little leakage or discomfort. The urine may be evacuated intermittently or allowed to drain into a proper receptacle, but it is preferable not to allow the bladder to become contracted by continuous drainage. With care and attention to antisepsis, a suprapubic drainage apparatus may be worn indefinitely. Perineal drainage has been used in a few cases, but never satisfactorily. In some cases patients, who were supposed to be beyond operative relief, have improved so wonderfully after urethral or suprapubic drainage, that in a few weeks (or months) they were sufficiently strong to warrant operative interference. Many such cases have ultimately been operated upon with success.

The treatment of the kidneys should go on, *pari passu*, with vesical drainage. The rules have already been laid down, viz.:

Large amounts of water, preferably by mouth, but if necessary subcutaneously, by rectum, or intravenously. The use of alkalies or internal urinary antiseptics, as the case may require. Chronic nephritis to have appropriate treatment, and arterial and cardiac conditions to receive the attention they require.

Preoperative.—As shown elsewhere in a brief description of the progress made in the treatment of prostatic hypertrophy and in the reduction of mortality, it is in the preliminary or preparatory treatment before operation where the greatest strides have been made. It is through this work that the mortality has been reduced from 25 per cent. to practically zero, except in the desperate cases. The treatment before operation varies with the condition of the patient. Most patients can be operated upon without delay; others require but a brief period of preparatory treatment, while some require weeks, and even months, of most pains-taking care to make it possible to carry out finally a successful prostatectomy. In hospitals where this is not recognized, the mortality still remains about 25 per cent.

We find that our cases may be conveniently classified as follows:

(a) *Patients with moderate hypertrophy of the prostate, who have had symptoms of moderate frequency and difficulty of urination, who have not been catheterized, and in which the bladder, after voiding, cannot be percussed above the symphysis.* In such cases it is safe to conclude that the residual urine is not high, probably not over 300 c.c. After a rectal examination and a study of the urine it is usually quite safe to carry out cystoscopy, without fear of suppression or uremia following emptying of the bladder. In such cases, when the patient enters the hospital, if the residual urine is more than 150 c.c., even though the phthalein shows a good kidney function and the physical examination is satisfactory, a retained catheter may or may not be used until the patient is operated upon, and this can usually be done without delay. During this period the patient is given water in abundance to keep the kidneys active. A mild antiseptic irrigation of the bladder two to three times a day is employed. If the circulatory system requires treatment, this is given, as will be described later, but if absent, the patient is operated upon within two to three days, unless complications prevent.

Some surgeons believe that a week or more of preparatory treatment should be given in every case, regardless of the conditions present. We feel that this is unnecessary, but a thorough knowledge is essential in selecting the cases for im-mediate operation. If the surgeon feels the slightest doubt, or if the slightest unfavorable symptoms appear, such as fever, leukocytosis, hematuria, marked pyuria, or any signs of uremia or circulatory failure, operation should be deferred. Delay is usually safe, haste may often be dangerous.

(b) *Patients with hypertrophy of the prostate, upon whom a catheter has been used, or who are leading a catheter life; in whom the kidney function is good, the residual urine not over 400 c.c., the cardiovascular and renal condition satisfactory,* may also be operated upon without delay of more than a few days, during which the physical condition of the patient is carefully studied. If the phthalein test or the presence of a continued fever shows evidence of renal impairment or pyelonephritis, opera-tion must be delayed while these conditions are combated by appropriate means. This applies also to vascular conditions, chronic lesions of the heart and arteries, high blood-pressure, etc., which require appropriate courses of digitalizing, diet, rest, etc.

(c) *Probably the most dangerous cases are those that come with high residual urine.*

This can often be surmised from the history, *e. g.*, marked frequency and difficulty of urination with a feeling of fulness and a sense of incompleteness of evacuation after urination; incontinence of urine, which is, really, a paradoxic incontinence with high residual urine; abdominal distention and discomfort in the pelvic portion; chronic uremia as exemplified by distaste for food, nasuea, vomiting, headaches, dizziness, eye changes, etc.; pronounced circulatory and cardiac changes. In such cases, there is usually a palpably enlarged bladder present. Not infrequently it can be percussed well toward the umbilicus and sometimes above, and if catheterized, residual urine between 500 and 4000 c.c. may be obtained, but to withdraw it at once is to court disaster. In such cases, after rectal examination of the prostate, the patient is sent into the hospital at once, and a careful physical examination given, in which the blood-pressure, cardiac condition, blood urea, etc., are determined. When the catheter is introduced, it is connected at once with the Shaw-Young irrigating decompressor apparatus, the vesical tension is determined, and the exit level placed 2 cm. below the determined vesical pressure. The irrigating apparatus is filled with 1 : 400 meroxyl solution or perhaps 1 : 8000 acriflavin or oxycyanid of mercury and every effort made to keep the bladder from becoming infected during the period of decompression. (See page 74.)

If, despite the high residual, the blood urea is not much above normal and the general condition of the patient good, the head of water against which the bladder empties may be reduced fairly rapidly by simply lowering the outlet tube gradually each day. In such cases, ordinarily starting with a pressure elevation of 2 cm. below the vesical pressure as determined, it is possible to reduce the pressure head about 5 cm. daily after the first twenty-four hours and when within 15 cm. of the bladder level, the pressure apparatus may be removed and continuous drainage through a catheter employed without danger. During this period water should be given in fairly large quantity, say 4000 c.c. daily, in order to keep the kidneys acting profusely. It has the additional advantage of washing out infections already in the urinary tract and combating new infections.

Where an abnormally high blood urea (say between 0.50 and 0.80 grams per liter) with incipient uremia is present it should be combated not only with water in abundance (5000 to 8000 c.c. daily), but the cardiovascular system should be supported with digitalis and the strength of the patient improved by light massage, slight exercise, and avoidance of confinement to bed. One advantage of the Shaw-Young apparatus is that the patient can move about in a wheel chair with this apparatus attached, as shown in Figs. 46, 47. When the patient is in bed, he should be allowed to turn from side to side and be propped up so that hypostatic congestion of the lungs is avoided. Vesical infection, which may be present, is best combated by means of continuous irrigation of the bladder, which is afforded by the apparatus. The bladder empties itself intermittently, and as soon as the contraction is over, one usually sees a varying amount of the antiseptic solution in the reservoir descend into the bladder from which it is expelled in part with the next voiding. This necessitates a refilling of the reservoir from time to time, so as to prevent too great dilution of the antiseptic solution. In numerous cases we have employed a solution of 1 per cent. meroxyl, but in rare instances irritability of the bladder is caused and definite chemical irritation, in which the cystoscope shows dilatation of the blood-vessels and general reddening of the mucosa with superficial changes in the mucous membrane. In very rare instances we have seen evidences of absorption, diarrhea, slight stomatitis, and other evidences of mercury intoxication, never however pronounced or serious, and which have always disappeared when the treatment was discontinued or a change of drug made. Such cases are usually patients who have a peculiar susceptibility to mercury, a condition which is experienced not infrequently by syphilographers and others while employing therapeutic doses of mercury.

With the solution of 1:400 meroxyl, excellent germicidal results are obtained and it is possible to keep the bladder sterile, even though the apparatus is maintained for two weeks or more. In very rare instances, we have found it desirable to use a strength of 1:600 owing to marked susceptibility to mercury, and occasionally we have substituted a solution of permanganate of potash but this has generally resulted in a bladder infection. Permanganate of potash, as Dawson has shown from this clinic, has a very pronounced desquamating effect upon the vesical mucosa when retained in the bladder for a protracted period. Dakin's solution is too irritating and the same applies to bichlorid of mercury and nitrate of silver, both of which have the added disadvantage of being reduced in the presence of urine. Acriflavin cannot be used in a solution stronger than 1:4000, and mercurochrome has the disadvantage that it masks the presence of blood. Meroxyl, which is not precipitated by urine, serum, pus, or blood, which is only slightly irritating, and is powerfully antiseptic, furnishes the nearest to an ideal drug for a germicidal solution to be used in this irrigating decompressor apparatus.

By this apparatus a number of lives have been saved, and many desperate cases carried successfully through preparatory treatment and prostatectomy.

B. U. I. 11,153, age fifty-eight, entered the hospital January 13, 1923, complaining of nausea and vomiting. He gave a history of complete urinary retention three years prior to admission, subsequent to which there had been frequency of urination. For six months before admission he had been voiding at twenty-minute intervals day and night with greatly reduced stream. He had noticed the presence of a tumor in the suprapubic region four months before. He had been having nausea and vomiting and headaches for three weeks before admission. The general physical examination showed cardiac hypertrophy and arhythmia, mitral insufficiency, and chronic bronchitis. Urologic examination showed the bladder to be 4 cm. above the umbilicus, the prostate was greatly enlarged, the urine was sterile, but contained an occasional granular cast and a trace of albumin; the blood urea was 1.56 grams per liter. A retention catheter was inserted and decompression apparatus attached. The bladder pressure was found to be 55 cm. The overflow level was set at 60 cm., fluids were forced and digitalis therapy begun. The pressure was lowered 5 cm. each day until the level reached 15 cm. where it remained until operation. There was an immediate decrease in blood urea and ten days later it was normal. Phthalein done on the tenth day had an appearance time of fifteen minutes, 30 per cent. first hour and 15 per cent. the second. On the fourteenth day after admission, the appearance time of the phthalein was nine minutes, 35 per cent. first hour and 25 per cent. second. The urine remained uninfected. Seventeen days after admission perineal prostatectomy by Dr. Young. The postoperative course was afebrile and uncomplicated, and the patient was discharged February 17th, eighteen days after operation, with fistula closed and voiding at normal intervals.

B. U. I. 11,375, admitted to the hospital March 4, 1923, complaining of frequency of urination. History of gradually increasing frequency of urination and decrease in size of urinary stream for one year. The general physical examination showed mitral insufficiency and stenosis, with cardiac hypertrophy. Urologic examination showed a greatly enlarged prostate with the bladder extending to the umbilicus, the urine was uninfected, the blood urea was 1.12 grams per liter. A retention catheter was inserted and decompression apparatus attached. Fluids were forced and the overflow level of the apparatus was reduced 5 cm. a day. Two days later the patient became irrational, although the blood urea had fallen to 0.85 grams per liter. The temperature was normal and the heart was holding out fairly well against the large quantity of fluid introduced. Two days later he was again rational and the blood urea had fallen to 0.44 grams per liter. Six days after admission phthalein had an appearance time of twenty minutes, 30 per cent. first hour and 10 per cent. second. The urine remained sterile until operation, which was successfully carried out twelve days after admission to the hospital.

Where the blood urea is very high, (say over 1 gram per liter) it should be recognized at once that the patient is in great danger of suppression of urine and uremia, and very active measures adopted. Not only should water be given by mouth in as large quantities as possible (with careful observation of the cardiovascular system and digitalis if necessary to prevent a breakdown), but water should be introduced per rectum, subcutaneously, and if the case is desperate, intravenously. We have not infrequently employed as much as 12,000 c.c. daily by these combined routes and have had the satisfaction of seeing patients who were so uremic that they were practically comatose, gradually emerge from their stupor as the kidney function improved and the excessive blood urea slowly disappeared, and their strength steadily increase until a successful operation was finally possible.

Cases with arteriosclerosis, high blood-pressure, or cardiac lesions require the greatest care during this period. It is not safe to reduce greatly the blood-pressure, even though high, lest the patient go into suppression. We have seen cardiovascular breaks occur when the amount of water taken was increased to combat ascending pyelonephritis.

B. U. I. 12,272, age seventy, admitted August 20, 1924, complaining of difficulty of urination. He gave a history of mild symptoms of lower urinary obstruction of one year's duration. Temperature 98.6° F., pulse 80, respiration 20, blood-pressure 160/100, white blood-cells 9700 on admission. The general physical examination showed chronic bronchitis and emphysema and slight hypertension with occasional extrasystole. Urologic examination showed benign prostatic hypertrophy with a residual urine of 500 c.c. Urine was uninfected but contained albumin and hyaline casts. Phthalein 15 per cent. first hour and 10 per cent. second. Blood urea was normal. The bladder was refilled with 1 : 500 meroxyl and the decompression apparatus attached. Pressure was gradually reduced over a period of ten days. During this time the patient's general condition appeared to be quite good. The urine was uninfected when the decompression apparatus was removed. Phthalein at this time was 15 per cent. the first hour and 15 per cent. the second hour. Two days after the beginning of free drainage, the patient had a severe chill and temperature rose to 102° F. He became toxic and the blood urea increased to 1.4 grams per liter. Fluids were forced to 5000 c.c. daily. On the day following the chill the pulse became quite irregular and the patient showed signs of cardiac decompensation. Digitalis therapy was instituted at once and fluids were restricted. In spite of the treatment for the cardiac condition, the patient gradually became worse and he died 4 days after the chill, the immediate cause of death apparently being myocardial failure. Autopsy showed chronic myocarditis, marked arteriosclerosis, benign prostatic hypertrophy, and extensive recent pyelonephritis.

This was a case suffering from extensive cardiovascular and renal disease in addition to kidney impairment resulting from back pressure. The bladder pressure was gradually decreased without the urine becoming infected. It seems that a mistake was made in this case by removing the decompression apparatus at this time as the urine promptly became infected and pyelonephritis was superimposed upon the existing kidney lesion. In attempting to combat this infection with forced fluids, the cardiovascular system was not able to stand the strain. Digitalis should have been given before the break occurred.

Had we, in this case, instituted an adequate course of preliminary digitalis, it is quite possible that the circulation would have withstood the forced water cure, which was necessitated by the advent of pyelonephritis. In such cases the infection of the urinary tract is one of the most important complications to be avoided.

Infection.—Before the adoption of our irrigating decompressor, vesical infection occurred in practically every case when catheter drainage of the bladder was kept up for more than a few days. Cystitis almost invariably resulted, and occasionally ascending infection to the kidneys (whether it reach there through the lumen of the ureters or by the lymphatics matters not).

When renal infection occurs, water is our most valuable and almost only means of attack. It is remarkable what can be accomplished by this simple means.

We may cite here a case in which there was a considerably enlarged prostate, complete retention of urine, marked impairment of the kidney function, and the blood urea was high. This patient was placed on continuous urethral catheter drainage. After two weeks he suddenly developed chills and fever and rapidly went into uremia, became unconscious, blood urea rose to 1.35, and both kidneys were palpable and tender. An active water cure was at once adopted, nevertheless for a short time his condition rapidly grew worse and his life was despaired of, but within four days the temperature and his general condition began slowly to improve. After a week he became rational; within three weeks the uremia and infection had disappeared and about five weeks later his condition was sufficiently good to carry out a perineal prostatectomy, from which he had an excellent result.

When infection is already present in these cases, but has not extended to the kidneys, it may be possible to get rid of it and make the bladder sterile by means of the irrigating decompressor. In many cases, however, this is not accomplished and occasionally pronounced infection of the urethra occurs regardless of the fact that the catheter is changed every three days. Our rule is to irrigate the urethra with some mild antiseptic solution and give it three to four hours' rest before again inserting a catheter, but despite this precaution, in some cases, in which prolonged catheter drainage is necessary, marked urethritis occurs. In rare instances the infection may produce peri-urethral infiltration and even abscess formation. This may occur either along the penile, perineal or prostatic portion of the urethra. It may involve the peri-urethral ducts and glands, including Cowper's, the prostate, and the seminal vesicles. It may penetrate beyond the confines of the urethra and prostate and invade the tissues beneath Buck's, Colles', and the pelvic fascia. The suppuration may even penetrate beyond into the perirectal spaces and from there infiltrate the thighs, buttocks, hips, perineum, scrotum, and even follow the course of Scarpa's fascia on the abdomen.

Peri-urethral infiltration is the most feared complication of the retained catheter and assistants should be instructed to be constantly alert and on the outlook for it. Daily palpation of the urethra, perineum, and scrotum along the retained catheter should be made and if induration, fluctuation and particularly crepitus (gas) is discovered, the catheter should be removed at once. The urethra and perineum should then be stripped by pressure, to evacuate and disclose the presence of abscess, and a rectal examination made to see if the infection extends to the prostate, seminal vesicles, or the tissues around them. The following case exemplifies well the danger of such infection.

B. U. I. 11,514, age sixty-five, admitted June 12, 1923. Case of prostatic hypertrophy with 450 c.c. residual urine, urine infected with staphylococci. Phthalein 30 per cent. in two hours; blood urea, 0.41. The patient was placed on continuous catheter drainage. After a few days, he developed a fever, the temperature varying between 100° and 103° F. for three weeks. There was considerable urethral suppuration, but examination failed to reveal any evidences of peri-urethritis, nevertheless on June 29th, suprapubic drainage was provided, although the blood urea was still normal. Seven days later, fluctuation was discovered in the region of the bulbous urethra. Examination at that time failed to reveal any evidences of peri-urethral or periprostatic infiltration on rectal examination. An incision was made, which opened up a small peri-urethral abscess within Colles' fascia, apparently not extending beyond. Vigorous antiseptic treatment was instituted and the water cure forced. The patient failed to improve, fever continued, and five days later examination showed an infiltration around the anus extending out upon the thighs, and rectal examination disclosed a periprostatic abscess. A second operation was carried out in which the spaces were widely opened, but the patient survived the operation only a few hours.

Our mistake in this case was in not performing a suprapubic drainage sooner. When the patient continued to have fever, in the absence of evidences of pyelitis and with no increase in the blood urea, suprapubic drainage would probably have avoided the generalized infection which subsequently occurred.

If the irrigating decompressor is not used, bladder irrigations should be given at least twice a day through the catheter, and 15 or 20 c.c. of mercurochrome (1 per cent.), meroxyl (0.5 per cent.), or argyrol (10 per cent.) left in the bladder.

The following case, in which there was marked cardiovascular disease, associated with a very poor phthalein, shows the danger of a very small peri-urethral infection:

B. U. I. 12,692, age sixty-seven, admitted August 5, 1924. Considerable hypertrophy of the prostate, residual urine 300 c.c., phthalein test 33 per cent. in two hours. Blood urea 0.53 gram per liter. Patient had a temperature of 102½° F. and continued to have fever, off and on, during his entire stay in the hospital. The urine was infected with bacilli and the cardiovascular condition was very bad. At the end of three weeks, as patient continued to have fever and occasionally chills, although no evidence of infection was discovered along urethra or in prostate, and neither kidney was tender nor enlarged, a suprapubic drainage was given under local anesthesia. The patient stood the operation badly and three days later crepitation was discovered on palpation of the bulbous urethra. Under local anesthesia an incision was made, evacuating a peri-urethral abscess in the perineum. The process had not extended beyond the triangular ligament. For a time the convalescence was very satisfactory. The perineal wound granulated well and the suprapubic drainage was satisfactory.

On September 3d, following the operation, pulse became irregular and dropped every third beat. Blood-pressure dropped from 112/64 before operation to 95/45 and he developed extrasystoles. He was given an active course of digitalis, but regardless of this gradually became weaker. On September 6th, a small abscess of the scrotum was opened. Following this the patient had no fever and drainage was excellent. The blood urea did not go above 0.49, but the patient gradually became weaker and died on September 17th. Impression: Cardiac death. It is probable, however, that had a suprapubic drainage been given earlier, before he was weakened by fever of one month's duration, he would have withstood the suprapubic operation with less shock and cardiac collapse would not have occurred. The occurrence of the peri-urethral infection demonstrates that urethral drainage was retained too long.

We cannot, therefore, lay too great stress upon the constant searching for infection, peri-urethral, perineal, periprostatic, vesical, and renal. With the onset of fever, every effort should be made to locate the source of the infection.

The treatment varies with the case: Water in large amounts by mouth when the kidneys are suspected, the cardiovascular system supported by digitalis to prevent decompensation; if a very pronounced urethritis is present, especially if accompanied by pain and intolerance to the catheter, suprapubic drainage should be afforded, and if peri-urethral infection is present, adequate drainage with a careful investigation of the periprostatic and perirectal spaces and evacuation if found infected, should be carried out.

On the other hand, the operation of suprapubic drainage is of a serious nature. As shown by statistics here and elsewhere suprapubic drainage is accompanied by mortality between 2 and 3 per cent., a mortality probably higher than prostatectomy itself.

A suprapubic puncture with trocar and cannula and the insertion of a catheter is a simple operation, but there is a real danger of extravasation, as shown by the fact that we have recently had 2 patients, thus treated, who came into the hospital with extravasation and perivesical infection. One of these patients died. The ideal is to give the patient adequate drainage of the bladder through an inlying urethral catheter without producing infection in the bladder or marked urethritis, and especially avoiding peri-urethral infection. That this can be done in almost all cases is shown by more than 1000 cases in which this method of treatment has been carried out at this Clinic.

The *cardiovascular system* presents a great problem in the surgery of the hypertrophied prostate. There is probably no branch of surgery in which the need of expert medical consultation, with internists versed in the problems of the urologist, is so necessary. In our experience the majority of medical men have little conception of the feasibility of operation in very old men with bad hearts and arteries.

Practically all of these cases with definite heart lesions, regardless of the character, and with hypertension (blood-pressure over 160), should be given a preparatory course of digitalis. Recently our procedure has been as follows: The patient is given 0.2 gram of powdered digitalis leaves twice daily for three days (which amounts to 1.2 gram). This is sufficient to completely digitalize the average patient. After this it is only necessary to give the patient about 0.2 gram daily in order to maintain the maximum effect of the drug and to obtain satisfactory digitalization. This therapy can apparently be continued indefinitely during the stay in the hospital without deleterious effect. Where the cardiac condition is urgent the drug may be given more rapidly and in desperate cases strophanthin may be indicated. The value of digitalis therapy is shown in the following case:

B. U. I. 12,792, age sixty-three, admitted September 15, 1924. Patient had led catheter life for two years. Examination showed moderately enlarged prostate, bladder filled with cal-

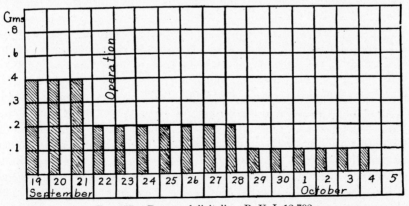

FIG. 277.—Dosage of digitalis. B. U. I. 12,792.

culi, one of which was shown with the x-ray to be in a diverticulum. Cystogram showed numerous diverticula. Phthalein test showed appearance time sixteen minutes, 39 per cent. in two hours, but the blood urea was good, 0.26 gm. per liter. Blood-pressure 152/102. Cardiac examination showed occasional extrasystole, but in view of high diastolic pressure and slight arythmia, it was decided to give a course of digitalis before operation. The dosage employed is shown in the accompanying clinical chart (Fig. 277). The patient was treated with inlying urethral catheter, but this was accompanied by marked pain, and as his condition was not too good, suprapubic drainage was afforded on September 22d. This operation was done under gas and oxygen anesthesia (without ether). The calculi were removed from the bladder and, with great difficulty, a large one from an intraperitoneal diverticulum, which it was thought wise to excise by intravesical diverticulectomy. The operation was difficult, consuming one and a half hours. Although the pulse varied between 120 and 145, the patient stood the operation well and had a satisfactory convalescence. As shown in chart, digitalis was continued for twelve days after operation and in our opinion made it possible not only for the patient to undergo the strain of a tedious operative procedure but also made it possible to force fluids to 5000 c.c. a day. Despite the presence of multiple diverticula, the temperature never rose above 100° F. On October 11th, phthalein test showed 20 + 10.

A serious difficulty in the preparatory treatment of prostatic cases with valvular cardiac lesions, hypertrophic decompensation, extrasystoles, etc., is that the limiting of the fluids, which is usually thought advisable in the treatment of the heart, is opposed to the plan of forcing fluids to improve the condition of the kidneys. Often a compromise between the cardiac treatment and the renal treatment must be arrived at or varied from time to time according to the predominance of the cardiac or the renal picture. By the use of digitalis it is possible eventually to use fluids in increasing amount. The circulation becomes capable of taking care of a larger amount of fluid introduced by mouth, rectum, subcutaneously, or intravenously. But one must recognize the limitations of this therapy, carefully follow the effect upon the heart and circulatory system and desist as soon as embarrassment is exhibited. Edema is often the first danger signal. It should be constantly sought for and fluids restricted immediately on its appearance. Changes of cardiac rhythm and pulse rate should also cause one to concentrate upon the cardiac therapy and in case digitalis has not been employed, it should be started at once.

High blood-pressure was formerly considered a serious contraindication to operation, but as a result of numerous cases in which operation was imperative, (complete retention, catheterization difficult and painful, etc.), and in which blood-pressure had mounted to 180, 200, and even 240, the results obtained have demonstrated that it is quite possible to carry out a prostatectomy even in the presence of extremely high blood-pressure. For a time these patients were treated by rest in bed and depressing drugs. These have been shown to be unsatisfactory, and at present we simply give them rest in bed and a restricted diet, water in moderation, until the blood-pressure becomes stabilized and generally somewhat lower. At the same time a supportive treatment of digitalis, as previously outlined, is given. The effect of this is to increase the cardiac reserve without having a pressor effect upon the blood-pressure. Recent experience seems to show that these patients undergo operation with little shock, while the blood-pressure almost invariably goes up considerably if an ether anesthesia is employed. No ulterior effects have been noted and patients with fearfully high blood-pressure have come through the operation successfully. During the past year we have had several cases in which, during operation under general anesthesia, the blood-pressure rose to 260, 280, and even 300 without fatal outcome. We now employ epidural sacral anesthesia in all such cases and in fact in most perineal prostatectomies and have had no such formidable increase in blood-pressure occur. Marked lowering of the blood-pressure in hypertension cases is certainly to be avoided, and, on this account, spinal anesthesia is, we believe, dangerous. Depressing drugs are also to be avoided during both preliminary and postoperative treatment. We are confident that in 2 cases in which cerebral thrombosis occured (following the use of aspirin, 12 gr., in 1 case, and eserin in the other), the use of these depressing drugs resulted in a slowing of the cerebral circulation and a consequent thrombosis.

Where high blood-pressure is present, a marked lowering of tension is apt to lead to serious curtailment of the renal function. Where the bladder has been greatly distended by chronic high residual urine, hypertension is usually present. If the bladder is emptied precipitately, a marked drop of blood-pressure sometimes occurs followed by partial or complete suppression of the urine.

The following case exhibits this:

B. U. I. 11,594, age fifty-one years. Admitted with complete retention. History of urethral stricture for twenty years. Increasing frequency and difficulty in urination for six months. Complete retention without relief for four days when admitted.

Examination.—Temperature 99° F. Pulse 80. Blood-pressure 135/90. Was mentally clear, but in extreme pain. General examination was negative. Rectal examination showed slight enlargement of prostate. Bladder palpated 3 cm. above umbilicus. Dense stricture in bulbous urethra was dilated with filiforms and followers. Fifteen hundred c.c. of foul urine withdrawn through catheter.

The catheter was strapped in with adhesive and patient put to bed. He immediately had a severe chill, temperature rose to 104° F., but fell to 100° F. in three hours. No urine was obtained after first catheterization. Blood-pressure began falling immediately after catheterization. Twelve hours later it was 50/30. Nine thousand c.c. of fluids had been introduced by various routes and the patient was developing generalized edema. Caffein and adrenalin had only slight temporary effect. Blood urea had increased from 24 to 84 mgm. per 100 c.c., the patient was conscious but extremely drowsy. At this time 400 c.c. of 10 per cent. glucose was given intravenously. The blood-pressure rose to 120/70 within thirty minutes; coincident with the rise in blood-pressure, urine began flowing from catheter. Urine was collected at half-hour intervals. The first few specimens showed a high specific gravity and a high urea content. There was a trace of albumin, a few red blood-cells, and cellular casts.

On the following day the blood-pressure was 125/70, and remained around this level throughout the patient's stay in hospital. The blood urea was normal on the third day; the phthalein normal on the sixth day. The temperature remained normal after the first day.

Such a marked circulatory shock as shown in this case is fortunately rare. We are not able to explain the mechanism producing the low blood-pressure. The chill and rise in temperature suggest that a transient septicemia might have been a factor; the sudden change in abdominal pressure might also have played a rôle. Whatever the cause, the suppression of urine was apparently secondary to the impaired circulation.

We cannot here enter into a discussion of the pressor effect of intravenous glucose, but it might be mentioned in passing that we have found it quite efficacious in selected cases.

Low blood-pressure, if marked and chronic, is often of graver importance than hypertension in prostatic cases. It may be associated with myocarditis and other chronic cardiac lesions and is frequently seen in patients of low vitality, anemic and undernourished. In such cases, effort should be made, by rest, diet, exhibition of iron and other supportive methods, to improve the blood-pressure, the arterial tension and the general condition of the patient, so that operation may be undertaken. The effect of adequate bladder drainage (generally through an inlying urethral catheter) is often little short of marvelous. We could cite many cases in which the patient is very aged, extremely weak, with marked cardio-vascular-renal disease, chronically uremic with senses befuddled and occasionally almost comatose, which have, as a result of drainage, forced water, appropriate medical treatment and rest, been so amazingly improved that eventually perineal prostatectomy was carried out successfully. The transformation secured in some of these cases is indeed one of the most amazing feats in medicine.

Diabetes mellitus is occasionally met with in the prostatic case and requires appropriate preparatory treatment. Here again the presence of pain and other imperative symptoms forces the urologist to operate, even in cases of very severe diabetes. Experience has shown, however, that under proper antidiabetic diet, and with the assistance of insulin, practically every patient can be brought into a satisfactory condition for perineal prostatectomy. Expert medical consultation is highly desirable in these cases and before operation is undertaken the optimum results of antidiabetic treatment should be secured; a stabilization of the body economy under diet and insulin and a nearly normal blood-sugar and alkali reserve. We have been surprised to find that wound healing has been, in the great majority of cases, just as satisfactory as in non-diabetics. One must recognize, however, the proneness to infection in these cases and mild antiseptic treatment should be assiduously applied.

Psychoses furnish a very perplexing problem in prostatic cases. The mental picture is occasionally very difficult to explain and the etiology impossible to interpret. The psychosis may be due to impaired renal function, chronic infection, and occasionally low grade septicemia. In some instances, however, chronic psychosis with marked disorientation persists, with little or no evident cause, as shown in the following case:

B. U. I. 11,883, age sixty-six, admitted November 5, 1923, complaining of frequency of urination three to five times every night. On physical examination, the condition of the patient was good; prostate only slightly hypertrophied, no residual urine, bladder capacity 100 c.c. Cystoscopy showed only a small median lobe, but there were numerous cellules in the bladder, indicating marked obstruction. Phthalein test showed appearance time of ten minutes and 60 per cent. in two hours. The urine was clear, contained no albumin or pus, and was sterile. The temperature was normal. Six days after admission, complete retention of urine occurred and catheterization was necessary. This was followed by temperature of 100° F. and the patient became irrational. The mental condition gradually grew worse, resulting in delirium. The patient continued to have a slight daily temperature. There was no evidence of local infection. The phthalein test remained good and the physical examination was entirely negative. The blood-pressure, which on entrance was 195/140, had dropped to 120/80 and possibly might have been partly responsible for his mental condition. The patient was treated by water in large amounts and continuous catheter drainage. The psychosis continued; medical and neurologic consultations furnished little light on the condition and, finally, two months after admission, patient's mental condition being still confused and unimproved, perineal prostatectomy was carried out under ether anesthesia. The blood-pressure rose to 230 during the operation, but the patient survived and made a satisfactory convalescence. During the second week he became rational. He was discharged one month after operation in excellent condition, and mentally quite clear.

Another case was reported by Shaw and Young[1]:

B. U. I., 11,795, aged seventy-seven years. Duration of obstructive symptoms five years. Complete retention on admission. No history of nervous symptoms and family had noted no mental change.

[1] Journal of Urology, 1924, xi, 373–394.

Examination.—Temperature 100° F., pulse 110, blood-pressure 140/90. Blood urea 30 mgm. per 100 c.c. The patient was rational, well oriented, and capable of giving an intelligent history. The general and urologic examinations were negative. Rectal examination showed a large, benign prostate. The bladder was palpated at the umbilicus.

He was cystoscoped immediately and 700 c.c. of infected urine withdrawn. A retention catheter was inserted and free drainage allowed. Six hours later he became confused and within twelve hours following bladder drainage was in a state of violent delirium, requiring a re-straining jacket to keep him in bed. The urinary output was normal, specific gravity 1.010 to 1.020. The blood urea had remained 20 mgm. per 100 c.c. The blood-pressure had not changed and the temperature was normal. The patient's condition remained unchanged for three days. At this time the blood chemistry was still normal—blood non-protein nitrogen 40.5 mgm. per 100 c.c., creatinin 1.67, uric acid 3.1, and chlorids 488. On the third day he became less restless, occasionally answered questions, but was much weaker. At this time the temperature suddenly rose from normal to 104° F. He gradually became weaker and died three days later. Autopsy revealed early bronchopneumonia and pyelonephritis. Examination of the brain was negative.

The shock to the nervous system in this case was unusually severe. While it can hardly be stated with absolute certainty that the symptoms were not a result of impaired renal function, the reaction was apparently unassociated with the retention in the circulation of any known urinary product.

With the onset of fever, an immediate examination should be made to eliminate the respiratory tract. The nose, tonsils, pharynx, and lungs should receive careful examination, x-rays being taken, if advisable. Early vigorous antiseptic applications to the nose and throat will often abort an infection which might easily result in pneumonia; in the presence of pulmonary involvement, most careful medical attention should be provided. During the course of both preliminary and post-operative treatment, these old men should be protected against drafts and exposure to cold. It is not uncommon to see patients near an open window with their necks, shoulders, arms, and upper chest covered only with a cotton night-shirt, and we are confident that pulmonary complications have come from such exposure.

Operative Treatment.—The pendulum has swung back and forth for many years, and it is still not at rest in this problem of what is the best operation for prostatic hypertrophy. We see no better way of discussing this many-sided question than to present a review of our experiences.

Coming from the medical school into the hospital at a time when the catheter was the sole treatment employed except for those desperate cases which could not be catheterized and which were given suprapubic drainage and a bag to wear for the rest of their days, the first surgical procedure which we saw proposed was that of castration—that remarkable discovery of Ramm and White, that castration produced atrophy of the hypertrophied prostate. Although some cases on the wards did definitely improve following castration, the majority had very little benefit.

The first prostatectomy done in this hospital was in July, 1898, upon a patient fifty-three years of age, who was brought into the hospital in May in uremic coma. The bladder was greatly distended, it was impossible to pass a catheter, and suprapubic drainage was done under local anesthesia. We then witnessed for the first time the marvelous improvement which often comes from drainage in a case of uremia due to prostatic obstruction. Within a few days the patient was conscious and in a month's time apparently normal with the exception of his prostatic obstruction, which persisted, necessitating the permanent suprapubic drainage. In July, 1898 we carried out in this case the first prostatectomy, here, through the suprapubic wound and enucleated in one piece a very large prostate which projected far into the bladder.   Great difficulty was encountered in enucleating the deeper portions, and, accordingly, a gloved finger was inserted into the rectum and found to give great assistance in pushing up the prostate.   This, we believe, was the first time in which suprapubic prostatectomy, combined with rectal assistance, was employed, and was also, we believe, the first two-stage prostatectomy recorded.[1]   The patient made a rapid recovery.

The remarkable improvement in renal function in this case led us to adopt continuous drainage, either by retained catheter or suprapubic tube, in all cases of large residual urine associated with renal impairment, and especially if uremia was present.   This was our first important step in lowering the mortality of prostatic operations.

The next important step in preparatory treatment was in the use of large quantities of water, and this point in technic was adopted as a result of the following case which we reported in 1898[2]:

A boy with a large appendical abscess was operated on by **Dr.** Halsted, and on the following day grew rapidly weaker, temperature rose to 105.8° F., the pulse to 156, but there were no signs of general peritonitis, and the condition was one of general septicemia.   Being in charge of the case in the country and having the responsibility, we realized that drastic measures were necessary and decided to try the effect of venesection and saline transfusion to wash out the poison from the blood.   Accordingly at 7 P. M., using cocain anesthesia, we opened the right basilic vein and allowed the blood to flow out, but the blood-pressure was very weak and we could obtain only about 2½ ounces.   We then injected normal salt solution, 1300 c.c. being inserted.   During this procedure the pulse steadily improved, and at the end had fallen from 160 to 130, and the volume had become fairly strong.   His temperature fell from 105.8° to 104° F., and his general condition was much bettered.

This improvement was very decided for an hour after the transfusion; the nausea ceased, and he slept for a short while, but very soon the pulse became more rapid, and at 3 A. M. was 146 and quite weak.   The patient was restless and the temperature was 104° F.   It was very evident that while the transfusion had been very beneficial it had not been sufficient, although he had received 700 c.c. subcutaneously and 1300 c.c. intravenously.   Preparations were then made for another transfusion and at 6.45 A. M. it was begun.   Twenty-five hundred c.c. of salt solution were introduced into the vein during a period of one hour and twenty-five minutes, and had the effect of completely washing out the blood infection.   The temperature and pulse dropped to almost normal, and after that there was never any concern about the boy's welfare.

Our conclusions were that this case demonstrated the wonderful possibilities of saline solutions, but that it was certain that a small amount would be utterly useless in most cases; that the curative effect was probably due to the dilution of the poison, and its rapid elimination by the excretory organs, and we recommended the method in acute uremia, eclampsia, coma, operative shock, etc.   It may be noted that the patient received 700 c.c. of salt solution subcutaneously and 3800 c.c. intravenously during a period of fourteen hours.   Thereafter we did not hesitate to use water in large amounts in all cases of impaired renal function or uremia and sepsis.

One of the most striking examples of the results of this method of treatment was the following:

A man, B. U. I. 144, aged seventy-six, was brought into the hospital with uremic coma, Cheyne-Stokes respiration, and a distended bladder, from which a catheter withdrew 580 c.c. of residual urine of very foul character filled with pus, bacteria, albumin, and casts.   This pa-

---

[1] Young: Transactions Virginia Medical Society, 1899; American Journal of Dermatology and Genito-urinary Diseases, 1900, iv, 17–19.

[2] Young: Maryland Medical Journal, Baltimore, 1898, xl, 71–74; Canada Lancet, Montreal, 1898–99, xxxi, 904–907.

tient was treated by intermittent catheterization, blood letting, transfusions, and infusions. He was bled twice, 75 and 400 c.c. being removed, and salt infusions were given beneath the breast and saline transfusions (1000 c.c.) into the veins. This was repeated several times during the next four days. In two days the patient, who had been apparently moribund, became conscious and was soon able to talk coherently. At the end of a week the uremic symptoms were entirely gone, and after that the patient's improvement was steady, so that at the end of six weeks operation was successfully performed to remove the prostatic obstruction and the patient lived several years afterward.

The results obtained in these three striking cases furnished the groundwork for the method of preparatory treatment which has since been carried out in our cases of prostatic hypertrophy.

In August, 1900, we assisted Guiteras in preparing a paper on "The Status of Prostatectomy in America" which he read before the section in Urology of the International Medical Congress, Paris, August, 1900. In this paper various methods of technic were given, and among them the suprapubic enucleation with assistance of a gloved finger in the rectum to push the prostate up toward the suprapubic wound, a method which we had been employing for two years. Mr. P. J. Freyer was present at this meeting. Several months later he carried out this very operation on several cases which he reported in detail in the British Medical Journal, July 20, 1901. This was followed by numerous publications in which he claimed that the method was original with him and he has been rewarded by the operation now being called Freyer's operation in the European literature. These facts were set forth in our chapter in Keen's Surgery.[1] As a matter of fact, Belfield, Fuller, and others had carried out radical suprapubic prostatectomy in this country many years before Freyer operated upon his first case.

In 1900, impressed by the enthusiastic papers of Freudenberg describing his success in the treatment of prostatic hypertrophy by means of the Bottini electro-cautery operation, we secured his instrument and operated upon a series of cases by this method. The Bottini operation was at that time carried out as follows: The bladder was filled with fluid. The instrument was introduced into the bladder, the beak turned downward and drawn up against the median lobe. The current was then turned on, heating the blade which was gradually drawn through the hypertrophied median lobe for a distance thought to be sufficient and regulated by a millimeter scale on the shaft of the instrument. The cautery blade was then returned to its sheath in the beak slowly, about one minute being consumed for each centimeter in the travel of the blade forth and back. The instrument was then rotated 90 degrees and a similar incision made (presumably through the right lateral lobe). The instrument was then turned to the opposite side, and a similar cut made for the left lateral lobe. These three cuts destroyed tissue for several millimeters in all directions and were usually sufficient to remove the obstruction to urination if complete and to allow voluntary urination. In some cases a retained catheter was employed, especially if hemorrhage was encountered.

One of our early cases was a patient aged fifty-five years in whom the cystoscope showed a pedunculated intravesical median enlargement. The usual Bottini technic was employed, the first cut being posterior and intended to divide the median lobe. The operation did not remove the obstruction to urination and at the end of a month it was necessary to carry out suprapubic cystostomy at which

[1] Young: The Surgery of the Prostate, Keen's Surgery, 1906, iv, 433.

time it was discovered that the posterior cautery incision had gone, not through the median lobe, but to one side of it. On passing a sound it was seen that the instrument slipped naturally into the groove to that side of the median lobe. Prostatectomy was carried out and the patient was cured.

Following this experience we[1] modified the Bottini technic for median lobe cases so as to place the cuts on each side of the base of the median lobe instead of trying to hold the instrument upon the summit of a pedunculated lobe, which had been shown to be impossible. This was accomplished by the following maneuvers: Introduce incisor, draw back up against anterior portion of the prostatic orifice, rotate instrument 180 degrees (hugging the prostatic orifice all the while). This will bring the beak into the sulcus at one side of the median lobe. Carry the rotation 45 degrees further and the beak will then lie obliquely across the base of the median lobe ready for the first cut. By reversing these movements, the cut on the other side of the median lobe may be similarly performed and then the two lateral cuts are made. This was designed to partially sever the median lobe from its attachment.

As cautery operations upon the prostate are again prominently before the profession, it seems advisable to present in full the study which we made in 1902 of the results and complications of the Bottini operation. We quote fully from the article published at that time[2]:

Although the electrocautery operation was brought out by Bottini as far back as 1876, it was not generally adopted until 1897, when Freudenberg presented to the profession a greatly improved instrument, and followed it up by numerous convincing articles. During the past four years this operation has been performed very extensively, and we are now in a position to look over our results, and discuss the shortcomings of the operation, as well as its merits.

Freudenberg's large collection of operated cases probably shows very accurately the value of the procedure. The statistics are as follows: 752 cases, in which the result was good in $86\frac{1}{2}$ per cent., a failure in $7\frac{1}{2}$ per cent., and the mortality 4 per cent.

These figures, if correct, undoubtedly show much better results than can be claimed for any other operative procedure. Castration, while peculiarly effective in a certain class of cases, has been woefully unsatisfactory as a routine procedure, and has justly been relegated to the list of operations historically interesting, but practically valueless.

Prostatectomy thoroughly performed is undoubtedly an operation of great value. There is no question that the statistics as to the value of this operation are entirely misleading for many reasons; principally because in most of the recorded cases (and in all until recently) the operation was entirely inadequate—merely a nipping off of the most evident intravesical projections, leaving the equally important points of compression in the deep urethra untouched. There is no question, however, that a thorough removal of the entire gland, which can generally be easily accomplished by enucleation with the finger, is a very successful operation and entirely satisfactory when perfectly accomplished.

There are, however, several varieties of prostate which are unsuitable for this operation, principally the small and the sclerotic varieties. This, however, is not the principal objection, but the fact that in the majority of instances we are confronted with patients too old and too feeble to safely undergo the shock of a satisfactory prostatectomy. It is for just this class of cases that the Bottini operation has proved such a blessing, and has achieved really wonderful results. On account of the success of the cautery operations in the otherwise hopeless cases it has become more and more the question whether it should not become the method of choice in all manner of cases. Since there are, however, a certain number of failures (10 per cent. or more)

[1] Young: Monatsberichte für Urologie, 1901, vi, 1–13, and A New Combined Electrocautery Incisor for the Bottini Operation for Prostatic Obstruction, Journal of the American Medical Association, 1902, xxxviii, 86–93.

[2] Young: Journal of the American Medical Association, 1902, xxxviii, 86–93.

and a certain mortality (between 4 and 8 per cent.) shown by the Bottini operation, it still remains questionable whether it should replace prostatectomy. To settle this point more extended investigation is necessary. It also behooves us to study the causes of failure and fatality in the Bottini operation, with a view of finding means of obviating both as far as possible.

Among the causes of death besides uremia, shock, sepsis, etc. (presumably unavoidable), we find recorded several not unavoidable reasons, principally from improperly placed or too lengthy incisions. In the first category are deaths from the cautery blade burning its way into the rectum, due, as has been shown by Freudenberg, to the fact that the beak of the instrument became caught in a postureteral pouch, which is separated by only a short space from the rectum. In the same class are those fatal cases in which the entirely useless anterior cut was made and penetrated (as might have been expected) into the space of Retzius. In the second category are a number of cases in which the operator has rashly made his incisions too long, resulting in the rupture of the urethra in front of the prostate, abscess, and sometimes fatal hemorrhage from division of perineal vessels.

The statement of certain writers that incisions of $4\frac{1}{2}$, 5, or 6 cm. in length were often necessary to remove the obstruction is absolutely without pathologic substantiation, and undoubtedly liable to lead to a great many serious blunders in the profession. Very rarely, even in the very largest hypertrophies, should an incision over $3\frac{1}{2}$ or 4 cm. be made, first, because it is unnecessary, and, second, because it is dangerous. Deaths from any of the causes outlined above are preventable, and should in the future be eliminated from the statistics.

In Freudenberg's statistics, after excluding the fatal cases (4.2 per cent.) we find 92 per cent. improved, 55 per cent. cured, 37 per cent. definitely improved, and 8 per cent. failures. Why should there not be a greater uniformity of results? Is the operative technic or the instrument at fault? Turning to the instrument, we find the one of Freudenberg much preferable to that of Bottini, as has been very frequently pointed out. But there are several very evident weaknesses in even the former instrument. In the first place, since there is the greatest difference as to size, shape, and condition among hypertrophied prostates, it is unreasonable to expect one single cautery blade to be suitable for all. An incision which is plenty deep enough for a medium-sized hypertrophy may be wholly inadequate for a very large one, and positively dangerous for the small fibroid forms. Then, again, one lobe is often very greatly enlarged, while another is only slightly so. Are we, then, to give each the same depth of cautery incision? We have in our collection of autopsy specimens several prostates with small but very obstructive middle lobe enlargements, where the ordinary Freudenberg and Bottini instruments would have penetrated beyond the capsule and perhaps into the rectum.

It is very evident, then, that an instrument with several easily interchangeable blades of graded sizes would be a decided improvement.

There are two other defects in Freudenberg's apparatus which, while apparently trivial, are of considerable importance. The first is in the shape of the beak of the instrument as now constructed. The traction necessary to hold the beak up against the prostate during an operation will often pull it into the urethra. This is due to the fact that the beak meets the shaft at such a wide angle, or at such a slope that even moderate traction causes it to ride over a median bar (for example) and slip into the prostatic urethra. The dangers of this accident are not small. Indeed, it has occurred several times, and has been responsible for several deaths, the cause being division of the membranous urethra, extravasation, hemorrhage, etc. In order to be certain that the beak of the instrument is against the prostate, and has not slipped into the urethra, Freudenberg has wisely advised that a finger be inserted into the rectum to determine its location before an incision is begun.

I have carefully followed this practice for the past two years, and have thus prevented several accidents, for in numerous instances we have found that a little steady traction (as in an operation) would draw the beak into the urethra. But this safeguard is not always sufficiently accurate, for while it is comparatively easy to feel the tip of the instrument turned downward toward the trigone, one cannot often feel the beak with sufficient certainty when the instrument is turned to make a lateral cut, as one of our own cases demonstrated to my sorrow (Freudenberg's instrument was being used). The forefinger of the right hand was inserted into the rectum, and the tip of the beak definitely located to be in the bladder. The rotation was made for a lateral cut, and with the finger still in the rectum traction put upon the instrument to draw the beak up snugly against the prostate. The beak was not felt to slip into the urethra, but before beginning the cautery incision another careful examination with finger (which was kept in the rectum during the entire operation) was made and did not reveal any slipping of the beak.   Despite all these precautions (which happened to be unusually carefully taken in this case) an incision of $3\frac{1}{2}$ cm. was followed by a gush of blood from the meatus, and a perineal section done under cocain revealed a ruptured membranous urethra, and extravasated blood behind the triangular ligament.   A timely operation saved his life, but it brought very forcibly to our mind the *need of a beak which would not slip into the urethra*, one more nearly at right angles to the shaft.

The form of Freudenberg's instrument is adhered to, the changes being in its having four interchangeable blades, a beak of different angle, a connecting handle with more extensive contact surfaces, and a few minor changes in construction.   By a very simple device, the mere elevation of a sliding bar on the rotary wheel, one blade may be removed and another inserted. The sliding bar working on a spring holds the rod containing a blade firmly attached to the screw mechanism by engaging the circular groove near its outer end.   We have had four blades constructed, the smallest having an elevation of 0.8 cm., the second 1.2 cm., the third 1.7 cm., and the fourth 2.1 cm.

Blade No. 3 corresponds to the one usually found in Freudenberg's instrument, and is the one most generally used, while No. 2 is useful in small hypertrophies, and No. 4 for the very large. Blade No. 1 (the smallest) was constructed mainly to complete the set, and without any idea of much practical value.   We have been surprised, however, to find it very useful in several cases, which will be given in detail further on.

During the past five months we have used this instrument on 16 cases, and have amply proved it to be practical, and one, we think, that has overcome many of the defects to be found in Freudenberg's instrument.   As to the efficacy of the Bottini operation, of which we were at first very skeptical, our experience (now of 41 operations) forces us to testify decidedly in its favor.   In these 41 cases we have had 3 deaths, all men in very bad condition before operation, and 2 with pyonephrosis.   Fifteen patients were over seventy years of age, 3 over eighty, and among these there have been no deaths, and all but one have been cured of the prostatic obstruction.   Of 13 patients who had to use the catheter, there is only one who still requires it, and this one is considerably improved.   Some of our cases are of too recent date to show the ultimate results, and these we will reserve for a later publication.   We are still, however, of the opinion (from an experience of 15 prostatectomies) that in certain cases, *e. g.*, men between forty-five and sixty-five, in good condition, and with easily enucleable enlargements, a complete prostatectomy is a very safe operation, and certain as to lasting results.

In closing we cannot too strongly urge that the Bottini operation should be performed in accordance with the character of the prostatic obstruction as found by exhaustive examination as previously outlined.   There is no doubt that a perfunctory performance of the operation with one blade for all cases, and one cut directed posteriorly and one laterally on each side, while perfectly satisfactory in a large number of cases, is insufficient in some and dangerous in others.

As shown by us in another paper, when a decided median lobe (more or less pedunculated) is present, the ordinary operation is entirely inadequate, as the posterior cut will generally pass to one side of the median lobe and leave it to continue its obstructive work.   If, however, the cuts be so made as to pass obliquely across the base on each side of this projecting lobe, we have shown that this lobe may be dropped back out of the way and a rapid atrophy induced by thus cutting off most of its blood-supply.   This has been abundantly proved in 5 cases, some of which were entirely unaffected by the usual three incisions and the prostatic obstruction immediately removed by the incisions described above.

We continued to use the Bottini operation for another year, but imperfect results and an occasional death caused us again to turn our attention to prostatectomy, having also been stimulated by publications by Sims, Murphy, Ferguson, and Bryson, who had presented papers on removing the prostate through the perineal route.   The suprapubic route had then lost favor, owing to the high mortality.

In studying the methods that had been proposed, the intravesical balloon, which Sims used to draw the prostate into the perineal wound, seemed to overcome the objection to perineal prostatectomy.   The rubber balloon, however, did not appear to us to furnish sufficient strength for the great traction which is necessary. We, therefore, set to work to construct an instrument of metal for this purpose. At first we used simply a steel sound, the end of which had been flattened and fenestrated as shown in Fig. 805.

The first case upon which we used this instrument was a man aged sixty-six years, who was admitted to the hospital October 11, 1902, with a moderately enlarged prostate. Under ether anesthesia an inverted Y incision was made in the perineum. The central tendon and recto-urethralis muscle were divided and the posterior surface of the prostate exposed by blunt dissection. The membranous urethra was then opened upon a sound and the single-bladed prostatic tractor, above described, was introduced and passed into the bladder with ease. The beak was then turned over the median portion of the prostate and traction made. It was found possible to draw the prostate well down toward the perineum. A curved transverse capsular incision was then made near the apex, and the lateral and median lobes of the hypertrophied prostate were removed in one piece. A rubber drainage-tube and gauze pack were provided and the patient made an excellent convalescence. Additional cases were operated upon by the same technic.

On January 10, 1903 bilateral capsular incisions were first used to preserve the ejaculatory ducts. The single-bladed tractor had in the meantime been provided with a spur to prevent its slipping out of the bladder when traction was made, but this was not entirely successful, and it then occurred to us to design a double-bladed tractor. This was made, as shown in Figs. 280, 281. This instrument with slight modifications is the instrument which we employ today.[1]

The description of the new prostatic tractor and the cases upon which we had used it was made in brief to the Southern Surgical Association in November 11, 1902. Several months later we published the details of the operation along with a report of 15 cases, which we had presented to the American Association of Genito-Urinary Surgeons on June 12, 1903.[2] In this paper we presented a pathologic study in which we described the relation of the ejaculatory ducts to the hypertrophied middle lobe and demonstrated that the ducts and the seminal vesicles may remain *in situ* while the middle and lateral lobes grew upward into the bladder, as shown in Figs. 278, 279. As a result, it was possible by the technic which we presented (bilateral capsular incisions) to remove the lateral lobes; and then enucleate the median lobe from the side and in front of the ejaculatory ducts without injury of these structures. The exposure of the prostate was through an inverted V perineal incision, a careful division of the central tendon and recto-urethralis muscle and a wide exposure by blunt dissection of the membranous urethra and prostate being made. When writing this paper we discovered, for the first time, several months after we had described and practised this operation on numerous cases, a paper by Proust[3] which had just appeared (1903). In this paper Proust exposed the prostate in much the same way that we had done, but the prostatectomy, which began with hemisection of the prostate and excision

---

[1] See description of this tractor in Transactions of Southern Surgical and Gynecological Association, November 11, 1902, vol. xv.

[2] See Transactions and also Young: Conservative Perineal Prostatectomy, Presentation of New Instruments and Technic, Journal of the American Medical Association, 1903, xli, 999–1009.

[3] Centralblatt für Harn und Sexual-organen, 1903, vi, 52–62 (abstract, in great detail).

of the floor of the urethra, ejaculatory ducts, and verumontanum along with the lateral lobes with scissors was in no way similar to our method, although published almost simultaneously. The charge that has been made by some that we copied the methods of Proust is therefore erroneous, as will be seen from Proust's thesis in 1903. In our paper we demonstrated that by means of bilateral capsular incisions it was possible to enucleate the lateral and median portions of the prostate without injury to the ejaculatory ducts. In 15 cases which we reported it was shown that spermatozoa had been found in some patients and that others had had complete return of normal coitus, and abundant ejaculations following the operation. In this paper our two-bladed rotating tractor was presented, and the following footnote was added: "Paris, France, July, 1903. Since the presentation of this paper and after my arrival in Paris, I found in the instrument shops, two "desenclaveurs," one by dePezzer and one by Legueu. The former is similar in some respects to our tractor, but it is very much smaller and is only used to depress the prostate while the prostatic urethra is incised. It is then removed, not being

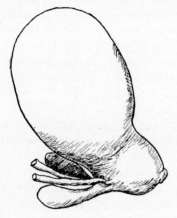

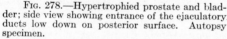

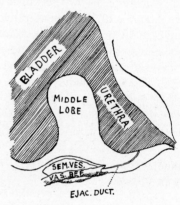

FIG. 278.—Hypertrophied prostate and bladder; side view showing entrance of the ejaculatory ducts low down on posterior surface. Autopsy specimen.

FIG. 279.—Sectional view, same case, showing middle lobe rising high into bladder and low position of ducts.

used to assist in the enucleation of the lobes, for which it is manifestedly too small to be of any service. The blades are not fenestrated and are only $\frac{1}{2}$ inch long. Neither author has published a description of his instrument, so far as we know." As we have been accused of copying dePezzer's instrument and failing to give credit we are reproducing here photographs of the two instruments side by side (Figs. 280, 281). The fact that they are similar, in that the two blades revolve upon a central staff, is evident. The fact that the one was designed in America and the other France, simultaneously and independently, is not remarkable. Further inspection will show, however, that our tractor was an entirely different instrument with large fenestrated blades and made sufficiently large and powerful as to be able to draw down the prostatic lobes so that they could be enucleated. DePezzer's instrument, on the contrary, is so small that, with its small non-fenestrated blades, it could not possibly have been used for this purpose. It was, in fact, removed by those who employed it before the enucleation of the prostate had begun. Legueu's and Albarran's desenclaveurs were used through the urethra and were totally different from our instrument. We had never heard of any of these instruments before this visit to Paris in the summer of 1903. All of these

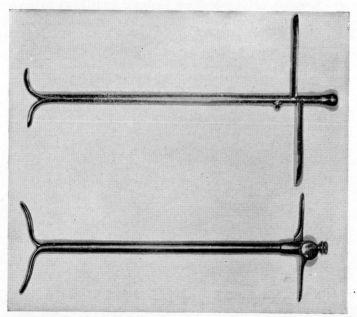

FIG. 280.—Showing similarity between dePezzer's "desenclaveur" and Young's prostatic tractor, devised independently in France and in America. DePezzer's instrument is much smaller, is not provided with an incline which brings the blades, which are not fenestrated, around to a level when opened out, and was removed by its author before the enucleation of the prostate was begun. It was simply used to steady the prostate while the urethra was opened in the median line. It was not used as a tractor to draw down and facilitate the enucleation of the lobes.

instruments have long since been abandoned. Our method of removing the middle lobe by means of our tractor was entirely different from that of Proust, who used

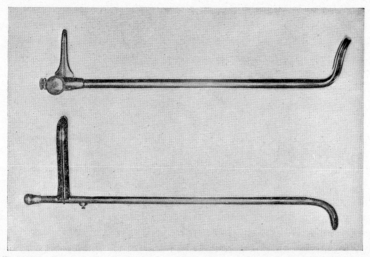

FIG. 281.—Young's prostatic tractor closed above, dePezzer's desenclaveur closed.

the finger for this purpose. In our operation the ejaculatory ducts were preserved and in Proust's they were excised and the vasa deferentia ligated. It is not necessary to go further to show the entire dissimilarity of the instruments and technic in the methods employed by us and by Proust.

Results of Operation of Conservative Perineal Prostatectomy.—The question can be best stated by discussing at length the results which were obtained in a study of 1049 cases in which we carried out our operation of conservative perineal prostatectomy. These have been analyzed as follows:

TABLE 69

SHOWING RELATION BETWEEN AGE AND MORTALITY AFTER PROSTATECTOMY

Age, years.	Cases.	Deaths.	Percentage.
30 to 34	1	..	
35 to 39	3	..	
40 to 44	2	..	
45 to 49	10	..	
50 to 54	52	2	3.8
55 to 59	140	1	0.7
60 to 64	217	6	2.7
65 to 69	264	10	3.7
70 to 74	213	6	2.8
75 to 79	113	6	5.3
80 to 84	28	2	7.1
85 to 89	2	2	
90 to 94	1	1	
Not given	3		
Total	1049	36	3.4

Age as a causative factor of mortality is graphically shown in Table 69. A glance at this table shows us that, with negligible variations, the mortality rate per cent. increases gradually in each decade of life, but up to seventy-five years of age it remains very low, 2.8 per cent. After seventy-five years the operation is definitely more dangerous, but it is interesting to note that, during the last series of 198 cases without a death, there were 18 patients over seventy-five years of age (6 over eighty)—all of whom went home well. Several successful prostatectomies in men over ninety years of age are recorded. One of our patients who had reached the age of ninety-three, died two weeks after operation, of cerebral thrombosis—apparently not associated with the operation.

In 1049 consecutive cases there were 36 deaths in the hospital, a mortality of 3.4 per cent. In the accompanying chart (Fig. 282) the death rate has been charted by the succeeding years, the number of cases and the deaths for each year being given, and from these the death rate, per cent., has been calculated and charted. This chart is interesting as showing a gradual decline in the mortality among our perineal prostatectomy cases from 8.4 per cent. in 1903 to 2.4 per cent. in 1919, and to zero since then. During the twenty years included in the chart there have been two long periods in which there were no fatalities, first in the year 1906–1907 and part of 1908 in which there were 128 consecutive cases without a death (4 patients being over eighty and 43 over seventy years of age), and the second from February 8, 1919, to October 15, 1922, during which there were 198 consecutive cases without a death. During this last period there were only 4 patients in which operation was not carried out, and 2 of these died in the hospital (vide supra).

The preoperative treatment by which these cases were prepared for a successful operation has been outlined. The postoperative complications may be grouped

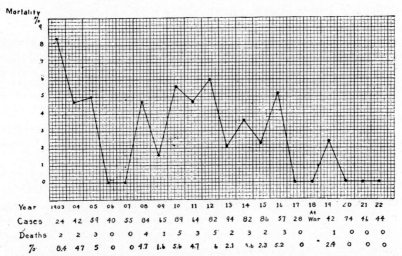

Fig. 282.—Chart showing annual mortality rate for the past twenty years. The number of cases operated on each year and the number of deaths among these cases is recorded, and mortality percentage is given on the bottom line. Seven years in which there was no mortality in our cases (personally operated) are shown.

under various heads which may be discussed after giving a classification showing the cause of death in the 1049 cases charted in Table 70.

TABLE 70

CAUSE OF 36 DEATHS AFTER PERINEAL PROSTATECTOMY IN 1049 CASES

Principal cause of death.	Cases.	Percent-age.	Complications.
Pneumonia..........	8	22	Old tuberculous lung, 1; myocarditis, nephritis, 1; pyelitis, uremia, 1.
Acute pulmonary edema............	1		Patient had recently recovered from pneumonia.
Uremia.............	7	20	Hydropyonephrosis, 1; hemorrhage from nose, 1; pneumonia, 1; hydronephrosis, double, 1.
Pulmonary embolism..	4	12	Clot in heart and vena cava, 1; nephritis, dilatation heart, mural thrombus, 1; coronary thrombosis, 1; thrombosis femoral vein, 1.
Cerebral hemorrhage..	3	8	Marked arteriosclerosis general, 1; grave fear of operation, great mental excitement, 1.
Cerebral thrombosis...	2	6	In one case, man, age ninety-two, thrombosis followed 12 grains of aspirin three weeks after operation.
Heart disease........	1	..	Myocarditis, dilatation of heart, pyelonephritis.
Endocarditis........	1	..	Bronchopneumonia.
Hemorrhage of wound	2	6	One case immediately after operation, due to insufficient packing; other case, secondary hemorrhage at end of week.
Hemorrhage from nose	1	..	Hemorrhage from nose came on suddenly three weeks after operation when wound was healed.
Sepsis..............	2	6	
Abscess of spleen.....	1	..	Bronchitis.
Tuberculosis of lungs..	1	..	Arrested case of pulmonary tuberculosis, ether anesthesia, should have been operated upon under epidural.
Extravasation of urine	1	..	We made mistake of incising orifice of the diverticulum and as a result perivesical extravasation occurred.
Cancer of intestine....	1	..	Patient died of intestinal complications; necropsy showed large unrecognized cancer of sigmoid.

Hindsight is better than foresight. It is easy now to look over the above list of fatal endings and see how many of them should not have happened; for example, in the last mentioned, the carcinoma of the sigmoid should have been discovered and no prostatectomy performed. In the case above it the extravasation came from an incision made in the neck of a diverticulum—a great mistake! The next, with tuberculosis of the lungs, should not have been given a general anesthetic, etc., etc.

And it is a fact, as shown by the two long periods which were without a fatality, that by exercising the greatest care almost every patient can be prepared to go safely through perineal prostatectomy.

Shock.—The prevention of operative shock is of great importance, and when we consider that about 40 per cent. of the patients are over seventy years of age and many of them very feeble, we realize that great care must be taken. Our patients receive water in abundance up to the time of going to the operating room. This does not seem to lead to nausea or vomiting and prepares against the loss of blood. By quick operation, careful hemostasis, ligation of bleeding arteries in the capsule of the prostate if possible, and thorough control of the bleeding after the drainage-tube has been introduced, either by packing within the capsule and vesical sphincter, by pressure against the capsule posteriorly or by an inflatable rubber bag, the patient should leave the table in good condition with the hemorrhage stopped. The operator should see to it that the hemorrhage is controlled, and in some cases we have put as many as twelve strips of gauze packing in order to secure this, but now that we have adopted the Davis inflatable bag all packing is done away with. One of the great advantages of the perineal route is that this is possible. Should the patient's pulse be very weak, an infusion or intravenous transfusion should be started before he leaves the operating room, and it is our invariable rule to give submammary infusions to every case on return to the ward. Should subsequent developments show that the packing has not been sufficient to stop hemorrhage, additional gauze should be introduced, preferably with a tubular packer which, when introduced deep into the cavity of the prostate, makes it possible to insert a large amount of gauze in the proper place without danger of injury to the rectum. In very feeble patients it is our rule to have blood matching done before operation, and if possible have a member of the family ready to give blood. Occasionally transfusion is resorted to with amazing results. Secondary hemorrhage, following removal of gauze on the first or second day after the operation or sometimes later, may lead to considerable shock, which should be handled by repacking, infusion, or blood transfusion, as necessary. In one of our cases hemophilia gave us a great deal of trouble.

As seen in the above chart there were two deaths from hemorrhage; one on the day after operation and another six days later. The first could have been prevented by more packing, which was very inadequately done in this case. The latter case was a secondary hemorrhage which could not be controlled even by suprapubic cystostomy and packing.

Pulmonary Complications.—As seen in Table 70 pneumonia has been the most frequent cause of death—22 per cent. A few of these were ether pneumonias, but since the introduction of nitrous oxid-oxygen anesthesia operation pneumonias have not occurred, but several patients have developed pneumonia in two or three weeks after the operation. The prevention of these complications is difficult.

It is important that the patient should be up and about, as it is dangerous for old men to be in bed, and on this account it is our rule to get them out of bed in a few days, and have the patient walking within a week or ten days. Great care should be taken to avoid chilling, exposure to cold, and association with others who have acute respiratory infections. The use of gargles and mouth-washes and oil in the nose is also of much help.

Uremia, which has been the cause of death in 20 per cent. of the cases, is a direct result of the serious impairment of the kidneys from back pressure or infection, which is generally present before operation, but may result from ascending infection after operation. One must take grave risks of uremia occurring, but by prolonged catheter drainage, gradual decompression, and the use of water in large amounts the patient can usually be brought into a condition safe for operation. It is absolutely essential, however, that the imbibition of water should continue after operation, and if nausea or refusal of the patient to drink should interfere, salt solution should be given by infusion, by rectum or by transfusion, and, if the onset of fever and localizing symptoms indicate that a pyelitis has supervened, the water cure should be forced with redoubled activity by every possible means. We have seen numerous cases in which this has occurred, and it is most extraordinary how it is possible to wash away acute renal infections and severe uremias.

Nausea and *hiccup*, on account of their interference with the "water cure," are of very great importance, and should be combated most vigorously. The use of a stomach-tube is often of great help, and when one drug will not work another should be tried, especially in cases of hiccup. In our opinion, there is no one specific.

Cardiovascular complications are of the next importance. Pulmonary embolism was the cause of death in 12 per cent. of the cases. It sometimes occurs as a result of endocarditis or other cardiac diseases, but, as a rule, the clot comes from the region of the wound. Two such cases followed the taking of enemata and 1 case followed a femoral thrombophlebitis. Phlebitis of the veins of the leg occurs rarely and should be treated by elevation of leg, ice-bags, and quiet. Intravenous mercurochrome or gentian-violet have been used in phlebitis.

Cerebral hemorrhage occurred in 3 cases. When we realize that fully 50 per cent. of the patients have arteriosclerosis and abnormally high blood-pressure, it is remarkable that it does not occur more often. Two of these patients were found to be hemiplegic immediately after the operation; one had a very high blood-pressure—over 220—and the other was a man who was extremely nervous and fearful of death. *Cerebral thrombosis* occurred in 2 cases. One, a man aged ninety-two, was up and about and almost ready to go home three weeks after operation. He complained of some pain in his wound, and was given aspirin, which was soon followed by stupor and death. Autopsy showed cerebral thrombosis. An explanation of death in this case was that the aspirin had lowered the blood-pressure and slowed up the pulse, so that thrombosis in the sclerotic cerebral vessels occurred.

Heart disease was immediately responsible for only two deaths, and when we consider that fully 50 per cent. of the patients were suffering from cardiovascular disease, and many of them with grave cardiac lesions, as stated previously, it is remarkable that there were not more. Surgeons have long been aware that cases with heart disease go through operation under ether anesthesia with remarkable facility, and on this account we have operated on many a patient when a cautious clinician has advised against operation. It is extremely important, however, to take every care, and to have the assistance of the best internist, because much can be done with digitalis, quinidin, and other drugs to get the patient in trim for operation and to carry him safely through the convalescence.

Infection.—There is no more important feature of the treatment than the prevention or combating of sepsis. As stated before, it is almost impossible to carry out frequent or long-continued urethral or suprapubic drainage without infection. The colon bacillus is the most common organism and is usually not very virulent. Efforts should be made to prevent cocci from being added to the infection, and this can usually be done. The colon bacillus may, however, produce very severe cystitis, prostatitis, epididymitis, and ascending renal infections. Of these, epididymitis is the most frequent and may be sufficiently severe to require incision and drainage, especially if the patient is feeble or if he continues to run fever or show evidences of considerable toxemia. The great majority of the cases, however, can be controlled by ice-packs and resolve without operation. Infection of the wound and bladder should be treated by mild irrigations, preferably of some of the newer antiseptics, meroxyl 1: 2000, acriflavin 1: 8000, mercurochrome 1 per cent., or Dakin solution (if accompanied by breaking down or sloughing of the wound). It is rare now to see the nasty perineal and suprapubic wounds, encrusted with urinary salts and accompanied by necrotic tissue, such as we used to see so frequently. Ammoniacal cystitis, with its rapid deposit of phosphatic calculi, is practically a thing of the past as a result of modern antiseptics. Hexamethylenamin is of slight value, unless given in large doses and in conjunction with sodium benzoate. Alkaline infection of the wound is rapidly cured by application of 1 per cent. acetic acid.

Infection during the preoperative period of drainage can now be prevented or controlled in most cases by means of our irrigating decompression apparatus, which has already been described.

Ascending infections of the kidney pelvis and cortex can usually be dealt with by internal hydrotherapy, submammary and intravenous infusions often being necessary. Occasionally a definite abscess forms or the condition becomes so serious that a hasty drainage operation is necessary.

The use of drugs intravenously to combat sepsis looms up as a method of the future. Full details of these intravenous methods are given in the section on Treatment in Chapter III.

Gastro-intestinal Complications.—Nausea, vomiting, distention due to obstruction, or severe obstipation present problems of the greatest importance and have required minute attention and vigorous treatment. The use of gas and epidural anesthesia has done away with almost all of the postoperative nausea and vomiting, and it is possible to have the patient drink water in abundance early. In this way uremic vomiting is prevented in most cases. Abdominal distention from obstipation or intestinal obstruction, or undue gas formation, is nothing like so common from perineal as from suprapubic prostatectomies, but it may be a most serious complication and every effort should be made to prevent its occurrence. A few doses of white oil before and immediately after operation, followed by a gentle purgative, is generally sufficient, but if the bowels become greatly distended, the use of pituitrin, supplemented by hot stupes, and other appropriate measures have usually been effective in our cases. Enemata, of course, would be useful, but owing to 2 deaths from pulmonary embolism following enemata, their use has been prohibited after operations on the pelvic organs and genitalia in our clinic.

Closure of Fistula.—This is usually spontaneous and within the first three weeks after operation. In our experience 23 per cent. closed within fourteen days, and a persistent fistula is extremely rare and does not furnish the bugaboo which has been held against the perineal operation by certain writers. As a matter of fact, it is not so common as a persistent suprapubic fistula in our experience, and is infinitely less disagreeable, as there is no continuous leakage as in suprapubic cases, but only the escape of urine at urination, the patient being dry the rest of the time. In a very exhaustive study of 450 cases we have found only 5 in which the fistula was present after a prolonged period; 3 of these were paupers, and had not received proper treatment after leaving the hospital. The use of the curet is of assistance in hastening the closure of fistulæ and a sound should be passed so as to be sure that no stricture or valve is present in the urethra. When the opening is small a gimlet, screwed into the fistula, makes a splendid curet.

Although we are insistent that the patient remain in the hospital until the fistula has been closed three or four days, 64 per cent. of the patients have left the hospital inside of four weeks, and only 5 per cent. have remained more than eight weeks. When we consider the great age and serious condition of many of these patients, this shows that the convalescence from perineal prostatectomy is comparatively short and simple.

The act of micturition, which is materially altered by the considerable impairment or derangement of musculature about the vesical neck or perineum after any form of prostatectomy, may not return to normal for several weeks or months. The bladder is usually contracted and urination on this account more frequent than normal. The weakness of the internal and sometimes of the external sphincter leads to a slight escape of urine on coughing, sneezing, or sudden movements, in some cases for several weeks after the operation. By retaining the urine as long as possible in a sitting posture and exercising the sphincter muscles by attempting to cut off the outflow of urine several times during each urination, it is possible in most instances to restore normal urination very promptly; in some cases more prolonged exercise must be undertaken.

Incontinence of urine occurs very rarely. In our 450 cases presented before the International Medical Congress in 1911 there was not a single case of complete incontinence—dribbling night and day. There were 3 cases of incontinence when the patient was on his feet, and in 1 of these the operative notes show that the muscular structures in the region of the triangular ligament were injured at operation, and this probably occurred in the other 2 cases. There were 4 other cases of occasional slight leakage, and cystoscopic examination showed that the prostate had not been completely removed and that an irregularly dilated posterior urethra was present in which urine collected and from which it occasionally escaped.

There is no question that the fear of incontinence of urine has been responsible for the unpopularity of the perineal route. But this came about as a result of the old-fashioned median perineal incision which passed through the external sphincter and triangular ligament and through which the prostatic lobes were removed piecemeal. It is remarkable that all of these cases were not incontinent, not only on account of the destructive injury of the external sphincter, but on

TABLE 71

Analytic Study of 1049 Consecutive Cases of Prostatectomy by H. H. Y., up to October 15, 1922

Ages.	Cases.	Residual urine.		Preliminary treatment.	Preliminary treatment. Duration, admission to operation.		Closure of fistula in 450 cases:		Of 450 cases: sexual powers. Answers from 251.
		C.c.	Cases.		Days.	Cases.	Weeks.	Closure, per cent.	
Under 50 years..	16	Under 50..	208	Continuous cath., 279.	4..	85	1	4.5	Normal before operation.......... 133
50–54..	52	50–99..	140	Intermittent catheter, 60.	5–9..	249	2	17	Erections normal........ 75 per cent.
55–59..	140	100–199..	168	Suprapubic drain, 11.	10–14..	88	3	30	Coitus normal .... 59 per cent.
60–64..	217	200–299..	108	Suprapubic aspiration, 1.	14–29..	114	4	16	Patients under 60 years.. 95 per cent.
65–69..	264	300–399..	41		2 months..	45	5	7	
70–74..	213	400–499..	27		3 months..	1	6	5	Deaths: Among these 1049 consecutive cases by
75–79..	113	500–699..	41		4 months..	3	7	2	H. H. Y. there were 36 deaths, a mortality of
80–84..	28	700–999..	21		6 months..	1	8	2.5	3.2 per cent. In this series over a period of
85–89..	2	1000–1499..	20		7 months..	1	3 months.	2.8	twenty years there were seven years in which
90–94..	1	1500–1999..	4		Less than 4 days...	462	Later	7	no deaths occurred.
N. I...	3	2000–2600..	1				Incont.	0	
Total...1049		4500..	1				Partial incont.	0.29	
Over 70 years...	144	C. R...	158						
Over 80 years...	31	No information...	111						

account of the fact that not infrequently deep prostatic lobules were left behind. Ever since our early publications on this subject we have insisted on a careful open operation back of the bulb, transversus perinei muscles, triangular ligament, and external sphincter, all of which structures should be seen and carefully avoided, and the urethra opened far back near the apex of the prostate well behind all sphincteric fibers. In an early paper we discussed the use of a long tractor through the urethra or the insertion of a tractor through the bulbous urethra in order to avoid an opening through the membranous and prostatic urethra, but the cases in which we tried this showed that the traction obtained was less perfect and the operation lengthened. The use of the long tractor has been continued in operations upon the tuberculous prostate and seminal vesicles, and Dr. Geraghty has recently advised its use in cases of prostatic hypertrophy with the object of completely avoiding the membranous urethra. Study of cases operated upon by this method shows nothing gained by this. Cecil has tried the same scheme with the same object, but we believe that if one is careful to see the anatomic structures and particularly to avoid injury to the transversus perinei muscles and triangular ligament (which injury occasionally has happened in our hands from faulty exposure), no difficulty will be experienced in reaching the apex of the prostate and making the incision at a point where no possibility of injury to the external sphincter is present. With this precaution the act of micturition after perineal prostatectomy is distinctly more perfect than after suprapubic prostatectomy because the internal sphincter is usually restored to normal after perineal prostatectomy, whereas, after suprapubic prostatectomy, it is usually widely dilated, and as shown by Hyman, Thompson-Walker, and others, generally forms a dilated gourd-like neck to the bladder, the urine of which fills the posterior urethra down to the external sphincter. The same thing can be said in regard to rectal fistulæ—they should never occur except in extremely rare instances as a result of suppuration. The rectum has been injured in something less than 1 per cent. of the cases, but practically all of them have been cured by our operation of rectal resection, which is similar, in part, to a procedure of Wildbolz. The injury of the rectum is certainly less common and less dangerous than cutting or tearing into the peritoneum, as in the suprapubic operation, which has a definite mortality of its own.

The general statistics of our 1049 consecutive cases are shown in Table 71.[1]

Sexual Powers.—Tabulation of the 1049 cases shows that many had diminution or absence of sexual powers before admission. Of those whose sexual powers were described as "normal" before operation, 80 per cent. retained them afterward. Of those in whom they were "diminished," less than half retained them after operation, but in this number were some who showed improvement over the condition before operation. Of those whose sexual powers were "absent" before operation, practically all remained in the same condition afterward.

Summary: Results Obtained in 198 Recent Cases.—As an evidence of what might be accomplished by the methods which we have outlined above, we present a brief analytic report of 198 consecutive cases on which we have personally operated recently during a period of three years and nine months. During this period there have been 198 cases, and we have had the good fortune to have no fatalities. The analysis of these cases is shown in Tables 72 and 73. These tables need very little explanation. It may be noted that 58 patients, 21 per cent., were

[1] Young: Surgery, Gynecology, and Obstetrics, 1923, xxxvi, 589–609.

over seventy years of age, that the blood-pressure was 160 or more in 55 cases, 20 per cent., that the two-hour phthalein was below 50 per cent. in 93 cases, 45 per cent., the blood urea over 0.50 gram per liter in 15 cases, 8 per cent., and some form of heart disease present in 96 cases, 49 per cent. Preparatory treatment with a catheter was carried out in over 60 per cent. of the cases, but suprapubic drainage was employed in only 4, or 2 per cent., of the patients. The average length of stay in the hospital was thirty-two days, and the average duration of the fistula twenty-four days; 14 per cent. being open on discharge. As the cases are recent the ultimate result is incomplete, and the 56 cases on which no information is cited are mostly recent cases. The fact that 198 consecutive cases, many of which were very old, feeble patients with markedly impaired kidneys and heart, can be carried through perineal prostatectomy without a death shows very effectively the benignity of this operation.

TABLE 72

ANALYSIS OF 198 CONSECUTIVE CASES OF PERINEAL PROSTATECTOMY WITHOUT A DEATH— FEBRUARY 8, 1919 TO OCTOBER 15, 1922

Ages.		Residual.		Blood-pressure.		Phthalein.		Blood urea.	
Years.	No.	C.c.	No.	B. P.	No.	Per cent.	No.	Grams.	No.
50–54	13	0– 49	40	100–109	5	0– 9	1	1.40–1.49	1
55–59	26	50– 99	31	110–119	12	10–19	2	1.30–1.39	1
60–64	48	100–199	37	120–129	24	20–29	10	1.20–1.29	1
65–69	50	200–299	21	130–139	29	30–39	17	1.10–1.19	1
70–74	40	300–400	11	140–149	41	40–49	36	1.00–1.09	1
75–79	12	500	4	150–159	24	50–59	55	0.90–0.99	1
80–84	6	600	6	160–169	19	60–69	46	0.80–0.89	1
No information	1	900	1	170–179	15	70–79	14	0.70–0.79	3
		1000	1	180–189	10	80–89	2	0.60–0.69	2
		1200	2	190–199	6	90–99	1	0.50–0.59	3
		1800	1	200–209	2	No information	12	0.40–0.49	10
		Complete		210–219	3			0.30–0.39	16
		retention	12	No information	6			0.20–0.29	20
		No information	29					0.10–0.19	6
								0.01–0.09	1

TABLE 73

ANALYSIS OF 198 CONSECUTIVE CASES OF PERINEAL PROSTATECTOMY WITHOUT A DEATH— FEBRUARY 8, 1919 TO OCTOBER 15, 1922

Heart.		Discharge.		Fistula closure.		Result on discharge.	
	Cases.	Days.	No.	Days.	No.		No.
Enlarged	34	10–14	5	5– 9	2	Well	165
Murmur	30	15–19	12	10–14	19	Improved	25
Enl. and Mur.	16	20–24	40	15–19	53	No information	6
Myocarditis	16	25–29	32	20–29	54		
		30–39	56	30–39	19	Ultimate results:	
		40–49	22	40–49	6	Cured	129
Preliminary treatment.	No.	50–59	9	50–59	8	Improved	10
None	52	60–69	8	75–79	1	Not improved	1
Catheter continuous	100	70–79	1	100–104	1	No information	56
Intermittent	6	Over 90	6	Average		Deaths after 6	
Suprapubic	4	No information	1	24 days		mos.	8
No information	34					Deaths before 6	
						mos.	2

Operative Indications Summarized.—While distinctly preferring the perineal route for reasons previously expressed, we readily admit that suprapubic prostatectomy is a very satisfactory way of removing the prostate in most cases, particularly those which project well into the bladder and present readily enucleable lobes. For the smaller prostate, for the larger prostate which does not project into the bladder, and particularly those with a tight fibrous prostatic orifice, the suprapubic route is certainly more difficult, more destructive, and less satisfactory. The small, fibrous prostate is not at all suited for the suprapubic route. The general operative indications and technic are given in a special chapter. Success in the surgery of enlarged prostates depends very largely upon the preoperative treatment, the indications for which may be summarized briefly as follows:

1. *Early Cases with Small Residual Urine.*—We have here the excellent prostatic risk, the phthalein being good and general condition presumably excellent. Such cases may usually be subjected to prostatectomy without delay.

2. *Cases with Large Residual, Previous Catheter Life, and Good Phthalein.*—When the patient has been systematically catheterized so that the renal condition is stable, these cases can usually be operated upon without delay, the general condition being presumably good.

3. *Cases with large residual urines which have not been catheterized*, even though the first phthalein may be good, are prone to go through a period in which the phthalein becomes progressively worse after the first catheterization. Such cases should, therefore, be given preliminary treatment with intermittent catheterization three or four times daily, or with a retained urethral catheter, generally with a decompression apparatus, until the kidneys have become accustomed to an empty bladder such as will be present immediately after prostatectomy.

4. *Cases Intolerant to Catheterization.*—Where catheterization is difficult, produces traumatism, hemorrhage, marked irritation, or is followed by urethritis or where an inlying catheter produces marked irritation, pain, urethritis, or drains poorly, suprapubic drainage may be preferable. The same is true where periurethritis or abscess along the course of the lower urinary tract is present. Vesical calculi or other conditions of the bladder which make urethral-catheter drainage unsatisfactory also warrant suprapubic drainage. Persistent fever, either from the bladder or kidneys, unrelieved by catheter drainage, may occasionally be improved by suprapubic drainage. In our experience suprapubic drainage is necessary in about 2 per cent. of the cases, but the indications may be more frequent than this. We believe catheter drainage is preferable in the great majority of cases for reasons set forth in the section under Treatment.

5. *Cases with severe complications*, such as acute infections of the urethra, bladder or periurethral and perivesical spaces, epididymitis, pyelonephritis, cardiovascular diseases, etc., usually require that the operation be delayed until appropriate treatment or operation be carried out and the patient put in the optimum condition for operation. Intravenous mercurochrome is often of great value.

It may be said, however, that practically all patients with prostatic obstruction sufficient to warrant operation can, by careful preparatory treatment, be brought into sufficiently good condition for prostatectomy, which is unquestionably safer than the catheter life as a routine procedure and far safer than a policy of non-intervention when large residual urine is present, even though the patient may be having very little discomfort. Periodic examination of the prostate should be carried out in practically all men past fifty-five or sixty years of age, especially in view of the insidious character of the disease and the frequent occurrence of carcinoma (20 per cent.) often without symptoms for a long period and until too late for a radical cure.

Conclusion.—1. Just as radical and satisfactory removal of the entire adenomatous prostate in one piece can be accomplished through the perineum as by the suprapubic route, with, however, complete conservation of important anatomic structures (vesical sphincter, ejaculatory ducts, etc.) as outlined above. As a rule we now prefer our original bicapsular technic, with separate enucleation of the lateral and median hypertrophied lobes, as giving the most conservative results, the quickest healing, the avoidance of stricture, incontinence, and injury to the sexual powers.

2. As a result of the great natural advantages of the lower operation—ability to do an open operation through visual inspection, to arrest hemorrhage and to apply sufficient packing for complete hemostasis, and with dependent drainage, and avoidance of sepsis and the inconvenience of distention of the bowels which so frequently follow suprapubic operation—a remarkably low mortality can be secured and prostatectomy brought within the ranks of those modern major surgical procedures which are practically free from danger.

CHAPTER VIII

NEOPLASMS OF THE UROGENITAL TRACT

A. TUMORS OF KIDNEY AND URETER

PATHOLOGY

Renal Neoplasms.—*Cysts of the kidney* are not properly classified as tumors, as they are considered to be the results of retention due to inflammatory changes or to congenital errors of development. The subject is a fascinating one, and many theories have been proposed, but it must be said that our real knowledge is very slender. Multiple small cortical cysts are a frequent finding at autopsy in cases of chronic diffuse nephritis. They are always in association with a fibrotic change in the interstitial tissue and are probably the result of occlusion of the tubules with distention above.

The typical benign cyst is solitary and usually of considerable size. The contents may be clear and watery, in which case the cyst is known as a "serous" cyst; or mixed with blood, when it is known as a "hemorrhagic" cyst.[1] In the gross one sees a thin-walled non-adherent sac, varying in size from a centimeter or two to a structure large enough to fill and distend the abdominal cavity. It may be located at any point on the surface of the kidney, but most often on the convex border, and at one of the poles. Harpster, Brown, and Delcher[2] have collected 93 cases from the literature and added 2, which shows incidentally that the condition is a rare one.

There has not been a case discovered among the 12,500 at the Brady Institute. In Harpster's series, 41 were at the lower pole, 18 at the upper pole, 7 in the midportion of the kidney, and in 29 the location was not stated. If we add the 29 cases of small cysts found by Cunningham[3] in autopsy records in Boston and Brooklyn, the totals are: In 124 cases, lower pole 50, upper pole 33, midportion 12, not stated 29. The distribution as to the two sides is about equal, *i. e.*, left 49, right 53, not stated 22. No bilateral case is recorded. Of Harpster's cases, 27 are in males, 55 in females, and in 13 the sex is not stated.

The cyst never communicates with the pelvis. It is lined with a delicate epithelium, either cuboidal or flat. There is no fibrous capsule in the serous cysts, the epithelium lying on a basement membrane of about the same thickness as that of a normal tubule, and directly in contact with the parenchyma (Fig. 283). In the hemorrhagic cysts, there may be a thick wall of organized blood-clot, and adhesions to the surrounding organs may be more marked. The large cysts may press upon the other abdominal organs, and produce symptoms.

In other cases the cysts are multiple, or single cysts may be multilocular The exact relation to polycystic kidney is not clear. Small cysts may show epithe

[1] Brin: Encyclopædie Française d'Urologie, 1914, iii, 1–74.
[2] Journal of Urology, 1924, xi, 157–175.
[3] Watson and Cunningham: The Diseases and Surgery of the Genito-urinary System, 1908, ii.

lial hyperplasia or even papillary projections[1] (Fig. 284). This question is more fully discussed under the heading of "Malformations of the Urogenital Tract."

The contents of serous cysts usually has a yellowish color and urea may be found in greater concentration than in the blood, suggesting that the lining epithelium has some relation to the secretory epithelium of the kidney. The reported studies of hemorrhagic cysts are unsatisfactory, in that they do not explain clearly why hemorrhage has occurred. Apparently the hemorrhagic cysts are somewhat more apt to be multilocular, and sometimes areas of a hemagiomatous character may be seen. The investigations of Rienhoff[2] are of especial interest in connection with speculations concerning renal cysts, polycystic kidneys, and renal neoplasms. In tissue cultures taken from early embryos he saw convoluted tubules, glomeruli, vascular endothelium, and connective tissue, all arising *in situ* from the undiffer-

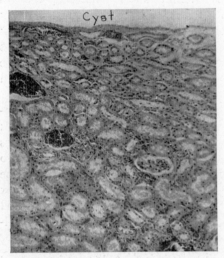

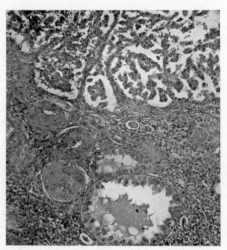

Fig. 283.—The walls of a simple cyst of the kidney showing the low cuboidal epithelium lining the cyst and the entire absence of any fibrous wall about it. J. H. H. Autopsy 6355.

Fig. 284.—The edge of a very small area of apparently typical papillary cystadenoma growth at the capsule of a kidney removed on account of chronic pyelonephritis. The whole area of tumor growth was only 8 or 10 mm. in diameter. The lesions of pyelonephritis are seen and also a small epithelial lined cyst. There were four or five other such cysts in the kidney. B. U. I. Path. 4886.

entiated mesenchymal cells of the primitive kidney. Thus any of these tissues might be represented in cystic or solid neoplasms or malformations of the kidney.

Adenomata are practically always small, giving no symptoms, and, therefore, not found except at autopsy. They are found in all portions of the kidney, more often near the capsule, and are lighter in color than the rest of the kidney. They are sharply demarcated, and usually consist of a mass of small tubules packed closely together, but no glomeruli. Sometimes a part or all of the cells lie in little groups which have no lumina, or the ducts may be dilated and show epithelial hyperplasia or papillary projections. They show no tendency to become malignant; at least, no transition stages between them and malignant tumors have been described. Fibromata, lipomata, myomata, etc., have been described, but many

[1] Nauwerck and Hofschmidt: Ziegler's Beiträge, 1893, xii, 1–28.
[2] Johns Hopkins Hospital Bulletin, 1922, xxxiii, 392–406.

of them, no doubt, fall in the group of teratoid or embryonic tumors to be described later. Hemangiomata, usually quite small, are perhaps not so infrequent as commonly stated. We have seen them on the outer surface of the kidney, and also in

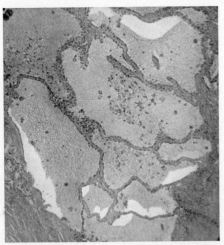

FIG. 285.—A small typical hemangioma found in the kidney at some little distance from the tumor growth illustrated in Fig. 309. Note the resemblance between this picture and certain stages of the blood-filled cysts illustrated elsewhere (Fig. 298). B. U. I. Path. 3671.

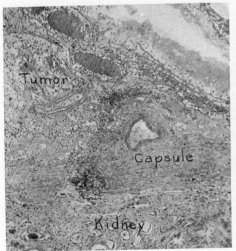

FIG. 286.—The edge of a small tumor 8 mm. in diameter lying just under the capsule of the kidney. The tumor shows the typical large, clear cells of the Grawitz tumor and also the blood-filled spaces lined by clear cells which are just as typical of these tumors, but are not seen in tumors of the adrenal. We have preferred to speak of this tumor as "nephroma." J. H. H. Autopsy 1466.

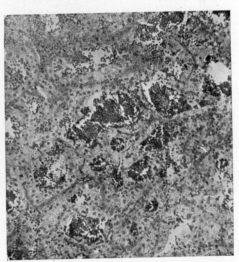

FIG. 287.—Typical area of blood-filled spaces lined with large clear cells in a nephroma. B. U. I. Path. 3157.

association with malignant tumors (Fig. 285). When on the pelvic surface they may give rise to severe hemorrhage.

The classification of *malignant kidney tumors* is a matter of the utmost difficulty. The common kidney tumor of adult life, described by Grawitz[1] as arising from bits

[1] Virchow's Archiv, 1883, xciii, 39–63; Archiv für Klinische Chirurgie, 1884, xxx, 824–834.

of adrenal tissue incorporated in the kidney during fetal life, and christened "hyper-nephroma" by Lubarsch,[1] is usually known by that name.   This conception of its

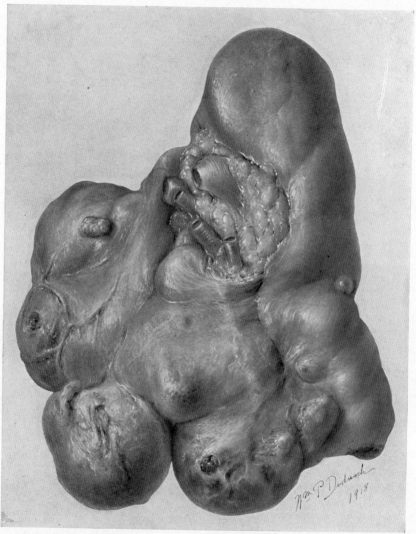

Fig. 288.—Malignant tumor of kidney removed at operation.   Front view showing pedicle with the enormous vessels which are present in these large tumors.   B. U. I. 6835.

origin, however, has been attacked, especially by Sudeck,[2] Stoerk,[3] Driessen,[4] Manasse,[5] von Hansemann,[6] and Wilson.[7]   Albarran[8] also does not accept the

[1] Virchow's Archiv, 1894, cxxxv, 149–223.

[2] Ibid., 1893, cxxxiii, 405–439.

[3] Ziegler's Beiträge zur Pathologischen Anatomie und Allgemeinen Pathologie, 1908, xliii, 393–437.

[4] Ibid., 1893, xii, 65–114.

[5] Virchow's Archiv, 1895, cxlii, 164–192.

[6] Zeitschrift für Klinische Medizin, 1902, xliv, 1–21.

[7] Journal of Medical Research, 1911, xxiv (new series xix), 73–90.

[8] Albarran and Imbert: Tumeurs du Rein, Paris, 1903.

PLATE X

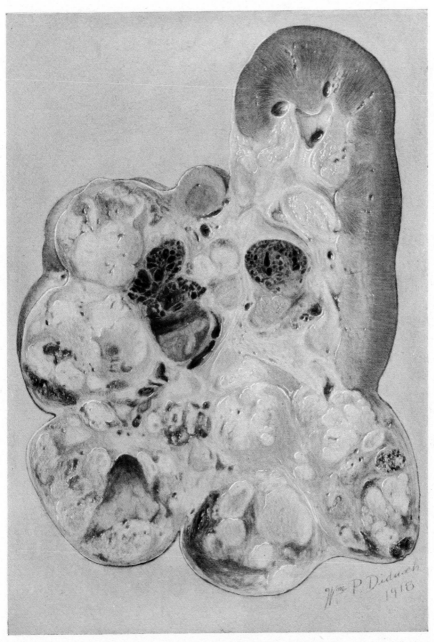

Malignant tumor of the kidney. Sectional view of the tumor, the external aspects of which are shown in Figs. 288 and 289. This tumor is a nephroma with clear cells and blood-filled cysts. Many of these blood-filled cysts are large enough to be easily visible to the naked eye as shown. Note the normal upper pole of the kidney (B. U. I. 6835; B. U. I. Path. 2894).

term "hypernephroma." We believe that the objections of these writers are well founded, but the alternate theories proposed by some of them have little proof. Indeed, the greatest uncertainty reigns as to the histogenesis of these tumors, and competent pathologists have described them as sarcoma, hypernephroma, angiosarcoma, endothelioma, and carcinoma. While the abandonment of a term in

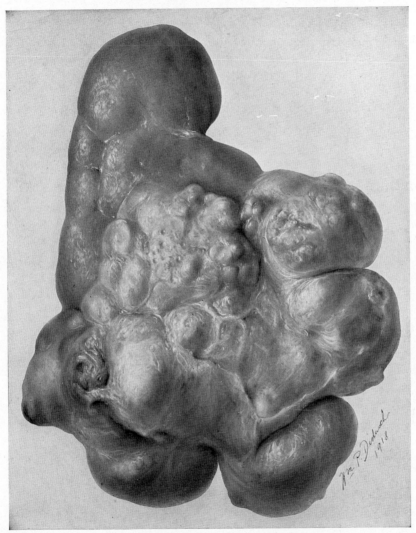

FIG. 289.—Same case as preceding picture. Posterior view of the tumor. The upper pole of the kidney not invaded. Hematuria and renal colic for eight years. Tumor composed of large clear cells with tubular arrangement in some places. Died two months after operation of metastases. B. U. I. 6835.

such wide use as "hypernephroma" is inconvenient, yet it should be abandoned, since it contains the unwarranted assumption that the tumor in question arises from adrenal tissue. Perhaps the appellation of "nephroma" would be best for the present, since it resembles the term in use, and commits us to no unproved theory.

These tumors may arise in any part of the kidney, and only a trifle more frequently in the upper pole. They are usually slow growing, and not invasive; therefore, they have a well-marked fibrous capsule. The kidney tissue is pushed aside, compressed, and undergoes pressure absorption. The tumors are usually opaque, of a yellowish tint, and show marked necrosis and hemorrhage.

A common finding is that of cysts, containing blood-clot or colloid material, and varying up to 1 cm. in diameter. We have seen them in a small, round, capsular tumor, less than 1 cm. in diameter (Fig. 286), and otherwise identical with the pure hypernephroma first described by Grawitz, which, by the way, was never a large tumor. This appearance has even led von Hansemann[1] to suggest the endothelial origin of these tumors. In numerous cases also careful examination while the tissue is immersed in fluid will detect papillary formations—occasionally the entire tumor is papillary. The tumors have a well-marked tendency to invade and obstruct the pelvis, and may, therefore, be difficult to distinguish

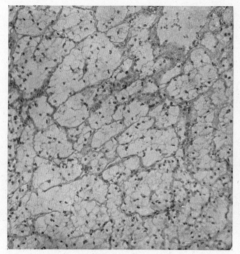
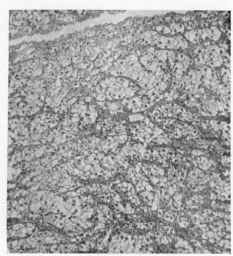

FIG. 290.—Renal neoplasm. This is a typical picture of the so-called Grawitz tumor. Note the small pyknotic nuclei, tremendously swollen cytoplasm, the absence of lumen, close relationship to blood-vessels. B. U. I. Path. 2812.

FIG. 291.—Another area of the same tumor showing slightly more stroma. B. U. I. Path. 2812.

from the true papillary pelvic tumors, which, of course, are capable of invading the parenchyma. Invasion of the renal vein, and later of the vena cava, is not infrequent, the artery being less often involved. The growth may extend down the ureter, even to the bladder, with or without involvement of the ureteral walls. There may be also involvement of the hylic or other perirenal tissues by direct extension which may include the neighboring organs, as the diaphragm, or liver, or the retroperitoneal tissues. There is a tendency to invade the pelvis and to be hemorrhagic. Hematuria, as a fact, is the commonest and usually the earliest symptom. Large cysts—quite different from the small blood cysts—occur in certain types of these tumors. If the papillary contents of the cyst becomes necrotic, it may resemble somewhat a solitary benign cyst on hasty external inspection.

Microscopically the most striking characteristic is the frequent presence of greatly distended tumor cells (Fig. 290). When unfixed sections are stained with

[1] Zeitschrift für Klinische Medizin, 1902, xliv, 1–21.

scharlach R, it is seen that this distention is mostly due to material staining with this dye, and, therefore, of a fatty, lipoid, or myelinic nature. This material is present in droplets, sometimes as large globules filling the entire cell, sometimes as innumerable fine droplets. A portion at least of the droplets is doubly refractile.

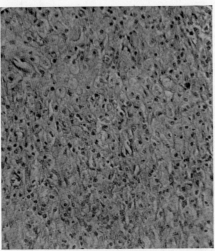

Fig. 292.—This picture shows granulation tissue from a case of pyonephrosis. Note the large swollen cells with clear cytoplasm. This phenomenon is seen in granulation tissue not only in the kidney but elsewhere. The section is of interest in that owing to these large cells an inexperienced pathologist made the diagnosis of "hypernephroma." B. U. I. Path. 3008.

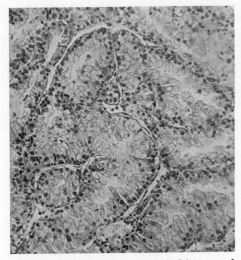

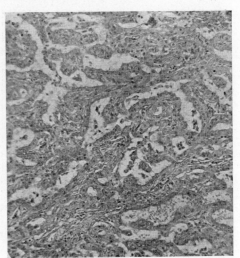

Fig. 293.—Nephroma. A typical instance of Grawitz tumor except for the presence of lumina in the cell cords which in this instance are not blood filled. B. U. I. Path. 4145.

Fig. 294.—Another example of the existence of lumina in a nephroma. In this case the lumina contained only a few red blood-cells. J. H. H. Autopsy 5008.

This lipoid material alone is not sufficient to fix the adrenal origin of the tumor, since the normal epithelial cells of the kidney, especially of the ascending limb of Henle's loop, contain a small quantity of a similar material,[1] and it is found in

[1] MacNider: Journal of Pharmacology and Experimental Therapeutics, 1921, xvii, 289–332. Löhlein: Virchow's Archiv, 1905, clxxx, 1–50.

many other tissues and tumors (Fig. 292).   Glycogen has been found in these cells, but adrenalin is absent.   Characteristically, the cells are found in alveoli, separated by fine trabeculæ, bearing capillaries, and recalling the arrangement of the

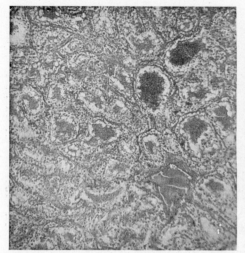

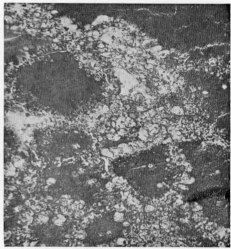

FIG. 295.—Another picture of blood-filled spaces in the typical nephroma. B. U. I. Path. 4943.

FIG. 296.—A further stage in the development of the blood-filled spaces which have here undergone a marked enlargement. B. U. I. Path. 3157.

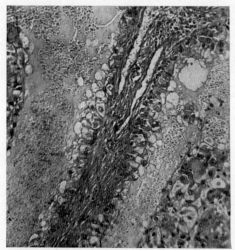

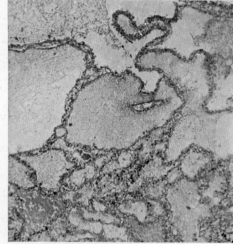

FIG. 297.—Higher magnification showing the blood-filled cysts and the tumor cells with clear swollen cytoplasm which line these spaces without any intervening membrane. B. U. I. Path. 4145.

FIG. 298.—A still further stage in the dilatation of the blood-filled spaces which have here reduced the tumor tissue to a mere network. These cysts are of long standing since the blood which they contain is not fresh. There are many hematin crystals. B. U. I. Path. 3631.

cortical part of the adrenal.   Often, however, the alveoli contain definite lumina (Fig. 293), and many of these lumina contain blood—sometimes a few corpuscles, sometimes a great quantity, giving rise to a cyst lined with a single layer of clear, glassy cells (Figs. 295 to 298).   Some of these cysts contain a colloid material, which may or may not be stained with blood pigment (Fig. 299). In some cases the cysts are crossed by strands consisting of a capillary surrounded by a layer of epithelial cells, in others definite papillæ are seen, projecting into cysts or into the pelvis. One must rule out pseudopapillæ, due to a necrotic process in a solid

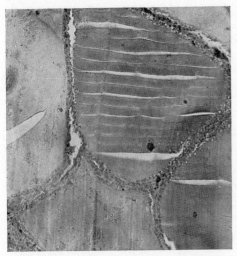

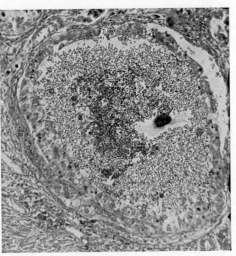

FIG. 299.—Final stage in the development of the blood-filled cysts. Here the cyst contents have taken on a colloid form which is quite clear and translucent and stained in varying degree with blood pigment. B. U. I. Path. 3631.

FIG. 300.—Nephroma showing a single blood-filled cyst lined with tumor cells. J. H. H. Autopsy 5008.

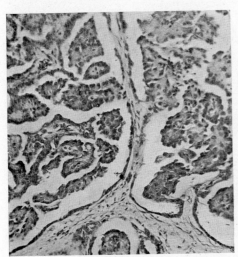

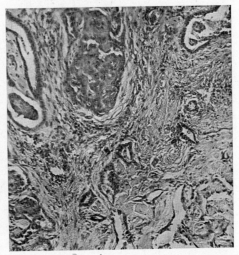

FIG. 301.—Renal neoplasm of the type known as "papillary cyst adenoma." Note the cyst-like spaces filled with complicated papillary arrangements covered by a single layer of flat or cuboidal epithelium. B. U. I. Path. 4229.

FIG. 302.—Another portion of the same tumor showing numerous narrow spaces lined with cells similar to those covering the papillæ. One is struck by the resemblance of these clefts to capillaries. B. U. I. Path. 4229.

part of the tumor, leaving intact only a thin layer of tumor cells nearest the capillaries. This picture caused some earlier pathologists to call the tumor "perithelial angiosarcoma." When papillæ project into cysts, they are more apt to be covered by a thin layer of epithelium—only one or two cells thick. Fusion and polymorphism are seldom seen.   This picture has been called "papillary cyst adenoma" (Fig. 301).   Papillæ projecting into the pelvis are more apt to be covered with a thick layer of epithelium, eight to twelve cells thick, showing basal, middle, and outer layers (Figs. 311, 312).   Fusion and polymorphism are frequently seen

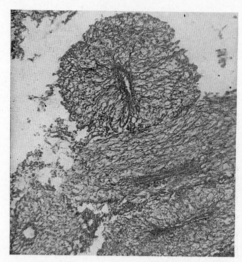

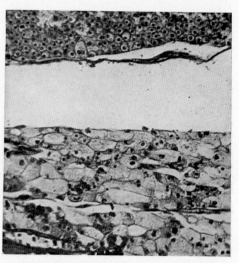

Fig. 303.—Papillary structures projecting into the pelvis in a tumor which elsewhere appeared to be a typical Grawitz tumor. B. U. I. Path. 3747.

Fig. 304.—Renal neoplasm.   Two adjacent areas of tumor tissue showing how the appearance varies with the degree of swelling of the cytoplasm of the tumor cells. J. H. H. Autopsy 2506.

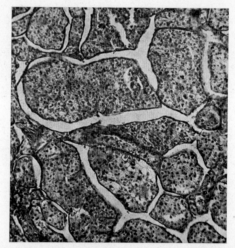

Fig. 305.—Malignant renal neoplasm or nephroma composed of large clear cells and especially characterized by the presence of very large crevices or sinuses lined with endothelium, but containing no blood and separating tumor cells into nests and cords.   Note the resemblance of this tumor to the normal structure of the coccygeal body and that of certain tumors arising from the carotid body.   B. U. I. Path. 4412.

exactly as described for papillomata of the bladder.   It is not always possible to distinguish, however; one occasionally sees papillary tumors in which the covering epithelium is between the two types described above, or in which it varies from place to place, as much as from one to fifteen cells in thickness.   Occasionally one sees solid nests of tumor cells separated by vast, sinusoidal capillaries, recalling the normal picture in the coccygeal body, and similar to tumors of the carotid body described by Paltauf[1] (Fig. 305).

The typical cell has a distended cytoplasm, as described above, a small to medium sized round nucleus, rather deep staining, and comparatively uniform, with few mitoses. There are often to be seen, however, areas of cells which differ only in having a cytoplasm which, being devoid of the lipoid globules, is small and dense. This distention of the cytoplasm with fatty material so universally considered to be characteristic of "hypernephroma" is almost surely not characteristic at all.

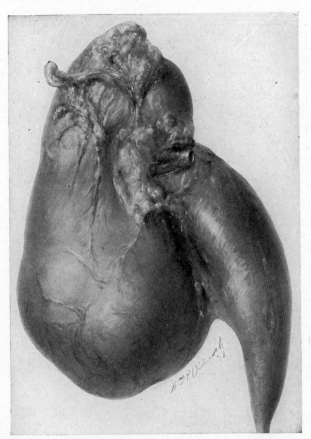

Fig. 306.—Malignant tumor of the kidney. Hematuria, renal colic for eight months. Removal incomplete, pedicle infiltrated. Death four months after operation. B. U. I. 6766.

It is apparently associated in some way with the kidney. The same phenomenon is seen in the normal cat's kidney. Inflammation and diuresis increase the amount of lipoid material in renal cells. Any type of tumor cell in the kidney may show this distention of the cytoplasm, and there is no reason to believe that the resulting resemblance to adrenal cells is anything but accidental. In other cases the cells are quite different, being larger, irregular, with large, irregular nuclei, showing many mitoses. These cells resemble those found in the papillary carcinomata of the bladder, and probably indicate that the tumor originated in the stratified

[1] Ziegler's Beiträge, 1892, xi, 260–301.

epithelium of the pelvis. Deep down, however, they may be arranged in alveoli, and contain globules of lipoid material.

Any or all of the above-described pictures may be found in a single renal tumor; therefore, it is of little use to try to distinguish definite varieties of tumors as clinical or pathologic entities. We know with certainty only that malignant kidney tumors usually show a number of definite different forms of growth, any combination of which may be present in a given case.

Unfortunately, we cannot always be sure, even, whether a tumor is primary in the kidney proper or in the pelvis. Some tumors, papillary at the pelvic surface,

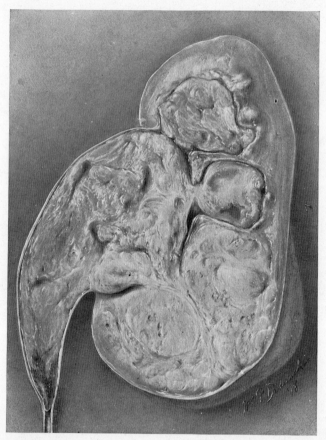

Fig. 307.—Same case as preceding picture. Tumor viewed in section. Note the extensive intra-pelvic growth which has reached 8 cm. down the ureter. The growth was composed of large clear cells, but the arrangement was in large part papillary. B. U. I. 6766.

and showing all the characteristics of papillary carcinoma, have in their depths alveoli of large clear cells indistinguishable from the picture described as "hyper-nephroma." Equivocal pictures are the rule, and since parenchymal tumors invade the pelvis, while pelvic tumors invade the parenchyma, in a tumor of any great size it is impossible to be sure where it has originally arisen. Exceptions are the squamous-cell epithelioma of the pelvis, and the single or multiple non-invasive papilloma of the pelvis, to be discussed later.

Carcinoma of the kidney is frequently described. Many of these tumors re-

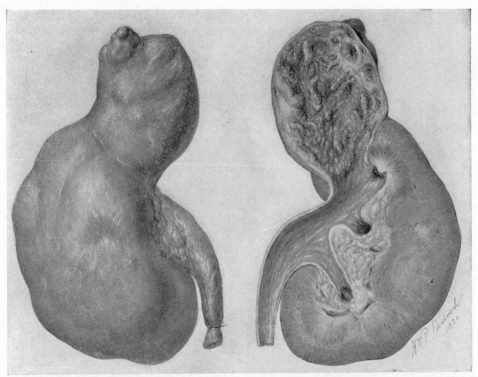

FIG. 308.—Operative specimen of malignant kidney tumor. Hematuria and renal colic for two years. Microscopically papillary cyst adenoma. Patient well two years after operation. B. U. I. 8432.

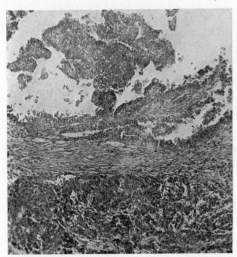

FIG. 309.—Renal neoplasm showing above the structure of papillary cystadenoma, while below similar tumor cells are massed closely together into a form which resembles a simple and rather undifferentiated carcinomatous growth. B. U. I. Path. 3431.

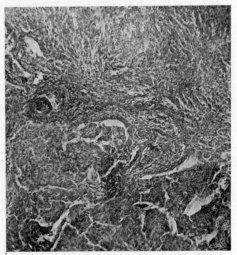

FIG. 310.—A picture taken in the midst of the invasive "carcinomatous" form of growth. B. U. I. Path. 3431.

semble the common tumor, or "nephroma," and have been called carcinoma on account of the presence of gland-like structures. In other cases the description leaves little doubt that the neoplasm was really a papillary carcinoma originating in the pelvis (Fig. 315). There are, however, some undoubted carcinomata of the kidney, usually adenocarcinomatous in type. The growth is invasive, and the fibrous capsule is absent or inconspicuous. A few cases have been reported in which an invasive carcinoma has grown throughout the entire kidney, causing a symmetrical enlargement of the organ. We have seen a case (Figs. 309, 310) in which the kidney was invaded widely by carcinoma-like strands, but which in its center had areas of "papillary cystadenoma."

Pelvic Neoplasms.—The tumors which arise from the renal pelvis are practically identical with those of the bladder, and the reader is referred to the section on Vesical Neoplasms for the finer details. They are, however, much rarer. *Benign papillomata* (Figs. 311, 312) are apparently of infrequent occurrence. Malignant changes appear to be the rule, and may take on any of the appearances described for the bladder. Thus they may be tall and pedunculated, or short and spreading.

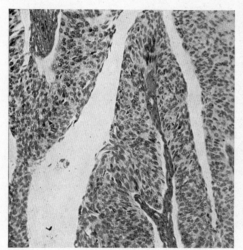
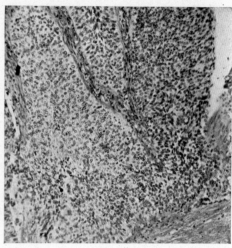

FIG. 311.—Benign papilloma of the renal pelvis. This tumor is indistinguishable from benign papilloma of the bladder. B. U. I. Path. 1546.

FIG. 312.—Benign papilloma of the renal pelvis showing base of the papillæ and absence of infiltration. B. U. I. Path. 1546.

Multiplicity is common, and there may be implantation in the ureter or bladder, or lateral spread, until the ureter or even the bladder become filled with tumor masses.

When the growth is low and spreading, infiltration is early, and after it has involved any considerable portion of the kidney, the pelvic origin may not be apparent. In other cases infiltration is absent or late, as in the bladder, and these are the ones where the pelvic origin is obvious, and which are found recorded in the literature.

Within the kidney the *papillary carcinoma of the pelvis* (Figs. 314, 315) is often identifiable by the cell picture, namely, large oval, vesicular nuclei, blue staining cytoplasm, and alveolar arrangement. But, as stated above, the picture may undergo certain changes apparently due to the influence of the kidney, so that the appearance is changed, especially by hydropic enlargement of the cells.

Epithelioma may also occur, of which the squamous-cell type appears to be somewhat more common (Fig. 316). Kretschmer has collected 43 cases, in 19 of which the microscopic description is complete enough to justify a positive diagnosis

of epithelioma.   The remarks made concerning the relationship of squamous-cell
epithelioma of the bladder to leukoplakia apply equally well to the renal pelvis.

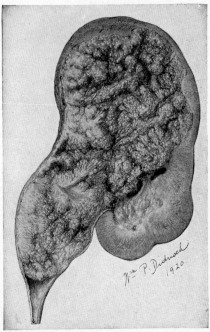

FIG. 313.—Operative specimen of malignant tumor of kidney.   Papilloma of pelvis with beginning
malignant change.   Hematuria and renal colic for one year.   Died ten years after operation, cause unknown.   B. U. I. 2582.

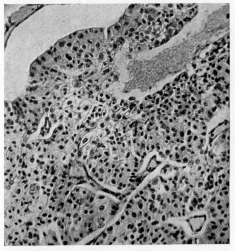

FIG. 314.—Papillary carcinoma of the renal
pelvis showing fusion of the papillæ as in
papillary carcinoma of the bladder. B. U. I.
Path. 4246.

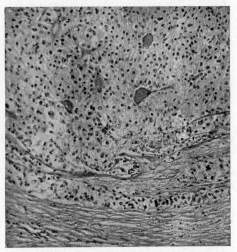

FIG. 315.—Papillary carcinoma of renal pelvis
showing a solid form of growth invading the kidney due to complete fusion of the papillæ. B. U.
I. Path. 4246.

Epitheliomata ulcerate early, and invade the subpelvic tissues, apparently equally
in all directions.   Thus the hylic fat and the renal parenchyma are both infiltrated,

and the peripelvic invasion is apt to produce obstruction and hydronephrosis. For the above reasons symptoms are usually produced before the tumor grows very large.

Adenocarcinoma of the pelvis is rare, and we have not found a case clearly separated from adenocarcinoma of the kidney.

Cavernous hemangiomata are rare. They are often associated with great hemorrhage, even when small, and this may give great difficulty in diagnosis. In other cases they are deep in the parenchyma. Venous varices also occur, but are not, properly speaking, neoplasms.

Whether the cases where various types of growth are present in the same tumor represent the simultaneous occurrence of distinct tumors, or the divergent effects of a single stimulus on different kinds of epithelia, is a matter for speculation, but not, at the present time, for dogmatic pronouncement. Suffice it to say,

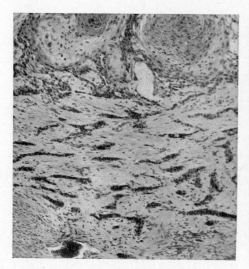 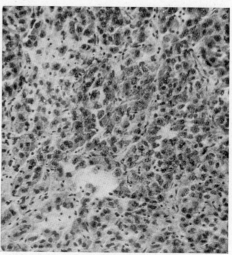

Fig. 316.—Squamous-cell epithelioma of the kidney pelvis, showing the marked invasive qualities.   J. H. H. Surg. Path. 17,921.

Fig. 317.—Renal neoplasm the nature of which is uncertain. It may be a nephroma the cells of which are not swollen, or an embryomatous tumor of some kind. The cells resemble carcinoma cells.   J. H. H. Surg. Path. 21,483.

for clinical purposes, that all kidney tumors giving symptoms are malignant, and should be treated, if there be no metastasis demonstrable, by immediate nephrectomy, with added ureterectomy, if the tumor is of the pelvic papillomatous type. Aside from efforts to discover if the latter is the case, it is unnecessary to try to distinguish clinically between the different types of growth.

We have given no systematic classification of renal tumors because we do not believe that it is possible to do so at this time. The desirable thing is to get rid of all unfounded preconceptions, in the hope that eventually the pathology of renal neoplasms and cysts may be placed on a sound basis. The following observations may be set down to indicate the complexity of the problem.

Along the vertebral ridge there develop, in the embryo, a number of organs, such as the coccygeal, aortic, and carotid bodies, the gonads, the kidneys, and the adrenals and other chromaffin tissue, in which the ectoderm plays no part, or only a secondary one. All of these organs, with their varying functions, spring from the mesoblast.   In all of them, the functioning cells are in exceptionally close relationship with the blood vascular system.   In the kidney the function of the organ is to remove substances from the blood-stream, and in all of the others we assume that the function, or one of the functions, is to pour some substance into the blood-stream.   Rienhoff's[1] observations show that the renal tubules develop in a manner analogous to that of the blood-vessels, namely, a solid cord condenses from the mesenchyme, and in this a lumen forms later.   The endothelium of the blood and lymph vascular systems also differentiates *in situ* from exactly the same kind of cells as those which give rise to the convoluted tubule.   In the primitive glomerulus apparently identical cells lying side by side become some endothelium, some epithelium.

The cells lining the lumina of the renal tubules assume epithelial characteristics, but also retain certain peculiarities of their own.   Cyst formation is not uncommon, papillary structures occur in the cysts, and the papillary adenomata, often small, are seen in every autopsy room.   The relations of these structures to renal neoplasms are not worked out.   In view of the above facts it is not surprising that the renal neoplasms should be peculiar, nor that they should resemble in certain ways the tumors of others of the organs mentioned.   Indeed, it would seem that there is perhaps something characteristic about tumors of organs associated in some close functional way with the blood-stream, for we see tumors very similar to the "nephroma" or "hypernephroma" arising in the adrenal, carotid body, and bone-marrow.   The rôle of the endothelium in these tumors has yet to be deciphered and it is only by retaining an absolutely open mind that we can hope to solve the riddle.

While malignant kidney tumors do not *metastasize* especially early, the fact that they are so often "silent" tumors, except perhaps for some hematuria, accounts for the not infrequent existence of metastases at the time the kidney tumor is first discovered.   The statement that the nephroma or "hypernephroma" is non-malignant has no basis in fact.   It is thought that metastases occur usually by the blood-stream, since the area of predilection is in the lungs.   The chest, therefore, should always be studied with the x-ray.   The next commonest site of metastasis is in the cervical glands (Fig. 321), usually on the left, suggesting transmission by the thoracic duct.   In later stages metastases may occur in any organ or tissue of the body.   The microscopic picture in the metastasis may resemble that in the primary tumor, or differ from it.   Thus, in a case of the "papillary cystadeno-carcinoma" type, the cervical gland metastases contained large clear cells of the type spoken of as "hypernephroma cells" (Figs. 318, 319).   Garceau admits that "carcinoma" may metastasize as "hypernephroma."   There seems to be a definitely marked tendency for the cells of the kidney tumors to assume this form more than those of other tumors, but one cannot always depend on it for diagnosis.

One may see the growth extending very far both up and down in the vena cava, even as far as the right auricle.[2]   Secondary results may be ascites and edema of the lower extremities.   Retroperitoneal growth may obstruct lymph- and blood-vessels, giving rise to unilateral varicocele, or more rarely to varicose veins or edema of one leg or both.

Embryonal Neoplasms.—The adult type of kidney tumor described above may

[1] Johns Hopkins Hospital Bulletin, 1922, xxxiii, 392–406.

[2] Pleasants: Johns Hopkins Hospital Reports, 1911, xvi, 363–548 (Lit.).

occur in children, but is very rare. The tumor usually occurring in infants is quite distinct in every way. It is essentially an *embryonic tumor*, practically

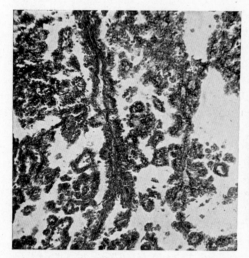

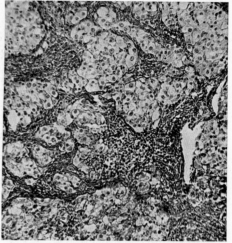

Fig. 318.—Typical picture of growth known as "papillary cyst adenoma." B. U. I. Path. 3671.

Fig. 319.—Section from cervical lymph-node showing metastasis from the tumor illustrated in the previous picture, B. U. I. Path. 3671. Papillary form is completely lost. Cells are swollen and indistinguishable from the picture commonly known as hypernephroma, B. U. I. Path. 3734.

always containing a multiplicity of tissues, and may be a complete teratoma or dermoid cyst. It may undergo malignant carcinomatous or, more rarely, sar-

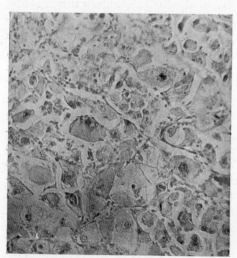

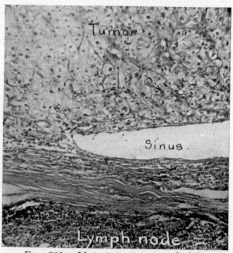

Fig. 320.—Renal neoplasm, nature uncertain. Composed of very large epithelial cells with great variety in size and shape of the nuclei. It is possibly an unusual form of papillary carcinoma. B. U. I. Path. 1414.

Fig. 321.—Metastasis to a cervical lymph-node from malignant kidney tumor. Note the large clear cells. Type of primary tumor not determined. B. U. I. Path. 2499.

comatous degeneration, and even if it does not, tends to recur after removal. These tumors usually are not, properly speaking, of the kidney, but arising in the retroperitoneal area close by, grow into the kidney, sometimes pushing it aside, and sometimes extending into the hilus in such a manner that they expand within

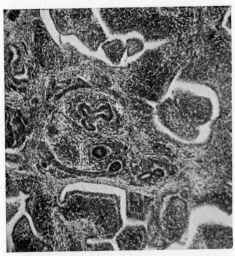

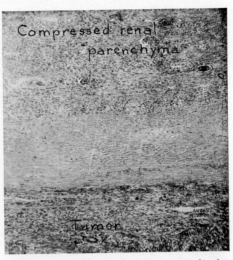

FIG. 322.—Embryoma of the kidney from a child. The growth comprises both mesothelial and epithelial elements. Note the small curved tubules which resemble very closely developing convoluted tubules in the embryonic kidney.   J. H. H. Surg. Path. 20,999.

FIG. 323.—The edge of the tumor showing how it has developed within the kidney, causing the parenchyma to be stretched out and atrophied over it in exactly the same way as occurs in hydronephrosis.   J. H. H. Surg. Path. 20,999.

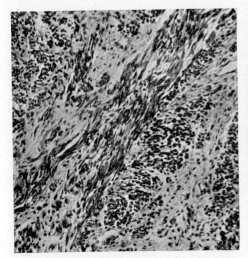

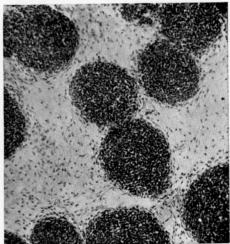

FIG. 324.—Another portion of the same tumor showing mesothelial elements with both smooth and striated muscle-fibers.   J. H. H. Surg. Path. 20,999.

FIG. 325.—Embryoma of the kidney showing rounded masses of condensed mesothelial cells in an edematous matrix of embryonic connective tissue. What these bizarre structures represent is uncertain, but they suggest the condensations which precede in the embryo the formation of various structures, such as myotomes, metanephros, etc.   J. H. H. Surg. Path. 24,945.

the kidney, causing the renal tissues to assume a form exactly like that seen in hydronephrosis (Fig. 323). Occasionally they arise in the kidney itself. They have little tendency to involve the pelvis, to undergo necrosis, or to become hemorrhagic, and, therefore, the symptoms are usually swelling and pain, without urinary manifestations.

The usual microscopic picture is an abundant connective-tissue stroma of embryonic type, beset with numerous acini or tubules lined with columnar or

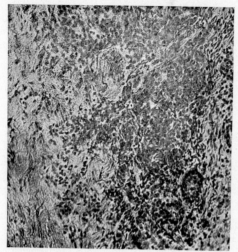

Fig. 326.—Embryoma of kidney showing small tubular formations in connective-tissue stroma. J. H. H. Surg. Path. 8099.

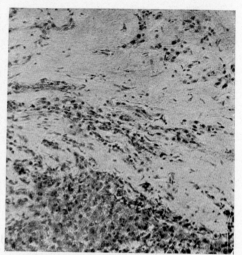

Fig. 327.—Embryoma of the kidney. Edge of the tumor growth showing strands which are apparently invading the surrounding tissue suggesting that the tumor has undergone sarcomatous degeneration. J. H. H. Surg. Path. 8099.

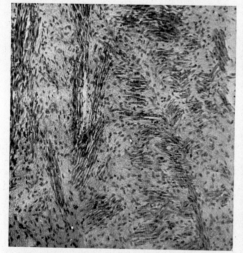

Fig. 328.—Embryoma of kidney showing area composed of smooth muscle. J. H. H. Surg. Path. 21,038.

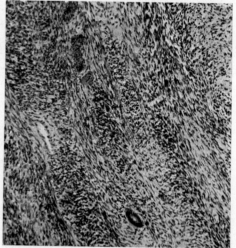

Fig. 329.—This tumor would be a pure leiomyoma were it not for the presence of small ducts like the ones shown here which fixes its embryomatous nature. J. H. H. Surg. Path. 21,038.

cuboidal epithelium. Occasionally the epithelial elements may be hard to find (Figs. 326, 329). Sometimes the stroma is more highly differentiated, with smooth (Fig. 328) or striated muscle (Fig. 324), or cartilage, while the epithelial elements may show large cysts, skin, hair, teeth, etc. Watson and Cunningham have found striated muscle in 42 of 100 cases. In other cases the connective-tissue strands may be separated by quantities of a gelatinous material, giving rise to the designation of myxoma or myxosarcoma. Malignant changes may occur, in the form of embryonal carcinoma (Fig. 330), epithelioma, or any of the various types of sarcoma.

In the gross these tumors are usually smooth and not adherent to the surrounding organs. Their attachments and extent in the retroperitoneal tissues are wide and difficult to delimit, especially at operation. The cut surface is not characteristic, varying with the particular tissues which predominate in the tumor. Cartilage-containing tumors are very hard. Hemorrhage and necrosis occur, but not as frequently as in the adult tumors (nephroma). Cysts are not uncommon.

Metastases may occur when malignant changes are present, and usually represent only the malignant portion of the tumor. Walker found them in 38 per cent. of 142 cases, and Watson and Cunningham in 21 per cent. of 100 cases. Owing to the large size which kidney tumors attain in children, serious pressure effects

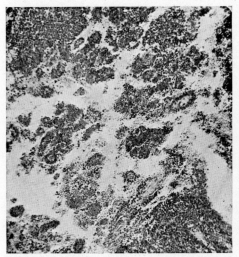
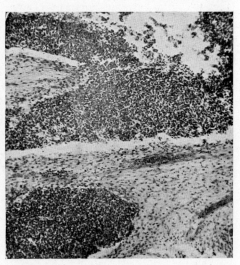

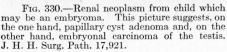

Fig. 330.—Renal neoplasm from child which may be an embryoma. This picture suggests, on the one hand, papillary cyst adenoma and, on the other hand, embryonal carcinoma of the testis. J. H. H. Surg. Path. 17,921.

Fig. 331.—Another area of the same tumor showing a more solid form of growth. J. H. H. Surg. Path. 17,921.

often occur. There may be intestinal obstruction, peripheral edema, ascites, and compression of the thoracic contents by upward pressure through the diaphragm. Even where there is no malignant change, local recurrence is very frequent, as it is so difficult to remove the tumor radically. The growth may be very slow for long periods, and suddenly assume the greatest rapidity. Tumors have been observed to double in size in two weeks.

These interesting tumors have given rise to a great literature in which a number of the most ingenious theories of their pathogenesis, mostly from the point of view of embryology, have been proposed. Unfortunately, none of them is susceptible of proof. It is unnecessary to discuss them here, and the interested reader is referred to the literature.[1]

[1] Wilms: Die Mischgeschwülste, Berlin, 1899; and Birch-Hirschfeld, Freitag, and Bruns: Ziegler's Beiträge, 1898, xxiv, 341–384. A symposium on renal tumors continues to page 414 (Graupner).

Other Neoplasms.—A tumor arising supposedly in the adrenal, containing embryonic nerve cells and fibrils, and known as *neurocytoma*, may invade the kidney in infants.

The kidney may be involved in a *lymphosarcomatous* process.

Dermoid cysts and *teratomata* of the kidney are described, but are very rare.

Metastatic growths in the kidney are uncommon, but perhaps oftenest from malignant tumors of the opposite kidney. They are seen occasionally in uterine cancer.

The kidney may be involved by extension or by pressure from neoplasms in neighboring organs or tissues. This is most frequent in the case of the embryonic retroperitoneal tumors and neurocytomata mentioned above. Rarer instances are carcinomata of the liver, biliary system, stomach, pancreas, or intestines. Retroperitoneal metastases from malignant tumors of the testicle may surround and press on the kidney, but seldom invade it. Hydronephrosis may be caused by pressure of an external tumor on the pelvis or ureter.

Neoplasms of the Ureter.—These tumors are rare. Albarran and Imbert found one tumor of the ureter to four of the renal pelvis. Jeanbrau[1] has collected only 30 cases of primary tumor of the ureter.

Pathologically, neoplasms of the ureter are like those of the renal pelvis and bladder. Cases have been reported of *papilloma*, benign and malignant, *papillary carcinoma, squamous-cell epithelioma*, and *sarcoma*. Jeanbrau adds a diagnosis of "papillary adenoma" for 2 cases in which a carcinoma had a definite glandular structure.

Papilloma may be single or multiple. As in the bladder, the multiple tumors are practically always malignant. These cases are difficult to distinguish in the late stages from cases in which a papilloma primary in the renal pelvis has invaded the ureter by extension along the surface or by implantation. Primary ureteral papillomata may invade the pelvis by extension along the surface.

Papillary carcinoma may be mainly a surface growth or may invade the ureteral wall early and extensively.

Squamous-cell epithelioma, as elsewhere in the urinary tract, is preceded by leukoplakia, which, although infrequent, may occur in the ureter.[2] The tumor is invasive and ulcerative, and leads to early obstruction.

The very few cases described as *sarcoma* are apparently, in some instances, embryomata, since one was called rhabdomyosarcoma. They usually occur in young subjects.

Owing to the small caliber of the ureter, obstruction, with consequent hydronephrosis, is an early complication. This may be due to a mass growing into the lumen, or to circumferential infiltration of the ureteral wall.

Metastasis is usually generalized, and, therefore, probably by the blood-stream. Neighboring organs, as the seminal vesicle and retroperitoneal tissues, may be involved by extension. Implantation of papillomata may occur in the bladder, or if the tumor has spread to the ureteral orifice, it may continue to spread into the bladder. Pedunculated tumors may project through the orifice into the bladder. (See Plate XI.)

[1] Encyclopædie Française d'Urologie, 1914, iii, 917–927.

[2] Kretschmer: Surgery, Gynecology, and Obstetrics, 1920, xxxi, 325–339. Mainfold: Journal of the Royal Army Medical Corps, 1923, xli, 365–368.

The ureter may be secondarily involved by metastasis or extension of neoplasms. We have observed 3 cases in which metastasis to the ureteral wall led to obstruction and hydronephrosis. In 2 the primary growth was in the bladder, and in the other, the prostate. In each the metastasis was in the lower third of the ureter.

Growths which may involve the ureter by extension from the outside include carcinoma of the bladder, carcinoma of the prostate which has reached the tip of the seminal vesicle, retrovesical sarcoma, carcinoma of the uterus and ovary, tumors of the pelvic bones, retroperitoneal tumors, carcinoma of the pancreas, carcinoma of the intestine, etc. The ureter may be compressed by various growths, as uterine fibroids, retroperitoneal metastases of testicular neoplasms, etc.

In a series of 43 cases of malignant renal tumors at the Brady Institute, the right kidney was involved nineteen times, the left twenty-two times, and in 2 cases the side was not stated in the record. The two sides, therefore, are involved with about equal frequency. The following table gives the age incidence:

TABLE 74

	Number.	Per cent.
20–29	2	4.6
30–39	4	9.3
40–49	10	23.2
50–59	16	37.2
60–69	9	20.9
?	2	4.6

This list comprises no cases of tumors in children, which have usually come with huge abdominal tumors, and have been operated upon in the department of general surgery.

SYMPTOMS

The cardinal symptom of kidney tumor is *hematuria*. It is one of the four important and serious conditions giving rise to hematuria, namely, tumor of the kidney, tumor of the bladder, tuberculosis, and urolithiasis. For this reason hematuria should never be neglected, but always traced to its source at all costs.

The hematuria from renal tumor may be slight or grave; a few microscopic red cells or large clots. It may even tend to be terminal, if unclotted blood collects in the base of the bladder. Occasionally blood-casts of the ureter may give a hint of the renal origin of the bleeding. In general, however, no definite and absolute conclusions can be drawn from the character of the hematuria.

Hematuria may be the only symptom for a long time, during which period the suspicions of patient and physician as to its serious import may be lulled to rest. It is often intermittent and the intervals may be long. If, however, the amount of bleeding is great, clots will form in the pelvis and ureter, giving rise to typical *renal colic*. If this does not occur, however, loss of weight and strength may be the next thing to give alarm, and rightly so, for this indicates an advanced stage of malignancy.

Diffuse, fixed, or constant renal *pain* is less frequent, but occurs in about one-third of the cases. Unlike the colic, it bears no special relation to bleeding.

Owing to the deep location of the kidney, a perceptible *tumor* is usually a late manifestation, although the thickness of the abdominal wall has much to do with our ability to palpate it.

If the tumor growth obstructs veins or lymph channels, obstructive symptoms may be seen, the most important of which is unilateral *varicocele* on the same side as the tumor. Compression or occlusion of the vena cava gives edema of one or both legs, oftenest both. Ascites indicates a grave condition, in that the portal vein must be already involved. We have seen a case, however, with ascites, in which at autopsy there was found a portal thrombosis having no obvious relation to the primary tumor in the kidney or to a single small metastasis which was present in a remote part of the liver.

Frequency of urination is noted occasionally even in the absence of infection.

Metastases may cause symptoms in various parts of the body, as cough, hemoptysis, dyspnea, headache, failure of vision, jaundice, etc. They are, of course, very important, since the presence of metastases contraindicates operation. Infection may supervene, with pyuria, fever, chills, etc.

The following table shows the incidence of the various symptoms in a series of 43 cases studied at the Brady Urological Institute:

TABLE 75

	Number.	Per cent.
Hematuria	36	83.7
Loss of weight	29	67.2
Renal colic	20	46.5
Diffuse renal pain	17	39.5
Tumor	13	30.2
Frequency of urination	7	16.2
Pyuria	5	11.6
Varicocele	4	9.3
Chills and fever	4	9.3
Previous removal or passage of stone	4	9.3
Headache	3	7.0
Weakness	3	7.0
Nausea and vomiting	2	4.6
Swelling of legs	2	4.6
Urgency of urination	1	2.3
Dyspnea	1	2.3
Pain in leg	1	2.3
Jaundice	1	2.3
Constipation	1	2.3
Epigastric pain	1	2.3
Urticaria	1	2.3
Pain in testicle	1	2.3
Impairment of vision	1	2.3
Pain in chest	1	2.3

It will be seen, therefore, that hematuria, pain, loss of weight, and tumor are the most important symptoms. The first symptom, *i. e.*, that which the patient described as the first noticed by him, was as follows:

TABLE 76

	Number.	Per cent.
Hematuria	19	44.2
Renal colic	9	20.9
Diffuse renal pain	5	11.6
Tumor	2	4.6
No symptom (condition discovered accidentally at insurance examination)	2	4.6
Pain in testicle	1	2.3
Loss of weight	1	2.3
Frequency and hesitancy	1	2.3
Varicocele	1	2.3
Epigastric pain	1	2.3
Not noted	1	2.3

The duration of symptoms before the diagnosis was made is as follows:

TABLE 77

No symptoms.... 1	} 0 to 1 month........ 2		
3 weeks........ 1			
5 weeks........ 1			
4 months....... 3	} 1 to 6 months........ 6	0 to 1 year........ 14...... 32.5 per cent.	
6 months....... 2			
7 months....... 2			
8 months....... 2	} 6 to 12 months....... 6		
10 months....... 1			
11 months....... 1			
1 year.......... 4			
13 months....... 1			
15 months....... 1	} 1 to 2 years......... 9............................ 20.9 per cent.		
18 months....... 2			
21 months....... 1			
2 years......... 3	} 2 to 3 years......... 5............................ 11.6 per cent.		
2½ years........ 2			
3 years......... 4	} 3 to 5 years.......... 5............................ 11.6 per cent.		
3½ years........ 1			
5 years........ 1			
6 years........ 1			
7 years........ 1	} 5 to 10 years......... 5............................ 11.6 per cent.		
8 years........ 1			
9 years........ 1			
12 years........ 1—Over ten years....... 1............................ 2.3 per cent.			
? .... 1— ? .... 1............................ 2.3 per cent.			

Two-thirds of the cases were allowed to go one year or over before diagnosis and proper treatment—which, no doubt, accounts for some of the unfavorable results. Unfortunately, however, some of those who came for treatment soon after the appearance of symptoms died of metastasis, the physical findings indicating that the tumor had been present for a long time during which it gave no symptoms whatever.

The *embryonic neoplasms* occur mostly before the age of seven, and very rarely after eighteen. There is no distinction as to sex. They are characterized by the fact that they usually cause no urinary symptoms. Pain is absent until the growth attains a large size. The *tumor* itself, therefore, is practically always the only local symptom. Malnutrition and anemia occur in the late stages, but may be the first manifestations. Hematuria is very rare; probably due to circulatory disturbances in the kidney from pressure. One case was seen in a man of fifty-seven.

The tumor may be of any size. The higher it is situated in the abdomen, the more difficult it is to discover. It is usually smooth, tender, and does not move with respiration unless entirely intrarenal. Pressure symptoms are frequent and variegated. One may mention enlarged veins in the abdominal wall, edema of the legs, scrotum, and lower abdomen, ascites, varicocele, diastasis of the recti, diarrhea or constipation, vomiting, intestinal obstruction, dyspnea, cyanosis, cardiac irregularity and insufficiency, and jaundice. Pain when present is dull and aching or dragging.

The duration of the disease is usually short—a matter of weeks or months—

especially after the tumor has begun to grow more rapidly. The prognosis is bad owing to the tendency to early metastasis and to recurrence.

The symptoms of solitary *renal cyst* are not characteristic. Indeed, there are only 7 cases in the literature in which a positive diagnosis was made before operation. Urinary symptoms and pain are practically always absent, so that the tumor itself is usually the initial symptom. It, of course, makes itself apparent much more easily if in the lower pole. If large, pressure symptoms may occur and there may be dragging pain.

Neoplasms of the ureter give rise to hematuria and the symptoms of ureteral obstruction. Since colic due to blood-clots is not infrequent in renal tumors, and since ureteral tumors often produce enlargement of the kidney (hydronephrosis), the symptom complex will usually be indistinguishable from that of renal or pelvic neoplasm.

DIAGNOSIS

When the tumor is large and located in the region of the kidney a diagnosis may sometimes be made by simple physical examination, especially as hematuria is usually present. In most cases the physical signs are less definite.

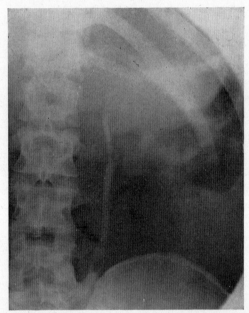

FIG. 332.—Pyelogram in a case of renal tumor. The growth has filled the pelvis to such an extent that it is practically entirely obliterated. Some of the vague shadows seen to the left side may be caused by thorium in portions of the flattened pelvis remaining. B. U. I. x-Ray 2305.

Cystoscopy and ureteral catheterization with functional tests are always indicated. The total renal function is usually not reduced, as one kidney is unaffected and capable of hypertrophy. In early cases the affected side will show no reduction, but usually there is definite impairment. As in all other operations on the kidney, it is essential to know the function of the sound side.

Careful ureteral meatoscopy should be done to determine if possible the side from which the bleeding comes. It is important to watch the jets of urine from each ureter, as ureter catheters will not infrequently produce traumatic hemorrhage, which may lead to a mistaken diagnosis of bilateral hematuria. In a few cases study of the divided urine will show microscopically tumor cells, which are a great aid in the diagnosis. In one case seen by us there was a yellow, worm-like mass protruding from the ureteral orifice, which slid up and down with ureteral peristalsis (Plate XI). When removed this proved to be made up not of pus but of large cells, with large, irregular, vesicular nuclei; undoubtedly tumor cells. The chest x-ray showed the lungs already studded with metastases.

Pyuria is more common in tuberculosis, but hematuria may obscure pus in both. The plain x-ray aids greatly in distinguishing from stone.

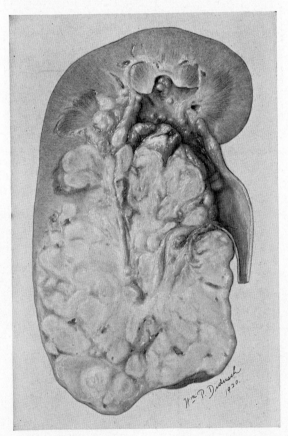

Fig. 333.—Same case as Fig. 332. Operative specimen of malignant kidney tumor. Hematuria and renal colic for four months. Microscopically papillary cyst adenoma with much infiltration. Note intrapelvic growth. Operation incomplete, metastases in aortic glands. Died three months after operation. B. U. I. 8600.

At this point one not infrequently still remains in doubt. The presence of a palpable tumor does not help greatly, as hydronephrosis sometimes simulates neoplasm, even to having hematuria as its first symptom. The *pyelogram* is the most important diagnostic agent here, and usually serves to clear up the uncertainties. Colston[1] has called attention to its value and published interesting records of some of the cases seen at the Brady Institute. The pyelogram is often of great assistance because of the very marked tendency of practically all renal neoplasms

[1] Journal of Urology, 1921, v, 67–87.

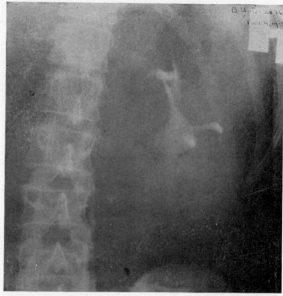

Fig. 334.—Pyelogram from a case of tumor of the kidney. The pelvis is very markedly distorted, invaded, and compressed by a large growth. The upper portion of the ureteral shadow is seen opposite the body of third lumbar vertebra, but no connection can definitely be made out between this and the pelvis. B. U. I. 2036.

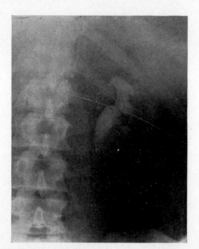

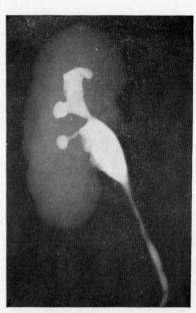

Fig. 335.—Pyelogram in a case of tumor of the kidney. The calyces are not affected, but the tumor is seen as a filling defect on the outer margin of the pelvis proper. It proved to be a benign papilloma of the pelvis. B. U. I. x-Ray 5032.

Fig. 336.—Same case as preceding picture. Pyelogram made by injecting operative specimen after removal. B. U. I. x-Ray 5032.

to invade the pelvis. This is equally the case whether the tumor originates in the parenchyma or in the pelvis. As a result the outline of the pelvis is irregular, with definite encroachments on parts of its circumference. In pushing into the

PLATE XI

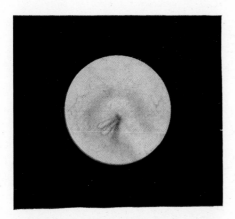

A. Ureteral papillomata projecting into bladder. B. U. I. 6454.

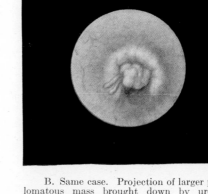

B. Same case. Projection of larger papillomatous mass brought down by ureteral peristalsis.

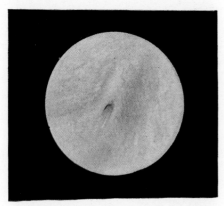

C. Tumor of kidney with prolongation down ureter. Orifice between urinary jets. B. U. I. 10,239.

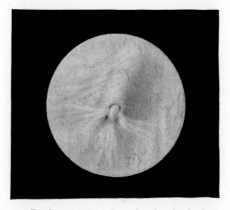

D. Same case. Jet of urine beginning, accompanied by end of ureteral tumor mass. B. U. I. 10,239.

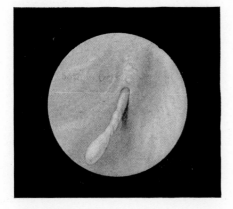

E. Same case. Full extent of projection of ureteral mass after which it slowly receded completely into ureter. B. U. I. 10,239.

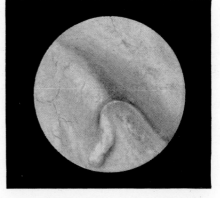

F. Tuberculosis of right kidney with shortened, thickened ureter and ureteral ridge; worm-like stream of pus. B. U. I. 5541.

cavity of the pelvis, the tumor very often leaves a thin, compressed, cup-like extension of the pelvis about the periphery of the tumor mass. This often gives a characteristic picture. In more extensive growths the pelvis may be reduced to a thin leaflet, scarcely casting a shadow except where it presents itself tangentially to the rays. These appearances must be distinguished from the erosions with enlargement of the calyces typical of tuberculosis, from the very irregular pelves of infection and from the elongated, complicated arrangements in congenital cystic kidneys. A previous operation on the kidney adds to the difficulty of making the distinction. The essential element, however, which is characteristic of neoplasm is compression of part or all of the pelvis. The varied character and appearance of the pelvic pictures and their diagnostic significance are shown in the accompanying illustrations from cases in our series (Figs. 332–342).

The plain x-ray may show the kidney outline enlarged and irregular. In a large hydronephrosis the pyelographic medium may be so diluted as to cast no

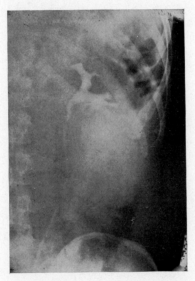

Fig. 337.—Pyelogram in a case of renal tumor. The upper calyces are normal, the middle calyces slightly distorted, while the lower calyx is represented by a very thin layer of thorium capping the tumor mass. Note the abnormal position of the ureter. B. U. I. x-Ray 2702.

shadow at all if the sac is not emptied before the injection is made. It is seldom that a tumor is so extensive as to block the pelvis completely.

The most careful study must be made for metastases. The most important feature is the chest x-ray, since the lungs are usually first affected. All suspicious nodules and glands must be carefully investigated, while jaundice, headache, loss of vision, etc., call for examination of the regions affected. In 1 case we have seen there was no sign of metastasis before operation, except slight headache and impairment of vision. The patient died within a year of cerebral metastasis.

The ureterogram may give evidence of involvement of the ureter, especially if it contains papillomatous masses. The catheter may dislodge papillæ, which can be identified microscopically. If these procedures fail, involvement of the ureter can usually be easily made out at operation. Aside from these measures, efforts to distinguish the different types of tumors are useless, since, in the first place, there are no dependable criteria, and, in the second place, the treatment is exactly the same, regardless of the nature of the tumor, in all cases.

The pyelogram is of the greatest value in ruling out solitary cysts and juxta-renal tumors of all kinds. Where they are in the kidney or closely related to it, the pelvis may be deformed, but the characteristic leaflet deformity will seldom be seen, since the pressure is from outside the pelvis, and not from the growth of a mass inside it. Hydronephrosis due to involvement of the ureteropelvic junction

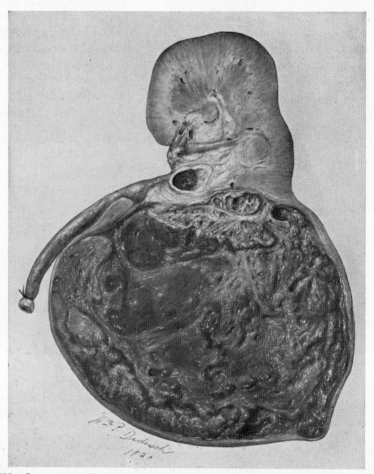

FIG. 338.—Same case as Fig. 337. Operative specimen of malignant tumor of the kidney. Note intrapelvic growth. Hematuria and renal colic for six months. Microscopically showed large clear cells, blood cysts, and also papillary cyst adenoma. Operation apparently complete. Died of metastases three months after operation. B. U. I. 9171.

by renal or pelvic neoplasms is rare, but should be kept in mind. If the pelvis is entirely normal in outline, but merely displaced, it is excellent evidence that the kidney itself is not involved in the displacing mass. The outline of the entire mass and its relation to the pelvic shadow is important in determining the portion of kidney involved.

In cases of *embryonal neoplasm* the patients usually come complaining only of abdominal tumor or of weakness and malnutrition, and the abdominal tumor is easily found at examination. The problem then is to differentiate from other forms of abdominal tumor, among which may be mentioned tumors of the intestine, enlarged spleen (malaria, leukemia, syphilis), retroperitoneal neoplasms or tuberculous glands, hydronephrosis, and tuberculosis of the kidney. If the tumor is

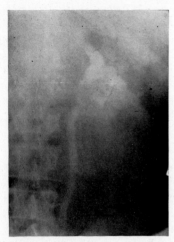

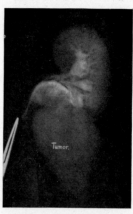

Fig. 339.—Pyelogram in a case of renal tumor. The lower calyx is involved, a tumor mass pushing into it and leaving only a thin layer of thorium about its periphery. The tumor in this case was comparatively small. B. U. I. x-Ray 4873.

Fig. 340.—Pyelogram of the same case of renal tumor shown in the preceding picture. Note the great distortion of the lower calyx, the filling defect in the pelvis proper due to an intra-pelvic tumor mass, and the normal upper calyx. This specimen also showed a partial venous injection due to the pyelovenous backflow described by Hinman and Lee-Brown (this picture was made by injecting the operative specimen after removal). B. U. I. x-Ray 4908.

small, it may be possible to localize it in the kidney region. When large, this is impossible. Tenderness is usually slight or absent. The consistence varies from

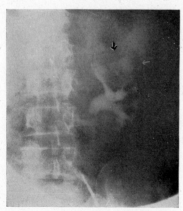

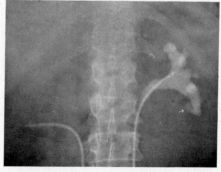

Fig. 341.—Pyelogram in a case of renal tumor. The tumor is at the upper pole and has distorted and distended the upper calyx. The middle and lower calyces are normal. Note the distortion of the ureter, due at least in part to the kidney being pushed downward by the tumor. B. U. I. x-Ray 3605.

Fig. 342.—Pyelogram in a case of a tumor of the lower pole of the kidney. This picture is unusual in that the filling defect of the pelvis ordinarily seen is represented only by the very small shadow extending mesially from the lower calyx, although the tumor was large enough to be palpable at the time. The very marked widening of the angle between the ureter and the lower calyx was another important point which helped to make the correct diagnosis. B. U. I. x-Ray 5135.

hard to fluctuant. Pressure symptoms depend purely on the size of the tumor, and are in no way characteristic. The urine is usually normal, and if pus or bacteria are present they will suggest some other lesion of the kidney. Very few pyelographic studies have been carried out in children, but this should often be done now that satisfactory children's cystoscopes (Nos. 10 to 15 F. in size) are available. Displacement of the pelvis is of no significance, but distortion or compression indicate that the kidney is involved. Examination of the blood is of assistance where splenic enlargement is suspected.

Solitary cysts are also difficult to diagnose. In women they are frequently mistaken for ovarian cysts. The urine is clear. The tumor is usually fluctuant. Pyelography should be done, though we are unable to give any statistics as to its diagnostic value. Hydronephrosis will be distinguished by its characteristic features. Complete closure of the pelvis indicates a closed hydronephrosis, and rules out simple cyst. Deformity or compression of the pelvis indicate at least that the kidney is involved. If this point can be determined, further distinctions are of less importance, since operation is at once indicated. Diagnostic puncture is never permissible. One should make very sure that one is dealing with a simple cyst, since so many cases of malignant neoplasms show cyst formation, the malignant nature of which may not be apparent before they are opened.

According to Hyman[1] there is an interesting combination of lesions occasionally seen, oftenest in children. There is progressive mental failure, and small yellowish-white nodules are seen on the skin, mostly of the face. Autopsy discloses superficial indurated plaques on the cerebral cortex, and in 80 per cent. of these cases of "tuberose sclerosis" of the brain and "adenoma sebaceum" of the skin, a renal tumor, of the Grawitz or "nephroma" type, is found.

The *ureter* has always to be considered. If in the presence of symptoms of malignancy its outline in a ureterogram is irregular and enlarged, we suspect that it is the seat of primary or secondary neoplastic growth. If we see a tumor mass projecting from the ureteral orifice, the ureter is probably involved, though occasionally a cylindrical mass from a renal tumor may grow all the way down the ureter to the bladder without involving its walls. Observation of the mass during peristalsis is useful. If its position relative to the orifice changes little or none during the peristaltic wave, it is probably attached to the ureteral wall near the orifice. If, on the contrary, it slides up and down for a considerable distance during peristalsis, as in a case observed by us (Plate XI), it cannot be attached in the lower part of the ureter, but must spring from its upper part or from the kidney.

The difficult cases are those in which the ureteral tumor is small and, while causing no change in the ureterogram, is the source of hematuria. Ordinarily palpation of the ureter at operation will disclose a thickening due to a mass in the lumen or to an infiltration of the ureteral wall. A small papilloma may escape observation even in this way, as in cases reported by Suter[2] and Culver,[3] which illustrate the difficulties encountered under these circumstances. In Suter's case the patient's hematuria was severe and came from the ureteral orifice. Examination was negative for renal tumor, but to avoid exsanguination exploration was carried out. There was no tumor, and nephrotomy disclosed a normal pelvis. The hemorrhage continuing, nephrectomy was performed in spite of the absence of positive findings. The ureter was negative to palpation at both operations. Still the hemorrhage continued, and when it was seen to come from the ureter of

---

[1] Journal of Urology, 1922, viii, 317–321.

[2] Urologic and Cutaneous Review, Technical Supplement, 1913, i, 62–65.

[3] Journal of Urology, 1921, vi, 331–339.

the nephrectomized side, ureterectomy was done, and the source of the blood at last disclosed in a pair of small, fine, unbranched papillomata in the upper third of the ureter. If, therefore, we find a normal kidney in a case where blood has been seen coming from the ureteral orifice, we may assume that the source of the hematuria is in the ureter, even if it is normal to palpation.

The following table shows the proportions of positive diagnostic findings in our series of 43 cases.

TABLE 78

Tumor:	Number.	Per cent.
Noticed by patient	13	
Not noticed, but found at examination	17	
Total	30	70.0
Positive pyelogram	25	58.1
Diminished phthalein on affected side	18	42.0
Shadow in plain x-ray	13	30.2
Cystoscopic bleeding	12	28.0
Diminished Doremus test on affected side	7	16.3
Varicocele: Unilateral	6	14.0
Bilateral	1	2.3
Edema of leg: Unilateral	1	2.3
Bilateral	1	2.3
Metastases	1	2.3
Mass of tumor tissue in ureter	1	2.3

Summary.—Kidney tumor is to be suspected when painless hematuria, shown to come from one ureter, is present. A palpably enlarged kidney or mass in that region is of import, but the diagnosis is generally made positive by the pyelogram which is often diagnostic, while the tumor is small and no mass or even renal enlargement palpable. Unfortunately, these cases usually reach the cystoscopist late.

TREATMENT

Malignant Tumors.—OPERATIVE.—*Nephrectomy*, as radical and as early as possible, is indicated. The wound should be large, giving a splendid exposure so that the operation may go wide of the tumor mass, removing, if possible, the fatty capsule, the glands, and sometimes the adrenal. Owing to the frequency with which the tumor invades the renal veins, the vascular pedicle should be seen or palpated carefully, and divided as far from the tumor as possible. In cases where an intravenous growth is found, withdrawal of this through an incision into the vein may be carried out before ligation is done. A remarkable case has been reported in which the operator even opened the vena cava, removed a considerable tumor growth, and then successfully sutured the great vein.

For tumors of moderate size and not too fixed the mass may be removed through an oblique extraperitoneal operation. Most of our cases have been treated in this way, but the recurrences have been so frequent that we are now inclined to attribute the poor results obtained either to non-removal of the fatty capsule, the glands of the pedicle and the adrenal, or to forcing tumor substance into the circulation.

For large tumors a transperitoneal exposure and primary ligation of the blood-vessels, before attempting to free the mass, is the method of choice. This considerably reduces the hemorrhage, and makes it possible to remove not only the fatty capsule and the adrenal but also a large area of adherent peritoneum, as well as the glands adjacent to the pedicle. The transperitoneal operation is, therefore, a much more radical procedure and should be the method of choice in almost all cases of malignant tumors of the kidney. (See Chapter XIV, in which we describe a new method with extensive excision of peritoneum and fat covering the kidney.)

Involvement of the ureter if present will usually be evident on palpation. Complete *ureterectomy* must then be done.

TREATMENT WITH RADIUM AND *x*-RAY.—Owing to the great frequency of recurrences and metastases after nephrectomy for malignant disease, the use of *radium* and *x-ray* must be seriously considered in all cases. If at operation there is doubt as to whether any tumor tissue or locally involved gland remains, radium should be applied *in situ*. Radium element in containers of various shapes and sizes may be employed either as a surface application or as buried needles, the laws governing the employment of radium being strictly followed and care being taken not to get a burn through important blood-vessels. Emanations of radium, if employed in the form of seed implantations or otherwise, require the same care. (See remarks on the use of radium in the sections on Neoplasms of the Bladder and Prostate.) Massive doses of radium may be used later through both lumbar and dorsal regions. The *x*-ray may likewise be used in the form of deep therapy with machines of high voltage. The object is to influence any glandular, bone, or visceral metastases that may have occurred, or to ward off metastasis from tumor cells left behind at operation. Owing to the debilitating effect of such treatment, it should be postponed ten days or more after operation.

Just what is to be expected from irradiation and the comparative value of the different methods cannot as yet be stated with any certainty. A few brilliant results make it incumbent upon us to give our patients every possible chance. Where the condition is manifestly hopeless, the use of radiotherapy is not only useless, but it is often very devitalizing and harmful. It is sometimes indicated to relieve pain. *Subsequent courses of radiotherapy* may be very advisable, on the doctrine of giving the patient every chance. Here again the limitations and indications have not been sufficiently standardized to warrant positive statements.

PALLIATIVE TREATMENT.—*Hematuria.*—If slight, or intermittent, no special attention need be paid to the loss of blood, especially in hopeless cases. If considerable or continuous and productive of a steadily increasing anemia, the use of horse-serum intravenously may be immediately successful. Blood transfusions may not only stop the hematuria promptly but also supply much needed blood. The usual careful study of patient's and donor's blood is to be made, and careful grouping and matching carried out. In one of our cases the blood of a brother was used without matching (in the early days of this work) and resulted fatally in a few hours. Various drugs have been suggested, but have never proved of much benefit in our hands.

Pelvic lavage through a ureter catheter may lead to an immediate cessation of the bleeding. Probably the best method is to wash out the pelvis with sterile water or a weak antiseptic solution and then to introduce a 1 per cent. solution of silver nitrate by gravity from a buret. Occasionally a much stronger solution— up to 5 per cent.—may be required, but is apt to cause severe reactions (pain, colic, prostration, etc.).

Adrenalin may occasionally stop the bleeding at once after intrapelvic injection of 2 or 3 c.c. of a 1:1000 solution. Tubes of radium or emanation, placed in a ureter catheter, might be employed to stop hemorrhage. So far it has not been used. In cases where nephrectomy is to be carried out it may be necessary on account of severe secondary anemia to employ some of the methods enumerated above in the course of careful preparatory treatment, before so extensive an operation can be considered. The function of the other kidney must, of course, be accurately determined, and its ability to assume the entire load must be carefully considered before removing the diseased organ.

If all other methods fail, it may be advisable in some cases to ligate and divide the ureter.

Pain.—Blockage of the ureter with blood-clots may cause severe pain which may be intermittent or continuous and require relief. Attempts to stop the hemorrhage should be carried out as above described. Anodynes may be necessary, the coal-tar derivatives being tried first, and opiates only as a last resort.

Solitary Cyst of the Kidney.—This is a very rare condition. Of the 48 cases collected by Kretschmer in 1920,[1] 11 were found at autopsy and 35 were operated upon (16 nephrectomy and 18 resection or excision), with 2 deaths, one of bronchopneumonia and one of erysipelas.

The kidney should be exposed through an extraperitoneal incision and the cyst removed by partial resection of the kidney. The sac of the cyst should be extirpated completely and the cut edges of the kidney wound approximated with catgut sutures. If the cyst (or cysts in multiple cases) be so large that no important portion of renal tissue can be saved, nephrectomy must be done.

Results.—The table given on page 536 summarizes the results of treatment in a series of 39 cases of malignant renal tumors.

One other case is of especial interest. The patient, who had had symptoms for three years previous to operation, felt perfectly well for six years following a nephrectomy performed in Boston. He then noticed a small swelling under the scar of the operation, which increased gradually for two years. When examined by us there was a large, fixed mass in the region of the kidney which had been removed—a local recurrence after six years. This indicates how conservative we must be in estimating "cures."

Figure 343, p. 537 shows graphically the length of time during which symptoms had existed prior to operation in 34 cases with satisfactory follow-up records.

From this it is evident that there is no constant relation between the duration of symptoms and the results; *i. e.*, a number of cases operated upon very soon after the onset of symptoms were not cured, while others in which the symptoms had existed a long time (five years, three and a half years, three years, two years) have had apparently good results. In 1 case, where hematuria was first noted three weeks before examination, a very large tumor, which had undoubtedly been present a long time, was found, and operation, while apparently complete, was unsuccessful.

Aneurysm of the Renal Artery.—This rare condition may well receive brief consideration at this point. According to Conroy,[2] but 32 cases have been reported, and autopsy statistics show that aneurysms of the renal artery comprise 1.2 per

[1] Journal of Urology, 1920, iv, 567–583.
[2] Annals of Surgery, 1923, lxxviii, 628–640 (Lit.).

TABLE 79

ANALYSIS OF 26 CASES OF NEPHRECTOMY FOR KIDNEY TUMOR

Nephrectomy 26.

Obviously incomplete, 7.

Of incomplete operations, 6 died.

3 months ⎫
4 months ⎪
5 months ⎬ After operation.
8 months ⎪
8 months ⎪
18 months ⎭

1 had radium treatment, is living, has "severe pain in feet," 1 year after operation.

Apparently complete, 19.

Of apparently complete operations, 10 died.

4 years ⎫
3 years ⎪
3 years ⎪
14 months ⎪ After operation, all of metastasis or recurrence except one who died
8 months ⎬ of postoperative hemorrhage.
7 months ⎪
4 months ⎪
2 months ⎪
4 days ⎪
"soon" ⎭

7 report themselves as entirely "well."

10 years ⎫
6 years ⎪
3½ years ⎪
3 years, 3 months ⎬ After operation.
2 years ⎪
1½ years ⎪
1 year, 4 months ⎭

(In the 1 case surviving ten years the tumor was a papilloma of the pelvis showing beginning malignant changes.)

One is living, and reports that he is not in good condition and has lost weight, although there is no sign of local recurrence and x-rays are negative for metastasis, 5 months after operation.

One was discharged from hospital in good condition and has failed to answer letters since.

No nephrectomy performed, 13.

The tumor was inoperable in 11.

Exploratory operation performed in 4.

Nephrostomy performed in 1.

Ureter ligated in 2.

No operation performed in 4 (of which 1 had deep x-ray treatment).

10 died: 5 years ⎫
3½ years ⎪
2 months ⎪
2 months ⎪
1 month ⎬ After appearing for treatment.
1 month ⎪
"a few weeks" ⎪
17 days ⎪
"soon" ⎪
"soon" ⎭

1 is living, tumor still present, but smaller after deep x-ray treatment. Four months after appearing for treatment.

1 died of collargol poisoning following a diagnostic pyelogram.

1 refused operation and was lost to view.

cent. of all aneurysms. On the other hand, there is no case recorded in the autopsy reports of the Johns Hopkins Hospital. The 32 reported cases include only 14 true aneurysms, the remainder being false or "dissecting aneurysms," usually following trauma. The true aneurysms are usually small, varying in size from that of a pea to that of an orange, and give no symptoms. Of 13 cases, 2 were located on the main trunk, 3 at the bifurcation, and 8 on one or another of the branches of the renal artery. The walls are often calcified and may give an x-ray shadow simulating renal stone.

The symptoms and signs of false aneurysm may come on soon after injury or be delayed, even for several months. The course is usually progressive, with fatal outcome unless operative intervention is successful. For this reason the size attained may be very great, in 1 case 25 by 20 cm., with a weight of 3490 gm. The complications are rupture into the pelvis, rupture into the peritoneum, and

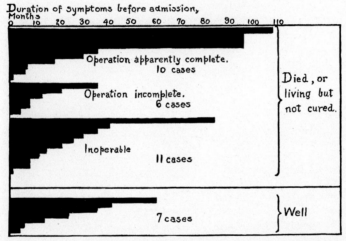

Fig. 343.—Diagram of 34 cases of malignant renal tumor, showing the relationship between duration of symptoms before admission and the results of operative treatment. Note that while the average duration of symptoms of the 7 cases *well* after operation is shorter than the average duration of symptoms of those *not well* after operation, yet in many of the cases where the result was unfavorable or the tumor so extensive that it was inoperable or that complete operation could not be done, the duration of symptoms had been very short. Each horizontal black line represents a single case.

destruction of the kidney. The common symptoms are pain and hematuria. The bleeding may be serious and even fatal. In 2 cases a throbbing sensation was experienced by the patient. Palpable tumor was present in 57 per cent. of the cases, but in only 2 was pulsation demonstrable, and in only 1 was a bruit heard.

In cases with rapid course, diagnosis from rupture of the kidney may be impossible, but this is of little importance, since operation is imperative in either case. In slower cases, renal neoplasm is simulated. The history and the comparatively rapid development of the tumor may give a clue.

The treatment is always by operation. In case of doubtful diagnosis, the sac may be nicked carefully, and if laminated clot is found, further investigation must be deferred until the pedicle is secured. In 1 case the sac was successfully removed and the artery sutured, but usually nephrectomy is indicated, and is much safer. The renal vessels must be clamped as early as possible in the procedure.

It should be stated that the renal arteries may be involved in the late stages of aneurysms of the abdominal aorta, with consequent infarct, atrophy, or compression necrosis of one or both kidneys, as illustrated in a case autopsied at the Johns Hopkins Hospital (J. H. H. Autopsy 2419).

NEOPLASMS OF THE BLADDER

PATHOLOGY

According to statistics gathered by Verhoogen,[1] bladder tumors comprise about 0.1 to 0.2 per cent. of hospital cases, 0.9 per cent. of autopsies, 0.39 per cent. of tumor cases, and about 3 per cent. of urologic cases. In our clinic bladder tumors are 4 per cent. of some 12,500 urologic cases. This indicates well enough that while comparatively rare, they are by no means exceptional. Another well-attested fact is that they are markedly more common in males than in females, the relation being given as from 92 : 8 to 66: 33, the average about 80: 20. The figures vary according to the preponderance of males or females in the practices of various authors.

In regard to age, 80 per cent. of 380 cases in our clinic were between forty and sixty-nine years old. Geraghty[2] gives the following figures:

TABLE 80

Age.	Papilloma.	Carcinoma.
10–19	1	0
20–29	5	0
30–39	13	3
40–49	23	10
50–59	18	33
60–69	11	28
70–79	2	15

In our series the youngest case was that of a boy of fourteen, who had a benign papilloma. In infants and children the embryomatous tumors appear to be more frequent, although Koll[3] has observed a papilloma in a child of thirteen months.

In general, bladder tumors may be divided for clinical purposes into: (1) Growths projecting well into the bladder, that is, papillomatous or pedunculated; (2) sessile growths, projecting less into the bladder, and spreading laterally along the mucosa, in a layer of varying thickness, from 1 mm. to 2 or 3 cm.; and (3) infiltrating growths. which penetrate all layers of the bladder and, as a rule, eventually invade the perivesical tissues. Infiltrating epithelial tumors always begin from a surface epithelial growth, pedunculated or sessile, while sarcomata, beginning as infiltrating growths of the bladder, may grow in such a manner as to show intravesical pedunculated or sessile masses.

Classifications of tumors are always unsatisfactory, but necessary. We have adopted the following grouping, which differs from that ordinarily used, (1) in that benign and malignant tumors are not separated, and (2) in that chondroma, myxoma, etc., are gathered under the general heading of embryoma. The most recent studies indicate that the fundamental processes concerned are the same in benign

[1] Encyclopædie Française d'Urologie, 1921, iv, 425–538.
[2] Cabot's Modern Urology, 1923, ii, 197–254.
[3] Quoted by Verhoogen (see Note [1]).

and malignant growths, and in the bladder especially we see this in the papillo-matous tumors.

B=benign.   M=malignant.

I. Tumors of Adult Tissue.
    1. Organoid.
        A. Epithelial:
            (a) Adenoma.
                Solid (B).
                Cystic (B).
        B. Mesothelial:
            (a) Angioma.
                Hemangioma (B).
                (Lymphangioma).
    2. Histoid.
        A. Epithelial:
            (a) Papillary tumors.
                Benign papilloma (B).
                Malignant papilloma (M).
                Papillary carcinoma (M).
            (b) Adenocarcinoma (M).
            (c) Epithelioma.
                Squamous-cell or epidermoid (M).
                Non-squamous (basal cell) (M).
        B. Mesothelial:
            (a) Sarcoma.
                Round-cell (M).
                Spindle-cell (M).
                Giant-cell (M).
            (b) Fibroma (B).
            (c) Lipoma (B).
            (d) Leiomyoma (B).
                (Lymphosarcoma.)

II. Heterotopic tumors.
    1. Embryoma:
        (a) Dermoid cyst (B and M).
        (b) Teratoma (B and M).
        (c) Rhabdomyoma (B).
        (d) Chondroma (B).
        (e) Myxoma (B).

III. Extravesical tumors.
    Retrovesical sarcoma.

Lymphosarcoma is included in parentheses because of some doubt as to whether it is properly a neoplasm, and lymphangioma because no example has been found in the literature.

I. Tumors of Adult Tissue.

1. **Organoid Tumors.**—A. EPITHELIAL.—(a) *Adenoma.*—Adenomata of the bladder are spoken of as *solid* and *cystic*. They are benign, but may play a part, not yet demonstrated, in the genesis of adenocarcinoma.

Small, slightly complicated glands, resembling those of the posterior urethra, occur rather commonly at the vesical orifice (posteriorly), in the mucosa over the trigone (subtrigonal glands, Fig. 345), and, more rarely, elsewhere in the bladder. In general, these structures are more common near the vesical orifice, and become more exceptional as one passes away from the trigone and base of the bladder.

Such glands may undergo a hyperplasia at any time in life, producing either a mass of small acini, without marked infolding of the epithelium (solid adenoma), or, if there is retention of secretion, a wholly or partially cystic one (cystic adenoma) (Fig. 344). A few goblet-cells are sometimes seen in these tumors, and the contents of the cysts may contain some mucus. This recalls the fact that the bladder is formed from the allantois, and therefore has close embryonic relations with the cloaca and hind-gut. The intestine sometimes opens into an exstrophied bladder.

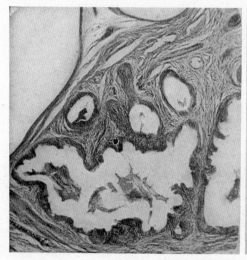 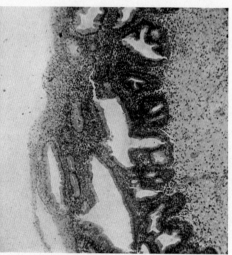

Fig. 344.—Benign cystic adenoma of the bladder. This tumor occurred on the posterior surface of the bladder in a boy of nine. Note the villous epithelial outgrowths and cystic dilatations resembling very closely benign hypertrophy of the prostate. B. U. I. Path. 3866.

Fig. 345.—Section of the bladder mucosa in the area of the trigone showing unusually well-developed subtrigonal glands. These glands are capable of undergoing hypertrophy like the prostate and may produce a large intravesical mass above the sphincter. B. U. I. Path. 1961.

In addition, since these glands resemble those of the prostatic urethra (suburethral or Albarran's glands) they also resemble the prostatic glands proper. It sometimes happens, therefore, that at the age of prostatic hypertrophy, they undergo an analogous change. Again, solid or cystic tumors may be produced, but microscopically one sees the complicated villous infoldings of the epithelium, as in prostatic hypertrophy. If this occurs in the subtrigonal glands, the tumor is usually considered a median lobe, and may often be pedunculated, acting as a ball valve, and giving rise to severe symptoms of obstruction while still small. Adenomata may rarely occur in women. This is explained by the fact that the same primitive gland groups appear in both male and female embryos, and in adult females their vestiges are still present (Johnson[1]).

In the gross, these tumors, of whichever type, appear as smooth, opaque, often yellowish-gray nodules which are usually sessile, but may be pedunculated. They

[1] Journal of Urology, 1922, viii, 13–33.

PLATE XII

VESICAL TUMORS

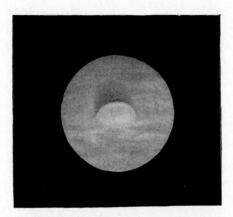

A. Small globular tumor of bladder just behind trigone. Resection, cure. Microscopic report, adenoma, benign. B. U. I. 8525.

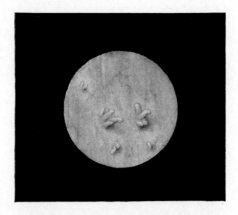

B. Multiple small benign papillomata of bladder. B. U. I. 7397.

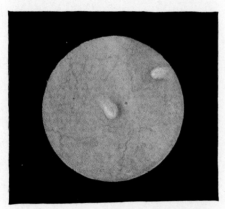

C. Small papillomata of bladder. Supposed to be benign. Fulguration. B. U. I. 11,114.

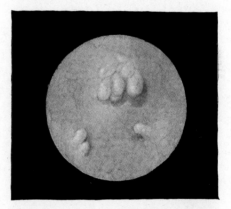

D. Recurrences in Case C after fulguration. Diagnosis, papillary carcinoma of bladder. B. U. I. 11,114.

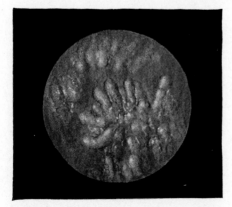

E. Papillary cystitis, simulating multiple papillary tumors, successfully treated with fulguration. B. U. I. 7533.

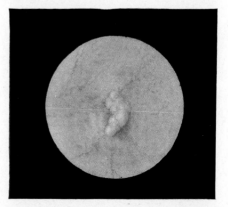

F. Small papillary carcinoma of bladder. Fulguration and radium applications. Subsequent multiple recurrences, same treatment. Final cure, followed two years. B. U. I. 5748.

are covered with essentially normal epithelium. The size is usually not large, seldom exceeding 2 cm. in diameter. The tumors are subepithelial, invasion of the muscularis not occurring (Plate XII, a).

B. MESOTHELIAL.—(a) *Angioma.*—Varices of the bladder occur frequently in conjunction with varicose conditions elsewhere, as in the pelvic veins and veins of the leg, but should be distinguished from true *hemangiomatous* new growths. The latter are extremely rare, and the description must be taken from the literature.[1]

The tumors have been small, sessile or pedunculated, and single or multiple. They were situated in the mucosa, mostly in the fundus of the bladder, and all made themselves known by abundant hemorrhage. Microscopically, they were capillary hemangiomata, the walls of the blood spaces being surrounded only by a single layer of endothelium and a very small amount of connective tissue. Scholl[2] reports and illustrates a beautiful example.

We have found no example of *lymphangioma.* The lymph varices occurring, for example, in filariasis, would have to be ruled out.

2. **Histoid Tumors.**—A. EPITHELIAL.—(a) *Papillary Tumors.*—Papillary epithelial tumors constitute the very great majority of all bladder tumors. Statistics as to the exact proportion are unobtainable, for the reason that simultaneously with the formulation of modern ideas of bladder tumor pathology, the introduction of intravesical methods of treatment deprived us of proper pathologic specimens in a large proportion of cases. It is certain, however, that papillary tumors, including benign and malignant papilloma and papillary carcinoma, comprise not far from 90 per cent. of all bladder tumors.

The pathology of the papillary tumors is more satisfactorily determined than in the case of many other tumors, especially in the urogenital tract. Briefly, there is, first of all, the *benign papilloma*, which is entirely intravesical. Every malignant papilloma probably begins as a benign papilloma, though the malignant change may occur almost as soon as the tumor appears. This tendency to assume a malignant form of growth is variable, and depends partly, but not entirely, on the age of the patient. Thus a young individual is more apt than an old one to have benign papilloma go for a long time without showing malignant changes, but is not sure to do so. In some cases benign papillomata may exist for years, be removed, and recur repeatedly, always in the benign form; in others, malignant changes appear as soon as the papilloma manifests itself. The average course is between these two.

Since the gross appearances are best interpreted in the light of the histology, it is best to study the histology first. The benign papilloma appears first as a very tiny excrescence on the surface epithelium. The initial stages have been best observed in the case of recurrences, where they were seen in the presymptomatic stage, as the result of routine cystoscopic re-examination. The epithelium covering this excrescence differs but slightly from that of the normal bladder, the cell layer may be a little thicker, or a little thinner, but the cells are of the usual type, are arranged in regular layers, and show no irregularities in size, shape, or staining. In the middle is a core of connective tissue, containing capillaries and lymphatics. It is manifestly secondary to the epithelial overgrowth, and contains no muscle, or tissues other than those mentioned. As the papilloma grows, its

---

[1] Broca: Gazette des Hôpitaux, 1868; Albarran: Tumeurs de la vessie, Paris, 1892.

[2] Surgery, Gynecology, and Obstetrics, 1923, xxxiv, 189–198.

increase is much more marked longitudinally, that is, at right angles to the original bladder mucosa, than it is laterally. There is produced, therefore, a papillary process having the same general microscopic picture as that described for the early stage. The papillæ may be long and slender or short and stubby. Soon,

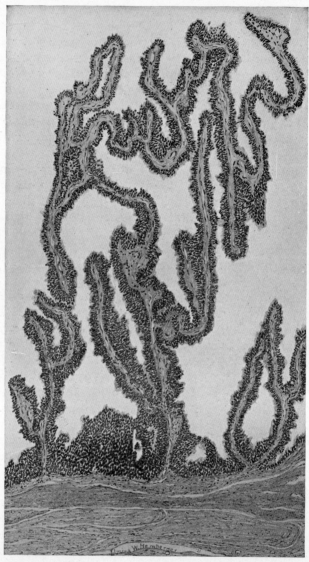

Fig. 346.—Microscopic drawing of benign papilloma of the bladder showing the very intricate branching which may occur. From the Pathologic Laboratory, Yale University Medical School, through the courtesy of Dr. M. C. Winternitz.

however, another characteristic feature appears, especially in tumors with long papillæ, namely, branching of the papillæ, so that very complicated tree-like structures are produced (Fig. 346).

Secondary changes within the papilloma may be produced by circulatory difficulties incident to its complicated structure, by infection, by trauma, or by various forms of local treatment. They include edema, congestion, hemorrhage, cellular infiltration, epithelial desquamation, and necrosis, which may be partial or include the entire tumor. These changes may alter the appearance of the tumor markedly, both gross and microscopic. The important points to be looked for are: (1) Uniform thickness of epithelial layer, thinner or only moderately thicker than normal bladder epithelium; (2) regular, orderly arrangement of epithelial cells, with definite basal layer, the middle layer of fusiform or "tailed" cells, with long axis at right angles to the basement membrane, and more superficial layers of a squamous type without cornification; (3) uniformity in size, shape, and staining of the nuclei; (4) absence of mitotic figures; (5) absence of fusion of papillæ, and (6) if the base of the papilloma is in the preparation, absence of any invasion of the bladder wall (Figs. 346–349).

Malignant changes in a *papilloma* are characterized especially by the following features: (1) Thickening, generalized or local, of the epithelial layer; (2) loss of the

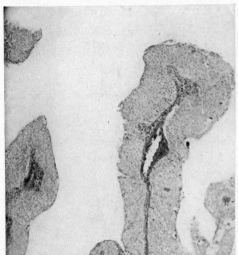

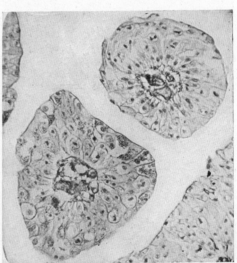

FIG. 347.—Benign papilloma of the bladder. Note the regular arrangement of the epithelial cells and the presence of basal and peripheral layers. B. U. I. Path. 3935.

FIG. 348.—Benign papilloma of the bladder. Higher magnification of two small papillæ. Note the absence of any tendency to coalescence. B. U. I. Path. 3938.

regular, orderly arrangement of the epithelial cells, often to be seen as the absence of the normal differences between the cells of the outer and of the basal layers and suppression of the middle layer of "tailed" cells; (3) lack of uniformity in size, shape, and staining of the nuclei, often with some very large, irregular nuclei, and some small pyknotic ones; nucleoli may be more prominent than normal; (4) fusion between the epithelial layers of adjacent papillæ (Fig. 350). This fusion produces sometimes rather puzzling pictures (Fig. 351). Since the space between the papillæ is obliterated, one sees in the preparation a thick layer of epithelial cells bounded on each side by a connective-tissue stalk containing capillaries. This picture is well represented in Figs. 353 to 355, and should be kept in mind, as it is essentially the same as the type of growth which eventually invades the bladder wall, and is then known as *papillary carcinoma*. We make this distinction to keep separate the growth projecting entirely into the bladder (malignant papilloma) and growths invading the wall (papillary carcinoma). Strictly speaking, the malignant papilloma is a carcinoma too. Little stress can be laid on the presence

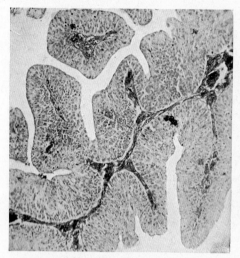

FIG. 349.—Another example of benign papilloma of the bladder. B. U. I. Path. 3938.

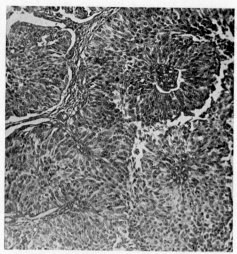

FIG. 350.—Beginning malignant change in papilloma of the bladder. The papillæ while still distinguishable are beginning to fuse and in some places the layered arrangement of the epithelium is lost. B. U. I. Path. 4911.

of mitotic figures. They are not an indication of malignancy, but rather, in a general way, of the rapidity of the growth going on in the tissue. In addition,

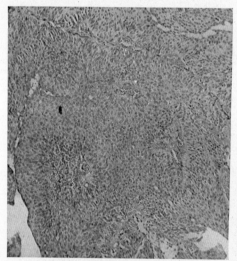

FIG. 351.—Papillary carcinoma of the bladder. This picture represents a more advanced malignant change. The general outlines of the papillæ can still be detected, but there has been extensive fusion, and excepting immediately around the connective-tissue cores the layered arrangement of the cells is lost. B U. I. Path. 3021.

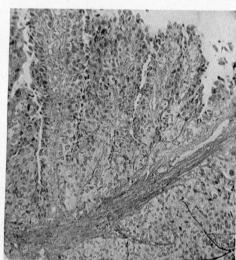

FIG. 352.—Papillary carcinoma of the bladder. In the upper part the papillary structures can still be seen, while in the lower part fusion has been complete and there is a solid carcinomatous growth. B. U. I. Path. 2172.

mitotic figures disappear from specimens of tissue if they are allowed to remain unfixed very long after death or removal. Therefore, the absence of mitotic figures is of no significance, the presence of one or a very few mitotic figures is of no importance, as these may be found in normal tissues, while the presence of a

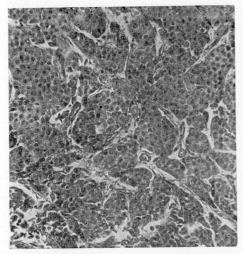

FIG. 353.—Papillary carcinoma of the bladder. Here in the depths of the tumor papillary architecture can no longer be made out. The type of cell is characteristic for this growth. B. U. I. Path. 2074.

FIG. 354.—Papillary carcinoma of the bladder. Higher magnification in which the epithelial character of the cells and variations in the size and shape of the nuclei are well shown. B. U. I. Path. 4910.

very large number of mitotic figures indicates a very rapid growth process in the tissue, suggesting, but not proving, malignancy. This suggestion is even stronger

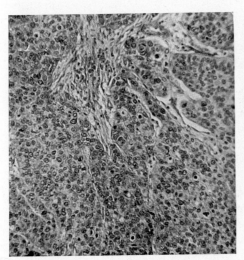

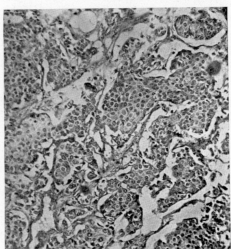

FIG. 355.—Another example of papillary carcinoma of the bladder showing many mitotic figures. B. U. I. Path. 2379.

FIG. 356.—Metastasis from papillary carcinoma of the bladder to a cervical lymph-node. The characteristics of the tumor growth are retained. B. U. I. Path. 3046.

if some of the mitotic figures are atypical, as when 3 or 4 centrosomes (indicating two or three planes of division instead of one) are present. Mitotic figures may be absent from preparations of malignant growths: (1) Because they have disappeared (by completion of the cell division) before the tissue was fixed, or (2) because they may be extremely infrequent in slow-growing tumors.

The degree and extent of the malignant changes in the papillary tumor bear little relation to the time when invasion of the bladder wall begins. Thus invasion may occur when there is only a small area of malignant change near the base of the papilloma, or the entire intravesical tumor may become malignant before any invasive process is demonstrable. Where invasion does occur, however, the tumor microscopically is exactly the same as that seen in malignant papilloma after fusion of the papillæ. Indeed, if fusion of the papillæ is complete at the base of the papilloma, it may be impossible to tell just where the invasive portion of the growth begins. The interpapillary spaces being eliminated, the cores of the papillæ now appear as fine strands or trabeculæ, enclosing elongated nests of tumor cells of the same type as those described in malignant papilloma. If, however, the section happens to be cut at right angles to some of these cores, we see simply a mass of tumor cells containing here and there small round areas of connective tissue and capillaries. Occasionally this tissue may be shrunken or degenerated, or may fall out of the section, leaving a hole resembling a lumen, and giving a fallacious appearance of an adenocarcinomatous process. This error can be avoided only by very careful study of a number of slides. The typical picture described may be altered in parts of the tumor, especially as follows: (1) At the edges, where invasive growth is occurring from the nests of tumor cells, the invasive masses may push into the normal tissue in such a manner that the cell nests are smaller, more elongated, and more compressed, and the connective-tissue trabeculæ between them much wider than in the original part of the tumor. In trabeculæ formed in this way muscle, fat, larger blood-vessels, etc., may be found. (2) In other parts of the tumor where, apparently, growth is rapid, the cell nests or strands may reproduce themselves in small and irregular forms, the connective tissue and vascular framework also being scanty and very irregular. In such places the typical low-power architecture may be scarcely recognizable, but its essential features and cell picture remain the same, and one can usually find the typical appearance somewhere else in the tumor.

The *gross appearance* can be correlated fairly well with the microscopic picture. Since this is so, it is well to consider it here, even though it is the cystoscopic appearance that is described. (The cystoscope is much the best way to examine the intravesical aspect of bladder tumors.) At operation or autopsy the surface appearance is altered by hemorrhage, trauma, etc., but, on the other hand, one is able to palpate invasions and extensions not seen at cystoscopy.

The early *benign papilloma* is a small, slightly irregular excrescence on the bladder wall, of practically the same color as the surrounding mucosa, and, in the absence of inflammation, without any halo of redness about it. This is because its epithelium is practically the same thickness as the normal epithelium, and its blood-supply about the same. In later stages it may be seen as a tree-like structure, the branches being fine, translucent, and uniform in size, or it may consist of short stubby papillæ, branching little or not at all. Its color is usually a trifle redder than that of the rest of the bladder, due probably to some trauma from the contractions of the bladder. Sometimes the branches are so closely packed together that it appears as a solid mass, but if a stream of water is directed at it, its structure may be revealed. These typical appearances can be altered in various ways.

If hemorrhage has occurred from the papilloma, adherent clots of blood or actual bleeding may be seen. If infection has occurred, shreds of pus may partially conceal the tumor, but it is remarkable how the benign papilloma resists infection. It may remain unchanged in the presence of a severe cystitis. Edema and cellular infiltration are, therefore, rare. If part or all the tumor becomes necrotic from infection, torsion of the pedicle, or therapeutic efforts, such as fulguration, cauterization, or radium, one sees the affected portion converted into a white, perfectly opaque mass. Sloughing of the necrotic tissue leaves a small clean ulcer, which heals quickly, or part of the tumor, reddened and edematous, may remain. In this case the surrounding bladder mucosa is inflamed, and edematous mucosal bullæ may make it difficult to outline the actual tumor. This is an important point, as persistent slough and inflammatory changes after fulguration indicate

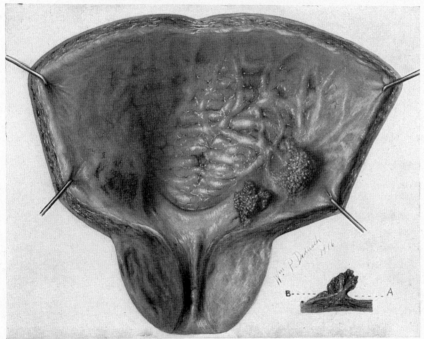

Fig. 357.—Autopsy specimen. Multiple papillomata of bladder. Invasion of bladder wall from pedicle is shown (B).

malignancy. If there is little or no infection, the slough may remain in place long enough to become encrusted with calcareous deposits.

Benign papillomata may be large or small, and almost always single at the beginning. In the larger tumors the size of the pedicle, excluding edema, bears rough relation to the size of the tumor. In some tumors a good-sized pedicle-like process raised up from the mucosa seems to bear a number of closely set, but separate papillomata. Papillomata appear to have the property of spreading by implantation, but the tendency to implant is much more marked in malignant cases, and is, therefore, of diagnostic significance. If a bladder containing a papilloma is opened, and the papilloma handled and removed, multiple implantations and recurrences of the tumor are apt to occur. Implantations in the intact bladder also occur at points opposite the original tumor or elsewhere. Multiple small papillomata may arise in the immediate neighborhood of the original tumor (Fig. 357). In severe, advanced cases large areas, even the entire interior of the bladder, may become covered by masses of papillomatous tumor—known as general papillomatosis of the bladder, which is always malignant. In one of our cases there were about 100 minute papillomata present. The mechanism of late recurrence, weeks or months after destruction of the original tumor, is not clearly understood. It may represent a tumor formation *de novo*, or the development of a tiny portion of the primary growth left behind.

Location.—Tumors of the bladder, both benign and malignant, occur in far greater frequency in the region of the trigone and ureteral orifices, than in all the other portions of the bladder put together, as shown in the chart (Fig. 358), upon which we have recorded the site as accurately as possible in 209 cases.[1]

Malignant changes are often totally imperceptible in the gross. When they are marked enough to be seen, the most characteristic feature is an appearance of

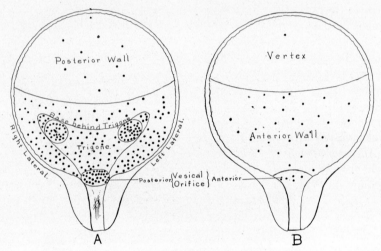

Fig. 358.—Chart showing frequency of location of vesical tumors. Diagram carefully prepared from 209 cases, benign and malignant bladder tumors. Note the infrequency of tumors on the vertex and high posterior wall. The relative infrequency on anterior wall. Great frequency in base, particularly in region of ureteral and prostatic orifices.

thickening of the papillæ—sometimes only slight—which is grayish and opaque, due to the relative increase in epithelial elements. Where the changes are more advanced, the fusion of the papillæ can be seen, and finally the tumor may be converted into an almost solid mass. In this process the pedicle becomes thickened; if invasion of the bladder wall occurs, it may become very thick, so that the tumor appears almost or quite sessile. The detection of early malignancies in papillomata is impossible by the eye alone, and in case of doubt a therapeutic test, to be described later, should be applied. Malignant papillomata recur and fragments become implanted in the bladder or in wound tracts like benign papillomata. Likewise, in a few cases, areas of considerable size may be covered by multiple malignant papillomata, apparently arising separately.

Invasion of the bladder wall is not easy to determine on gross ocular examination. One looks for marked thickening of the pedicle, and, in the zone surround-

[1] Young and Scott: New York Medical Journal and Medical Record, 1923, cxviii, 262–268

ing the intravesical tumor, for thickening, usually rather nodular, in the mucosa. This picture is often obscured by inflammatory changes in the early stages, but the inflammatory changes themselves, especially if localized about the tumor, suggest infiltration. Later, as the growth becomes more extensive, the enlargement is observable as an actual encroachment on the bladder cavity, and the irregular thickening of the bladder wall is seen in the form of rather papular elevations of the mucosa, which are opaque, and markedly congested and reddened. If the area is palpated, it is markedly indurated. Necrosis is common in the larger tumors, leaving ulcerations of various sizes, usually with grayish base, covered with shreds of mucopus, and elevated, irregular borders. The invasion may extend in various directions, to the prostate, vesicles, or other perivesical tissues, with induration and fixation. Any type of tumor may become invasive, so that a diagnosis of "infiltrating" or "invasive" carcinoma is not complete from a pathologic point of view. If microscopic specimens are obtained, it will be found that a great majority of all infiltrating carcinomas of the bladder are papillary carcinomas. The intravesical portion of the tumor will usually be present, at least in part, but occasionally, in late cases, it will be entirely sloughed away. Infiltrating tumors are usually single, but sometimes the tumor invades the walls of the bladder throughout its entire extent. This result is more apt to follow in the case of multiple malignant papillomata covering wide areas, spreading horizontally along the bladder surface with, at first, no tendency to invade the bladder wall. This is truly a transition between malignant papilloma and papillary carcinoma, since the papillary processes are completely fused, and the growth is low and sessile in appearance, yet invasion does not occur until late.

(b) *Adenocarcinoma* is rare, not over 1 or 2 per cent. of all bladder tumors. Its mechanism of origin is not known, but it is possible that it arises from small gland groups in the bladder like those concerned in adenoma. Verhoogen adopts this explanation. It is remarkable that the histology of some of them resembles closely that of prostatic carcinoma in the arrangement of the epithelial cells, and in the absence of the ordinary cellular and nuclear stigmata of malignancy. (Irregularity in size, shape, and staining.)

Microscopically, the tumor may be seen projecting into the bladder, but invasion of the bladder wall is seldom if ever absent. There may be good-sized masses or nests of cells, with a moderate amount of rather clear protoplasm and oval, not especially irregular, nuclei. In the cell masses are numerous open spaces, usually rounded, resembling gland lumina (Fig. 359). The cells bordering these spaces often show regular circumferential arrangements. Many of these spaces are separated only by tumor cells, no connective-tissue trabeculæ or capillaries intervening, which arrangement recalls the "pseudo-acini" in the "alveolar carcinoma" type of growth seen in carcinoma of the prostate. In other areas the lumina may be lined by a single layer of cuboidal cells resting directly on a thin basement membrane. Elsewhere actively invasive growth, consisting of small nests and strands of rather undifferentiated cells without lumina, is seen. The amount of stroma varies greatly, but is usually greater in the invasive portions. Geraghty believes that this type of tumor is closely related to papillary carcinoma, that is, that certain papillary carcinomata develop pseudo-acini or gland-like spaces so that the designation *papillary adenocarcinoma* would apply (Fig. 361).

In other cases the picture is dominated by multiple, small, irregular, rounded or polygonal acini, often massed closely together, but separated from one another by connective-tissue stroma. This stroma may be scanty or abundant; when abundant the tumor is very hard and leathery. This type is less apt to show

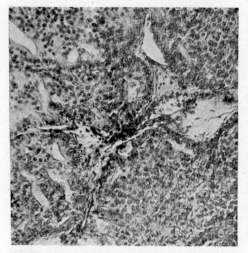

FIG. 359.—Adenocarcinoma of the bladder. Many of the lumina are not separated by connective-tissue trabeculæ. B. U. I. Path. 4719.

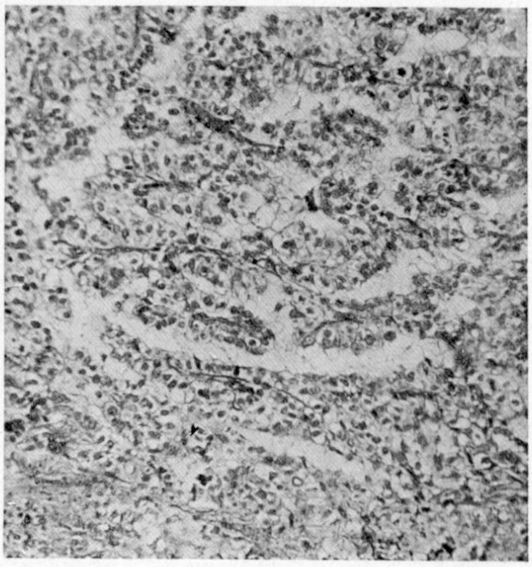

FIG. 360.—An unusual tumor of the bladder, probably best described as a tubular adenocarcinoma. B. U. I. Path. 2551.

masses projecting into the bladder. The cells and their nuclei are apt to be smaller and more compact than in the first type. Again, there is little irregularity in size, shape, and staining of the nuclei and undifferentiated invasive growth around the

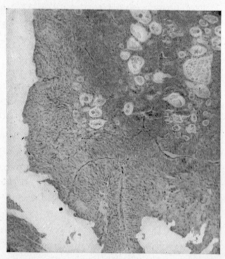

FIG. 361.—Papillary carcinoma of the bladder showing a very unusual picture in which apparently through localized degeneration of tumor cells many spaces or pseudo-acini have been produced. Compare this picture with those of adenocarcinoma (Figs. 359, 360). B. U. I. Path. 2742.

periphery is common. This is in marked similarity to prostatic carcinoma and some of these tumors very likely do originate in the prostate.

Very rarely one sees a tumor resembling a rectal tumor, with gland-like structures lined with cylindric epithelium and goblet-cells, and filled with mucus (Figs. 362–364). These tumors have been described as "colloid cancer."

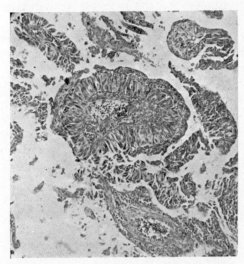

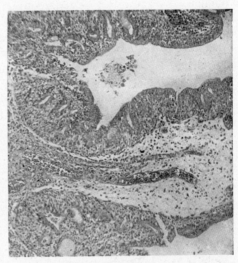

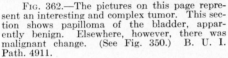

FIG. 362.—The pictures on this page represent an interesting and complex tumor. This section shows papilloma of the bladder, apparently benign. Elsewhere, however, there was malignant change. (See Fig. 350.) B. U. I. Path. 4911.

FIG. 363.—At the edge of the malignant papilloma was found this adenomatous structure, apparently benign. B. U. I. Path. 4911.

They are, no doubt, due to the retention in the bladder of small bits of epithelium of the intestinal type owing to developmental abnormalities at the time the division

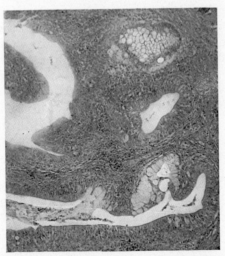

FIG. 364.—Another area in the adenomatous structure showing goblet-cells which resemble closely intestinal epithelium. This adenoma is probably entirely independent of the papillary carcinoma and represents a fetal inclusion of a bit of the cloacal epithelium. B. U. I. Path. 4911.

of the cloaca into the rectum and urogenital sinus occurs. In support of this theory is the fact that this type of tumor is more common in exstrophy of the bladder.

In the gross, adenocarcinoma is practically always found on the base of the bladder, often on the trigone or near the vesical orifice. The tumor may project for some distance into the bladder, and may even have a thick pedicle, but no papillary structure can be made out. More often it appears sessile, though the edges may roll out, giving a mushroom appearance. This point is made to show that a pedunculated tumor does not necessarily arise as a papilloma. As stated above, infiltration is the rule and can usually be seen as a thickened, roughened area in the bladder wall around the tumor, indurated to the touch. In the same way ulceration is common. There is nothing to distinguish the ulcers in the gross from other malignant ulcers of the bladder.

(c) *Epithelioma.*—The designation of "epithelioma" is reserved for certain types of bladder tumor, though it should be remembered that papillary neoplasms are, strictly speaking, epitheliomatous in character, since they develop from the preformed epithelium of the bladder. It should not be surprising, therefore, that certain similarities are found, or that in some cases it is not altogether easy to make the distinction.

Epitheliomata, so-called, are characterized by a growth consisting of strands or columns growing down from the epithelium and penetrating the subepithelial layers. The picture resembles very closely that seen in epitheliomata of the skin. In spite of the character of the growth, the tendency to invade the muscular coat is at first slight; the tumor tends to heap up somewhat on the surface, and to spread horizontally along the mucosa. Ulceration is the rule, even in early cases. There is no papilla formation, and therefore relatively little intravesical growth. Eventually the bladder wall is invaded, the perivesical tissues attacked, and metastases occur. Epitheliomata may occur in any part of the bladder, not especially the base.

Microscopically one may see, in a good preparation, the normal mucosa coming up to the edge of the neoplasm, where it commences to throw out strands of somewhat altered epithelial cells, downward into the deeper tissues. The surface of the growth itself is often ulcerated. The strands grow irregularly in every direction, just as in the skin, and at their tips may be very attentuated. The thickness of the stroma between the strands varies greatly, depending on the direction the epithelial growth has taken—in other words, the framework is not a definite secondary formation, like the connective-tissue cores in papillary tumors, and therefore lacks all uniformity. There is usually a round-cell infiltration of the stroma, increased by infection, but always present, and indicating, by its intensity and extent, the tissue reaction to the neoplasm. If the epithelial strands have reached beyond the zone of cellular infiltration it may be assumed, as in the skin, that malignancy is fully established, and that the tumor has outstripped the protective mechanism of the organism. In early cases the neoplastic cells stop sharply at the muscular layer. As growth continues the tumor heaps up on the surface and may produce good-sized sessile or even mushroom-like masses. Central ulceration is then the rule. In other cases lateral growth is more pronounced, and one may see tumor masses pushing out under normal epithelium.

Cells forming these tumors may be of the *squamous* type; or of the less differentiated type—the *basal cell* epithelioma of Krompecher. In the squamous-cell type one sees the cells becoming larger and paler toward the centers of the nests or strands, and intercellular fibrillæ (prickle-cells) may sometimes be seen, while at the centers the nuclei are lost, epidermization occurs, and typical epithelial pearls are formed (Figs. 364–368). In other cases epidermization is not complete, and cells may be desquamated into a central cavity while the nucleus can still be identi-

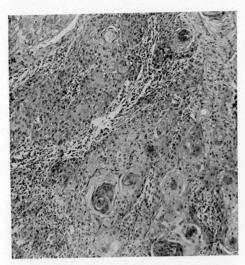

FIG. 365.—Squamous-celled epithelioma of the bladder (epidermoid carcinoma). The absolutely typical architecture of this growth is well shown. It differs in no way from squamous-celled epithelioma of the skin. B. U. I. Path. 2866.

FIG. 366.—Higher magnification of the same type of tumor. The cell characteristics and a small pearl are well shown. B. U. I. Path. 2668.

fied. Such cells break down eventually into a granular débris, different from the concentric, keratinized layers of the pearl, but the picture is definite and charac-

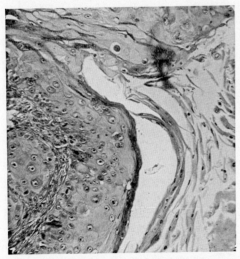

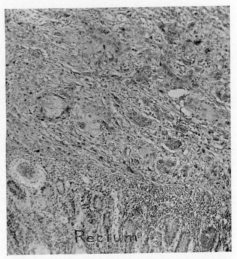

FIG. 367.—Higher magnification of the edge of a large pearl showing very well the process of epidermization and desquamation. B. U. I. Path. 2668.

FIG. 368.—Squamous-celled epithelioma arising in the bladder invading the rectum. The entire wall of the rectum except the mucosa has been invaded. B. U. I. Path. 4413.

teristic. Why squamous-cell epithelioma should occur in the bladder has long been a subject for debate, but most authorities agree that a pre-existing leukoplakia is probably necessary for its formation.   Hinman and Gibson[1] feel that leukoplakia is always the result of chronic inflammation, epidermization being the response to chronic inflammation in different kinds of epithelium in various parts of the body. Verhoogen, on the other hand, maintains that the leukoplakia may be congenital, citing cases of young infants where leukoplakia was found with no trace of inflammation.   Geraghty has seen leukoplakia of the kidney pelvis with sterile urine.

In the other type of epithelioma the tendency to epidermization is slight or absent (Figs. 369, 370).   The strands of neoplastic cells are often solid, with no marked differentiation between the central and peripheral cells.   In other cases there may be a central degeneration going on to necrosis, or consisting only in a shrinkage of the cells so that spaces are left between them.   These pictures are well illustrated in the accompanying photomicrographs.

In the gross, epithelioma is usually a flat tumor, projecting little into the bladder cavity.   In the cases showing lateral growth one may see numerous small heaped-

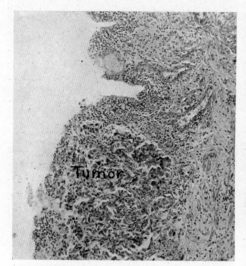

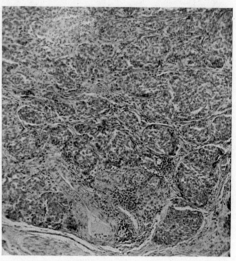

Fig. 369.—This section shows the edge of a very small basal cell epithelioma of the bladder which at the time of removal was still superficial and had not invaded the muscularis. B. U. I. Path. 4163.

Fig. 370.—The center of the same basal cell epithelioma of the bladder. At the bottom can be seen the beginning of the muscularis which is nowhere invaded. B. U. I. Path. 4163.

up masses of tumor tissue, opaque and yellowish, apparently resting on the surface of the vesical mucosa, which is otherwise normal.   Where the growth is more coherent one may see a flat, wafer-like mass, or a mushroom-like projection.   With these, ulceration is to be expected; the remaining tumor tissue gives the ulcer a thickened, elevated edge.   Invasion of the bladder wall causes thickening and induration.

B. MESOTHELIAL TUMORS.—(*a*) *Sarcoma* of the bladder is rare; no exact figures as to its occurrence are available.   Verhoogen states that sarcomata form less than 5 per cent. of bladder tumors, and this is surely a generous estimate. Geraghty found two possible sarcomata in 180 cases at our clinic, and Albarran two in 89 cases of bladder tumors.   They may occur at any age, but are apparently more frequent in the very young and in the aged than in middle life.

[1] Journal of Urology, 1921, vi, 1–50.

Sarcomata begin, of course, beneath the epithelium. They may, however, push the mucosa before them and project into the bladder as sessile growths. A certain amount of mushrooming may be present, and occasionally pedunculation may occur. The growth is usually single, though multiple tumors are reported. Invasion of the bladder wall is usually early and may be extensive, and may occur without any intravesical growth. The tumors may occur in any part of the bladder. The commonest sarcoma in the bladder region is the retrovesical sarcoma. Invasion of the bladder by it or by other sarcomata is possible, but the extensive growth elsewhere, which has occurred before the bladder invasion, will be made out.

Microscopically, sarcoma of the bladder may be round-, spindle-, mixed-, or giant-celled, with the familiar appearance of each. Malignancy is shown by invasiveness, metastases, and cellular changes; irregularity in size, shape, and stain-

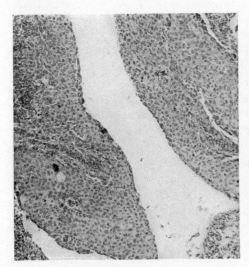

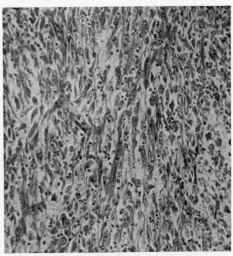

Fig. 371.—Typical papillary carcinoma of the bladder. B. U. I. Path. 4797, 4607.

Fig. 372.—Another section from the same tumor shown in the preceding picture. This illustrates beautifully how papillary carcinoma may, in rare instances, assume a type of growth almost indistinguishable from spindle-cell sarcoma. It emphasizes the necessity for examining microscopically all parts of a tumor. B. U. I. Path. 4797, 4607.

ing of the nuclei, multinuclear cells, and abundant and atypical mitoses. Central necrosis is common. In some cases of spindle-cell sarcoma the strands of tumor cells are separated by a quantity of semifluid, gelatinous material. Such cases are known as myxosarcoma, but they suggest an embryomatous nature. In a case seen by us (B. U. I. No. 11,325, B. U. I. Path. 4607 and 4797), the intravesical tumor removed at operation showed a beautiful picture of spindle-cell sarcoma. The nuclei were quite large, and the cytoplasm took a definite blue tinge of hematoxylin. Later, however, the patient, in whom the tumor recurred rapidly, passed a small fragment of typical papillary carcinoma (Figs. 371, 372). No autopsy could be obtained. The interpretation of such a case is obscure, and Verhoogen[1] calls attention to similar cases. He believes that the carcinoma cells, when packed together in the tissues in a certain way, may be elongated and take on the fusiform

[1] Encyclopædie Française d'Urologie, 1921, iv, 425–538.

shape suggesting spindle-cell sarcoma. One must, therefore, be very conservative in making a final diagnosis of sarcoma of the bladder, especially if it be the spindle-cell type.

(b) *Fibroma* is also a rare tumor of the bladder. No case of it has occurred in our clinic. It is described (Verhoogen[1]) as a tumor, usually single and not very large, with a definite tendency to form a pedicle, which may be long and slender.[2] A very few large specimens are described. The bladder wall is never infiltrated. The consistence may vary from hard to quite soft. Microscopically, the tumor is composed of interlacing bands of fibrous tissue, often with a few lymphocytes and plasma cells. Necrosis and ulceration do not occur, as a rule, but there may be cyst-like spaces due to central degeneration. In the presence of such cysts, one would have to rule out an embryoma carefully, by noting the absence of any epithelial lining. In the soft tumors the cells are separated by quantities of semifluid, mucoid material (myxofibroma). Calcification may occur.

Certain authors have interpreted as fibromyomata structures about the vesical orifice which will be found described under contracture of the vesical orifice, median bar, hypertrophy of the trigone, and benign prostatic hypertrophy.

(c) *Lipoma.*—Only a few cases of lipoma are recorded in the literature. They are small, sessile, multiple, and of a yellow color. Microscopically, they show ordinary fat cells, usually larger than normal, with a fibrous capsule. Apparently they cause no symptoms, all having been found by chance in autopsies.

(d) *Leiomyoma.*—A very few cases of leiomyoma of the bladder have been described. They apparently originate in the muscular coat, and as they grow, may push into the bladder cavity, or in the opposite direction, into the perivesical tissues. They often contain much fibrous tissue, some having been called fibro-myoma. Likewise there may be numerous dilated blood-vessels, and Kidd and Turnbull[3] have called one such tumor an angiomyoma. Ordinarily the microscopic picture is like that of uterine myomata, with interlacing bundles of smooth muscle. Sarcomatous changes may occur. The intravesical types may be pedunculated. Some myomata become very large, one (Pollailon) weighing 3 kilograms, and another (Kouznetski) 9 kilograms. While often covered with normal vesical mucosa, superficial ulceration may occur. Dilated vessels are often present, giving rise to hemorrhage. Of 740 cases of bladder tumor in the literature, 19 were myomata. On the other hand, there is no case in our series of over 500 bladder tumors. Concetti[4] reports 6 myomata among 41 cases of bladder tumor in children, suggesting a greater frequence in early years.

Intravesical prostatic lobes containing considerable smooth muscle should not be mistaken for myomata. Certain other bladder tumors may, however, also contain a few muscle-fibers.

Tumors containing striated muscle are probably embryomatous, and are described under that heading.

(e) *Lymphosarcoma.*—Lymphosarcomatous nodules may occur in the bladder, but seldom form an important feature of the general disease, though they may rarely cause obstruction. The microscopic picture is typical of the disease.

[1] Encyclopædie Française d'Urologie, 1921, iv, 425–538.
[2] Koll: Journal of Urology, 1923, ix, 453–460.
[3] Surgery, Gynecology, and Obstetrics, 1923, xxxvi, 467–472.
[4] Archives de médecine des enfants, 1900, iii, 129–158.

II. Heterotopic Tumors.—1. EMBRYOMA.—(*a*) *Dermoid cyst.* (*b*) *Teratoma.* (*c*) *Rhabdomyoma.* (*d*) *Chondroma.* (*e*) *Myxoma.*—Under this heading have been included all tumors which apparently arise from embryonic tissue. The most complete embryomata are the teratomata, which may show a large cyst, where it may even be possible to distinguish the opposite poles of the embryo (dermoid cyst), multiple small cysts (cystic teratoma), or a solid structure (solid teratoma). All of these tumors are distinguished by the presence of a multiplicity of tissues, representing at least two of the embryonic germ layers.

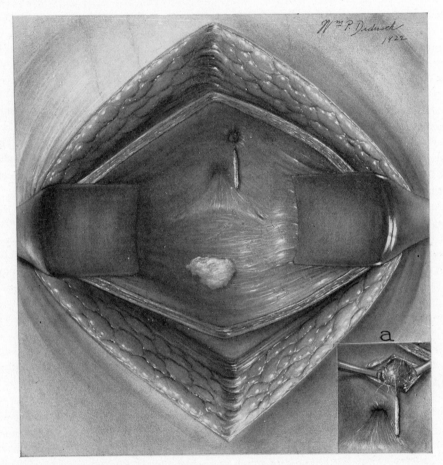

FIG. 373.—Dermoid cyst of anterior wall of bladder. Slender calculus formed around hair projecting into bladder cavity. *a*, Excision of prevesical cyst. B. U. I. 8808.

Dermoid cysts are very rare, but may occur at any age. They may arise in the bladder wall itself, having been observed on the trigone, or in the tissues in the immediate neighborhood of the bladder. In a case observed by us the cyst originated anterior to the bladder behind the symphysis pubis.

Sooner or later the cyst communicates with the bladder by a fistulous opening, and discharges its contents into the cavity. In 1 case strands of hair grew out into the bladder and on these slender calculi swung from the cystic orifice (Fig. 373).

Microscopically, skin, with hairs and sebaceous glands, is practically always present. There may be also embryonic connective tissue, often edematous, fat, smooth and striated muscle, cartilage, bone, teeth, intestinal and other types of epithelium, often with papillary arrangement, etc. The cystic cavity contains desquamated epidermis, a greasy material suggesting vernix caseosa, and hairs. The presence of these in the urine, especially hairs, is diagnostic. Malignant degeneration, usually of the embryonal carcinoma type, may occur. Hairs projecting into the bladder may become encrusted with calcareous material, and thus form the nuclei of stones.

Cystic teratoma is rarer. In the Encyclopædie Française d'Urologie it is stated that Blick, Thomson, Bryant, and Delpech have described cases. In each of these the tumor was polypoid and showed no malignancy. The cysts were lined with columnar epithelium. In some the differentiation into various tissues was more pronounced, resembling, except for the multilocular character, dermoid cysts. The stroma is of embryonic connective tissue, which in the more differentiated cases may show muscle, cartilage, etc.

Solid teratoma is also rare, but we believe that under this heading should be put those tumors showing a mixture of fibromatous or sarcomatous stroma with glandular epithelial structures. These tumors recall the embryomata occurring in the kidneys of infants, formerly known as adenosarcoma or sarcocarcinoma.

Any teratomatous tumor may undergo malignant degeneration, usually in the form of embryonal carcinoma, and but rarely sarcomatous. Blecher and Martins (1913)[1] have described a tumor containing syncytial masses, analogous to chorio-epithelioma of the uterus, ovary, and testicle. The observation is unique.

Other tumors containing or composed entirely of tissues foreign to the normal bladder are probably teratomatous in origin. According to Rokitansky, we may assume that one tissue overgrows the others, dominating the entire picture. Thus in the bladder there may be rhabdomyoma, chondroma, myxoma, etc. Tumors of striated muscles (rhabdomyoma) are exceedingly rare in the bladder, only a very few cases having been reported. Two cases have been described as *chondroma*, but it is likely that they were mixed tumors (teratoma) containing a large proportion of cartilage. The exact position of the *myxomata* is doubtful. As we have seen, both myxofibroma and myxosarcoma have been described, also myxomatous infiltration of leiomyomata. Most of the tumors thought to be true myxomata have been described in infants. They are rounded, often lobulated, usually pedunculated, and markedly soft and translucent. The structure recalls that of embryonic connective tissue, with fusiform and stellate young fibroblasts in a plentiful gelatinous matrix. With this structure, it is reasonable to place them among the embryomata. They have no doubt much in common with the myxoid tumors occurring elsewhere, of which the most familiar is the retroperitoneal myxoma. Like them, they do not, as a rule, metastasize, but tend to recur unless very radically removed.

III. **Extravesical Tumors.**—*Retrovesical Sarcoma.*—Many tumors arise in the tissues adjoining the bladder, which it is not necessary to discuss, but one of them, the *retrovesical sarcoma*, is associated with no particular organ, and, in its symptoms and diagnosis, concerns mostly the bladder. It is found in the space behind the bladder, above the prostate, and between the seminal vesicles. Histologically, it is usually a small round-cell sarcoma, but may be spindle-celled. In its growth it

[1] Quoted by Verhoogen, Encyclopædie Française d'Urologie, 1921, iv, 425–538.

pushes the bladder forward, the rectum backward, and usually the prostate downward. Depending on its exact manner of growth, the seminal vesicles lie on its posterior surface, are squeezed between it and the bladder, or are completely surrounded by it. Layers of growth may be sent down around the prostate. The ureters may be surrounded and pressed upon, causing obstruction. Actual invasion of all these structures is, however, late, and often they can be found intact in the midst of large growths. The same is true for the bladder wall itself. It is usual to see the bladder pushed forward by a large, rounded growth, the mucosa entirely intact. Microscopic section shows the various layers still present, though the muscle may be atrophied. In late stages the tumor cells creep between the muscle bundles, and may push out beneath the mucosa where the appearance and subsequent course are like sarcomata originating in the bladder wall. It is usual, however, for a large mass to develop, and even push entirely around the bladder and project up above the brim of the pelvis before the cavity of the bladder is actually invaded. The encroachment of the mass, when extensive, makes it impossible for the bladder to expand, so that the capacity is reduced and urinary frequency results. If the vesical orifice is pressed upon or pushed forward against the symphysis, difficulty or retention will also occur.

The above observations as to the effects on bladder function also apply to other intrapelvic, extravesical tumors, as osteosarcoma of the pelvis, large carcinomata of the rectum or uterus, hydatid cysts, etc.

Secondary Effects of Bladder Tumors.—Aside from metastasis and the cachexia of malignancy, bladder tumors produce their effects in the following ways: hemorrhage, obstruction (of ureter or of vesical orifice), necrosis, ulceration (leading sometimes to fistulous communications with other organs), encrustation or stone formation, infiltration of the bladder wall with loss of elasticity and of contractility of the bladder, and the development of extravesical masses with pressure on bladder, ureter, or urethra. In addition, infection is common, and adds its effects to the others.

Hemorrhage is characteristic of bladder tumors practically without exception. The vessels developing in tumors are all of the capillary type, and very thin walled even when of abnormally large caliber. Rupture of such vessels is easy, especially as the tumor undergoes some trauma every time the bladder contracts. Hemorrhage is also increased by ulceration. The bleeding from bladder tumors may be very severe, even leading to a fatal anemia. It is usually venous, but may be arterial, and the spurting vessel may be seen with the cystoscope, as in one of our cases.

Obstruction.—Bladder tumors can cause obstruction in four ways: (1) By an intravesical mass pressing upon or filling the ureteral or vesical orifices, causing stricture; (2) by infiltration about the ureteral or vesical orifices, causing stricture; (3) by metastatic foci infiltrating the walls of, usually, the ureter, causing stricture; (4) by pressure of extravesical masses on ureter, bladder, or urethra, and (5) by invasion of and elevation of the trigone, sufficient to obstruct the vesical orifice.

The second mechanism is the usual one, the first fairly common, while the third, fourth, and fifth are rare. The ureter is usually not obstructed by a non-infiltrating mass unless it is very large, or unless a number of pedunculated tumors press themselves together just over its orifice. Even quite small tumors, however, can obstruct the vesical orifice when they grow near it, and fill its lumen or fall into it like ball-valves.

Since tumors, on the whole, are much more common in the base of the bladder and in the region of the trigone, they often, when they become infiltrating, cause a stricture of the ureter. This is usually unilateral, or if bilateral, one side is affected some time before the other. The results are the characteristic ones of supravesical obstruction, fully described in the section on Obstructive Uropathy. Such obstructions are always partial at first. Hydronephrosis and hydro-ureter are caused and the function of the affected kidney is reduced. As shown in the section on Infections of the Urogenital Tract, obstruction favors infection, so that a kidney obstructed by a bladder tumor may become the seat of pyelitis, pyelonephritis, or pyonephrosis even when there is no primary infection of the bladder. In such cases the bladder is usually secondarily infected. When the bladder is infected early, usually as the result of instrumentation, the renal infection may be secondary thereto. Sometimes ulceration occurs about the ureteral orifice, so that the ureter comes to open directly into the base of the ulcer. In such cases some degree of infection and obstruction is the rule. In like manner the urethra can be obstructed by a growth surrounding its opening into the bladder. For this to occur, extension into the prostate must take place at least for a little distance, and the mechanism and results thereof will be found discussed under the heading of Neoplasms of the Prostate.

Metastasis to the ureter occurs, but is rare. We have observed one such case at autopsy, and others are reported in the literature. The metastasis and its resultant obstruction may be at any point along the ureter, but the majority of instances have been in the lower third. Implantations may occur in the urethra (see below), but we find no record of an actual metastasis to the wall of the urethra.

When large extravesical masses develop as the result of extension with involvement of the perivesical tissues, pressure phenomena may be produced. The bladder capacity may be reduced even to practically nothing by pressure from the outside. The ureter, seminal vesicle, and vas deferens may be obstructed. This obstruction usually occurs, under these conditions, before actual invasion. Since these phenomena usually occur in late cases where the bladder wall is also extensively involved, they are best studied in cases of retrovesical sarcoma, where the picture is not complicated by any intravesical involvement.

Necrosis of intravesical growths may remove part or all of their substance (Figs. 374, 375). If there is no invasion of the bladder wall, the ulcer left may be small, and may heal over rapidly. A very few cases of spontaneous cure of benign papilloma in this manner are recorded. If the bladder wall is involved, necrosis of the surface portions is almost inevitable, and this results in ulcers which show no tendency to heal, but, on the contrary, usually get larger as the growth extends. The presence of necrotic tissue, or of sloughing ulcers, is almost always soon complicated by infection. The infection then takes firm root on the ulcerated surface, and cannot be removed as long as the ulceration persists. Ordinarily the advancing tumor mass precedes the ulceration, forming a barrier, but in some cases, where the neoplasm has invaded the rectum, sigmoid, cecum, small intestine, uterus, or vagina, fistulæ may form into these organs.

The necrosis usually results from circulatory disturbances with anemia—the common mechanism in neoplasms. Often infection plays an important rôle in the process, sometimes causing thrombosis with consequent anemia. Pedunculated tumors may undergo torsion, or be traumatized by instruments or calculi. Treatment by fulguration, radium, or x-ray often leads to necrosis. The necrotic mass is usually sloughed off and expelled in the urine, where it may help in diagnosis. Sometimes small portions of papillary tumor are actually broken off without being necrotic. If the slough is not expelled, it is because it is too large, or because it remains adherent to its original site. In either case it may persist for a long time, undergoing partial autolysis, but not digestion, since proteolytic organisms are usually not present in the bladder. Such degenerated masses become infiltrated and encrusted with calcareous material, and may become the nuclei of good-sized stones. Calcareous infiltration also occurs in the mucopurulent material or small tags of slough adhering to ulcerations. In this way the entire surface of a malignant ulcer may become encrusted.

Pain and frequency may result from infection when there is no invasion of the bladder wall, but otherwise do not usually occur until invasion takes place, unless

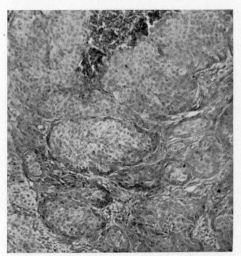

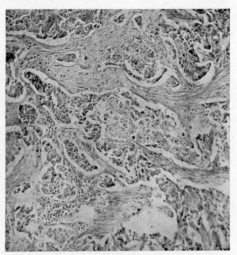

Fig. 374.—Papillary carcinoma of the bladder. A large mass of tumor cells, the center of which has undergone necrosis. This process precedes the ulceration which is so common in these tumors. B. U. I. Path. 4552.

Fig. 375.—Epithelioma of the bladder. This picture is given to contrast with the preceding and illustrates the much greater tendency to generalized necrosis in epithelioma. B. U. I. Path. 4038.

the intravesical tumor itself becomes large enough to interfere with bladder function. The infiltration of the mucosa destroys its elasticity; the infiltration of the muscular layer destroys elasticity and contractility as well. Pain then results whenever the bladder becomes distended; pain and the irritation therefrom cause urinary frequency sometimes even while the actual capacity of the bladder remains good. Ulceration and infection increase pain and frequency. As the infiltrated area increases, the bladder capacity is actually reduced, and may reach an extreme minimum when the entire extent of the wall is transformed, as it is in some cases, to a thick, indurated, inelastic layer of tumor tissue.

Extension of Bladder Tumors.—A bladder neoplasm may originate in a diverticulum. The tumor may be concealed from view in its cavity, or it may fill the cavity entirely, and project through the orifice into the bladder proper. In the latter case one may see cystoscopically only a small portion projecting, and be deceived as to the size and extent of the tumor.

Extension may occur in any direction, but since tumors are most frequent in the base of the bladder, it usually involves the structures bordering on this area first. Growth may occur by extension into the urethra with ulceration and stricture. The prostate is not infrequently involved. Within the prostate, the vesical neoplasm grows in much the same manner as the prostatic carcinomata; that is, it produces enlargement and induration of the prostate, is confined by Denonvillier's fascia, and extends upward into the seminal vesicles. It is not so hard as we usually find a prostatic cancer to be. It retains its histologic characteristics, however, and pathologically can seldom be mistaken for primary prostatic carcinoma. The seminal vesicles may be involved directly from the bladder. In the vertex of the bladder extension may be toward the peritoneum, but it is rare for the tumor actually to involve the peritoneal surface. If it does so, it may invade adjacent coils of intestine, which may result in intestinal obstruction or enterovesical fistula. In the male the rectum may be involved after extension through the prostate or seminal vesicles. The prevesical space may be filled with a neoplastic mass, and the anterior abdominal wall and pubic bones may be invaded. In women the anterior vaginal wall and vault are most often affected, owing to their proximity to the base of the bladder, but the uterus too may be invaded. Vesico-vaginal or vesico-uterine fistula may result.

Operation often has an important influence on extension. Implantation may occur in a wound tract, with development of neoplastic masses there. This was especially common when papillomata were operated on suprapubically, the implantations developing in the scar both intravesically and also prevesically beneath the recti muscles or the skin. If an operation has been unsuccessful in removing all of a tumor, it may grow through a persistent suprapubic fistula or a partially healed wound. In any case, a mass, usually indurated, appears at the site of the incision, with later extension to the skin and ulceration. Under such conditions a bladder fistula is always present, even if there has been closure before the extension to the skin was complete. The ulceration may be extensive, and with the constant flow of urine and the infection these advanced cases may present the most distressing picture.

Implantation in the bladder and in surgical incisions has been discussed. It may also occur in the urethra with papillomatous tumors. It is remarkable, however, that such implantations occur only in the prostatic urethra, never in the membranous, bulbous, or penile urethra. This recalls a similar fact in connection with chronic renal bacteriuria, where chronic posterior urethritis is common, but where anterior urethritis is seldom seen. The fate of these implantations in the posterior urethra is similar to that of the bladder tumors; they assume malignancy, if not already possessed of it, and infiltrate the subjacent tissue, in this case, the prostate. In addition the intra-urethral part of the tumor may cause obstruction and difficult urination. In one case (B. U. I. 4204) a man of fifty-six with a papilloma, which was treated by cystoscopic instrumentation (partial removal), rapidly developed numerous implantations in the bladder and urethra which soon showed malignancy and ended fatally.

Metastasis of Bladder Tumors.—Metastasis from bladder tumors is moderately late, as a rule, depending, however, somewhat upon the biologic characteristics of the particular growth. Thus the more rapidly growing tumors will be more apt to metastasize, as they are to invade and to ulcerate. Metastasis does not usually occur until the tumor becomes invasive, but in rare instances it may happen in the case of a malignant papilloma where no invasion can be demonstrated. Frequently, however, bladder carcinomata cause death from hemorrhage, renal damage, infection, or cachexia before any metastases become apparent. Metastasis is apparently usually by the blood-stream, as noteworthy growths in the regional lymphatic nodes are seldom seen. They may be involved, however, especially late in the disease, and in a few cases metastasis appears in the inguinal glands. The explanation of this occurrence is obscure, as it is in prostatic carcinoma. Ureteral metastases may be by way of the lymphatics. There is no marked site of predilection for metastases from bladder neoplasms, but any tissue of the body may be involved. Search for metastases must, therefore, be thorough. The metastases ordinarily preserve the characteristics of the original growth, but since papillæ are absent, it is often impossible to distinguish metastases of papillary carcinoma—the common tumor—from those of certain other epithelial growths. The cystoscope, however, enables us to avoid all doubt in answering such questions.

Buerger has called attention to certain cases in which metastases to the bladder wall occur. One sees in sections a malignant papilloma, with no infiltration at its base, but deep down in the muscularis a few nests of typical tumor cells. If the original tumor were destroyed by local treatment, these local metastases would be responsible for local recurrence, which would then have the characteristics of infiltrating carcinoma. In a similar manner, actual metastasis may occur, rarely, to the prostate, so that there would be a layer of normal tissue between the carcinomatous mass in the prostate and the original tumor in the bladder.

Secondary Involvement of Bladder by Neoplasms.—The bladder is fairly frequently involved by neoplasms arising in adjacent structures.

Carcinoma of the prostate rather infrequently invades the bladder. In our series of 593 prostatic carcinomata note was made of invasion of the bladder in 34 cases. This, however, does not represent all cases, as cystoscopy was often not done owing to the pain, hemorrhage, and aggravation of symptoms caused by it in cancer of the prostate. The invasion usually occurs in the trigonal region, where a mass from the prostate pushes up into the bladder. This mass may be of good size, and often ulcerates, so that grossly it may resemble a primary bladder tumor. In such cases the involvement of the prostate and vesicles will usually be far advanced, but sometimes only the microscope will make clear the real origin of the tumor. In the bladder prostatic carcinoma shows not infrequently a somewhat different histologic picture from that seen in the prostate. It is no longer infiltrating a fibromuscular organ, but growing freely into the bladder cavity. The amount of stroma will, therefore, be reduced, the proportion of epithelium increased. Obviously, there will be a family resemblance to adenocarcinoma of the bladder, and sometimes it is only by following the tumor down into the prostate in sections that its prostatic origin can be determined. In the gross one has to judge by the relative extent of the tumor in the prostate and vesicles as opposed to the bladder.

The rare carcinoma of the urethra (usually squamous-cell epithelioma) may involve the bladder by direct extension through the prostate. Carcinoma of the rectum may involve the bladder after invading the prostate or seminal vesicles. Carcinoma of the intestine also may invade the bladder, usually through its peritoneal aspect.   If pathologic material is available, the diagnosis will usually be easy on account of the characteristic histologic picture.   These tumors are oftenest adenocarcinomata or papillary growths, with cylindrical cells, many of which contain mucus—"goblet cells."   If masses of mucoid material are present, they are sometimes known as "colloid carcinomata."   The microscopic picture of rectal neoplasms is similar.   It is probable that many of the colloid carcinomata of the bladder which have been described are really intestinal tumors which have invaded the bladder.   Invasion of the bladder is usually accompanied by the formation of enterovesical fistula.   The more scirrhous types of intestinal tumors are less apt to invade the bladder; they usually cause intestinal obstruction, with its characteristic symptoms, before they invade other structures.

Papillary tumors of the ureter and renal pelvis show the same tendency to become implanted as those of the bladder, and we may, therefore, see papillary tumors of the bladder, identical in every respect with primary vesical growths, which are really implantations from higher up.   These tumors, fortunately rare, may easily give rise to serious diagnostic error.   Their course is the same as that of primary bladder tumors, but, of course, the original growth in the kidney or ureter will practically always dominate the picture in the later stages.

Carcinoma of the cervix uteri may invade the bladder, causing large intravesical growths and vesicovaginal or vesico-uterine fistula, but this is a late event, occurring when the primary growth is far advanced.   We have described a case of carcinoma of a vesical diverticulum[1] with a large organized blood-clot projecting into the bladder which was mistaken for a bladder tumor.

SYMPTOMS OF BLADDER TUMORS

The symptoms of vesical neoplasm are not pathognomonic, but there are certain features about their sequence which may properly allow, in many cases, a strong presumptive diagnosis before cystoscopy is done.   The principal symptoms, in order of their importance, are:

Local:
   Hematuria.
   Urinary Frequency.
   Pain.   Constant or dysuria.
   Difficult Urination.
   Retention of Urine.
   Passage of Tumor Fragments.
   Incontinence of Urine.
   Mass in bladder region.
   Pilimictio.
With infection, the following may be added:
   Pyuria.
   Ammoniuria.
   Fever.
With stone formation:
   Passage of calculi.

[1] Young: Transactions American Association, Genito-Urinary Surgeons, 1909, iv, 121–125.

Constitutional:
　Anemia.
　Loss of weight and strength.
　Cachexia.

With renal complications and local extension:
　Renal pain.
　Renal mass (hydronephrosis).
　Uremia.

Enterovesical fistula:
　Fecal urine.
　Pneumaturia (fetid).

Uterovesical and vesicovaginal fistula:
　Incontinence of urine.
　Dyspareunia.

Rectal involvement:
　Pain.
　Difficulty of defecation.

Intestinal involvement:
　Peritoneal pain.
　Intestinal obstruction.

Metastases cause various symptoms according to their location.

Hematuria.—This is by far the most frequent symptom of vesical neoplasm, and in a very large majority of cases is also the first symptom noted. In 541 cases cited by Clado,[1] Geraghty,[2] and Verhoogen[3] hematuria was the initial symptom in 404, or 75 per cent. It occurs at some time during the course of the disease in practically all cases. Hematuria is usually observed promptly by male patients, except those of very careless habits, but is frequently ignored by females, who may mistake the blood for menstrual blood. There is no type of tumor which may not cause hematuria, although it is stated that myoma and fibroma are less likely to do so. In the typical case, hematuria from bladder tumor is distinguished from that of urinary calculi, and of tuberculosis by being neither preceded nor accompanied in the beginning by frequency, pain, or any other symptom. This may not, however, distinguish it from the hematuria of renal neoplasm or "essential" renal hematuria. In addition, hematuria from vesical neoplasm is typically intermittent. The intervals at first may be very long, even months or years, but usually tend to grow shorter as the growth advances. The bleeding is sometimes terminal or more marked in the last portion of the urine. This is due to the disturbance of the tumor by the contraction of the bladder, but is in no way characteristic. In general, malignant tumors bleed more than benign. The amount of blood lost is very variable; there may be only enough to make the urine smoky, or large quantities may pour out, so that the urine clots in the glass, and the patient is rapidly exsanguinated. In such cases the clotting may occur in the bladder, causing great pain and difficulty of urination, or retention. The blood may be retained in the bladder by some obstruction long enough

[1] Traité des Tumeurs de la Vessie, Paris, 1895.
[2] Cabot's Modern Urology, 1923, ii, 197–254.
[3] Encyclopædie Française d'Urologie, 1921, iv, 425–538.

to be dark brown when passed (the "coffee-grounds" appearance). Casper[1] cystoscoped 142 cases of bladder tumor immediately after the first hematuria. All but three were small, early tumors. This is a most potent argument in favor of immediate cystoscopic investigation of all hematurias, and indicates that bleeding is an early symptom in most tumors. In a very few hematuria does not occur until late, when extensive involvement has occurred, and it is probable that a good many of these cases are non-papillary tumors.

In one of our cases violent arterial bleeding came from an elevation no larger than a match head. It was stopped by fulguration, but two months later the cystoscope showed for the first time a papilloma now grown to 5 mm. in size. In several other cases continuous (venous) bleeding from one vessel in a small papilloma was seen.

Pain is a very inconstant symptom in early cases, but is practically always present in later stages. Pain is due to actual infiltration of the bladder walls, either by neoplastic tissues or by inflammatory products, or to some obstruction to urination. In the latter case the pain will be confined to the time of voiding, and is called, therefore, dysuria. In the former case the pain will be accentuated by distention of the bladder or by contraction of its muscles, and may, therefore, be a dysuria, with painless periods between voidings, or a constant pain. Constant bladder pain is practically always accentuated on voiding, though there may be a short period of relief afterward when the bladder is quite empty. Pain on voiding is usually stinging, burning, or lancinating, and is very frequently referred to the end of the penis or along the urethra. The constant pain is more apt to be of an aching character, and is less often referred, but felt over the suprapubic region and in the groins. Radiation to the thighs and legs usually means metastatic involvement of the sacral nerve roots.

Pain is unreliable as a symptom of bladder tumor because non-invasive growths do not cause pain unless there is infection or obstruction. Indeed, they may be grasped with forceps or burned with the fulgurating wire without causing pain, showing that they possess no functioning sensory nerves. In addition, a few infiltrating growths do not cause pain, probably because they destroy the nerve-fibers as they advance. We have shown that tumor tissue itself contains no nerve-fibers.[2] Infiltration usually causes pain, however, by destroying the elasticity of the bladder wall. If infection supervenes, there will be pain as in any cystitis (*q. v.*). If the pain is very severe, and intractable to the ordinary methods of treating cystitis, it probably means that infiltration is present in addition. If the intravesical tumor acts as an obstruction to the vesical orifice, there will be pain, as in any infravesical obstruction (*q. v.*).

In infiltrating ulcerated growths cystitis may be considered as always present. Its effects, in the production of pain, are mingled with those of the tumor itself invading the bladder wall. In such cases, therefore, pain is very rarely absent, and may be of the most severe and distressing character.

Frequency of urination occurs as the result of: (1) Cystitis; (2) irritation due to infiltrating tumor growth; or (3) diminished bladder capacity due to the encroachment of intravesical or extravesical masses upon the bladder cavity. As a rule,

---

[1] Deutsche Urologische Gesellschaft, 1909, abstracted in Zeitschrift für Urologie, 1909, iii, 579.

[2] Young: Journal of Experimental Medicine, 1897, ii, 1–12.

it is fairly late, unless an early cystitis has resulted from instrumentation. Its onset bears no constant relation to the onset of hematuria—a distinction from tuberculosis. Besides its lateness, the fact that it can occur from such different causes makes it of little diagnostic value. It is, however, closely related to pain, being seldom absent when pain is present.

Difficulty of urination indicates either infiltration and stricture of the vesical orifice, or the presence of an intravesical tumor acting as a ball-valve. (Assuming, of course, that other causes of obstruction, not related to vesical neoplasm, are ruled out.) Intravesical tumors do not often act as obstructions, so that, ordinarily, difficulty of urination is a late symptom and indicates an advanced stage of disease, with probable involvement of the prostate and the walls of the vesical orifice.

Retention may be the extreme stage of difficulty due to neoplastic stricture of the vesical orifice, or it may be an acute affair, due to sudden occlusion of the orifice by an intravesical tumor or blood-clot. In neither case is it pathognomonic of bladder tumor. When chronic obstruction, with perhaps repeated attacks of retention, is due to infiltration about the orifice, the anatomic and functional changes produced in the upper urinary tract (dilatation of bladder, functional damage to kidneys, hydronephrosis, hydro-ureter, etc.) are the same as those produced by other forms of infravesical obstruction.

Passage of Tumor Fragments.—While usually a late symptom, and not constant enough to be reliable, the passage of tumor fragments is a very characteristic one. They are usually described as bits of "flesh." In some cases they are passed over long periods, and the total quantity of material expelled may be very large. The passage of fragments, like that of blood-clots, may be accompanied by difficult urination, pain, and tenesmus.

Incontinence.—In a few cases infiltration about the orifice does not occlude the orifice, but destroys the contractility of the sphincter, so that partial or complete incontinence may occur. This is a late symptom. This true incontinence, however, is rare, and one more often sees a paradoxic or overflow incontinence due to obstruction by tumor growth at the vesical orifice, with dilatation of the bladder; or the patient may describe as incontinence an extreme frequency, in which he feels the necessity of voiding almost constantly. This is the result of severe cystitis and contraction of the bladder due to infection, infiltration of the bladder wall, or ulceration, or all three together.

Mass in Bladder Region.—In advanced cases, with extravesical extension, a mass may appear in the lower abdomen.

Pilimictio is very rare, but is an interesting symptom, and absolutely pathognomonic of dermoid cyst in the bladder or communicating with it. (See Fig. 373.)

Pyuria.—The presence of pus in the urine is an indication of infection, with cystitis. Uninfected bladder tumors do not cause pyuria.

Ammoniuria indicates an infection with urea-splitting organisms, and usually accompanies severe, extensive, ulcerating conditions.

Fever is not marked in cystitis alone, but usually indicates an extension of the infection to the kidneys, perivesical area, or blood-stream.

The *passage of small calculi* occurs in bladder tumor cases when there is encrusted cystitis, usually on an ulcerated area or adherent slough. While in no way characteristic, it is a fairly common event, and can be taken to mean ulceration.

Anemia, Loss of Weight and Strength, Cachexia.—Anemia, in the early stages, depends upon the hemorrhage from the tumor. Slight but persistent hemorrhages over long periods may produce serious secondary anemia, as in hemorrhoids. In such cases, however, there will be active blood regeneration from activation of the bone-marrow, and if the hemorrhages are somewhat less plentiful and persistent, the red blood-count will be maintained and the patient will not suffer from anemia. In acute, large hemorrhages this reaction of the bone-marrow is not present, since it takes some time to develop, and the patient may become very anemic from the loss of a much smaller total quantity of blood than in the chronic cases. In late stages anemia may be a part of the general malignant *cachexia*, or may result from wide-spread infection and intoxication.

Loss of weight and strength occurs in the later stages, due to severe local complications or metastasis. Pain, loss of sleep, and mental depression may play a part. It is often remarkable, however, how the weight, strength, and general health are maintained even in the presence of large tumors, especially if they be intravesical. Geraghty describes a patient who had an extensive bladder tumor for eleven years. The general health and nutrition were good until death, which resulted from myocardial insufficiency.

The so-called malignant cachexia, therefore, is not to be looked for in bladder tumor as a help in diagnosis. In the later stages infection is always present, usually severe, and the picture is complicated by the bacterial intoxication and by renal insufficiency.

Renal pain indicates ureteral obstruction or renal infection, often both. Uninfected hydronephrosis from obstruction due to vesical neoplasm is rare.

Renal Mass.—The development of a mass in the renal region indicates hydronephrosis (usually pyonephrosis) or perinephric abscess. In very rare instances the vesical tumor is simply a prolongation of a primary renal or ureteral tumor.

Uremia supervenes when the changes due to vesical neoplasm act on already damaged kidneys, or, more usually, when the renal infection is bilateral, so that the unobstructed kidney is damaged by pyelonephritis. Bilateral ureteral obstruction from vesical neoplasm can occur, but is rare.

Enterovesical Fistula, Ureterovesical Fistula, Vesicovaginal Fistula.—The symptoms due to these conditions are obvious enough, and require no discussion.

Rectal Involvement, Intestinal Involvement.—Here, too, the symptoms are obvious.

Metastases.—Since there is no marked site of predilection for metastases from vesical neoplasms, there is no particular area to be considered routinely in this connection. A thorough history may bring to light certain suggestive points, as headache, failing vision, hemoptysis, nerve-root pains, etc. Pathologic fracture may sometimes be the first sign of bone involvement. The bones, however, are involved late and very seldom in comparison with prostatic carcinoma.

In *résumé* we may say that the typical case of bladder tumor is characterized by the appearance of hematuria out of an entirely clear sky. This hematuria is usually intermittent, but we have seen very minute papillomata bleed steadily for a week or more (and sometimes violently). Pain, frequency of urination, pyuria, and all other symptoms are absent not only at first, but usually for some time thereafter. Such a history always points to neoplasm, usually of the bladder, but if not of the bladder, of the kidney. We cannot condemn too much the policy of treating such cases expectantly—a procedure that is all too common. Hematuria is never negligible, and its cause should invariably be investigated. The three-glass test or the urethroscope may show that it is urethral. Generally cystoscopy is indicated at once, and will quickly tell whether the blood is coming from either ureter, a vesical tumor, or the prostatic orifice.

Pain and frequency of urination are usually the next symptoms to appear. As time goes on, infection is more apt to occur, with its accompanying pyuria.

All the other symptoms can be considered together as rare, non-characteristic, or late.

While the syndrome described above is the typical one, it must be remembered that in a very considerable number of cases the symptom-complex is ambiguous, and only the cystoscope can give the diagnosis. If any suspicion exists, such examination should not be delayed.

Diagnosis of Bladder Tumors

General.—For practical purposes the diagnosis of bladder tumors is made principally by the cystoscope. Not only in the detection of tumors, but in the determination of the features upon which the type of treatment to be used depends, and in the observation of the response to treatment, we rely largely on this instrument. It is in the detection of infiltrating growth that it may fail, and here rectal or vaginal examination is most important.

For centuries there was practically no knowledge of bladder tumors. Later they were known only as they appeared at autopsy, and the diagnosis was impossible in any but very advanced cases. In the early days of the Johns Hopkins Hospital (1889 to 1899) suprapubic drainage was all that was attempted except in pedunculated small papillomata. With the advent of the cystoscope all this was changed, and it is since that time that all of our knowledge of bladder tumors, especially in the early stages, has been accumulated.

The symptomatology is of little value except as it causes suspicion and leads to cystoscopy. Hematuria is the cardinal symptom. There is nothing characteristic about the hematuria. The fact that more appears in the last portion may mean that the tumor is being squeezed by the contraction of the bladder, or only that some of the red cells have settled in the base of the bladder. In many cases the blood is uniformly distributed in the urine. Worm-like clots suggest a supravesical origin, but they will be accompanied by renal colic.

Examination of the urine should not be omitted, although it tells us comparatively little. One looks especially for microscopic blood, which may be present when there has been no frank hematuria. Its significance is the same. The presence of pus and bacteria indicates infection. The presence of pus and blood without bacteria suggests tuberculosis. The only decisive things which may be found in the urine are tumor fragments and hairs. Hairs, if they really come from within the bladder, are diagnostic of dermoid cyst. Tumor fragments, unfortunately, are often completely necrotic, so that usually no certain diagnosis can be made, but they should be sectioned and studied microscopically. Occasionally one can at once decide that a tumor is present, whether it is benign or malignant, and to what type it belongs. Squamous-cell epithelioma may give off flakes resembling those of leukoplakia, but under the microscope the characteristic malignant structure can sometimes be seen. Other things which may appear in the urine and resemble grossly tumor fragments are leukoplakia flakes, bits of necrotic mucosa, especially after operations, toxic damage to the bladder, as by turpentine or urotropin, or diphtheritic cystitis, agglomerations of pus, mucus, necrotic tissue, calcareous particles, etc., occurring in any sort of ulcerative cystitis, inspissated blood-clots, etc.   In severe cystitis the urine may be very foul, and even have a fetid odor.   Vegetable fibers, bits of partially digested meat, or other fecal components indicate enterovesical fistula.   To make certain, one can inject a colored solution, as gentian-violet, into the rectum, or give charcoal or lycopodium spores by mouth.   The appearance of any of these articles in the urine leaves no doubt of the presence of fistula.

In some cases where there is doubt about the character of cells appearing in the urine it is helpful to make a careful preparation as follows: The urine is centrifugalized, the supernatant fluid poured off and replaced with 4 per cent. formalin solution.   After about one-half hour centrifugalization is repeated, and in the same manner graduated strengths of alcohol are allowed to act on the cells in the centrifuge tube.   They are finally embedded in paraffin or celloidin.   Sections are then made and stained by the ordinary technic, usually with hematoxylin and eosin.   In this way the cells are much better preserved and in certain cases a definite diagnosis of neoplasm is made possible.

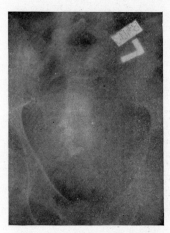

FIG. 376.—x-Ray of a case of carcinoma of the bladder with ulceration and incrustation. The calcareous material casts an irregular shadow, seen in the picture. B. U. I. x-Ray 2048.

In the *physical examination* nothing will be found in early cases.   In late cases, with extravesical involvement, a palpable, usually tender mass will be found in the lowermost abdomen, extending up from within the pelvis.   It is flat to percussion, and usually irregular, firm and fixed, though there may be slight mobility.   Tenderness in the costovertebral angle, or a palpable mass in the loin, indicate renal complications.

A history of nerve root pains suggest x-ray study of the skeleton, as bony metastases can be detected in this way.

Rectal and *vaginal examination* reach about the same portions of the bladder. They are valuable in diagnosis since they disclose infiltrating growths in the base of the bladder, when the induration of the bladder wall can be palpated directly. Non-infiltrating growths cannot be detected in this way unless they are large. Extension to the prostate, seminal vesicles, and rectum in the male and to the vagina and uterus in the female can be determined.

Since a great majority of all tumors occur in the base of the bladder, infiltration will usually be detected on rectal or vaginal digital examination.   In the male one must be sure to reach up into the intervesicular space in order to palpate the trigonal and basal regions of the bladder.   Prostatic carcinoma also causes an induration in this region, the intervesicular plateau.   When present, however, the involvement of the prostate itself and of the vesicles will give the diagnosis.   One should keep in mind the possibility of infectious pericystitis with induration.

Bimanual examination may be added in the female, and is, in a few cases, useful in the male. Retrovesical sarcoma is felt as a mass high up and anterior to the rectum. The prostate is usually palpated below it, and the seminal vesicles may or may not be palpable. The mass is usually firm and rubbery, but may be soft and fluctuant, or have soft areas. It may extend upward so that it can be palpated suprapubically, when bimanual examination may help.

x-Ray examination is ordinarily of little assistance in the diagnosis of bladder tumors. It may, however, help to rule out other lesions. Definite findings are present when there is any calcareous material in the bladder either in the form of a calculus or of incrustation on an ulcerated surface. Calculi may occur as a complication of bladder tumor, but the latter condition is much more common. An

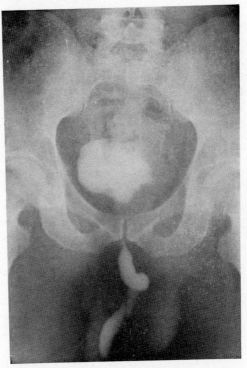

Fig. 377.—Cystogram showing filling defect caused by a large carcinoma of the bladder with ulcerated intravesical mass. The urethrogram shows nothing abnormal.

example of the irregular, rather moth-eaten shadows thrown by encrusted ulcers is shown in Fig. 376.

The *cystogram* is helpful only in case of a rather large intravesical mass which may give a filling defect, as shown in Figs. 377 and 378. One cannot depend on this diagnostic measure, however, since no defect will be visible if the mass is small, and even larger masses may fail to be evident in the cystogram. Where there is extensive involvement of the bladder wall, a cystogram will show a contracted bladder, and in the occasional case where large extravesical masses are present, the distortion of the bladder caused by them will be shown, but the cystogram itself will give, of course, no indication as to the nature of the extravesical mass. Tumor masses may also show in air cystograms.

These preliminaries are important and necessary, but it will be seen that the conclusions which can be drawn from them are not definite and final. They simply lead up to cystoscopy.

The two commonest obstacles to cystoscopy in vesical tumors are contracted and irritable bladder and hemorrhage. If the bladder is contracted and painful, morphin, or even anesthesia may be essential. Nitrous oxid may be used, or novocain injected epidurally through the sacral hiatus.[1] Persistent hemorrhage may require postponement of the examination. The use of an evacuation cystoscope is almost essential where there is much bleeding. We have devised a special irrigating cystoscope with very large inlet and outlet (Fig. 636).

With skill and patience, however, satisfactory cystoscopic examination can be obtained in practically every case. The exceptions will usually be cases so far advanced that the diagnosis is obvious, and intravesical treatment out of the question.

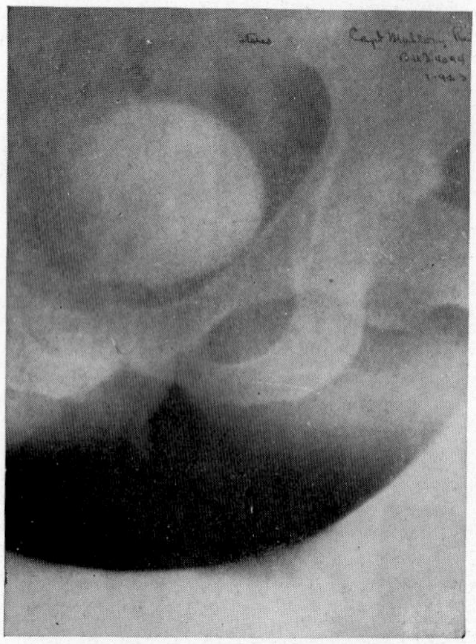

FIG. 378.—Cystogram in extensive carcinoma of the bladder. The large mass projecting into the bladder is well seen as an irregular defect in the bladder shadow. B. U. I. x-Ray 4094.

The bladder capacity tells us the extent of the contraction and loss of elasticity of the bladder, and may indicate infiltration of the wall. The residual urine, if present, gives an idea of the extent of any obstruction to the vesical orifice which may be present. We feel that one can inspect tumors, especially the papillary ones, better with a water-filled bladder and an indirect telescope, but others obtain satisfactory results with air cystoscopy.

Cystoscopic.—Cystoscopically, one classifies tumors according to appearance and form of growth. This classification has nothing whatever to do with the pathologic classification, but it appears to be indubitably true that it is of much greater clinical value, as regards prognosis and selection of treatment. This is undoubtedly because the course and malignancy of a tumor depend more on its biologic characteristics, that is, its rapidity of growth and its invasiveness, than they do on the type of cell of which it is composed. We may distinguish, therefore, the following:

1. Papillomata.
   A. Single.
   B. Multiple.
2. Papillary, non-infiltrating tumors, showing tendency to lateral spread.
   A. Single.
   B. Multiple.
3. Tumors with intravesical mass, showing infiltration of the bladder wall, and usually ulceration.
4. Tumors which are entirely infiltrating, with little intravesical portion.

[1] For this purpose the following formula will be found useful: Water, 30 c.c.; novocain, 0.6 gm.; sodium chlorid, 0.1 gm.; sodium bicarbonate, 0.15 gm.; adrenalin (1 : 1000), 0.5 c.c. The entire amount is injected. See DeButler d'Ormond, L'Anesthesie Régionale en Chirurgie Urinaire, Paris, 1921 (Doin).

5. Pedunculated tumors which are not infiltrating and not papillary.

6. Sessile tumors which are not infiltrating and not papillary.

1. *Papillomata.*—These tumors are usually quite definite cystoscopically, and have a distinct pedicle and overhanging edges. The papillæ of which they are composed may be long, thin, and branching, or short, stubby, and comparatively simple. While in general, the longer, thinner, and paler the papillæ, the more likely is the tumor to be benign, yet it is impossible to assure oneself from cystoscopic examination that a papilloma is benign. This is a cardinal point in the diagnosis, and should be remembered by all cystoscopists. We can, however, apply a therapeutic test, which is most valuable in the detection of malignancy. It consists in applying the fulgurating spark. The benign tumor melts away quickly, and the area left heals over smoothly. The malignant tumor may respond in various ways. It too may seem to be thoroughly destroyed by the fulguration, but at the next examination will be almost as large as ever. It may resist the spark, so that it is impossible to destroy it, and at the next sitting a necrotic portion of the tumor remains in place, and there are edema and congestion about it.

On the first examination multiplicity of the tumors, short, stubby, coalescent papillæ, necrotic areas, and a zone of inflammation, characterized by bullous edema and congestion about the tumor, are all signs of malignancy. Single papillomata may be benign or malignant; multiple papillomata are almost surely malignant. If these phenomena are well developed, it may not be necessary to apply the therapeutic test of fulguration. On the other hand, papillomata which are not obviously malignant are not characterized by necrosis, and show an extraordinary resistance to inflammatory changes such as edema, congestion, and leukocytic infiltration. Thus one may see a papilloma with pale, thin papillæ unaffected in a bladder which is everywhere else the seat of an acute cystitis.

There is a type of tumor which marks a transition between Groups 1 and 2, in which a number of short simple papillary structures, either unbranched or branching very slightly, arise from separate, but very closely spaced roots, usually covering a sharply demarcated area. This is known as the "villous" type. Histologically, the papillæ show the typical structure of benign papilloma. It is uncertain whether this represents an unusual form of growth of a single papillary tumor, or is really an instance of multiple papilloma formation. The prognosis and treatment are the same as for ordinary benign papilloma.

In papillomata one must be on the lookout for beginning infiltration of the pedicle or bladder wall. It is often impossible to see the pedicle, but there is a fairly definite relationship between the width and the height of the tumor which is maintained when the pedicle is not infiltrated, that is, the tumor tends to remain somewhat globular, whatever its size. If it has attained considerable width, but is comparatively low, as though flattened along the bladder wall, it is almost surely malignant and has an infiltrated pedicle. The distinction cystoscopically is that it may be difficult to see all of the globular tumor in one position of the instrument—at every turn one sees its rounded edge—while in the other case the entire tumor may come into view in one field, lying along the bladder wall. In a few cases one may be able to see the thickened, shortened pedicle. Marked cystitis, in which the pain and frequency are perhaps out of proportion to the lesions seen, irregularity, edema, and slight ulceration about the tumor, also suggest infiltration. While this may be scarcely more than infiltration of the pedicle, it is of the utmost moment, as it is certain that any tumor which infiltrates the pedicle will soon go on to infiltrate the bladder wall.

2. *Papillary, Non-infiltrating Tumors, Showing Tendency to Lateral Spread.*— This group of tumors is a definite entity cystoscopically, although it is only lately that it has been separated. It is of considerable importance, as it comprises about 15 per cent. of bladder tumors, and the cases offer difficult therapeutic problems.

One may see this type of growth spreading laterally from a central papillomatous tumor, or it may commence with its own characteristic growth. The surface is irregular, but definite papillæ are not seen. The growth is low, flat, and the edge is not overhanging, but rather slopes down to the mucosa, as though the most recent areas, on the edge, had not attained the same height as the central portion of the tumor. Such a tumor may be single, there may be several of about the same size, there may be many small ones scattered over a circumscribed area, or there may be a number of such areas each containing a multiplicity of tumors. The areas may grow and fuse until a large proportion of the bladder is covered. Infiltration is late—this is a characteristic feature—and ulceration is uncommon. There is never any large mass projecting into the bladder cavity. Consequently, when infiltration does occur, it does not give the deep, usually single ulceration of Group 3, but is more apt to involve almost the entire extent of the bladder wall, and give the picture described under Group 4.

Occasionally one may see a very early stage of epithelioma simulating the above picture, but ulceration will usually be present. Later the epithelioma invades at an early stage, and is usually seen in the ulcerated form described under Group 3.

3. *Tumors with Intravesical Mass, Showing Infiltration of the Bladder Wall and Usually Ulceration.*—Tumors falling in this group at the time of the first examination may represent later stages of any of the histologically malignant types. They usually begin as papillomatous tumors, though circumscribed sessile tumors, after they infiltrate, give the same picture (the low sessile form of papillary carcinoma, Group 2, epithelioma, or adenocarcinoma).

The stigmata of very early infiltration have been given in the discussion of papillomata (Group 1). Later the same appearances are intensified. As to the projecting part of the tumor, sessile growths may show sufficient intravesical growth to roll up into a mushroom-like mass, just as do skin cancers (Fig. 379). Pedunculated tumors, on the other hand, may become large and thick, due to extensive infiltration of the pedicle, edema, etc. This is of minor importance, however, as the indications for treatment are the same for each.

The prognosis, too, depends on the extent of the infiltration, the rapidity of growth, and the presence of metastases, not on the character of the intravesical part of the growth. In rare cases a tumor may retain its papillomatous character even after it is ulcerated and very large, almost filling the bladder. The ulceration may be large or small, shallow or deep, but is usually single and described as craterlike. The base is grayish and necrotic, and may be sprinkled with calcareous deposits. The lobulated and rolled-up borders distinguish it from inflammatory ulcers. There is a zone of inflammatory edema and congestion about the tumor, which is usually marked by greater intensity even when the whole bladder is the seat of cystitis. The projecting portions of the tumor are usually also inflamed, and one may see on the surface tags of adherent exudate. The commonest loca-

PLATE XIII

Bladder Tumors, Cystoscopic Views

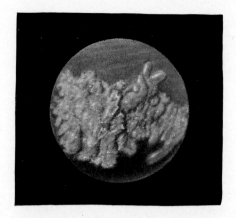

A. Papilloma of bladder, benign.

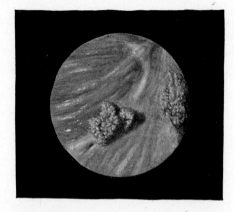

B. Multiple papillomata of bladder, benign.

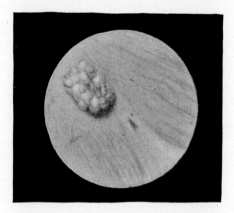

C. Small malignant tumor of bladder, papillæ fused, pedicle short. Bladder not infiltrated.

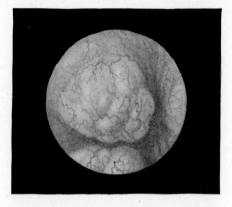

D. Malignant tumor of bladder, sessile, non-villous, broad pedicle.

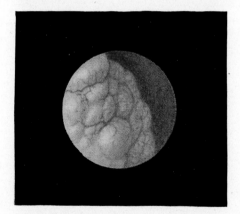

E. Close-up, lateral view of same tumor.

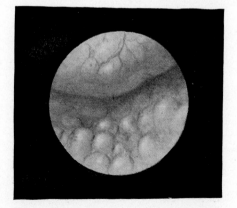

F. Marked bullous edema of bladder mucosa near malignant tumor.

tion is on the base of the bladder, and in this case the impression of infiltration is often confirmed by the palpation of an indurated area per rectum or vaginam. In late stages the infiltration may extend laterally in the substance of the bladder wall until it involves most of that organ, as well as invading the perivesical tissues.

Occasionally there may be doubt as to the malignant nature of an ulcer, the same problem which sometimes arises in skin ulceration. The characteristics given above, especially the thickened border, indicate malignancy pretty definitely, but in other cases they may be sufficiently indefinite so that it is only by a series of repeated cystoscopic examination that we may arrive at the proper diagnosis.

4. *Tumors which Are Entirely Infiltrating, with No Intravesical Portion: Mural Neoplasms.*—Tumors falling under Group 4 are not very common, but may give rise to confusion, and even be mistaken for severe cystitis. Oftenest they are the

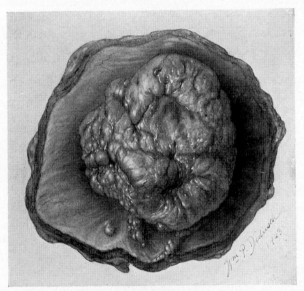

Fig. 379.—Operative specimen, papillary carcinoma with extensive resection of bladder wall. Large intravesical mass. Some lateral spreading at lower edge. B. U. I. 11100.

late stage of the multiple sessile low form of papillary carcinoma (Group 2). In this form there is never any great amount of tumor tissue projecting into the bladder and when infiltration begins over a broad area, with perhaps wide-spread ulceration, the picture is rather different from that usually associated with bladder tumor. In addition, the very extensive infiltration of the wall produces an extreme degree of contracted bladder, which is very painful, making cystoscopy difficult. Patient cystoscopy will usually disclose some characteristic tumor tissue, and the degree of induration felt per rectum or per vaginam will suggest that there is something more than an inflammatory process present. A sarcoma originating in the depths of the bladder wall may give a similar picture, but is a very great rarity.

5. *Pedunculated Tumors which Are Not Infiltrating and Not Papillary.*—These tumors are very rare. One must carefully rule out a papilloma in which the papillary structure is masked by fusion or otherwise. If really in this group, the

tumor is probably one of the unusual types, as fibroma, myoma, myxoma, or sarcoma.

6. *Sessile Tumors which Are Not Infiltrating and Not Papillary.*—Very few tumors fall in this group. The only ones at all likely to be seen are the rare benign adenomata, cystic or solid. These are rounded, usually yellowish-gray in color, and cysts may be visible. Unless cystitis is present from some other cause, there is usually no inflammatory reaction, and no hemorrhage or ulceration.

In *retrovesical sarcoma* the bladder mucosa is usually unaffected, but it may be possible to make out the convex mass impinging on the cavity. In some cases the cavity is reduced to a narrow semilunar slit, which can be seen with the cystoscope.

Dermoid cysts may appear as intravesical tumors or as ulcerated areas. A striking feature is the presence of hairs, which may be seen hanging from the tumor, and often encrusted with calcareous material. In one of our cases (B. U. I. 2566, 8808) hairs 2 inches long frequently appeared in the urine, and at intervals one of these would be encased in a slender calculus. The cystoscope showed an opening on the anterior wall of the bladder, and from this hung a hair encased in a calculus 1 inch long (Fig. 373). Subsequently the dermoid cyst was removed suprapubically.[1]

Lesions Simulating Bladder Tumor.—Certain other diseases produce pictures in the bladder that may lead to confusion with vesical neoplasms.

Chronic cystitis may produce ulcers and masses of granulation tissue which simulate new growths. The absence of definite intravesical masses, and of thickened, indurated edges for the ulcers, usually makes the diagnosis, but sometimes doubt may exist until the cystitis improves under ordinary methods of treatment. We have seen a case (B. U. I. 10,392) in which a small, flat, slightly reddened area with a small, superficial ulceration was seen in the vertex of the bladder. It did not respond to treatment, and was excised with the diagnosis of ulcerative cystitis. On section, it proved to be an early basal-cell epithelioma. The total thickness of the growth, which was superficial, was about that seen in cases of submucous cystitis.

Solitary ulcers, like that described by Fenwick, sometimes have a thickened edge suggesting carcinoma. The induration is less than that which would be expected in a malignant ulcer of similar appearance. The response of the ulcer to simple treatment is the final test.

After large doses of radium, either on the surface of the bladder or as implantations, very chronic ulcerations, which persist for from four to twelve months, may be caused. The edge may be somewhat thickened, and the ulcer is surrounded by a zone of inflammation, often bullous in type. Sometimes it is impossible to determine whether any neoplastic growth persists. One watches, however, for any change in the nature of a progression, that is, increased thickening, or increase in the size of the ulcer, since a pure radium burn, while chronic, does not increase after it is once established. Eventual healing is good evidence of the absence of neoplasia.

Tuberculous cystitis, like pyogenic cystitis, may rarely simulate tumor. The superficial, moth-eaten tuberculous ulcer is usually characteristic. The discovery of the bacillus in the urine makes the diagnosis certain.

Hypertrophy of the Prostate.—Occasionally an intravesical median lobe will

[1] Young: Journal of Urology, 1922, viii, 361–429.

give a picture very suggestive of vesical neoplasm. Such a lobe is usually pedunculated, congested, and inflamed as a result of cystitis. Good sized ulcers may occasionally occur on these lobes. One sees the surface reddened, irregular, covered with bullæ which may suggest edematous papillæ, and with perhaps enlarged vessels which give rise to hemorrhage. Indeed, hematuria may be the first symptom in such a case. The diagnosis is helped by noting the position of the mass. If the cystoscope rests in one of the lateral sulci, the tumor may seem to arise well to one side of the orifice. By imparting to the cystoscope motions which cause the beak to move toward the anterior wall (up) and toward the tumor (across) it will usually be possible to get it into the other sulcus, when the tumor will appear on the side opposite to that which it formerly occupied. This does not rule out a pedunculated neoplasm springing from the posterior lip of the vesical orifice. One searches carefully and may discover an area of mucosa on the mass free enough from the inflammatory changes to indicate by its smoothness that it cannot be neoplastic tissue. The presence of lateral lobe hypertrophy is not decisive, as this condition may coexist with vesical tumor. Sometimes the most careful study will fail to produce an absolutely certain diagnosis, in which case it is well to operate suprapubically, prepared to treat whichever condition is present. In one case of enlarged prostate, in which a catheter had been long used, and accompanied by a marked cystitis, the cystoscope showed intravesical masses covered with edematous papillomata and polyps. A diagnosis of tumor was made, and suprapubic drainage given. Six months later the "tumors" had disappeared and the cystoscope showed median and lateral lobes covered with smooth mucous membrane. By prostatectomy benign adenomata were removed. In other cases catheter drainage and irrigations have cleared up the cystitis—and simultaneously the diagnosis.

Rarely a *vesical calculus*, if covered with blood-clot and mucopus and especially if fixed at some point on the bladder wall (by adhesion or by extension into a small diverticulum), may simulate intravesical tumor. Investigation of the consistence of the mass with the tip of the cystoscope or with a wire, or the *x*-ray, will give the diagnosis.

Intravesical extension of *carcinoma of the prostate* may give an ulcerating, fungating mass in the bladder. This is usually a late phenomenon, so that extensive involvement of the prostate, and probably also the of seminal vesicles, will suggest the proper diagnosis. *Vice versa*, a bladder tumor invading the prostate may be mistaken for prostatic carcinoma. Clinically, the distinction is of little importance, since, whatever the origin of the tumor, such a case is beyond any radical treatment.

Implantations from papillary *tumors of the renal pelvis* are exactly like bladder tumors. This rare event may easily cause mistakes, as it would scarcely be advisable to catheterize the ureters and do a pyelogram in every case of bladder papilloma. Persistence of hematuria after destruction of a bladder growth should lead to immediate investigation of the kidney. Suter[1] reports such a case in which nephrectomy did not suffice, as the tumor proved eventually to be a tiny papilloma in the ureter—after nephrectomy had been done.

Bilharziosis of the bladder may give rise to appearances indistinguishable cystoscopically from neoplasm. Since the process is a proliferative granuloma, due to the presence of ova, good sized tumors may be produced. They are usually

[1] Urologic and Cutaneous Review, Technical Supplement, 1913, i, 62–65.

sessile, and may show hemorrhage and ulceration. The small yellowish nodules known as bilharzia bodies may be seen. The history, if it includes residence in infested areas (the disease is very common in Egypt, Arabia, and Turkey) is important, but the discovery of the ova in the urine is pathognomonic. One must remember, however, that malignant changes often supervene in chronic vesical bilharziosis.

Pelvic tumors may simulate grossly invasive vesical neoplasms, or retrovesical sarcoma. If osteosarcoma, the *x*-ray picture will be typical. Uterine tumors may press upon or invade the bladder. A urachal cyst may give a suprapubic tumor suggesting a bladder origin. Its movability, and the absence of any intravesical involvement, will give a clue. In the same way, large diverticula which do not empty on catheterization may be taken for tumors. Cystoscopic examination and cystogram clear up the diagnosis.

Hydatid cysts may simulate closely retrovesical sarcoma when they lie in the rectovesical culdesac, and are not very uncommon in this position. The history is valuable. Other cysts in the liver, etc., may be palpable and suggest the diagnosis. The tumor itself may give a cystic feel, though not invariably. Diagnostic puncture is not considered justifiable, but if any of the fluid does in any way become available, watery clearness and the *absence of all protein*, except perhaps a trace of globulin, is absolutely *diagnostic*. If infected, the contents is purulent, and if the lining has been disturbed at all, typical hooklets will be seen. In some cases the diagnosis will be very difficult, and if any suspicion exists, and the tumor fails entirely to respond to radium and *x*-ray, exploration may be necessary. One should be prepared to carry out the excision or marsupialization demanded in the treatment of this disease.

TREATMENT OF BLADDER TUMORS

There is no subject in urology concerning which opinion has varied more from time to time than in tumors of the bladder. For many years operative attacks consisted almost entirely in excision of a pedunculated tumor with or without a small portion of adjacent bladder mucosa. Then resection of the entire bladder wall surrounding the malignant tumor of the bladder came into vogue. In the early days of the Johns Hopkins Hospital these two methods alone were employed, but most cases arrived too late for anything more than suprapubic drainage.

In 1913 we made our first systematic study of the results which had been obtained at this hospital and it seems advisable to quote from this so as to compare it later with the methods which we now employ.[1]

A review of these 117 cases of vesical tumor, 83 per cent. of which were malignant, shows that excision, as usually carried out, is utterly inadequate and followed by prompt recurrence in both benign and malignant cases. The cautery is an extremely valuable agent in conjunction with suprapubic or intraperitoneal operations, and when it has been thoroughly applied, even in apparently hopeless cases, some brilliant cures have been obtained. Carcinoma of the bladder, except in very extensive cases, is best treated by suprapubic resection of the bladder, leaving a wide area of healthy wall around the tumor, ureter transplanted if necessary, and the peritoneum excised when the tumor involves that portion of the bladder. Intraperitoneal operations are rarely necessary (except in tumors of the vertex and posterior wall), as an excellent view of the bladder can be obtained by an extensive median incision, wide separation of the recti muscles, upward displacement of the peritoneum, a long incision into the bladder, and good retraction. The use of 50 per cent. resorcin, or alcohol, to kill any tumor particles which may have dropped

[1] Young: Journal American Medical Association, 1913, lxi, 1857–1861.

into the bladder, also seems desirable, but a better plan is to cauterize the tumor thoroughly before beginning the resection of the bladder.

For benign tumors the treatment with the high-frequency spark seems thoroughly satisfactory, but should be vigorously applied. In extensive cases the fulgurating sound, or the application of a strong spark through an open endoscope or cystoscope, the bladder being filled with air, may be very helpful. In apparently hopeless cases, destruction of the tumors and their bases and adjacent portions of the bladder wall by means of Paquelin, hot-air, or electric cauteries may occasionally give unexpected cures and brilliant results. Before applying treatment an adequate specimen should usually be obtained by means of the cystoscopic rongeur for microscopic diagnosis.

Only three years ago many authorities considered it almost impossible to cure benign papilloma of the bladder, and in many clinics abroad operations on cancer of the bladder were practically discontinued. The demonstration of the marvelous efficacy of high-frequency electric applications is one of the most brilliant and valuable additions to surgery in recent years, and the proof that resection of the bladder wall offers a good chance of cure in cancer shows that the surgery of vesical tumors, far from being a hopeless field, is indeed one of great promise.

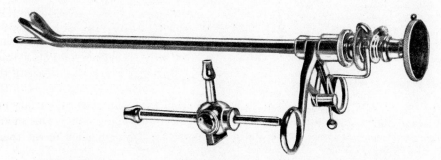

FIG. 380.—Young's cystoscopic rongeur with automatic centering device to keep cystoscope from moving with inner tube and thus greatly assisting accurate grappling of objects.

The cases were again systematically studied ten years later,[1] and an effort was made to obtain an accurate idea of the ultimate result in the 380 cases which formed the basis of the report.

Among these there were 28 in which the tumor was clamped and excised, with only 11 per cent. cured, demonstrating positively the futility of this technic. In 14 cases in which destruction of the tumor with the Paquelin or electric cautery was carried out, 9 patients are dead; 5 are alive, 2 recent cases and 3 in which a considerable time has elapsed since operation and with apparent cure. As all of these cases were malignant and extensive, the results obtained were fairly good.

Resection of the bladder with tumor had been carried out in 51 cases. All were malignant and 14 (27 per cent.) were apparently cured five years after operation. There were 55 per cent. alive and well at the last report.

There were 37 cases treated by fulguration through the cystoscope. Of these, 27 were benign and all were apparently cured; 10 cases of malignant papilloma were unimproved.

We treated 103 cases by radium and fulguration through the cystoscope. Of these, 25 were diagnosed benign and 78 malignant papilloma; 46 per cent. of these patients were reported alive and well. There were 22 per cent. alive with recurrence and 15 per cent. dead with recurrence; 10 per cent. were dead without recurrence.

Carcinoma of the bladder treated by implantation of radium through suprapubic cystostomy, 15 cases. Reports showed that 9 patients were dead, 3 have been lost sight of, and only 2 in which there was a definite improvement. The following conclusions were drawn:

Both papillomata and carcinomata are much more frequent in the region of the trigone

[1] Young and Scott, W. W.: New York Medical Journal and Medical Record, 1923, cxviii, 262-268.

and ureteral orifices and adjacent lateral walls of the bladder and vesical neck. The anterior wall is less frequently involved and the vertex and upper posterior wall are still more rarely involved.

The vertex, anterior, upper lateral, and posterior walls are most suitable for resection and excellent results may be expected by radical removal of a wide margin of bladder wall, but good results may be obtained by resection in the base of the bladder and region of ureters. When the vesical neck and prostate are involved deep cauterization is far more effective than excision, but it is dangerous.

Fulguration is the method of choice in benign papilloma, but in large tumors radium is of great assistance in causing a rapid disappearance of the tumor, and, owing to the potential malignancy of all vesical papillomata, radium should generally be applied, if possible. In malignant papillomata radium, applied with an operative cystoscope and held firmly in position with a clamp fastened to the table, is of the greatest value and gives more brilliant results. Here again the conjoint use of fulguration and radium is advisable. The same treatment is sometimes completely effective in papillary carcinomata, and four small and two large tumors of this type and one small infiltrating cancer have been apparently cured by it.

Where the tumor is definitely malignant or very extensive, and particularly if infiltrating, it should be attacked suprapubically; great care being taken not to touch the tumor or break off any papillary processes. Alcohol or resorcin 20 per cent. should be applied to destroy any fragment that may have dropped into the bladder or wound.

If resection can be carried out successfully with a wide area of healthy bladder wall, whether extraperitoneal or transperitoneal or with transplantation of a ureter, it should usually be done, but the operation should not be so extravagantly extensive as to face a very high mortality rate.

The position of radium implantation is still *sub judice*. Fulguration, radium, the electrocautery and careful radical resection have transformed the situation, so that now about 95 per cent. of the benign and 75 per cent. of the malignant papillomata, about 50 per cent. papillary carcinomata, and somewhere near 25 per cent. of the infiltrating carcinomata are probably curable by one or more of the methods above referred to. There is no phase of surgery in which during the last ten years more gratifying advance has been made than in that of tumors of the bladder.

High-frequency Electric Treatment of Bladder Tumors.—This most valuable method came as a result of a paper by Edwin Beer[1] who reported cases in which he had destroyed vesical papillomata by "fulguration." This was quickly confirmed by Keyes,[2] both using instruments for the application of high-frequency current made by Reinhold Wappler. The method has been modified variously and is now called fulguration, electrocoagulation, diathermy, etc. The apparatus came as a result of the introduction by Dr. Oudin of the high frequency induction coil. This work by a medical man has been the basis of much of the progress which has since been made in wireless telegraphy, telephony, etc. In the early work the unipolar current of Oudin was alone used. Subsequently the bipolar current of d'Arsonval has been much employed. We have not the space to describe the various instruments which are employed for high-frequency electric treatments in surgery. The cold cautery, diathermy, the radio-knife, etc., have in themselves a large literature.

In the treatment of bladder tumors the high frequency applications may be made by means of a cystoscope or directly through a suprapubic wound. Using the ordinary catheterizing cystoscope, an insulated wire is introduced into the bladder through the catheterizing tube and brought into contact with some portion of the tumor to be treated by means of the ureter catheterizing mechanism. The wire is connected externally with the high frequency apparatus and at a given

---

[1] Journal of the American Medical Association, 1910, liv, 1768–1769.

[2] Transactions of the American Association of Genito-Urinary Surgeons, 1910, v, 193–199, and discussion, 199–206.

PLATE XIV

CYSTOSCOPIC VIEWS

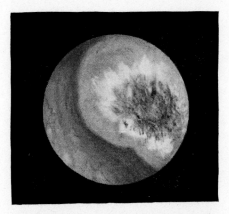

A. Malignant papilloma after fulguration.

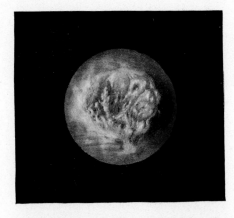

B. Result of radium applications, almost complete destruction of tumor, large slough.

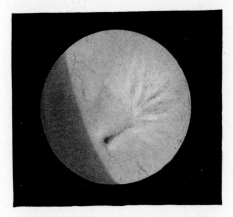

C. Vesical scar, pale mucosa at site of tumor destroyed by fulguration.

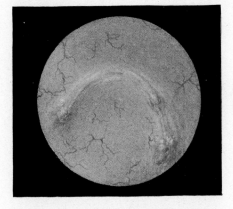

D. Submucous cystitis, characteristic elevated linear area, congested in places.

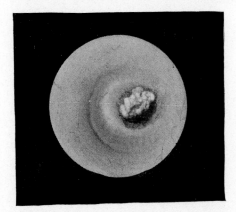

E. Small calculus protruding from end of ureter.

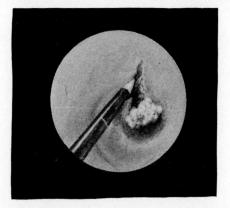

F. Enlargement of ureteral orifice by fulguration to facilitate passage of stone.

signal the current is turned on and the high frequency spark is applied to the surface of the tumor or plunged into it under cystoscopic guidance.

The point to which the application is made will depend on the position and character of the tumor. Where it is possible to make the application at or near the base of the tumor so as to destroy at one time the base and external portions of the tumor this should be done. In many cases it is only possible to reach that part of the tumor which is in proximity to the cystoscope, but by progressive fulguration as much of the tumor as possible is destroyed at one séance.

With local anesthesia of the bladder and urethra the operation is very little more painful than that of ordinary cystoscopy. A large dose of morphin hypodermically may be of assistance and in some clinics antipyrin per rectum is also used. Spinal and sacral anesthesia has occasionally been employed and in rare instances general anesthesia, but, as a rule, local anesthesia suffices, and the operation can be carried out with so little discomfort that fairly large areas and occasionally the entire tumor may be destroyed at the first sitting. Where tumors are multiple it may be desirable to destroy as much of each tumor as possible at the first sitting. Subsequent treatments are given as frequently as convenient or tolerable by the patient. We often make applications two or three times a week and endeavor to make each as thorough as possible. Not infrequently thirty minutes are consumed in one treatment and large areas of tumor tissue are completely destroyed. The effect of the treatment is to produce coagulation of the tissues, which turn white as a result of the application. This process extends deeply into the tumor, cutting off the blood-supply of the region attacked and also of regions depending upon it for their blood-supply. In some instances we attempt to introduce the electrode deeply into the tissues so as to increase the effectiveness of the destruction.

As long as the electrode touches only the tumor the patient feels no pain, and it is only when the current is passed through normal bladder mucosa that any painful sensations are felt.

Various difficulties are encountered in carrying out this treatment. The insulated wires are prone to become short circuited and ineffective and the insulation covering the terminal portion may become separated and allow the current to be dissipated in the bladder fluid. Removal of the electrode and cutting off the end will correct this defect and allow the application to continue. Larger and better electrodes have been produced, but require a single large catheter-bearing or operating cystoscope such as the Wappler posterior cystoscopes, which admit a No. 10 wire.

Radium Treatment.—In 1913 Pasteau and Degrais[1] and Schüller[2] reported a few cases of cancer of the prostate and bladder in which truly striking results had been obtained by the use of radium introduced through the urethra through the ordinary coudé gum catheter. As stated elsewhere, this led us in 1914 to procure 100 mg. of radium element and to begin clinical experimentation. It soon became evident that for accurate work much more exact methods and special instruments would be necessary, and in the shops of the Brady Institute we set about to design and construct an instrument to meet the varied needs in vesical tumors. The accompanying illustrations show the different models so well that very little description is necessary (Figs. 382–390).

[1] International Congress of Medicine, London, 1913, Section XIV, Urology, Part II, 28–29.
[2] Ibid., 115–117.

The first cystoscopic radium applicator was made by Paschkis.[1] This instrument was unknown to us until it was brought to light in a publication by Thomas[2] at a meeting of the American Urological Association several months after we had constructed and presented our cystoscopic radium applicator. The instrument of Paschkis employed a straight cystoscope similar to ours. The radium was carried in a short beak which was fastened to the shaft of the instrument by a screw. There was no provision for external fixation of the instrument in proper position against a tumor in the bladder, as shown in Fig. 381. He apparently did not employ

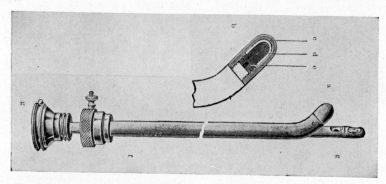

FIG. 381.—Paschkis' cystoscopic radium applicator. This is the first made, but no means of fixing instrument in position so as to hold radium firmly against selected portion of tumor is provided.

any clamp externally to hold the instrument in place. Nevertheless, the priority for having made the first cystoscopic radium applicator belongs to Paschkis. The instrument was evidently inconvenient and the absence of any mechanism for holding the radium against a tumor for a protracted period largely negatived its value. No report of further use of this instrument has been made.

The small straight cystoscope which is used in our cystoscopic rongeur was used as a basis around which to construct the various radium instruments. Radium

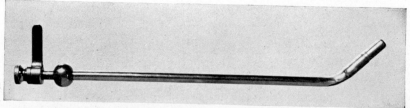

FIG. 382.—Young's cystoscopic radium applicator (No. 1), with obturator in place ready for introduction. One hundred or 200 mg. of radium are carried in the metal beak which is held by friction in cup of shaft. Note ball at outer end for fixation with clamp attached to table when radium has been placed in desired position by means of cystoscope.

instrument No. 1 (Figs. 382 and 383) carries radium in its beak. A platinum capsule 1 mm. thick is placed in a gold capsule which, in turn, is inserted into the tubular end of the beak, where it is held by friction. The instrument is passed through the urethra with an obturator, which is then withdrawn. The bladder is washed out and the cystoscope introduced (Fig. 383). With the beak turned away from the tumor careful inspection of the tumor is made for the purpose of

[1] Wiener klinische Wochenschrift, 1911, xxiv, 1562–1564.
[2] Thomas, B. A.: Transactions American Urological Association, 1915. ix, 141–225.

determining the point of application. This having been decided by means of the external handle the radium-carrying outer sheath is turned until the beak containing the radium is placed against the tumor. It is generally desirable to use sufficient pressure to force the beak well into the soft substance of the tumor at which point it is fixed and held by means of a clamp attached to the table externally

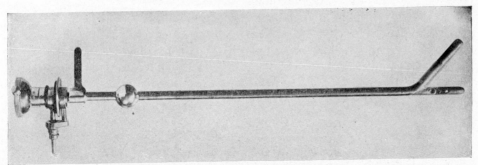

FIG. 383.—Young's cystoscopic radium applicator No. 1, with cystoscope introduced for inspection of bladder and placing of radium as desired.

(Fig. 384). The patient is requested to remain motionless for one hour, and during this time the cystoscope may be removed so that the bladder may empty itself, or if it is desirable for the bladder to contain fluid to prevent too great contraction upon the end of the instrument, it is partially evacuated occasionally by the temporary removal of the telescope. As a rule, when the patient has been given

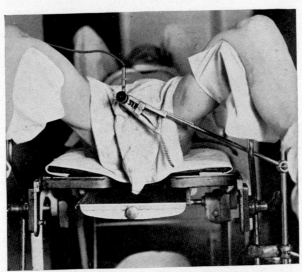

FIG. 384.—Young's cystoscopic radium applicator in use, showing clamp fixing instrument in proper position.

morphin, gr. $\frac{1}{6}$ or $\frac{1}{4}$, and the urethra and bladder anesthetized with 4 per cent. procain, no difficulty is experienced by the patient in undergoing treatment of one hour's duration. Where the bladder is very intolerant it may be necessary to shorten the duration of the treatment.

Radium instrument No. 1 has proved very satisfactory for most tumors of the bladder. It is especially good for those in the region of the trigone and base of the bladder (where fully 70 per cent. of all tumors are located), for the vesical neck, prostatic orifice, and immediately adjacent portions of the bladder wall. For very large tumors we have employed a similar instrument which contains two capsules of 100 mg. of radium each, placed tandem in the beak. This makes it possible to give twice the dosage in the same time.

For tumors well out on the lateral walls of the bladder or on the upper part of the anterior wall this instrument was not entirely satisfactory, as the tip of the radium capsule and not its length was presented to the tumor. For these tumors

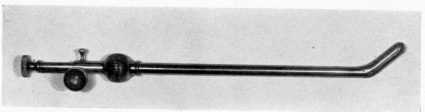

Fig. 385.—Young's parallelogram radium applicator, closed, with obturator, ready for introduction. (Instrument No. 2.)

radium instrument No. 2 was designed (Figs. 385, 386). This instrument carries a capsule of radium within its beak which is made up of two hollow halves which when separated by the external operating mechanism carry the radium out to a position parallel to the shaft and about 2.5 cm. distant from it, as shown in Fig. 386. This instrument may be loaded with one or two tubes of 100 mg. each of radium which are placed within a thin silver capsule. This slips, in turn, into a semcircular container which is attached by a pivot to the inner blade and slides up and down a slot to which it is attached in the outer blade. The mechanism is easily understood by reference to the accompanying illustrations. This instrument can be

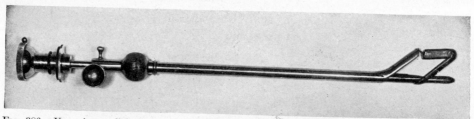

Fig. 386.—Young's parallelogram cystoscopic radium applicator opened out for use. (Instrument No. 2.)

used in place of instrument No. 1 without opening the blades. When closed the tubes of radium lie within the beak of the instrument and in exactly the same position as in instrument No. 1. It has the advantage that two tubes of radium (200 mg.) may be used instead of one, as in No. 1. With these two instruments tumors in almost every part of the bladder can be thoroughly treated with radium.

For tumors well back on the posterior wall of the bladder, however, it seemed desirable to be able to apply radium transversely to the axis of the cystoscope. For this purpose we first constructed instrument No. 3 (Fig. 387). By means of a thumb screw externally and wires which run within the outer sheath of the instrument, the capsule containing the radium is turned upon a pivot in the handle of the instrument and then may be applied transversely upon tumors, as shown in Fig. 388.

When tumors were on the anterior wall of the bladder immediately above the prostatic orifice we found difficulty in reaching them with any of the three pre-

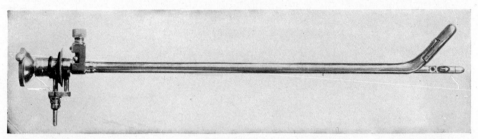

Fig. 387.—Young's rotating transverse cystoscopic radium applicator after introduction into bladder, but not opened out.   (Instrument No. 3.)

viously described instruments, and for this purpose have designed instrument No. 4, the mechanism of which is shown in Figs. 389, 390.   As seen here, the radium is also carried transversely to the shaft of the instrument by means of a screw mechanism externally.

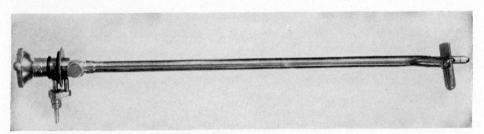

Fig. 388.—Young's rotating transverse cystoscopic radium applicator.   Used for tumors on anterior and posterior wall.   (Instrument No. 3.)

With these four instruments it is possible to apply radium to any portion of the bladder and generally with ease and accuracy.   It is important to chart exactly the location at which the radium has been applied so that a different spot may be selected at each subsequent treatment.   In some cases we find it possible to give a

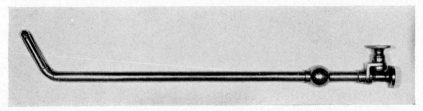

Fig. 389.—Young's triangular transverse cystoscopic radium applicator, closed for introduction.   (Instrument No. 4.)

treatment three times a week and generally for an hour.   The number of treatments required depends upon the character and size of the tumor, but owing to the fact that radium is buried in the soft substance of the tumor the effect is more pronounced than in carcinoma of the prostate where the tumor is reached through the intermediary of the rectal and urethral mucosa.   From 600 to 1000 milligram-hours is usually all that is required, and for smaller tumors and particularly when fulguration is used simultaneously to facilitate the reduction of the tumor mass, 400 milligram-hours may suffice. The treatment and charting of a case is shown in Figs. 391 and 392.

In our first report[1] the results obtained in 45 cases of tumors of the bladder which were treated by radium alone or a combination of radium and fulguration were given. Of these, 15 were papillomata and 30 were carcinomata. Of the papillomata, only 2 were treated with radium alone, 1 receiving 350 milligram-hours

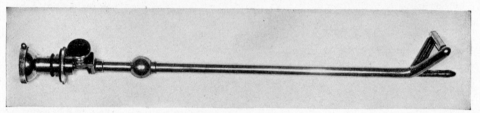

Fig. 390.—Young's triangular transverse cystoscopic radium applicator. For tumors on anterior and posterior walls. (Instrument No. 4.)

and the other 50 milligram-hours. Both tumors disappeared three weeks after radiation. In 13 cases of papillomata a combination of radium and fulguration was employed. In 7 cases the actual effect of the radium cannot be stated. The tumors disappeared, but it is probable that they might have responded to fulguration alone. In the remaining 6 radium played an important rôle. These were all papillary pedunculated tumors presenting cystoscopic appearances similar to those of the type of tumor which usually responds to fulguration. Specimens obtained

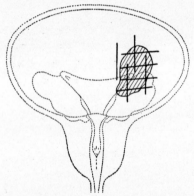
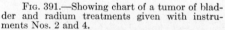
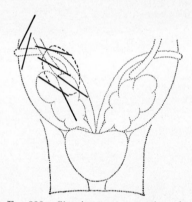

Fig. 391.—Showing chart of a tumor of bladder and radium treatments given with instruments Nos. 2 and 4.

Fig. 392.—Showing treatments given through rectum to base of tumor in bladder—also to pelvic glands.

with our cystoscopic rongeur showed that 2 of them contained malignant areas. They did not disappear following radium treatment, but responded rapidly to fulguration, the tumor disappearing in three treatments. There was thus pointed out for the first time the wonderful co-operative effect of radium and fulguration in hastening the disappearance of vesical papillomata. Tumors which would not disappear under either treatment were rapidly destroyed when both methods were employed alternately.

[1] Young and Frontz, W. A.: Journal of Urology, 1917, i, 505–541.

Since the publication of these radium cystoscopic applicators other instruments have appeared in the literature, several of which are almost identical with our instrument No. 1. Hinman presented a flexible tube which could be passed retrograde into a catheterizing cystoscope, and carried on the inner end a small tube of radium element, which could be applied thus to a vesical tumor.

Shortly after this Barringer, Buerger, and others presented similar instruments for applying radium element upon or into the substance of vesical tumors.

More recently Muir has devised a very ingenious tube to be employed with a catheterizing cystoscope for the insertion of glass tubes containing radium emanations into tumors of the bladder.

In 1915 Kelly and his associates[1] began to employ radium in the treatment of bladder tumors through a tubular endoscope, the bladder being filled with air with the patient in the genupectoral position.

In 1917 we employed our ordinary urethral endoscope most satisfactorily in the following case: A woman aged about seventy presented a very large malignant papilloma of the trigone. It measured fully 2 inches in diameter, but the adjacent bladder was apparently healthy. By means of our endoscope 200 mg. of radium were inserted by means of a needle into the tumor near the base (Fig. 393). The endoscope was then withdrawn and the needle allowed to remain in the urethra for six hours, during which time the inner radium-bearing end was buried in the base of the tumor. This procedure was done three times and the patient was then discharged. She returned six months later and examination showed that the tumor had completely disappeared. Subsequent examinations two and four years later showed a small papilloma in another portion of the bladder. This was destroyed by fulguration and application of radium with instrument No. 1. Since this time the patient has remained well.

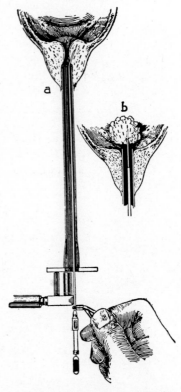

FIG. 393.—Showing implantation of radium through Young's urethroscope (a) into carcinoma of prostate; (b) into tumor of bladder, with rigid implanter, as shown, for implantation of seeds at neck of bladder through prostate or into tumors of bladder.

In 1922 Neill[2] devised an excellent instrument for introducing radium emanation seeds into bladder tumors through the Kelly tubular cystoscope (Fig. 394). He was able to use the same method in men with a longer endoscope, the patient being placed upon our urologic operating table with the head greatly depressed, thus allowing the bladder to fill with air by negative pressure (Fig. 396).

The advantage of the endoscopic method of applying radium emanation in seeds or element in small needles is that more accurate instrumentation is possible and we believe that in the future these open-air methods will be much more frequently employed.

[1] American Journal of Obstetrics and Diseases of Women and Children, 1919, lxxx, 1–7.
[2] Journal of the American Medical Association, 1922, lxxix, 2061–2063.

Application of Radium Through a Suprapubic Wound.—If radium element is used, the needles should not contain more than 1 mg. each and should be placed so that each needle is at the center of a cubic centimeter of tissue area.   Having

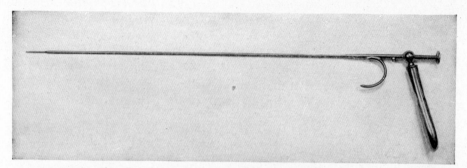

Fig. 394.—Neill's endoscopic needle for introducing radium emanation seeds into vesical tumors.

thoroughly exposed the tumor the operator plans his procedure so as to cover the entire area and the adjacent mucous membrane for a distance of at least 5 mm. around the extreme outer limits of the tumor.   If the tumor is a fairly flat growth,

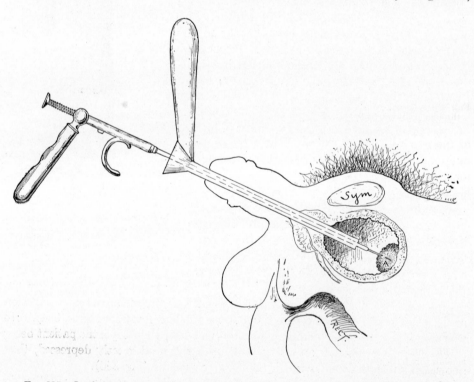

Fig. 395.—Implantation of radium emanation seeds into tumor of bladder with Neill's needle.

the radium is buried directly into it, the needles being about 1 cm. apart and placed sufficiently deep so that the emanation will reach well beyond the deeper confines of the tumor.   It should not, however, penetrate more than 1 cm. for fear of injuring adjacent organs.

As seen in Fig. 397, the radium is carried in a small pointed capsule of platinum, the outer end of which carries an eyelet through which a strong linen thread is placed. It is introduced by means of a special carrier, the threads emerging from slots on each side are utilized to hold the radium in the carrier while it is introduced into the tumor. As soon as it has been buried to the proper depth it is forced out

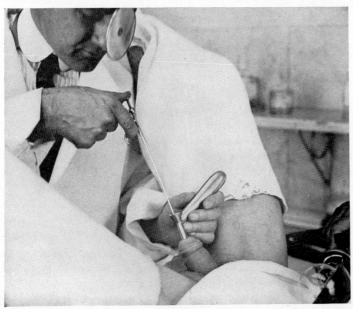

Fig. 396.—Actual implantation treatment of radium emanation being carried out within the bladder through Kelly open-air cystoscope in exaggerated Trendelenburg position on Young's table. Neill.

of the carrier by means of a plunger and the carrier then withdrawn, leaving the radium buried in the tumor and with the linen threads emerging from the wound for its extraction. Great care is taken to see that these points are firmly placed because they may easily emerge from the soft tumor tissue unless care is taken.

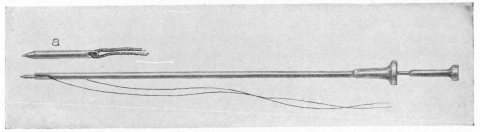

Fig. 397.—Young's injector for radium needles: a, Platinum needle containing 1 mg. radium element, threaded with strong linen (magnified). Below, reduced picture of needle in place, thread in slots, plunger in position to drive needle into tissues.

Before beginning an operation of this kind sufficient radium points should be at hand to cover completely the tumor and the adjacent tissue. We frequently employ from 20 to 30 of such needles, each containing 1 mg.

Where the tumor projects into the bladder more than 5 mm. it is usually desirable to remove the outer portion by means of an electrocautery before implanting the radium. If this is not done the mass may be too thick to be sufficiently irradiated by the radium. The tumor should usually be removed flush with the bladder by means of a long, flat, electrocautery or cold cautery blade, care being taken to remove it in one piece and to avoid dropping particles of the tumor into the bladder. It may be desirable to destroy the whole surface of the tumor before attempting to remove it, so that no live tumor tissue will be lost in the bladder or wound to set up implantations. If particles are dropped into the bladder they should be carefully removed and 95 per cent. alcohol poured into the bladder to destroy any remaining tumor particles.

Having destroyed the tumor with the cautery flush with the bladder, the burned area is then thoroughly implanted with radium needles 1 cm. apart and sufficient in number to cover the area of the tumor and for a distance of at least 5 mm. beyond the confines of the neoplasm. For this purpose the outer radium points are inserted at the boundary of the tumor into the adjacent normal tissues. The operator having thoroughly covered the surface of the tumor with radium implantations and being certain that each point is firmly bedded in the tissues so that it cannot easily escape into the bladder, the threads leading to the platinum points are carefully collected, counted again, fastened with a ligature, and brought out through the wound when the bladder is closed. Tube drainage with a mushroom catheter is also provided. The length of stay for these platinum points varies, but we have frequently not removed them for three days, during which time each point of 1 mg. will give 72 milligram-hours, and if 20 are used, 1420 milligram-hours will be the dosage which has been given to the base of the tumor—a fairly considerable radium treatment. In some instances, in addition to the points of 1 mg. each, we have introduced needles containing 10 or 12 mg. in the center of the tumor mass when we thought deeper penetration and a larger dosage were required. This has been particularly the case when the region of the vesical neck, prostate, and urethra was also involved, in which case we frequently implanted radium deeply into the substance of the prostate. As a rule, the use of large doses of radium into the bladder is a mistake, as too great necrosis is produced and painful sloughing cicatrices may be produced. The ideal result is to obtain disappearance of the tumor cells without much necrosis of the bladder wall and without the production of an ulcer which will not heal promptly.

The advantage of the use of radium screened with platinum is this: Marked ulceration is thus avoided by the cutting out of the alpha and beta radiation and the consequent more uniform radiation of the entire area with the gamma rays.

The use of emanation points has become wide-spread in recent years. At first we employed doses of 2 and sometimes of 3 millicuries, but some very disagreeable experiences have shown us the danger of using such large amounts. In one case with a flat adenocarcinoma of the trigone and right lateral wall of the bladder 8 glass seeds of $2\frac{1}{2}$ millicuries each were permanently implanted into the tumor masses which were elevated only a few millimeters above the surface of the bladder. As a result of this treatment the patient developed a most extensive and deep ulceration of the region of the trigone and vesical neck which caused fearful pain and refused to heal. In order to relieve the patient's agony it was necessary to do a second suprapubic operation and excise a large area, but this failed to give much relief and he eventually died as a result of overtreatment. Since then, having learned our lesson, we now never employ emanation seeds greater than 1 millicurie and prefer those of $\frac{1}{2}$ millicurie. When this small dosage is used it is necessary to insert them at intervals of about 8 mm., and if the tumor mass is very deep it may be desirable to put them in two layers. They may be introduced by means of the instrument of Neill or that of Muir.

Results.—At our request Dr. W. W. Scott and Dr. R. W. McKay have made a comprehensive study of all the cases of bladder tumor in the files of the Brady Urological Institute. Their study comprises 534 cases. These have been analyzed as to their pathology and the treatment employed. Every effort has been made to discover the ultimate results by physical examinations and cystoscopy wherever this has been possible, and in other cases by letters to the patient and, in many cases, to the patient's physician. In most instances it has been possible to get a fairly accurate idea of the results of treatment employed. The following table has been prepared to show the different types of therapy which have been used, the number of cases under each group, and the pathologic character of the tumors in which this treatment has been employed.

TABLE 81

VARIOUS TYPES OF BLADDER TUMORS AND THEIR TREATMENT. 534 CASES

Treatment.	Number of cases.	Benign papilloma.	Malignant papilloma.	Papillary carcinoma.	Infiltrating carcinoma.	Papilloma not classified.	Designated only as bladder tumor.	Adenocarcinoma.	Dermoid cyst.	Benign cyst.
Fulguration alone	51	33	2	4	5	6	1			
Radium plus fulguration	142	31	57	25	23	4	2			
Radium urethral route (cystoscopic), or urethral route plus another	49	2	6	5	36					
Application of radium by means other than urethra	12	..	1	1	10					
Suprapubic implantation of radium (needles and emanations)	28	..	2	4	21	..	..	1		
Resection	64	..	3	15	44	..	..	..	1	1
Cauterization alone	35	2	7	12	13	1				
Operative measures other than resection, cauterization, suprapubic application and implantation of radium	43	2	4	4	32	1				
x-Ray alone or combined with some other form of therapy	32	1	5	9	17					
Cases not treated	78	1	9	9	55	4				
Total	534	72	96	88	256	16	3	1	1	1

Comment.—It is only fair to say that in some cases the treatment employed has not been considered ideal or the most appropriate. In a number of instances the feeble condition of the patient due to old age or prolonged suffering made impossible the more radical procedures indicated. Other cases were complicated by the presence of previous operative scars, or pathologic conditions of the heart, lungs, kidneys, and lower urinary tract which precluded the use of more appropriate or ideal therapeutic measures. It is also freely admitted that in much of the early work the treatment was not such as is considered correct or even justifiable at present.

TABLE 82

AGE AT ONSET IN 534 CASES OF BLADDER TUMOR AND TREATMENT USED

Treatment.	Number of cases.	Age not given.	10–19 years.	20–29 years.	30–39 years.	40–49 years.	50–59 years.	60–69 years.	70–79 years.	80–89 years.
Fulguration alone........................	51	3	1	5	8	12	10	8	4	
Radium by cystoscopic applicator and fulguration................................	142	9	..	2	10	30	41	34	15	1
Radium applied cystoscopically or this method plus another.........................	49	4	..	1	2	7	14	11	10	
Radium applied by means other than cystoscopic method........................	12	2	..	..	1	3	3	1	2	
Suprapubic implantation of radium into vesical tumor................................	28	2	..	..	2	2	11	7	4	
Suprapubic resection of bladder with tumor..	64	1	..	..	2	9	20	28	4	
Suprapubic cauterization of tumor...........	35	..	..	1	4	4	8	15	3	
Other operative measures...................	43	3	..	..	2	9	10	13	4	2
x-Ray alone or combined with other therapy..	32	6	..	..	3	6	7	7	2	1
Cases not treated.........................	78	3	..	..	9	13	19	16	16	2
Total.............................	534	33	1	9	43	95	143	140	64	6

It is interesting to note that the majority of the benign and malignant papillomata appear between forty and fifty-nine years of age, while the bulk of the carcinomata occur between the ages of fifty and sixty-nine.

Treatment.—The cases have been studied according to the classification given in the previous tables.

A. Cases Treated by Fulguration Alone. 51 cases.

Here again it must be noted that we do not pretend that the treatment employed was ideal, but in some instances dictated by the exigencies of the case, such as hemorrhage, bad physical condition, etc.

The ages of these 51 patients were as follows: Ten to nineteen, 1; twenty to twenty-nine, 5; thirty to thirty-nine, 8; forty to forty-nine, 12; fifty to fifty-nine, 10; sixty to sixty-nine, 8; seventy to seventy-nine, 4; age not given, 3; total, 51.

The cystoscopic diagnosis, confirmed in many cases by the removal of a piece of tissue and microscopic examination, was as follows: Benign papilloma, 33; malignant papilloma, 2; papillary carcinoma, 4; infiltrating carcinoma, 5; papilloma not classified, 6; designated only as bladder tumor, 1; total, 51.

The results as shown by examination of patients and questionnaires are given in Table 83. The time interval between admission of patient and last report is stated in successive columns. Those patients who are reported alive and well have been divided into two groups: (1) Those in which a cystoscopic verification of the absence of tumor has been obtained; and (2) those in which the reported cure is based on absence of symptoms.

As 65 per cent. of these tumors were benign papillomata which are more suited to treatment by fulguration, we have prepared Table 84 of these cases alone.

Comment.—Only 6 deaths in this group can be attributed directly to the failure

TABLE 83

RESULTS OF FULGURATION ALONE IN BLADDER TUMOR. 51 CASES

	Less than one year.	One year.	Two years.	Three years.	Four years.	Five years.	Six years.	Seven years.	Eight years.	Nine years.	Ten years.	Eleven years.	Twelve years.	Total.
Alive and well:														
(1) Cystoscopic..............	..	3	3	2	1	3	1	..	3	..	1	..	..	17
(2) Symptomless.............	..	2	..	1	1	1	1	2	1	2	..	..	..	11
(3) Recurred, retreated, well....	..	1	..	1	..	..	..	..	..	..	..	1	..	3
Recurred, unimproved...........	..	1	..	1	..	..	..	..	..	..	..	..	..	2
Recurred, dead.................	6	..	..	..	..	..	..	..	..	..	..	..	..	6
Dead, other causes.............	2	..	..	1	..	..	1	..	..	1	..	..	1	6
Not followed	6	..	..	..	..	..	..	..	..	..	..	..	..	6

TABLE 84

RESULTS OF FULGURATION ALONE ON BENIGN PAPILLOMA OF THE BLADDER. 33 CASES

	Less than one year.	One year.	Two years.	Three years.	Four years.	Five years.	Six years.	Seven years.	Eight years.	Nine years.	Ten years or over.	Total.
Alive and well:												
(1) Cystoscopic.............	1	3	2	1	..	3	1	..	1	..	..	12
(2) Symptomless...........	..	3	1	1	..	1	1	2	2	1	..	12
(3) Recurred, retreated, well..	1	1	..	..	..	..	..	..	..	..	1	3
Recurred, unimproved........	..	..	..	..	..	..	..	..	..	..	..	0
Recurred, dead...............	..	..	..	..	..	..	..	..	..	..	..	0
Dead, other causes...........	1	..	..	1	..	..	..	..	..	..	..	2
Not followed.................	4	..	..	..	..	..	..	..	..	..	..	4

of the method of therapy employed. Of these, 5 occurred in cases of extensive infiltrating carcinoma and one in an extensive papillary carcinoma. In 2 other cases, one of them papillary carcinoma, frequent recurrences made it necessary to classify them among the unimproved. Another patient having a papillary carcinoma died from a ruptured bladder following cystoscopy.

A study of Table 84, showing the results of fulguration alone on benign papilloma, is most encouraging. In this series of 33 cases there is not a single death due to tumor. In 3 cases there were recurrences, but in each instance the new growths responded to fulguration. These findings demonstrate most conclusively that fulguration alone will destroy benign papilloma of the bladder.

B. Cases Treated by Radium with Our Cystoscopic Applicator and Fulguration. 142 cases.

The ages of these patients were as follows: twenty to twenty-nine, 2; thirty to thirty-nine, 10; forty to forty-nine, 30; fifty to fifty-nine, 41; sixty to sixty-nine, 34; seventy to seventy-nine, 15; eighty to eighty-nine, 1; age not given, 9; total, 142.

It is interesting to note that 50 of these patients (30 per cent.) were under fifty years.

The type of tumor as diagnosed cystoscopically or microscopically was as follows: Benign papilloma, 31; malignant papilloma, 57; papillary carcinoma, 25; infiltrating carcinoma, 23; papilloma (not classified), 4; designated only as bladder tumor, 2.

The following table gives the results obtained, and the time which has elapsed since beginning treatment:

TABLE 85

RESULTS OBTAINED BY RADIATION AND FULGURATION IN BLADDER TUMORS. 142 CASES.

	Less than one year.	One year.	Two years.	Three years.	Four years.	Five years.	Six years.	Seven years.	Eight years.	Nine years.	Ten years.	Total.
Alive and well:												
(1) Cystoscopic.............	..	17	6	5	2	1	1	..	2	..	..	34
(2) Symptomless............	1	7	4	3	2	..	3	2	..	1	3	26
(3) Recurred, retreated, well...	..	3	3	2	1	1	..	1	..	..	..	11
Recurred, unimproved	1	13	4	3	..	..	..	1	..	..	1	23
Recurred, dead	5	13	7	2	1	..	..	..	..	..	..	28
Dead, other causes............	1	4	1	..	1	1	1	..	..	2	..	11
Not followed..................	9	..	..	..	..	..	..	..	..	..	..	9

In view of the fact that 57 (over 40 per cent.) of the tumors in this group were malignant papilloma it seemed advisable to prepare the following analysis of these 57 cases.

TABLE 86

RESULT OF RADIUM CYSTOSCOPICALLY PLUS FULGURATION IN MALIGNANT PAPILLOMA. 57 CASES.

	Less than one year.	One year.	Two years.	Three years.	Four years.	Five years.	Six years.	Seven years.	Eight years.	Nine years.	Ten years.	Total.
Alive and well:												
(1) Cystoscopic.............	..	3	4	2	2	1	1	..	1	..	..	14
(2) Symptomless............	1	3	2	..	2	..	1	2	..	1	3	15
(3) Recurred, retreated, well...	..	2	2	2	..	..	..	..	..	..	..	6
Recurred, unimproved..........	..	5	2	..	..	..	..	..	..	..	1	8
Recurred, dead................	..	2	4	..	..	..	..	..	..	..	..	6
Dead, other causes............	..	2	1	..	1	..	1	..	..	..	..	5
Not followed..................	3	..	..	..	..	..	..	..	..	..	..	3

Summary.—About 50 per cent. of these cases are well one year or more. The majority of these patients had either malignant or benign papilloma. Table 86, showing the results of this form of therapy in cases of malignant papilloma, is especially interesting in that 62 per cent. of them are well, 24 per cent. are unimproved or dead due to recurrence, and 14 per cent. are dead due to other causes or not followed. (Many were very old men.) The combination of radium plus fulguration gives very satisfactory results in the treatment of malignant papilloma of the bladder, especially the early cases, and should certainly be tried before any more radical measures are considered.

The 31 cases of benign papilloma which were treated with a combination of radium and fulguration applied by means of a cystoscope showed uniformly good results and demonstrated conclusively that the addition of radium to fulguration caused the tumor to disappear more rapidly. This is particularly true in some of the larger benign papillomata which may be quite resistant to fulguration, but after treatment with radium will often melt away with subsequent fulgurations. It is only fair to say, however, that such tumors are usually entirely curable by means of simple fulguration. Radium, however, is quite necessary in the malignant papillomata and, as shown in Table 86, the result obtained is excellent, 35 of the 57 cases of malignant papilloma having been apparently cured by this treatment.

C. Cases Treated with Cystoscopic Radium Applicator Alone or Plus Other Methods of Application. 49 cases.

In this group we have collected cases of bladder tumor which were treated by means of our cystoscopic radium applicator either alone or combined with radium introduced without the cystoscope through the rectum or vagina (with the hope of having effect upon the tumor through the rectal and bladder walls) and a few cases in which the radium was applied through the urethra without use of a cystoscope. These cases have been treated by radium alone. The results, therefore, are attributable to radium alone.

The ages of the patients were as follows: Twenty to twenty-nine, 1; thirty to thirty-nine, 2; forty to forty-nine, 7; fifty to fifty-nine, 14; sixty to sixty-nine, 11; seventy to seventy-nine, 10; age not given, 4.

The type of tumor as made out by cystoscopic or microscopic examination was as follows: Benign papilloma, 2; malignant papilloma, 6; papillary carcinoma, 5; infiltrating carcinoma, 36. It is noteworthy that only 2 out of the 49 cases were considered benign and the majority were infiltrating carcinomas, and, therefore, most resistant to treatment and with the worst possible prognosis.

The treatment employed in 30 of the cases consisted of application of radium by means of one of our cystoscopic radium applicators. As a rule, either 100 or 200 mg. radium element was employed, and an effort was made to place the radium in close contact, often buried by pressure in the substance of the tumor and held there by means of a clamp externally for a period of an hour. In 19 cases, in addition to radium cystoscopically applied, treatments were given through the rectum and occasionally through the urethra and vagina by means of simple applicators without the use of a cystoscope. Where the tumor was situated in the region of the trigone or at the vesical neck, this additional treatment through the rectum was considered extremely valuable. The results obtained by these methods are shown in Table 87, page 596.

TABLE 87

RESULTS OBTAINED BY CYSTOSCOPIC APPLICATIONS OF RADIUM OR PLUS SIMPLE RECTAL AND
URETHRAL APPLICATIONS.   49 CASES

	Less than one year.	One year.	Two years.	Three years.	Four years.	Total.
Alive and well: (1) Cystoscopic........	2	2	..	2	..	6
(2) Symptomless.....	..	..	..	..	2	2
Recurred, unimproved....	..	..	1	..	..	1
Recurred, dead..........	16	11	4	..	..	31
Dead, other causes.......	2	..	..	..	..	2
Not followed.............	7	..	..	..	..	7

Summary.—There are 49 cases in this group and 8 patients are well, 4 of them
three years or more.   Of these, 3 were infiltrating carcinomas, 3 were papillary
carcinomas, and 2 malignant papillomas.   In addition, there were 2 patients with
benign papillomas who were cured at the time of their departure, but are not classified among those well, as 1 died from another cause a year later and the other was
not followed.   The high mortality in this group can be attributed to the fact that
15 per cent. of the tumors were infiltrating carcinomas.   The satisfactory cases
mentioned above indicate that occasionally carcinomas respond to the surface
application of radium alcne.   However, recent observations in this clinic lead us
to believe that more rapid results are obtained by the combination of radium plus
fulguration than by the use of radium alone.

D. Cases Treated by Application of Radium by Means Other Than Cystoscopic
Applicators.   12 cases.

The ages varied between thirty and eighty.

None of the tumors was diagnosed benign, and 10 were of the infiltrating carcinoma type.

The method of radium application was as follows: Massive doses through abdominal wall, 3 cases; application through fresh suprapubic wound or a fistula, 7;
applied only through rectum, 1; applied through rectum and suprapubic fistula, 1.

The results obtained were uniformly bad.   Practically all of these cases were in
desperate condition with very extensive tumors, and generally with metastases when
admitted to the hospital.   Radium was used simply as a last resort, and although
some of the patients improved symptomatically, 9 died in less than one year and
the others during the first year after admission.

E. Cases Treated by Implantation of Radium Into the Vesical Tumor Through
Suprapubic Operation.   28 cases.

The ages of these patients were as follows: Thirty to thirty-nine, 2; forty to
forty-nine, 2; fifty to fifty-nine, 11; sixty to sixty-nine, 7; seventy to seventy-nine,
4; age not given, 2.

The diagnosis, confirmed by cystoscopic or microscopic examination, was as
follows: Malignant papilloma, 2; papillary carcinoma, 4; infiltrating carcinoma, 21;
adenocarcinoma, 1.

Methods Employed.—Suprapubic cystotomy, wide exposure of bladder with
protection of adjacent structures, careful avoidance of tumor so as to break off

no particles, and implantation of needles of radium element or emanations in 14 cases, and in the other 14 cases removal of the upper portion of the tumor by simple cauterization of the outstanding tumor growth, followed by implantation of radium needles or emanations. The time the radium needles were allowed to remain varied, and the total amount of radium hours differed, according to the size or character of the tumor. Except in early cases radium needles containing 1 mg. radium element or emanation were employed one to each centimeter of area involved. In the case of the needles, these were removed generally after forty-eight hours, and not infrequently after seventy-two hours. The emanation "seeds" remained *in situ*. In a few cases emanation seeds containing 2 or 3 millicuries were used, but subsequent experience showed that the dosage was too great, and in recent years no permanent implantations larger than 1 millicurie have been used. In extensive cases spears containing radium element of 10 or $12\frac{1}{2}$ mg. were employed, generally 5 in number. They remained in the bladder at least twelve hours, and not infrequently twenty-four hours. By these combined methods a very large amount of intravesical radiation within the area of the tumor and immediately adjacent was obtained in most of these cases.

The results of this treatment are shown in the accompanying table:

TABLE 88

RESULTS OF SUPRAPUBIC IMPLANTATIONS OF RADIUM IN BLADDER TUMORS. 28 CASES

	Less than one year.	One year.	Two years.	Three years.	Four years.	Total.
Alive and well: (1) Cystoscopic........	..	2	..	..	..	2
(2) Symptomless.......	..		..	..	1	1
(3) Recurred, retreated, well............	1	..	..	..	..	1
Recurred, unimproved....	..	..	1	..	..	1
Recurred, dead..........	10	10	2	..	..	22
Dead, other causes.......	..	1	..	..	..	1
Not followed............	..	..	..	..	..	0

Summary.—In this group of 28 cases, 3 patients are well, one year or more. One patient who had an infiltrating carcinoma is well four and a half years, while another is symptomless over a period of more than a year. There is one case of papillary carcinoma well more than a year, while in another case there was a recurrence which responded to radium plus fulguration. One patient died from Streptococcus hemolyticus septicemia shortly after operation. Fully 75 per cent. of the tumors in this group were non-resectable infiltrating carcinomas. The results obtained should not discourage further attempts at this form of therapy.

F. Cases Treated by Suprapubic Resection of the Bladder and Tumor. 64 cases.

The ages were as follows: Thirty to thirty-nine, 2; forty to forty-nine, 9; fifty to fifty-nine, 20; sixty to sixty-nine, 28; seventy to seventy-nine, 4; age not given, 1.

The type of tumor in these cases, confirmed by cystoscopic or microscopic examination, was as follows: malignant papilloma, 3; papillary carcinoma, 15; infiltrating carcinoma, 44; benign cyst, 1; dermoid cyst, 1.

The table below shows the results of treatment:

TABLE 89

RESULTS OBTAINED BY RESECTION OF BLADDER TUMORS. 64 CASES

	Less than one year.	One year.	Two years.	Three years.	Four years.	Five years.	Six years.	Seven years.	Eight years.	Nine years.	Ten years.	Total.
Alive and well:												
(1) Cystoscopic.............	..	2	3	1	..	..	2	1	..	..	..	9
(2) Symptomless.............	..	3	1	1	1	2	1	..	1	2	1	13
(3) Recurred, retreated, well...	..	..	1	1	..	..	..	..	..	..	..	2
Recurred, unimproved..........	2	2	..	..	..	..	..	..	..	..	..	4
Recurred, dead................	21	5	..	..	..	1	..	1	..	..	..	28
Dead, other causes.............	..	..	1	1	2	1	..	..	..	..	..	5
Not followed..................	2	..	..	..	..	..	..	..	..	..	..	2

Summary.—The location of the tumors in the 64 cases of this group was as follows: Anterior wall, 12; posterior wall, 15; lateral walls, 19; ureteral orifices and part of trigone, 14, and vesical orifice, 8. In 6 cases the tumors were resected with the cautery. The ureters were transplanted in 14 cases, while a transperitoneal resection was necessary in 8 cases. The bladder was mobilized as much as possible in 5 cases, while partial mobilization was necessary in 4 other cases.

The results of this form of therapy are most encouraging. There are 22 patients well one year or more, 10 of them more than five years. Of these, 9 had infiltrating carcinomas, 9 papillary carcinomas, 2 malignant papillomas, 1 a benign cyst, and 1 a dermoid cyst. There are 2 additional cases, 1 an infiltrating carcinoma and the other a malignant papilloma, in which the tumor recurred, but in each instance the new growths responded to radium plus fulguration.

There were 5 postoperative deaths. Of these, 2 were due to pulmonary emboli and 1 to thrombophlebitis. These findings emphasize the importance of most careful manipulation on the part of the operator.

There is no doubt that resection, where possible, is the most satisfactory form of treatment in cases of infiltrating carcinoma.

G. Cases Treated by Suprapubic Cauterization of Tumor. 35 cases.

The ages of these cases were as follows: Twenty to twenty-nine, 1; thirty to thirty-nine, 4; forty to forty-nine, 4; fifty to fifty-nine, 8; sixty to sixty-nine, 15; seventy to seventy-nine, 3.

The diagnosis, as verified by suprapubic operation and generally microscopic examination, was as follows: Benign papilloma, 2; malignant papilloma, 7; papillary carcinoma, 12; infiltrating carcinoma, 13; papilloma (not classified), 1.

The treatment consisted generally in careful exposure of the tumor with protection of the surrounding structures, every effort being taken to avoid breaking off fragments. In many cases the tumor was immediately destroyed as completely as possible with the cautery; in others the pedicle was cut across with the cautery and the tumor lifted out bodily without touching the bladder or adjacent structures. The base of the tumor was generally burned quite deeply with the cautery, and in some instances this burning was evidently quite extensive, but was intentionally so on account of the deep invasion. Where the tumor involved the region of the prostate, the cautery was usually passed into the prostatic orifice, an effort being made to destroy the invasion as much as possible. Suprapubic drainage was used.

The results obtained are shown in the following table:

TABLE 90

RESULTS OF CAUTERIZATION ALONE IN BLADDER TUMORS. 35 CASES

	Less than one year.	One year.	Two years.	Three years.	Four years.	Eleven years.	Fourteen years.	Total.
Alive and well:								
(1) Cystoscopic............	...	...	1	1	1	...	...	3
(2) Symptomless..........	...	1	1	1	1	...	...	4
(3) Recurred, retreated, well	...	...	...	...	...	...	2	2
Recurred, unimproved........	...	2	...	1	...	...	...	3
Recurred, dead..............	9	8	3	...	...	1	...	21
Dead, other causes..........	1	...	1	...	...	...	...	2
Not followed................	...	...	...	...	...	...	...	0

Summary.—There are 3 cases in which particularly deep burning was necessary. The patients died shortly after operation, 2 from thrombophlebitis, and another from septicemia. We are confident now that a serious mistake was made in these cases in applying the cautery for so prolonged a period. As a matter of fact, the poor results obtained by this group are, we think, sufficient to warrant the assertion that cauterization of the superficial growth plus radium is superior to deep cauterization.

H. Cases Treated by Other Operative Measures. 43 cases.

The ages of these patients were as follows: Thirty to thirty-nine, 2; forty to forty-nine, 9; fifty to fifty-nine, 10; sixty to sixty-nine, 13; seventy to seventy-nine, 4; eighty to eighty-nine, 2; ages not given, 3.

The methods of procedure employed in the treatment of these cases were as follows:

TABLE 91

RESULTS OF OTHER AND VARIED METHODS IN 43 CASES OF BLADDER TUMORS

Cases.

Suprapubic drainage..	22
Curettage of tumor...	3
Suprapubic fulguration and drainage...........................	2
Removal by torsion and forceps...............................	1
Incomplete resection..	2
Excision and curettage of base..........	1
Excision of tumor.........................	4
Excision of tumor in diverticulum....................	1
Tumor twisted off with clamps......................	2
Punch operation for obstruction.....................	1
Perineal prostatectomy and curettage of tumor.................	1
Suprapubic exploratory.............................	1
Ureterostomy for obstruction.......................	1
Suprapubic operation for extravasated urine..................	1
Total...	43

The type of tumor as shown by cystoscope, operative exposure, or microscopic study was as follows: Benign papilloma, 2; malignant papilloma, 4; papillary carcinoma, 4; infiltrating carcinoma, 32; papilloma not classified, 1.

In explanation of the very varied methods which have been employed in this group, it may be stated that many of them were emergency operations to afford necessary relief (suprapubic drainage). Many of the patients were too advanced in years or the tumor was too extensive to warrant more than palliative treatment. This was particularly true where simple drainage or curettage was carried out.

Summary.—Only three possible cures occur in this group. One was a benign papilloma that was twisted from the bladder wall and did not recur over a period of sixteen years. The second case was a malignant papilloma that recurred a few months after it was excised, but was destroyed by fulguration. In the third case the tumor was fulgurated and then excised. There was no recurrence during the six years the patient lived.

In the light of our present knowledge it is quite evident that these 3 cases would have responded to fulguration alone or radium plus fulguration.

The extremely bad results obtained in this group are due to a combination of circumstances. In the first place, 80 per cent. of these tumors were infiltrating carcinomas in a more or less advanced stage of growth, and, therefore, practically hopeless from the start. Second, many of these patients came to the clinic before the more advanced forms of therapy in bladder tumors had been developed, hence the great diversity in methods of procedure.

I. Cases Treated by *x*-Ray Alone or Combined with Other Therapy. 32 cases.

The ages were as follows: Thirty to thirty-nine, 3; forty to forty-nine, 6; fifty to fifty-nine, 7; sixty to sixty-nine, 7; seventy to seventy-nine, 2; eighty to eighty-nine, 1; age not stated, 6.

The type of tumor as recognized by cystoscopic or microscopic examination was as follows: Benign papilloma, 1; malignant papilloma, 5; papillary carcinoma, 9; infiltrating carcinoma, 17.

The methods of procedure employed in these cases were as follows: *x*-Ray alone, 9; *x*-ray plus cystoscopic application of radium, 12; *x*-ray plus cystoscopic application of radium and fulguration, 10; *x*-ray plus fulguration, 1.

The use of the *x*-ray is a recent development. Until three years ago no machine of sufficient power was at hand for such treatment. During the past three years the majority of infiltrating carcinomas which could not be resected have had *x*-ray treatment in addition to radium in some form. In the 9 cases in which *x*-ray alone was used, the vesical condition was so extensive or the introduction of a radium instrument so painful that *x*-ray alone was used in the forlorn hope of obtaining relief.

The results of the treatment are shown in Table 92.

Summary.—Only 6 patients in this group are well, 4 less than a year, and 2 one year. Of these, 2 had malignant papilloma, 3 papillary carcinoma, and only 1 an infiltrating carcinoma. With the exception of the infiltrating carcinoma these cases would have responded just as well to radium plus fulguration. Of the 9 cases receiving *x*-ray alone, not one was cured; however, these were apparently hopeless cases.

x-Ray seems to be more effective if the tumor receives a number of surface applications of radium previous to its use. In a number of cases of hemorrhage

TABLE 92

RESULTS OF *x*-RAY ALONE AND COMBINED WITH SOME OTHER FORM OF THERAPY

	Less than one year.	One year.	Two years.	Three years.	Four years.	Five years.	Six years.	Seven years.	Total.
Alive and well:									
(1) Cystoscopic.....	1	2	...	...	...	...	...	...	3
(2) Symptomless....	3	...	...	...	...	...	...	...	3
Recurred, unimproved.	6	4	...	1	...	1	...	1	13
Recurred, dead........	13	...	...	...	...	...	...	...	13

which persisted during *x*-ray treatment, it has been necessary to use radium in order to stop the bleeding. *x*-Ray certainly tends to diminish the intensity of any pain due to nerve involvement.

It is extremely difficult to predict in advance just how a patient is going to react to *x*-ray therapy. Some patients stand a large number of treatments without any apparent general reaction, while others react violently. There were two deaths in our series that could be attributed to this form of therapy.

We can but conclude, therefore, that deep *x*-ray therapy affords little benefit in the more advanced cases of infiltrating carcinoma of the bladder.

J. Cases Not Treated. 78 cases.

The ages were as follows: Thirty to thirty-nine, 9; forty to forty-nine, 13; fifty to fifty-nine, 19; sixty to sixty-nine, 16; seventy to seventy-nine, 16; eighty to eighty-nine, 2; age not stated, 3.

The type of tumor present was as follows: Benign papilloma, 1; malignant papilloma, 9; papillary carcinoma, 9; infiltrating carcinoma, 55; papilloma not classified, 4.

Many of these cases were perfectly amenable to simple fulguration or radium treatment, but they either left for treatment elsewhere or refused treatment. Many of the infiltrating carcinomas were beyond hope of relief. It has been impossible to follow 23 of these cases, but of the other 55 cases 30 died within a year and 22 during the second year.

This group is simply interesting as showing the very rapid ending which generally occurs in such cases.

The following 8 cases are selected with an idea of briefly illustrating the practical application of the more important forms of therapy in bladder tumors.

Benign papilloma on trigone. Destroyed by fulguration alone. Followed six years. Apparently well.

B. U. I. 7397. W. P., male, age fifty. The patient came to the clinic December 21, 1918, complaining of frequency, slight dysuria, and hematuria. About one year previous he first noticed a little blood in urine and shortly afterward he began to gradually develop frequency and dysuria. Six months later a diagnosis of bladder tumor was made elsewhere and the growth was fulgurated four times. For the next two months the patient felt much better, however, after that, the frequency, dysuria, and hematuria gradually returned. Cystoscopic examination by Dr. Geraghty showed on the midline of trigone a slightly pedunculated, non-infiltrating papillary tumor about 1.5 cm. in diameter, having many long healthy looking, pink papillæ projecting from its short pedicle. This tumor was typically a benign papilloma. The growth was completely destroyed by seven fulgurations, the last treatment occurring on February 11,

1919. A cystoscopic examination two months later showed three tiny villous tumors that were immediately destroyed by fulguration. Examinations during the next year did not show any recurrence. Letter, January 12, 1925, no recurrence of symptoms.

Malignant papilloma of left corner of trigone, 2 by 3 cm. Cystoscopic application of radium and fulguration. Followed five years. Apparently well.

B. U. I. 8131. R. M. K., male, age forty-eight. Admitted September 18, 1919. History of hematuria eighteen months. Examination showed prostate normal, a large tumor in left half of bladder, in region of ureteral orifice, apparently about 3 cm. in diameter, surface irregular with a few small villi, no ulceration, pedicle short, base could not be seen, obscured by tumor. Right half of trigone normal. Diagnosis, malignant papilloma. Treatment, cystoscopic application of radium and fulguration, 400 mgh. radium given and seven fulgurations. October 16, 1919: Tumor appears to have completely disappeared. November 15, 1919: Cystoscopy; no tumor present, ulceration slight. July 19, 1920: Free from symptoms. Cystoscopy showed smooth white scar, no recurrence. After this patient was seen frequently and was always cystoscopically negative. March 18, 1924: Practically free from symptoms, cystoscopy negative.

Papillary carcinoma involving left half of trigone, ureter, and a portion of vesical orifice. Treatment, cystoscopic application of radium. Followed thirty months. Apparently well.

B. U. I. 10,961. M. L., male, age sixty-six, admitted August 16, 1922, complaining of hematuria, frequency, and pain in back. Five months previous, following a fall, he first noticed blood in his urine. Since then he has had constantly increasing attacks of hematuria. Cystoscopy showed a lobulated papillary carcinoma springing from the left half of trigone, involving the left ureter and a portion of vesical orifice. Cystoscopically no induration about the base of tumor could be made out, nor could the growth be felt per rectum. In view of these evidences of only superficial induration at the most, the patient was treated by the cystoscopic application of radium. After receiving 1600 mgh. of radium he was allowed to go home for six weeks and on return only a very small portion of tumor remained. Following the application of 500 mgh. radium this disappeared. A cystoscopic examination one year later showed no recurrence of tumor. Letter, January 12, 1925: Patient symptomless. Duration since treatment started, thirty months.

Papillary carcinoma of trigone and left lateral wall. Suprapubic cauterization, removal of tumor mass, and implantation of radium emanation tubes and needles. Followed three and a half years. Apparently well.

B. U. I. 9722. A. C., male, age seventy-two. Admitted May 25, 1921, complaining of frequency and difficulty of urination for one year and hematuria of seven months' duration. Cystoscopy showed a large, irregular vesical tumor, the surface of which was covered with mucous, on the left lateral wall and extending to the midline of trigone posteriorly. Rectal examination, prostate and seminal vesicles negative. June 1, 1921, operation, Dr. Geraghty, gas and ether. Suprapubic excision of bladder tumor with electric cautery and implantation of radium. On opening the bladder an irregular, shaggy tumor was found on the left lateral wall which extended down to prostatic orifice and from there backward along the midline of trigone to the posterior wall of bladder. The growth covered an area of 5 by 6 cm. Finger inserted in the vesical orifice showed definite invasion, the tumor seeming to be deeply infiltrating. The projecting tumor tissue was destroyed with cautery until flush with the bladder wall. Palpation showed deep infiltration and accordingly ten tubes of radium emanation 1.6 mc. each were implanted in the area of the tumor around the periphery and two 20 mg. needles of radium element were then inserted into the center of the growth. Bladder closed with drainage. Convalescence satisfactory. January 1, 1925, letter: No recurrence of symptoms. Patient considers himself cured. Has gained in weight, general health excellent.

Infiltrating carcinoma of vertex of bladder. Transperitoneal resection of upper half of bladder. Followed six years. Cystoscopically well.

B. U. I. 3286. A. P. Y., male, age sixty-eight, admitted September 17, 1912, complaining of painful and difficult urination of seven months' duration. Tumor of bladder diagnosed cystoscopically two months ago and fulguration given elsewhere. Cystoscopy showed irregular, globular tumor about 1½ inches in diameter along the anterior wall running up along the vertex, surface covered with a gray exudate, no other tumors present. Operation, H. H. Y. September 20, 1912, ether anesthesia. Transperitoneal resection of upper half of bladder. Median line suprapubic incision. The upper anterior wall and whole vertex of the bladder were hard, evidently invaded by a malignant tumor. Transperitoneal resection therefore carried out with wide area of bladder wall. About one-half of bladder was thus removed, forming large cap of tumor and bladder wall. Base of bladder, trigone, and region of prostate not involved. Bladder closed with catgut, peritoneum closed with catgut, suprapubic drainage.

October 24, 1912. Patient discharged from hospital, suprapubic wound healed, patient voiding freely. June 10, 1916. Cystoscopy: no recurrence, slight prostatic bar. April 28, 1917. Cystoscopy: no recurrence. June 20, 1918. Cystoscopy: no recurrence. February 26, 1921. Letter: Patient apparently well. Almost nine years.

Transperitoneal resection and transplantation of ureters. Apparently cured. Small papillary recurrences. Treated with radium, cystoscopic implantation of radium emanation. Finally cured. Followed three years.

B. U. I. 10,969. M. G., female, sixty-one, admitted November 10, 1922, with history of urinary frequency of fifteen years' duration, hematuria of six months. Bladder tumor recognized and treated by fulguration during past two months. Cystoscopy showed necrotic tumor about 5 cm. in diameter on left lateral wall, extending nearly to the left ureter. The tumor projected considerably into the bladder. Treatment: Radical resection advised but refused. A cystoscopic application of radium then employed, 1100 mgh. December 11, 1922, patient consented to operation. Resection of large infiltrating papillary carcinoma of bladder, by Dr. Geraghty. Anterior wall of bladder exposed through median suprapubic incision. Palpation revealed a hard tumor mass which was felt anteriorly as far as the midline and extended a considerable distance to the left, involving most of the left lateral wall as far up as the vertex. Peritoneum was apparently quite adherent and therefore opened and an area of peritoneum 5 cm. in diameter excised with bladder tumor. Peritoneum was closed and bladder opened and tumor resected with wide area of healthy bladder wall. This included the anterior wall, vertex, left lateral wall, portion of trigone, and left ureter which was divided and transplanted at the upper angle of the wound. Bladder closed with catgut suture, with drainage. Microscopic diagnosis: Infiltrating carcinoma. Convalescence "stormy," eventually satisfactory recovery. February 26, 1923. Suprapubic wound has been healed for two weeks. Cystoscopy showed two small papillary recurrences in region formerly occupied by left ureter. Two days later, one glass seed containing 2 mc. radium emanation was inserted through Kelly cystoscope into each small papillary recurrence. July 24, 1923. Cystoscopy: Bladder negative, no recurrence. October 16, 1923. Cystoscopy: No recurrence. October 19, 1924. Cystoscopy: No recurrence. Duration since operation two years.

Papillary carcinoma region of right ureter, 2 by 3.5 cm., removed with electrocautery, which included the base. Recovered. Followed three years, apparently cured.

B. U. I. 7502. A. C. C., male, age sixty-eight. Admitted January 13, 1919 with hematuria of five years' duration. Cystoscopy showed an irregular, papillary, infiltrating tumor springing from the bladder wall back of and external to the left ureteral orifice, base appeared to be quite broad, prostate negative. February 17, 1919. Operation, H. H. Y. gas, ether. Suprapubic cystotomy, destruction with electrocautery of papillomatous tumor, 2 by 3.5 cm. in size. Tumor covered the right ureteral orifice reaching almost to the median line of the trigone and from there extended upward along to the right lateral wall. It was a soft papilloma and projected about 1 cm. into the bladder lying close against the wall with a pedicle apparently about 1 cm. in diameter. The bladder around looked healthy. Cauterization was very thorough, the entire tumor being destroyed, excising only a small point which was removed by means of cautery for microscopic study. The cauterization was continued into the muscle tissue beneath the mucous membrane proper extending at least 5 mm. The terminal portion of the ureter was involved in this cauterization. A small median prostatic lobe was removed with cautery. Microscopic examination of the tissue removed showed papillary carcinoma. Convalescence good. November 17, 1919. Returned for observation. Cystoscopy negative. January 8, 1921. Cystoscopy negative. November 13, 1922. Letter: No recurrence of symptoms. Time followed, almost four years.

Papillary carcinoma 4 cm., in diameter. Treatment: Radium applications, 400 mgh., deep x-ray therapy. Apparently cured.

B. U. I. 12,568. Male sixty-eight, admitted June 8, 1924. Onset two and a half years before, history of frequency, difficulty, and hematuria, catheter life for one month. Prostate was slightly hypertrophied, cystoscopy showed sessile papillary tumor, 3 by 4 cm. in size, in region of left ureteral orifice, trigone, and left lateral wall of bladder. Tumor had a broad base, surface only moderately elevated and was covered with small villi. At the lower angle there was considerable adherent mucus. Treatment: Cystoscopic application of radium, 400 mgh., 4 applications directly against tumor, 100 mgh. radium element used each time. A complete course of deep x-ray therapy also given. July 3, 1924. A most remarkable result has been obtained. Fairly large tumor, definitely papillary carcinoma has entirely disappeared, under radium and x-ray therapy. (Dr. J. A. C. Colston.) September 30, 1924. Patient returned for examination. Feels very well. Cystoscopy showed mucous membrane in region previously occupied by tumor to be perfectly normal, no scar present. February 17, 1925. Patient returns for observation. General condition excellent. Cystoscopy shows no recurrence of tumor, slight papillary cystitis along left lateral wall, no tumor present.

Summary.—The age of onset varied between fifteen and eighty-three years of age. The majority of the benign and malignant papillomas appeared between forty and fifty-nine years of age, while the bulk of the carcinomas occurred between the ages of fifty and sixty-nine.

The types of primary tumors of the bladder in this series were classified as follows: Benign papilloma, 15 per cent.; malignant papilloma, 18 per cent.; papillary carcinoma, 17 per cent.; infiltrating carcinoma, 48 per cent.; papilloma not classified, 3 per cent.; growths designated only as tumor, 3 cases, adenocarcinoma, dermoid cyst, and benign cyst, 1 case each.

The importance of the ability on the part of the examiner to classify properly the various types of bladder tumor cannot be too greatly emphasized.

This knowledge can only be obtained by a thorough and conscientious study of the literature on the subject in addition to frequent cystoscopic and pathologic studies, both gross and microscopic, under competent instructors.

Once the tumor is properly classified the method of attack is usually quite clearly indicated.

Benign papillomas practically always respond very well to fulguration alone. However, these tumors show a rather marked tendency to recur, making necessary frequent cystoscopic examinations for some years after the destruction of the initial growth.

Malignant papillomas frequently respond to fulguration alone, but the operator can save himself considerable time and the patient much discomfort if the tumor is thoroughly radiated cystoscopically before fulguration is attempted. Under this combined form of therapy the tumors rapidly melt away. The tendency to recur makes frequent cystoscopic examinations necessary for a considerable period after the destruction of the growth.

Papillary carcinomas, especially the smaller ones, usually respond to the surface application of radium plus fulguration.

It is interesting to note here that the adherence of the slough to the surface of the tumor seems to be in direct ratio with the malignancy of the growth. There are a few cases in this group in which the tumors have responded very well to x-ray therapy after having previously received a number of surface applications of radium. If these methods fail the tumor should be resected if possible, or if its location is unfavorable for this it should be cauterized superficially and then implanted with radium needles or emanations.

The method of choice where the patient's general condition permits and where the location of the tumor is favorable, in dealing with infiltrating carcinomas of the bladder, is resection. These growths are, as a rule, slow to metastasize and where resectable offer a good prognosis. If resection is impossible it is advisable to try radium plus fulguration or radium plus deep x-ray. If there is no improvement under these forms of therapy suprapubic cauterization of the tumor with implantation of radium needles or emanations should be tried.

Although deep x-ray alone has not been effective in our series from the standpoint of tumor destruction, it has done much to diminish the intensity of any pain due to nerve involvement. In some cases in which there was a marked tendency to hemorrhage it has been necessary to use radium in conjunction with the deep x-ray therapy in order to check the bleeding.

NEOPLASMS OF THE URETHRA

PATHOLOGY

All neoplasms of the urethra vary in type according to the portion of the urethra in which they arise. Those in the most distal portion and fossa navicularis approach the types springing from the external surface of the glans. For this reason neoplasms of the penis should be considered in conjunction with those of the urethra. The distinction between the two becomes difficult in later stages, since tumors of the glans may extend into the urethra, and tumors of the urethra may spread to the surface of the glans.

Polyps of the urethra are not, properly speaking, neoplasms, and have been discussed in the section on Infections of the Urethra. They may, however, resemble small papillomata, and, in addition, various pedunculated tumors occurring in the female urethra or about the meatus are also sometimes spoken of rather indiscriminately as polyps. These distinctions, in so far as they can be made, will be discussed in the succeeding paragraphs.

Papillomata may occur at any point in the urethra, but are much commoner in the terminal urethra and fossa navicularis. Here they bear resemblance to the papillomata of the glans. Like those on the glans, papillomata of the urethra are often associated with chronic inflammation. This is also true of polyps, and it becomes necessary to define these two terms. The distinction is not always easy clinically or even pathologically. In general, one may say that the polypoid formations are those in which there is a proliferative reaction to chronic inflammation, involving both epithelium and connective tissue, and in about equal proportions. Thus we have polyps in the form of rounded or pointed excrescences, cylindric, or even pedunculated outgrowths. Microscopically there is a fairly abundant stroma, often edematous or infiltrated with leukocytes, and covered by an epithelium which is essentially normal. Not infrequently downgrowths occur, solid or with lumen, but there is no invasion, the basement membrane is preserved, and the regular, layered arrangement of the epithelial cells is not altered. Even when cylindrical forms are assumed, polyps do not branch. The true venereal warts and condylomata, both flat and acuminate, are properly considered as polypoid formations, though when the excrescences are very numerous, it may be difficult to make a certain diagnosis on clinical observation.

In papillomata, on the other hand, the epithelium has taken on an excessive growth, and the supporting stroma is secondary. The papillæ branch and downgrowths of the epithelium are the exception. The growth is more rapid than with polyps. The papilloma, therefore, is a true neoplasm, and continues to grow, independently of the stimulus, inflammatory or otherwise, which may nave caused it. Polypoid formations are always preceded by inflammation, while papillomata, even in the urethra, may begin in the absence of inflammation. It is probable, however, that growths originally polypoid may become papillomatous, and even undergo malignant change. Transition forms are, therefore, to be expected.

Papillomata are commonest in or near the fossa navicularis, but may be found at any point along the urethra. They may be single or multiple. They are much rarer than the simple inflammatory polyps. They differ from those of the bladder in that they are covered by the type of epithelium found in that part of the urethra from which they spring. In the deeper portions of the urethra, however, the epithelium is often stratified, the result of alteration from pre-existing chronic inflammation. In the fossa navicularis, especially when the tumors project from the meatus, there may be epidermization.

Adenomata, or "glandular polyps," are practically confined to the prostatic urethra. They consist of a sessile or pedunculated mass, covered by a simple and essentially normal epithelium. They have a connective-tissue framework, with blood and lymph channels, but the greater portion is composed of glandular or tubular structures, which vary from small lumina with simple cuboidal or columnar epithelium to large distended acini containing papillary outgrowths resembling those seen in prostatic hypertrophy and like them covered by a double layer of epithelium. They may arise from any point in the prostatic urethra, from the verumontanum, or, as in case described by Randall,[1] from within the prostatic utricle. There has been much discussion in the literature as to their origin. Some have suggested that they arise from prostatic tubules, but it seems more likely that they take origin from the short, simple submucous glands of the prostatic urethra—the same from which prostatic hypertrophy is supposed to arise by Motz, Tandler, and others. It is noteworthy that these little pedunculated adenomata, showing marked papillary epithelial overgrowth, have been found in men as young as thirty years, whose prostates were otherwise normal. They may properly be regarded as true neoplasms, and Bürckhardt[2] has seen them in uninfected urethras.

In the general consideration of these benign urethral growths, one must keep clinical and pathologic aspects distinct. Since it is practically always impossible to distinguish the pathologic features on clinical examination, many authors have made groupings based entirely on the naked-eye appearance in the patient. Thus Randall would call all such growths polyps, reserving the qualifying adjectives of fibrous, villous, and glandular until after the microscopic examination is made. In the same way Player and Mathé[3] speak of pedunculated polyps, sessile polypoid mass, and edematous excrescence, without reference to the histologic picture. In the 68 cases reported by them, 26 were located at the vesical orifice, 40 in the prostatic urethra, and only two in the bulbous urethra. Of Randall's 14 cases, all were in the prostatic urethra except one, which was in the membranous portion. Five took origin from the verumontanum itself, and one (an adenoma) from within the utricle.

Cysts may occur in the urethra. They are usually retention cysts, of the pros-

---

[1] Surgery, Gynecology, and Obstetrics, 1913, xviii, 548–562.

[2] Frisch and Zuckerkandl: Handbuch der Urologie, 1906, iii.

[3] Journal of Urology, 1921, v, 177–209.

tatic or urethral glands, due to inflammation, and not properly neoplasms. Larger cysts, arising from Cowper's glands, usually appear first in the perineum. They are described in the chapter on Malformations of the Urogenital Tract.

In women, the variety of lesions spoken of as polyps is greater than in men, and some of the lesions so included are true neoplasms. Thus besides the inflammatory polyp there may be myoma, angioma, neuroma, adenoma, or sarcoma. Cysts of Skenes' glands may project at the urethral orifice. The etiology of the small vascular tumors (caruncles) is obscure. They are thought by some to be inflammatory polyps in which the vessels become varicose due to circulatory changes, possibly consequent upon child-bearing, and comparable to hemorrhoids. Some such lesions have been described as true angiomata. True papillomata also occur in women, but are rare.

Malignant neoplasms of the urethra are practically always epithelial in origin. We prefer to divide them, as does Imbert,[1] into those of the pendulous urethra and those of the deep urethra. The importance of this distinction lies not in the types of tumors concerned, but in the course and extension, and the accessibility to diagnosis and treatment.

True papillomata may undergo a malignant change, just as in the bladder. The papillæ coalesce, the cells lose their layer formations and become uniform, and strands of neoplastic cells invade the subjacent tissues. Culver and Forster[2] describe and picture a beautiful example of such a case. This form of tumor occurs where papillomata are most frequent, namely, in the pendulous urethra.

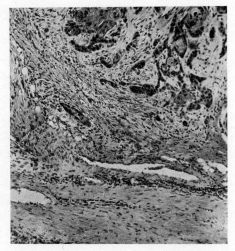

FIG. 398.—Squamous-celled epithelioma of the membranous urethra. This section shows the tumor invading the prostate. J. H. H. Autopsy. B. U. I. 9874.

Epithelioma may develop from epidermized papillomata, near the meatus, or may arise as a flat growth on the surface of the urethra. Microscopically, it may be either basal or squamous celled. Imbert states that the basal-cell type is more common. Intermediate types are seen. Where the squamous-cell type arises at any point distant from the meatus, it is assumed to be preceded by leukoplakia. Leukoplakia of the urethra is commonest in areas of chronic inflammation associated with stricture, and, in accordance with this, we find that epithelioma of the urethra often follows stricture. In Imbert's series 60 per cent. of the cases had histories of stricture, some of them over many years.

Extension of malignant tumors of the urethra takes place both along the urethra and into the deeper tissues. Neoplasms of the pendulous urethra may extend until they involve its entire length, appear at the meatus, and involve the glans. The corpus spongiosum and later the corpora cavernosa are invaded. The skin may be invaded, with formation of single or multiple fistulæ. The urethra may be

[1] Encyclopædie Française d'Urologie, 1921, v, 739–792.

[2] Surgery, Gynecology, and Obstetrics, 1923, xxxvi, 473–479.

obstructed, by pedunculated masses or by circumferential constriction, and then becomes dilated above the growth.

In the deeper urethra, the lateral extension of the growth may carry it into the bladder. The perineum, triangular ligament, and prostate are invaded (Fig. 398). The commonest site of origin is in the deep bulbar or outer membranous urethra; the points where one often finds stricture. The neoplasm may cause obstruction, or add to that produced by pre-existent stricture, usually by circular contraction, as in this region pedunculated masses are less common. Urinary extravasation is common, presumably beginning where the friable or necrotic tumor tissue

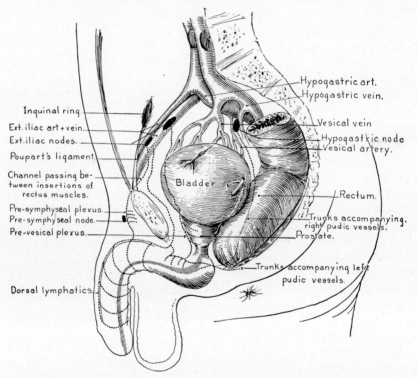

Fig. 399.—Diagram showing course taken by lymphatic channels draining urethra. From the penile portion channels form part of the dorsal lymphatics, but in their subsequent course they do not enter the inguinofemoral nodes. Some drain to a small channel passing between the insertions of the right and left rectus muscles to enter the external iliac node. There are anastomoses beneath the symphysis with the lymphatics of the bulbar and membranous portions. The bulbar lymphatics drain mostly into trunks accompanying the internal pudic vessels to enter the hypogastric nodes. At the apex of the prostate there are anastomoses with the prevesical lymphatic plexus and with the prostatic plexus and doubtless with the lymphatics of the ejaculatory ducts and vasa deferentia.

involves the urethra above the point of greatest obstruction. Fistula formation is also common, either with or without extravasation. These fistulæ often form before the diagnosis is made, in which case doubt may remain as to whether the tumor was primary in the urethra, or whether it began as malignant degeneration of the epithelium lining the fistulous tract. It is probably for this reason that many cases of urethral carcinoma have not been reported in the literature.

Metastasis occurs as in other forms of epithelioma, and is usually late. Regional metastasis is to the iliac or inguinal nodes, or both. If the growth is posterior to the suspensory ligament, there is little chance of metastasis to the inguinal nodes. From the urethra lymphatic drainage goes to the external iliac, hypogastric, and sacral groups of nodes, so any of these may be involved (Fig. 399). In two cases cited by Imbert, there were metastases to the testes, and in another to the bladder.

In women, carcinoma of the urethra is about as frequent as in men, although stricture is rare. The type is different, however, the squamous-cell form being rarer, the basal-cell commoner. Invasion of the vulva, vagina, and bladder is common.

Neoplasms Arising in Cowper's Glands.—A number of malignant tumors have been described as probably arising in Cowper's glands, but in none of them is this origin certain. We agree with Imbert that the distinction is impractical, and that tumors of the urethra and of Cowper's glands must be considered as one subject. Histologic evidence is lacking, since all of the neoplasms described have been typical epitheliomata, which are more likely to have arisen from the urethra. One might expect, from the structure of Cowper's glands, an adenocarcinoma of colloid or mucous type, but we have not found reference to any such tumor.

Benign cysts may arise in Cowper's glands as the result of developmental anomalies, or later occlusion of the duct. They are considered in the chapter on Malformations.

SYMPTOMS OF URETHRAL NEOPLASMS

Papillomata and Adenomata.—Since most of these tumors are associated with inflammation, the symptoms will be superimposed upon those of chronic urethritis (*q. v.*) and may be nothing more than perhaps an increase in the discharge and other manifestations. Hematuria may occur, especially after instrumentation. If the neoplasm is external to the triangular ligament the blood appears at the meatus between urination. When posterior to the external sphincter it fills the prostatic urethra and then forces its way through the internal sphincter into the bladder. While usually not pronounced, E. G. Davis[1] has seen a case in which hemorrhage from a pedunculated tumor in the prostatic urethra was sufficient to flow back through the sphincter and fill the bladder with blood-clot. In the outermost portions of the urethra, the tumor may project through the meatus and be seen by the patient. Elsewhere in the pendulous urethra, the mass of the tumor may be evident through the penile tissues. Urinary difficulty may develop, but seldom occurs until after the mass has been noticed. In the deep urethra, the reverse is true, as there are no characteristic symptoms until the mass of the tumor is great enough to obstruct the urethra.

In women papillomata and other tumors usually appear at the meatus, the urethra being so short, where they cause pain, dysuria, and often dyspareunia.

Malignant Tumors.—The clinical picture in malignancy varies greatly with the location of the tumor. In the pendulous urethra the mass of the tumor itself is practically always noted by the patient before it is very extensive. There will be either a protrusion from the meatus, or an induration along the urethra. Later urinary difficulty may ensue, with frequency and small stream, as in Culver's case. In neglected cases there may be fistula formation.

The symptom-complex in carcinoma of the deep urethra (bulbo-membranous) is not characteristic, and for this reason the diagnosis has apparently never been

---

[1] Surgery, Gynecology, and Obstetrics, 1923, xxxvii, 194–197.

made in an early stage. Ordinarily, there are the symptoms of stricture. They may have been present for a long time, even for years, so that they attract no particular attention. Even when the patient has been free from such symptoms for some time before the onset of the neoplasm, he has usually had an old urethritis and stricture at some time so that he is thought to have simply a recurrence. The other characteristic features of deep urethral carcinoma, namely, urethral discharge, perineal induration, extravasation of urine, and fistula formation, are equally characteristic of stricture. The only symptoms which might possibly lead to suspicion are hematuria, which may be rather more common and profuse than is to be expected in stricture, and pain, which may be more independent of voiding than in stricture. Epithelioma of the prostatic urethra is practically indistinguishable from cancer of the prostate.

In women there is usually an ulcerated mass in the region of the meatus, with pain, dysuria, and bloody discharge.

Since most malignant tumors of the urethra are epitheliomata, the age is the usual cancer age, and no cases have been reported in exceptionally young individuals.

As to sex, Culver and Forster have collected 122 cases in females and 74 in males. The statistics in regard to males are less reliable on account of the confusion resulting from the presence of fistula in many cases, as mentioned above. While rare, therefore, carcinoma of the urethra is not among the rarest tumors.

The prognosis is poor in cancers of the deep urethra in males. The tumor has usually become extensive before diagnosis; operation is impracticable. In cancers of the pendulous urethra prognosis is better, and a number of cures are recorded. In females operation is possible, but is often followed by incontinence or fistula.

DIAGNOSIS OF URETHRAL NEOPLASMS

Papillomata.—In the fossa navicularis these tumors can be inspected directly. The distinction from multiple polyps or condyloma acuminata is not particularly important, as the treatment is the same in each. Palpation may disclose induration which may indicate a malignant change, and biopsy should always be done. The remainder of the urethra should be inspected with a urethroscope for additional tumors.

Large papillomata farther within the urethra may sometimes be palpated from the exterior, but for these, as well as for those in the posterior urethra, direct inspection with the urethroscope or endoscope is by far the best, and indeed the only accurate method of diagnosis, since it is easy to remove a fragment with forceps for microscopic examination. One should keep in mind the possibility of implantation from papillomata of the bladder, ureter, or renal pelvis, especially in the posterior urethra near the bladder.

Adenomata.—Since these tumors are confined to the prostatic urethra, they can be diagnosed only by the urethroscope or cystoscope.

It is usually impossible to distinguish adenoma from papilloma, or even from inflammatory polyps or diffuse polyposis, on ocular examination. This is of little importance, since the treatment is the same for all. The point that is of importance, however, is that these growths, of whatever type, maintain urethral infections. The symptoms are increased, and new ones may be added, as hematuria, pain, irritation of the verumontanum with sexual hyperesthesia, and in late cases obstruction. It is, therefore. essential never to omit endoscopic examination in any case of rebellious chronic urethritis.

In women the tumors usually appear at the meatus and are quite evident. A piece should be obtained for microscopic examination whatever method of removal is adopted.

Malignant tumors in males are comparatively easy to diagnose if in the pendulous urethra, and extremely difficult to diagnose in the deep urethra. In the pendulous urethra induration is the principal feature which indicates malignancy. If a portion of the tumor appears at the meatus, the diagnosis is simplified, and in case of doubt a piece for microscopic examination can be easily obtained. When the lesion is deeper, it may be confused with intra-urethral chancre, tuberculosis, or peri-urethral abscess. The absence of Treponema pallidum, and failure to respond to specific treatment will rule out syphilis. Tuberculosis is usually associated with lesions elsewhere in the urogenital tract which, with the finding of the bacilli, will make the diagnosis. Peri-urethral abscess is usually painful, there may be fever, the evolution is rapid, and fluctuation may be expected. The endoscope will show, in case of neoplasm, papillary outgrowths or an indurated, ulcerated surface.

In the deep urethra the clincal picture resembles so closely that often associated with stricture that Imbert was only able to find three cases in the literature in which the diagnosis was suspected before operation. In each of these the endoscopic picture was the deciding factor. In one there was a pedunculated, red, raspberry-like outgrowth, while in the other two the urethra was bounded by an indurated, whitish tissue showing irregular unhealthy ulcerations. The four things which may mark the onset are increased difficulty of urination, perineal induration, extravasation of urine, and fistula formation. These may appear in any order. When extravasation occurs early, it may dominate the picture and obscure the malignancy—presumably localized—so that incision and drainage may be done without disclosing the new growth. Lavenant describes such a case in which the wound healed, only to reopen four months later, with obvious signs of malignancy. The only points which can be made are: A man in the cancer age, with a history of previous stricture, usually much treated; a rather sudden increase in the urinary difficulty without adequate cause; a perineal induration without quite the tenderness and fever to be expected from peri-urethritis; a little more hemorrhage than is common with stricture, a little more pain independent of voiding. Instruments when passed may penetrate the friable neoplastic tissue and seem to fall into a cavity. Such a case might be suspected of urethral cancer, and should be endoscoped.

Other lesions, as carcinoma of the prostate, tuberculosis, etc., can usually be ruled out by rectal examination. Ordinarily, incision is made on the diagnosis of extravasation or abscess, and the finding of friable masses of neoplastic tissue in the depths of the perineum is the first hint of malignancy.

We have seen only one proved case of carcinoma of the bulbomembranous urethra, which may well be abstracted here, as it is perfectly typical:

B. U. I. 9874, age fifty-eight, married. Thirty-eight years before admission the patient fell upon his perineum, and injured himself so that about two-thirds of his penis was amputated, and a traumatic stricture persisted. The difficulty in urination was intermittent, and always temporary, so that sounds were passed only a few times during the thirty-eight years. One week before coming to the clinic, urinary difficulty of unusual severity began, and terminated in complete retention. When first seen, a sound was passed which met an obstruction at a depth of 2 inches. This was passed without much difficulty and 1600 c.c. of urine removed. There was no perineal induration at this time. Later a false passage was made, but twenty days after the first instrumentation, a Kollmann dilator and then a cystoscope were introduced. The trigone was reddened, there was slight trabeculation, and some bleeding from the urethra. The prostate, palpated against the cystoscope, was slightly larger than normal, but not indurated. Fifteen days later (thirty-five days from the first visit) the urethra was again dilated, and a small indu-rated area was found in the perineum, which had already opened and was discharging a little pus, but no urine. Thirty-six hours later all the urine commenced coming through this fistula. It will be noted that this was *after* complete dilation of the urethra. When seen a day later (thirty-eight days from the first visit) there was also an extravasation of urine, the tumefaction involving the perineum and posterior part of the scrotum. The same day a perineal urethrotomy was done and the extravasation freely incised. No note as to any unusual finding was made, except that "the tissues were much scarred." Some small bits which were removed and sec-tioned showed only chronic inflammation. Following this operation the patient did well and the wound seemed to be closing normally for two weeks. At that time (fifty-two days from the first visit) there was a striking change for the worse. The patient began to feel ill, the tem-perature rose to 101° F., and the wound looked less healthy. The perineal induration began to increase. It was thought that part of the infected area was not draining and that the process was spreading, so that a second operation was performed thirty-six days after the first operation and ninety-four days from the first visit. When the fistula was enlarged the finger entered a cavity which appeared to be filled with necrotic tissue. A quantity of this was curetted out, and it proved to be a grayish, homogeneous material suggesting neoplastic tissue. A frozen section showed squamous-cell epithelioma. The course was then rapidly downward, with increasing cachexia, and the patient died forty-five days after the second operation and one hundred thirty-nine days from the first visit. Autopsy showed that the growth had replaced the membranous urethra with a large cavity. The distal part of the urethra was free, as was the juxtavesical portion. The tumor had invaded only the perineal tissues and the apical third of the prostate. (See Fig. 398.) It will be seen that the diagnosis was not made until the second operation. Probably the sudden onset of severe obstruction in a man of fifty-eight, who had had his stricture for thirty-eight years with very little trouble from it, should have given a clue.

The following recent case is probably another of carcinoma of the deep urethra:

B. U. I. 12,555, age forty-six, denies venereal disease. Has congenital phimosis with prepuce tightly adherent to glans. Nine years before admission there had been an abscess of the ventral surface of the penis, which required incision. It was probably due to the phimosis, and any connection with the tumor which appeared later is doubtful. Health was perfect for eight and a half years, but the external meatus gradually became contracted, and the final illness began with fever, chill, and perineal pain. The meatus was dilated, but a perineal abscess appeared, to be followed later by another. Both were incised, drained pus and urine, and within two weeks cauli-flower-like masses of tumor tissue appeared in each fistula. When the patient at this time came to us he was semicomatose and the findings were as stated above with the addition of enlarged and indurated inguinal glands. The prostate was normal on rectal examination. A biopsy showed squamous-cell epithelioma. Unfortunately no autopsy could be obtained.

In women the induration will indicate malignancy, and ulceration is usually early.

TREATMENT OF URETHRAL NEOPLASMS

Benign urethral neoplasms are best removed by fulguration. With those near the meatus, application may be made directly, while if deeper within the urethra, a tubular endoscope is necessary. In the deep urethra, the tubular endoscope or a telescopic urethroscope with catheter channel can be used. Care must be taken not to use too strong a spark, as sloughs and even stricture formation are possible.

Very delicate polyps in the posterior urethra may be destroyed by the silver nitrate stick, but usually this is ineffectual, as its escharotic action is too superficial.

Removal by means of urethral forceps is usually incomplete, and, therefore, not to be recommended. Such removal may, however, be practised as a preliminary to fulguration, in order to obtain specimens for microscopic study.

Malignant urethral tumors are seldom diagnosed early enough to allow radical treatment. If in the penile portion, an amputation of the penis must be done, extensive enough to give the tumor a wide berth. The inguinal glands should also be removed. If in the deep (bulbous or membranous) urethra, no treatment offers any hope except the most radical extirpation of the corpora and bulb of the urethra. A satisfactory perineal fistula can be made even if the entire membranous urethra is removed. The inguinal glands should be removed, but it is unnecessary and undesirable to excise the testes. If peri-urethral abscess, extravasation, or fistula has occurred, there is little hope for any good result of operation. Radium and deep x-ray treatment may be given, but little is to be expected from them.

NEOPLASMS OF THE PROSTATE AND SEMINAL VESICLES

PATHOLOGY

Prostate.—Benign hypertrophy of the prostate is regarded by some as a true adenomatous tumor, by others as a senile hyperplasia of normal elements. It seems to us impossible to arrive at a final conclusion on this point, and in view of the clinical importance of prostatic hypertrophy, we have not included it among the tumors, but have devoted a separate chapter to its consideration.

Cysts of the prostate are seldom true neoplasms. They are usually retention cysts, due to occlusion of prostatic ducts by inflammatory fibrosis, and do not attain a size greater than 1 or 2 cm. in diameter. Very rarely the utricle becomes the seat of a cyst. Cases in which more of the Müllerian duct than usual has persisted in the male may have good sized cysts, projecting through the prostate and up alongside the seminal vesicles. Dilated, persistent Müllerian ducts may extend all the way from the verumontanum to the epididymis. In some of these, ciliated epithelium like that of the Fallopian tubes has been noted. Further discussion will be found in Chapter III and Chapter IX.

CARCINOMA.—In the prostate it is not possible to distinguish different kinds of carcinomata. It will be found that there are several different types of growth, which cannot represent different tumors, since various combinations of them may be found in an individual case. All prostatic cancers are adenocarcinomatous in nature. The following types of growth have been found definite and recognizable by us:

1. *Extra-acinous growth*, consisting of a multiplication of small acini (adenocarcinoma of the prostate). Specimens differ in the quantity of stroma separating the small acini.

2. *Extra-acinous growth*, similar to the above, except that the new-formed glandular structures are elongated (tubular) and branching. The amount of stroma varies, but is less apt to be plentiful than in Group 1. This is the type of growth often seen in soft carcinomata which are missed at rectal examination.

3. *Intra-acinous growth*, in which the tumor cells proliferate in and fill preformed acini, often with the formation of pseudo-acinous spaces, with no stroma between

them (the alveolar carcinoma of Geraghty). These spaces may tend to be small and round, or larger and more tube-like (Fig. 401).

4. *Undifferentiated invasive growth*, consisting of small masses and strands of tumor cells, without lumen, pushing into the surrounding tissue.

Before discussing these types in detail certain peculiarities of prostatic carcinomata may be mentioned. As a rule, they are very slow growing, in accordance with which we find insidious onset, long course, late metastasis, and few mitotic figures. In addition, the cells usually depart very little if at all from the normal in size, shape, or staining. They are, therefore, quite different from the general run of carcinomata elsewhere in the body, and the ordinary cellular criteria of malignancy do not apply. The microscopic diagnosis, therefore, is specialized, and experience in this particular field is necessary for accuracy.

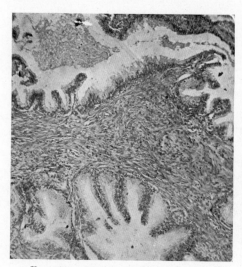
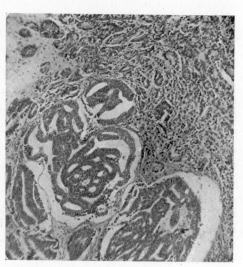

FIG. 400.—An area of typical benign hypertrophy in a prostate which is elsewhere the seat of carcinoma. These two processes may exist in any stage side by side. B. U. I. Path. 2770.

FIG. 401.—Carcinoma of the prostate. This picture shows well the two common forms of growth in carcinoma of the prostate, the small closely packed alveoli lined with a single layer of epithelium and the masses of larger cells growing into and filling preformed spaces. In the latter one sees the development of clefts or pseudo-acini. B. U. I. Path. 3060.

Group 1 includes the most frequent and familiar picture of prostatic carcinoma. It is spoken of as the adeno-carcinoma type. It consists, essentially, of a number of gland-like structures, lined with cells which may be in a double row but more often a single row, smaller than normal acini, with no intra-acinous projections, and usually packed closely together. The cells may be indistinguishable from normal cells, or they may be slightly larger, or slightly smaller with very clear cytoplasm, and nuclei somewhat smaller, rounder, and darker staining than normal. Mitotic figures are very rare, and there is no irregularity of size, shape, or staining of the nuclei. There is seldom necrosis, and it is never extensive (Fig. 403). The small acini comprising the tumor growth may be very close together, separated by only the finest hair-line of stroma, with few capillaries, or the stroma may form thicker layers between the acini. Both these forms are shown in the accompanying photographs (Figs. 401, 405, 412).

Group 2 merges into Group 1; the description of the finer details is the same. It is worth while to separate the group, however, in order to distinguish those cases in which all of the small new formed glandular elements are markedly elongated, and show very complicated branchings.

From the description given, one might imagine that there are certain cases in which the diagnosis as to the actual existence of carcinoma remains in doubt, and this is indeed true. When portions of the prostate suffer compression, as in inflammatory fibrosis, or in the outer layers in prostatic hypertrophy, the architecture is distorted, the acini and tubules compressed or elongated. In such areas pictures suggesting malignancy are sometimes found. On the other hand, small acini may develop in areas of ordinary hypertrophy, the exact significance of which is still a matter of dispute. Albarran and Hallé[1] first called attention to these pictures, and interpreted them as precancerous lesions, calling them "epithelioma

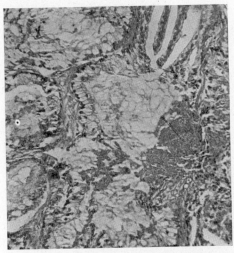

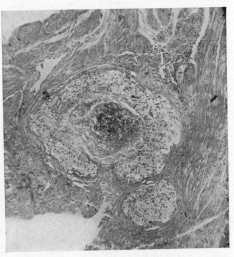

Fig. 402.—An unusual form of carcinoma of the prostate. A portion of this tumor shows the typical adenocarcinomatous and intra-acinous forms of growth, but in the area shown the tumor cells are columnar and distended with mucus (goblet-cells). The lumina of the acini are also filled with this mucus. B. U. I. Path. 2071.

Fig. 403.—An area of intra-acinous growth showing necrosis at its central point. While necrosis is rare in prostatic carcinoma, it may occur. B. U. I. Path. 2202.

adenoïde." We believe that the distinction is best made by noting the distribution of the small acini. If there are a few of them here and there, merging gradually into more normal tissue, there is probably no malignancy. If, on the contrary, the small acini are arranged in a definite group or groups, well demarcated from normal tissue or benign hypertrophy, and with the individual acini all about the same size and the same distance apart, the diagnosis is of probable malignancy. Such small areas of carcinoma do arise, undoubtedly, in hypertrophied lobes, and may be found while still small and early. A beautiful example has been recently described by Shaw[2] (Figs. 404, 405). Figure 406 shows a carcinoma nodule surrounded by benign hypertrophy. The usual site of origin of prostatic carcinoma, however, is in the posterior lobe or lamella. The best plan to follow, when carcinoma is

[1] Annales des Maladies des Organes Génito-urinaires, 1898, xvi, 797–801.

[2] Journal of Urology, 1924, xi, 63–73.

suspected, is to cut a number of additional sections, which will usually clear up the diagnosis if malignancy is really present. In the photographs are shown various examples. In general, it is not strange that certain cases are doubtful, since the

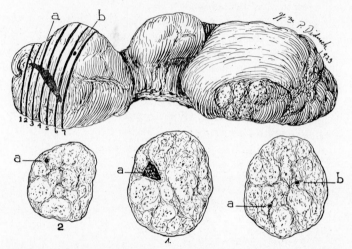

Fig. 404.—Schematic drawing showing location and extent of carcinomatous areas as determined by examination of serial sections. The cross-sections below were taken at the levels of the correspondingly numbered lines in the upper figure. There is everywhere a fair margin of hypertrophied tissue between the carcinoma and the surface. B. U. I. 10,648.

cell picture in prostatic carcinoma differs from the normal so much less than that of most other carcinomata.

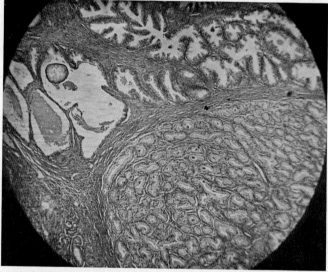

Fig. 405.—Low-power photomicrograph showing carcinoma (lower right) adjoining benign glandular hypertrophy. Several small cysts are present in the left portion of the field, one containing a corpus amylaceum. Same case as Fig. 404.

Group 3 represents, according to Geraghty, the intra-acinous proliferation of tumor cells, and this theory explains well the observed pictures. Most striking is the invasion of the dilated acini of cystic hypertrophy, which may produce tre-

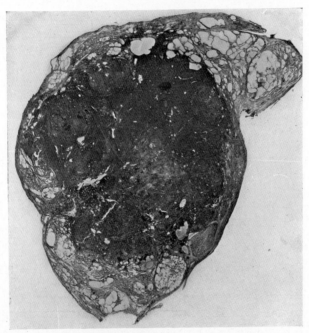

FIG. 406.—Low-power magnification of cross-section of a prostatic "lobe" removed at operation. The dark area centrally placed in the lobe is carcinoma. Note that it is everywhere surrounded by a zone of benign hypertrophy. From Mr. Henry Wade.

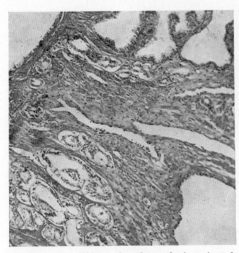

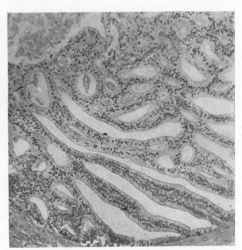

FIG. 407.—This section shows the invasion of a hypertrophied lobe by carcinoma. In this case the tumor instead of invading the acini and forming large masses of cells has retained the form of the small, closely packed acini (adenocarcinoma) and has invaded the trabeculæ between the hypertrophied acini. (See also Fig. 141.) B. U. I. Path. 3086.

FIG. 408.—This is an extreme picture of the intra-acinous form of growth. A large space has been almost filled by the tumor cells except at the center where an open space is seen (upper left corner) filled with debris. Note that the tumor strands nearest the outer part have become invaded by capillaries which have not, however, reached the most distant parts. B. U. I. Path. 2387.

mendous masses of tumor cells, or, in earlier stages, a thick lining of tumor cells all about the acinus, outlining but not filling it. As the tumor cells grow into the acinus, they throw out processes, which fuse at the tips, leaving walled-off spaces between them (Fig. 408). These spaces are known as pseudo-acini. In spite of this tendency, the processes never become very long, and papilliform structures seldom develop, even when the epithelial mass grows freely into the open space of a large cyst. The cells in these intra-acinous groups sometimes have larger, more vesicular nuclei than is the rule in Groups 1 and 2, and a few more mitoses are seen, but there is never the irregularity common in typical malignancy, as in papillary carcinoma of the bladder. When the intra-acinous growth is in question, the problem of diagnosis may arise. The appearance of thickened cell layers may be given in non-malignant acini by tangential cuts, but the experienced eye will detect this easily. The real criterion is a mass of cells thicker than the normal two-layered lining of the acini, with no connective-tissue core as in the papillæ of benign hypertrophy, with a slightly more irregular arrangement of the cells than normal. Sometimes a mass of such cells can be seen growing into an acinus from a duct, a large part of the epithelium of the acinus still remaining normal (Fig.

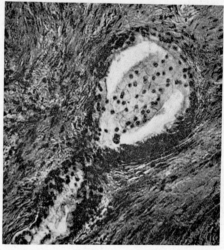

FIG. 409.—Section from a case of carcinoma of the prostate. A prostatic acinus is seen into which has grown a strand of carcinomatous cells. This strand is connected with the epithelial layer on each side, but in the places where it does not touch the epithelial layer the epithelium is of absolutely normal appearance. Either the contact of the growth replaces the normal cells or else stimulates them to take on a malignant form of growth. B. U. I. Path. 1434.

409). The presence of pseudo-acini is another point which makes the diagnosis more certain. In normal or benignly hypertrophied epithelium, the cell division takes place in a plane parallel to the basement membrane, so that the regular arrangement is preserved, while in carcinoma the division takes place at right angles to the basement membrane, as well as in other planes, so that a heaped-up mass is produced.

Group 4 includes growths which have become frankly invasive, and no longer depend on the formation of new acini or on growth along preformed gland spaces. There are masses and strands of cells, from thick to only a single cell in width, pushing into the adjacent tissues. They can often be seen taking advantage of lymph-spaces. The fibrous tissue reaction may be marked, giving the growth a very firm consistence (scirrhus).

The infiltrative growth may comprise the major part of the tumor mass—the massive cancer (of the French) or solid cancer (of the Germans). It is, however, never the primary growth, as in every case there will be found areas of the type of growth described under Group 1 or 2, or Groups 1, 2, and 3.

In the same way, we believe that the growth described under Groups 1 and 2 represent the primary type, since we may see them composing the entire mass of the tumor, while in Group 3, although the intra-acinous growth may preponderate greatly, some areas of Group 1 or Group 2 will always be found.

There are certain other observations bearing on the relations between the group-types. The outstanding clinical characteristic of prostatic carcinoma is hardness; it is upon this that the diagnosis is made, and when it is not present, the diagnosis is often missed. This hardness is due to the presence of fibrous connective tissue, which represents either the original framework of the prostate, a secondary development of a supporting framework for the neoplastic tissue itself, or a proliferative tissue reaction about the advancing growth. It is probable that

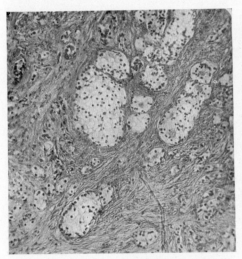
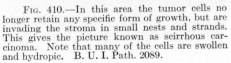
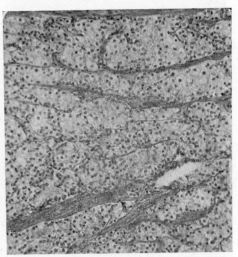

FIG. 410.—In this area the tumor cells no longer retain any specific form of growth, but are invading the stroma in small nests and strands. This gives the picture known as scirrhous carcinoma. Note that many of the cells are swollen and hydropic. B. U. I. Path. 2089.

FIG. 411.—An unusual infiltrating form in which the predominance of tumor cells over connective tissue is very marked. These cells also are swollen and hydropic, and such a tumor as the one illustrated is not hard, but quite soft to the touch, even softer than benign prostatic hypertrophy. B. U. I. Path. 2798.

all of these are represented in varying proportions in each case. The infiltrative growth seems to produce the greatest amount of fibrous reaction, indeed, some cases have been called scirrhous carcinoma. This is not always true, however. If the intra-acinous growth predominates, and produces the very large masses sometimes seen, it is clear that these masses, containing no stroma whatever, are soft. If group-types 1 or 2 predominate, there may be abundant fibrous stroma, or practically none, as shown above, and accordingly the consistence varies. If an obviously soft area, however, is surrounded by zones containing much fibrous tissue, it is the hard areas which dominate the picture. The really soft carcinomas, of which we have seen several examples, may be of three types: first, an infiltrating growth in which the cells, apparently growing faster than usual, collect in masses or separate the connective tissue and muscle fibers so much that no firm stroma is present (a picture which may be called medullary carcinoma, Fig. 411); second, large areas of glandular or tubular carcinoma (group-types 1 and 2) in which the elements are close together, separated only by the minimum possible amount of stroma (Figs. 412, 413); or third, large areas of intra-acinous proliferation, where no stroma is present (Fig. 408). In order to lend its quality of softness to the whole prostate, any of the growth types mentioned must dominate the picture, and comprise the great majority of the tumor present in the regions palpated.

Since all of the group-types are related, they often represent different stages in the growth of a single tumor. Thus when carcinoma invades or spreads through a hypertrophied lobe, it often grows rapidly along the tubules, leaving the slower extra-acinous or infiltrative growth behind. We therefore see ducts and acini filled with tumor cells, with the typical picture of Group 3, while the stroma is uninvaded and unchanged from its previous condition. In another case there may

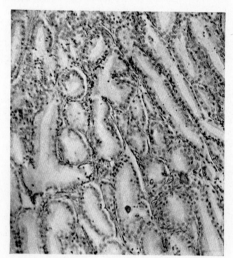 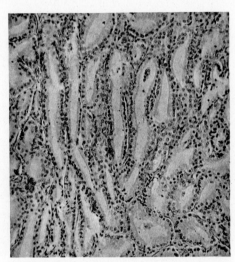

FIG. 412.—Section from a case of carcinoma of the prostate showing an excellent example of the type of growth in those prostates which are not stony hard. It is seen that a minimum amount of stroma is present and that the carcinoma is growing in a tubular form. The entire growth may be of this type, in which case the prostate will be as soft as in the ordinary benign prostatic hypertrophy. B. U. I. Path. 4024.

FIG. 413.—Another section from the same case shown in the preceding picture. The almost exclusively epithelial nature of the growth is well shown. This is the type described in the text as Group 2. B. U. I. Path. 4024.

be definite cancerous gland-like structures, surrounded and distorted by masses of infiltrative tumor and fibrous reaction, giving rise to the picture spoken of as scirrhous adenocarcinoma.

We have observed a few cases in which large spaces—apparently originally cystic acini—were completely filled with typical intra-acinous growth. Here and there, however, a number of short connective-tissue strands, containing capillaries, had commenced to penetrate between the pseudo-acini around the edge of the mass. None had reached anywhere near its center. In other groups, the growth of stroma was more complete, so that each pseudo-acinus was surrounded by a fine strand of it. We may conceive, therefore, the possibility of a transformation of intra-acinous growth (alveolar carcinoma) into something indistinguishable from the supposedly more primitive type of adenocarcinoma (Group 1).

The intra-acinous type of growth may show pseudo-acinous formation according to two types which are apparently fairly distinct. In one, the pseudo-acini are all round, in whatever plane they are cut, and, therefore, apparently spherical; in the other they are more irregular in shape, and tend to assume elongated forms, like slits or clefts, sometimes branching, in the tumor tissue. The first type is more often associated with, in the adjoining tissues, the glandular type of adenocarcinoma (Group 1) while the second is often associated with the tubular type (Group 2).

The intra-acinous type is conspicuous in large acini, but in small acini follows the same fundamental rules, where it is just as important from the point of view of histologic diagnosis. It is shown as a small acinus in Fig. 409. In larger acini, if they are not filled, the central spaces may contain desquamated and degenerated cells, or débris, just like those of benign hypertrophy.

In résumé, therefore, we may emphasize from our histologic study that all the group-types of carcinomatous growth in the prostate are closely related, usually appear together, and therefore must be considered as manifestations of a single kind of cancer. The type which predominates determines the conformation and consistence of the growth. Prostatic carcinoma may be soft, so that it is not safe to depend entirely for diagnosis on the hardness of a prostate to rectal touch. Prostatic carcinoma is slow growing, metastasizes late, and seldom shows necrosis. Large necrotic areas in a prostatic tumor are prima facie evidence that it has originated elsewhere, probably in the bladder.

In the gross, the appearance and feel vary markedly according to the nature and distribution of the tumor. In the usual form, the induration is marked, and is most evident on the posterior (rectal) surface. This is because the most frequent site of origin is in the posterior lobe. There is an irregularity, amounting even to nodularity. The growth is usually confined by Denonvilliers' fascia, and travels upward into the region of the seminal vesicles, the base of which may show the same induration as the prostate. The intervesicular notch is often obscured by fibrous tissue or extension of the new growth. In the early stages the vesicle and ampulla may be little, if at all, invaded. Later the entire vesicle may be involved, and indurated glands, containing metastases, may be found along the lateral walls of the pelvis near the outer border or tip of one or both vesicles. These glands seldom attain any great size, and vary from one to three palpable round masses, from 4 to 15 mm. in size. In cases of carcinoma unmixed with any hypertrophy the prostate may be of normal size, or even somewhat smaller. In later stages it may be enlarged, but large carcinomatous prostates usually contain hypertrophy as well.

On the vesical side enlargements in the region of the "median lobe" are usually due to hypertrophy. As pointed out by us in 1905, the mucosa of the bladder and urethra are remarkably free from invasion in carcinoma of the prostate. Direct extension to the bladder is late, and usually farther back on the trigone than the median lobe. An ulcerated fungating mass may result. Invasion of the adjoining bladder wall is indicated by an indurated nodularity, as in bladder tumors.

On section, the diagnosis of carcinoma is easy if much fibrous reaction is present, as the gland cuts like leather, and may even impart a gritty sensation through the knife. The growth is usually most marked in the posterior lamella, which may be much thickened. If hypertrophy is present, one often sees the enlarged lateral lobes, with the soft elasticity and the typical spheroidal surface appearance of benign hypertrophy, lying anterior to a hard, thickened, carcinomatous posterior lamella, as we first pointed out in 1905.[1]   At the same time we showed cancer was characterized by increased thickness in the retro-urethral portion of the prostate and could be detected by a finger in the rectum and a cystoscope in the urethra.

Hypertrophied lobes may be in part or entirely invaded by intra-acinous growth (Fig. 414).   In this case they may retain their general architecture.   The consistence is sometimes almost unchanged, or there may be increased induration.

The finer details of the surface depend on the nature of the growth.   In the usual indurated form of carcinoma, the cut surface is smooth and does not bulge out convexly, but remains flat.   It is grayish in color, with the translucency of fibrous tissue, and beset with irregular dots and streaks of yellowish, opaque material (the tumor cells).   There are no rounded spheroids, as in hypertrophy, and no cysts.

If hypertrophied tissue is invaded by intra-acinous growth, there is usually an increase in induration, causing the surface to bulge less.   Otherwise the picture may

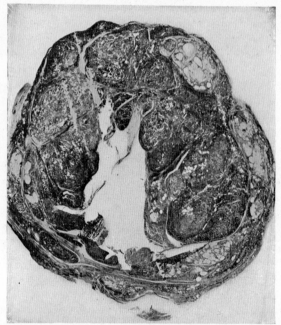

Fig. 414.—Low-power magnification of a cross-section of a prostatic "lobe" removed at operation showing both carcinoma and benign hypertrophy.   From Mr. Henry Wade.

be little changed, as the neoplastic cells simply take the place of the hypertrophied prostatic cells already present.   Later, when the growth has spread beyond the preformed acini, and the fibrous reaction has increased, the appearance becomes like that of ordinary carcinoma described in the previous paragraph.

If a soft type of growth is present, the appearance may be very misleading. The typical spheroids of hypertrophy are missing, but this is also true in certain cases of benign prostates.   The surface may be uniformly grayish, or may contain dots of opaque yellowish substance.

In certain rare cases, the growth is so cellular that it is soft and semifluid, even though no necrosis may be present.   We have seen one such case (B. U. I. 9100) which fluctuated like an abscess, but the material which exuded on incision was

[1] Young: Journal American Medical Association, 1906, xlvi, 699–704; Johns Hopkins Hospital Reports, 1906, xiv, 485–628; see Case II, p 564, also p. 527.

grayish, jelly-like and obviously not purulent (Fig. 426). The tissue consisted of papillary projections growing into a blood-filled cyst.

With all these considerations in mind, it is seen that the naked-eye diagnosis of prostatic carcinoma may often be difficult. The soft forms, and those composed mostly of intra-acinous growth may be missed, while, on the other hand, fibrous prostates the results of chronic inflammation, and acutely inflamed prostates, with diffuse cellular infiltration but without abscess, may simulate carcinoma. A normal posterior lobe does not rule out carcinoma, as we have seen that malignancy may occasionally arise in hypertrophied lateral lobes. Even the most experienced observer will occasionally be in doubt, and the only safe way, when there is any question at the time of operation, is to make a frozen section.

Even with the greatest care, some cases of the very tiny, early growths will be missed. Fortunately, they are usually the ones centrally placed in hypertrophied lobes, and simple prostatectomy often removes them completely.

NEOPLASMS OF MESOTHELIAL ORIGIN (SARCOMATA).—Tumors of the prostate of mesothelial origin are rare. The figures given in the older literature are misleading, since they were deduced at a time when most carcinomas of the prostate were not recognized. Proust and Vian[1] published an excellent article in 1907, giving details of 34 cases collected from the literature in which microscopic notes were available. We[2] have added another case. The subject is confused in two ways, first, because all varieties of tumors of mesothelial nature have been commonly grouped under the heading of "sarcoma of the prostate," and second, because mesothelial and embryonic tumors of the types described are not specifically associated with any organ, but may arise in it or near it. Thus some would consider only tumors arising in the prostate proper, while others include all tumors involving the prostate. As we have seen, a mesothelial tumor may arise in the bladder, or in the retrovesical connective tissue, as well as in the prostate itself. Whatever its origin, it may surround the prostate, invade it, or even destroy it, and for this reason it is impossible, in the late stages where the tumor is very extensive, to say just where the tumor originated. Pathologic studies must therefore be confined to those cases where the tumor is still sufficiently circumscribed so that there can be no doubt of its prostatic origin.

Such cases comprise only a small group, surely not over 1 or 2 per cent. of all malignant prostatic tumors. They are decidedly less common than those in which the tumor is distinctly retrovesical and supraprostatic. The distinction can be made in the earlier stages by rectal examination. Among the 593 cases of prostatic neoplasm in our series, only 2 of the non-carcinomatous ones apparently began in the prostate. There was no operation or autopsy in either case. All our other mesothelial tumors were obviously of retrovesical origin. The tumors which have been described in the literature include sarcoma (large round-cell, small round-cell, spindle-cell, mixed cell, and lymphosarcoma), "angiosarcoma," "myxosarcoma," "adenosarcoma," chondroma, rhabdomyoma, and fibromyoma.

All of these tumors are usually rounded, smooth, and of fairly firm consistence, but may be lobulated, firm, or fluctuant, or may show areas of varying consistence. On section they are grayish and homogeneous, except where there are hemorrhages or necrotic areas. These necrotic areas may account for the softness, or it may be

---

[1] Annales des Maladies des Organes Génito-urinaires, 1907, xxv, 721–778.

[2] Young: Cabot's Modern Urology, 1924, i, 802–804.

due to a loose structure with varying quantities of gelatinous intercellular substance. There may be projections into the bladder, usually covered by intact mucosa, but they are rare. The rectum is seldom invaded, but may be pressed upon by the growth so that no feces can pass. Since the development of these tumors is centrifugal, and they do not, as a rule, invade adjacent tissues, annular stricture of the rectum like that found in carcinoma of the prostate does not occur. The mass may push up behind the bladder, or downward into the perineum. When perineal extension occurs, there is often a constriction in the tumor corresponding to the level of the triangular ligament. The seminal vesicles and ureters may be surrounded and compressed, but are invaded late if at all.

Within the prostate, the growth may involve only one lobe, or one lobe more than the rest. The prostatic architecture may be completely destroyed, or remnants of gland structure may persist. There is much more tendency to invade the urethra than in carcinoma, and sessile or pedunculated nodules may occupy its lumen and cause obstruction.

Microscopically, the true sarcomata show a uniform cell type, or at most a mixture of round-cells of varying size, and perhaps spindle-cells. While intercellular fibrillæ are usually present, the total amount of supporting tissue is small. There may be varying amounts of gelatinous intercellular substance, producing a stellate appearance of the cells. When this substance is abundant and present throughout the tumor, the term "myxosarcoma" is sometimes employed. The round-cell types are most common. In a number of the cases described in the literature, small glandular structures are mentioned and assumed to be remnants of the prostatic glands. It may be that some of these tumors are really embryomatous, the gland structures being part of the tumor. Hemorrhage and necrosis are common, in contradistinction to carcinoma.

The picture in lymphosarcoma is the typical one of that disease.

Among the tumors with multiple tissues are mentioned "angiosarcoma." It is impossible to tell from the descriptions given whether these are really of endothelial origin, or merely have a factitious perithelial appearance due to necrosis of the parts distant from blood-vessels. There are also tumors with mixtures of glands and embryonic stroma, with masses of cartilage, and with smooth and striated muscle. It is probable that they are all embryomatous. No true teratoma has been described. The general growth characteristics and manner of spread of all these tumors are similar to those of the sarcomata. In a case of Verhoogen,[1] there were a number of good sized calculi within the tumor.

Regional lymphatic metastasis is stated to be rare, and there is no special predilection for bone. Metastasis is probably by the blood-stream, and tends to involve the internal organs, the lungs being often attacked.

In the end stages of these tumors, the large mass may occupy the entire pelvis, compressing rectum, urethra, bladder, and ureters, and projecting up into the abdominal cavity. Growth is usually retrovesical, but prevesical masses are described. The perineum and scrotum may be bulged out, and scrotal edema may occur. Surgical wounds may heal, but implantation may occur, and rapid growth after operation with enormous projecting fungating masses is described.

SECONDARY EFFECTS OF PROSTATIC CARCINOMA.—The secondary effects of prostatic carcinoma may be grouped as those due to obstruction, extension, and

[1] Encyclopædie Française d'Urologie, 1914, iii, 425–538.

metastasis. Carcinoma may attain an extensive growth in the prostate and seminal vesicles without causing any urethral obstruction, especially if not complicated by hypertrophy. In other cases, the fibrosis occurring with carcinoma may constrict the vesical orifice or prostatic urethra, or may give rise to obstructing bars at the vesical orifice. The effects on the upper urinary tract are the same as in any prostatic obstruction, and are described in the chapter on the Obstructive Uropathy. This obstruction may occur early or late, but is usually late, and sometimes may be absent even in very extensive and fatal cases. The frequency with which obstruction of the ejaculatory ducts occurs is difficult to determine. In nearly all of our radical operations, the ampullæ have been found filled with cancer cells.

The most striking fact about the extension of prostatic carcinoma is that it finds an effective barrier in Denonvilliers' fascia. The line of extension is first and most frequent to the seminal vesicles, second along the membranous urethra, third to the bladder (late), and last to the rectum (rare).

Extension to the seminal vesicles is comparatively early, considering the slow growth of these tumors. The base is first involved, later the entire vesicle. Secondary spread to the bladder and rectum from the vesicles may occur, but is rare. The type of growth found in the vesicles is usually the invasive type, though there may be some of the intra-acinous type in the cavities of the vesicle. When the growth reaches the tip of the vesicle, it may include and obstruct the ureter, giving rise to hydro-ureter and hydronephrosis.

Extension along the membranous urethra is not uncommon. The wall is infiltrated, but stricture is infrequent, on account of the wide caliber of the urethra at this point. Later the growth passes on to involve the triangular ligament, Cowper's glands, and urethral bulb. If the growth reaches the cavernous tissue of the bulb, it may spread through the entire extent, and even include the corpora cavernosa, giving rise to an extraordinary condition of carcinomatous priapism. The bulbous or penile urethra may be strictured. The growth may extend to the peri-urethral tissues in the perineum and base of the penis.

Extension to the bladder has been discussed. Extensive infiltration of the bladder wall is rare.

Late in the disease, Denonvillier's fascia may be penetrated, and the rectal wall involved in the growth. While the growth is usually low and flat, intrarectal masses may appear, when ulceration is common—in distinction to the prostatic and vesicular growths. The necrosis, however, is seldom extensive enough to cause recto-urethral fistula. Stricture of the rectum may be caused, both by pressure from without and growth within the rectum.

Prostatic carcinoma is almost invariably, except in the earliest stages, associated with changes in the surrounding areolar tissue, which take the form of an increasing fibrosis, and enlargement and dilatation of the blood-vessels, especially the veins. These changes are very important from a diagnostic point of view, since they are often present while the growth is small and confined entirely to the prostate. Indeed, thickened perineal tissues, with abnormally large and congested veins, have sometimes, when seen at operation, been the first indication of malignant disease of the prostate, even when the rectal examination was negative.

METASTASIS FROM PROSTATIC CARCINOMA.—Cunéo and Marcille[1] have investigated the lymphatics of the prostate. They find that the prostate itself has a rich

[1] The Lymphatics (Delamere, Poirier, and Cunéo), 1904 (London, English translation).

lymphatic network, leading into a series of sinuses about its periphery (Fig. 415). These large vessels can often be seen plainly in sections, especially near the vesical orifice. Collecting vessels run backward, outward, and upward along the sides of the rectum and the internal surface of the levator ani and ischiococcygeal muscles, to the lymph-nodes about the internal iliac artery. These nodes are in close relation to the sacral plexus. Other collecting vessels run up along the seminal vesicles and vasa deferentia and along the lateral surface of the bladder, to empty into the external iliac nodes. Another connection is by way of the membranous urethra, and indirectly to the internal iliac group. There are a few small inconstant nodes

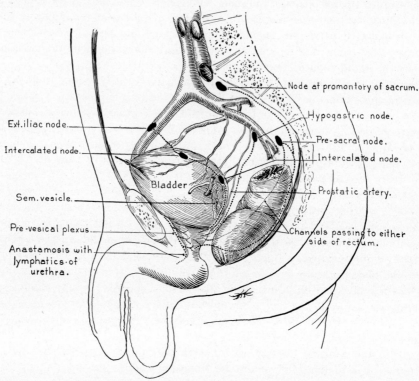

FIG. 415.—This diagram shows the lymphatics of the prostate which drain by a number of channels. The prevesical plexus drains into the external iliac nodes. Other channels pass alongside the rectum to enter the presacral nodes, often reaching as high as a node at the promontory. Other channels accompany the prostatic artery to enter the hypogastric nodes. Still other channels pass up the posterior surface of the bladder to enter the external iliac nodes. In the course of these channels are small, intercalated nodes in the region of the tips of the seminal vesicles. These nodes can sometimes be palpated on rectal examination.

lying along or above the seminal vesicles. Some of the nodes draining the prostate lie as far up as the bifurcation of the aorta. Metastases from prostatic carcinoma commonly occur first along this system, and any or all of the nodes mentioned may be involved. There are no exact data as to the time at which metastasis occurs, or the proportion of cases in which it occurs, because all of these nodes, excepting the small paravesicular nodes, are so deep that they cannot be investigated. Therefore, we remain in ignorance of their condition until large palpable masses are produced, nerves pressed on, or bones invaded. Bumpus[1] believes they are much

[1] Surgery, Gynecology, and Obstetrics, 1921, xxxii, 31–43.

more common and earlier than we have until now suspected. In 100 autopsies in carcinoma of the prostate, Kaufmann found only 27 cases with involvement of the pelvic glands. We found only 11 in our first 40 cases.[1] A characteristic effect of these metastatic masses is pressure upon the sacral plexus, causing pains in the legs. Later the veins may be compressed, causing edema of the legs. The lymphatic channels determine the course of local extension, which in advanced cases is in the form of a constricting collar encircling the rectum, starting from the prostate, and passing around obliquely upward.

Metastases to other lymph-nodes may occur, as the retroperitoneal, cervical, axillary, femoral, inguinal, etc. These involvements are usually late. It is possible that the inguinal nodes are affected only after all the intrapelvic ones are involved, and a collateral lymphatic circulation through the inguinals set up.

Aside from these regional lymphatic metastases, it is probable that metastasis also occurs by the blood-stream. Pauchet describes strands of carcinoma cells within small blood-vessels in the prostate. The distant metastases of prostatic carcinoma are usually somewhat later than the regional ones, but may be earlier, as observed by us.[2] Von Recklinghausen[3] first noted a remarkable predilection for bones, especially the vertebral column and pelvis. In fact, metastatic growths in bones always suggest a prostatic origin, even if there have been no local symptoms. The usual picture is that of a condensation process, with destruction of the architecture, but actual laying down of new bone, with increase in size. This is well illustrated in the x-ray photograph shown in Fig. 425. Bumpus states that very rarely marked bone destruction may be seen. The spine and pelvis are usually first attacked, and radiographers are accustomed to inspect the body of the fifth lumbar vertebra for the first signs of bony metastasis. The femora and ribs are also involved rather frequently, and other bones more seldom. Once bony metastasis has commenced, it is common for the process to become very wide spread. Whether this is by intramedullary extension, or by the formation of innumerable new metastatic foci is not clear, but it is likely the latter, since bone boundaries seem to have little effect on the process. One may see the entire spine and pelvis occupied by a diffuse infiltration, with a characteristic spottiness in the x-ray. While the bones may become large, the metastases, like the parent tumor, grow slowly and do not undergo necrosis. Consequently nerve involvement may be late or absent. There is reason from x-ray evidence to believe that almost always the involvement of the pelvis is due to true osseous involvement, and not to extension from regional lymph-node metastases. The bony lesions begin centrally in the bone, and are most common at points removed from the sites of the lymphnode groups.

Lymphatic or bony metastases may develop and give the first symptoms of prostatic carcinoma, in the form of pain or even of pathologic fracture of a long bone, urinary obstruction being absent.

More rarely, other organs are involved. We have seen 1 case in which a single metastasis in the liver was the only one found at autopsy. Metastasis to the wall of the ureter may occur, usually in the lower third, causing obstruction with hydro-ureter and hydronephrosis. The route in such cases may be lymphatic. We have seen two of these ureteral metastases from prostatic carcinoma. Rarely

[1] Young: Johns Hopkins Hospital Bulletin, 1905, xvi, 316–321.

[2] Ibid.: Annals of Surgery, 1909, l, 1144–1233.

[3] Festschrift, Rudolph Virchow, Berlin, 1891, 1–89.

there is a general peritoneal carcinomatosis. Skin nodules may occur. There is also the possibility of metastasis in tissues near the prostate; thus a bladder lesion may in some cases be a metastasis and not an extension. This phenomenon is probably not as frequent or important as in bladder neoplasms.

Seminal Vesicles.—A few cases of primary neoplasm of the seminal vesicles have been described, but in all the reports we have studied the tumors were mesothelial (sarcoma, embryoma) and the point of origin was difficult to determine accurately. We have found no case of proved carcinoma of the vesicles, though there is no reason why it might not occur. Benign tumors also are missing from the literature.

The vesicles are frequently the seat of secondary involvement by cancers of the prostate and bladder, and occasionally of the rectum. The pathologic picture in the first two has been described under the respective headings. Retrovesical and prostatic sarcomata surround and compress the vesicles, and less often invade and destroy them.

SYMPTOMS

Carcinoma.—The age at which the symptoms of prostatic carcinoma appear is quite definite, all statistics being in agreement except Thompson's.

TABLE 93

Age.	Thompson, 1860, 12 cases, per cent.	Young, 1909, 111 cases, per cent.	Bumpus, 1921, 361 cases, per cent.	Deming, 1922, 100 cases, per cent.
40–50	17.0	1.8	2.7	3.0
50–60	25.0	22.5	21.6	17.0
60–70	42.0	45.5	51.2	45.0
70–80	17.0	27.0	22.1	25.0
80–90		3.6	1.2	10.0

These figures of course tell us nothing about the age at which the disease actually begins, but it is evidently very rare before forty years of age. We know that prostatic carcinoma is, at first, and probably for a long time, symptomless. We can get a general idea of the rapidity with which it progresses by studying the average period of survival, especially in untreated cases, after the first onset of symptoms. In 100 cases from our clinic carefully followed by Deming,[1] 48 were dead an average of 2.54 years after the beginning of symptoms. Thirteen were alive, but with marked symptoms, an average of 3.6 years from the onset. Twelve were alive, with diminishing symptoms, an average of 4.4 years from onset, and 5 were almost symptomless, an average of six years from onset. All these patients received radium treatment. Bumpus[2] found the average survival, from onset of symptoms, to be an average of 2.73 years in 16 patients in whom metastases were demonstrated, and 3.4 years in 71 patients in whom no metastases were demonstrated. These patients received no treatment. These figures, however, are not conclusive as to the total duration of the disease. We know that in certain cases, the symptoms begin much earlier than in others, owing to the location of the growth, or to a complicating benign prostatic hypertrophy. In other cases, symptoms occur only

[1] Surgery, Gynecology, and Obstetrics, 1922, xxxiv, 99–118.
[2] Ibid., xxxii, 31–43.

in the end stages of the disease, as shown by the presence of extensive palpable involvement, metastases, etc., at the time symptoms are first noted. The figures on this last type of case would tend to cut down the average time of survival for the whole. Really early cases of uncomplicated carcinoma of the prostate are seldom discovered, and then only as a result of routine rectal examination. Most of such cases in our clinic have been operated upon radically, but we have seen an interesting case in which a small indurated nodule of carcinoma about 1 cm. in diameter was found in one lobe. Operation was refused. One year later the nodule had increased only to 2 cm. in diameter, and at the end of the second year, while it involved the entire lobe, it had not crossed the median line, entered the seminal vesicle, nor passed the prostatic capsule. The tumor may grow more rapidly in its later stages, and some tumors, no doubt, grow faster than others. Yet it is evident that prostatic carcinoma is, on the whole, a slow-growing tumor and that at first it usually causes no symptoms. It is also very probable that in many cases the carcinoma exists for a long time—possibly years—before it is discovered or even makes itself known to the patient. For this reason it is important for all physicians to familiarize themselves with the features of early carcinoma of the prostate, and to practice rectal examination on all male patients past middle life with a view of discovering the early cases.

Until comparatively recently, carcinoma of the prostate was not recognized. After Albarran and Hallé had discovered 14 "malignancies" in a series of 100 supposedly benign hypertrophied prostates, many other authors confirmed their findings that the disease was quite common. We[1] found carcinoma comprising 21 per cent. of the total number of cases of patients applying for treatment for prostatic enlargement which proved to be either carcinoma or benign prostatic hypertrophy. Other figures are: Oliver Smith, 16 per cent.; Davis, 20 per cent; Moullin, 25 per cent.; Kümmel, 20 per cent.; Pauchet, 20 per cent.; Wilson and McGrath, 15.5 per cent.; Freyer, 13.4 per cent.[2] In our clinic there have now (January 1, 1924) records of 2643 cases of benign prostatic hypertrophy and 593 of prostatic carcinoma. The carcinoma cases are thus 17.01 per cent. of the total. They also furnish 4.7 per cent. of all the urologic cases seen. We may say that, roughly and for practical purposes, 20 per cent. of all men over 60 will have symptoms due to prostatic trouble, and that of these 20 per cent. will have cancer; in other words, 4 men in every hundred who live to be sixty years of age will have cancer of the prostate.

Even after symptoms commence, long periods sometimes elapse, as in so many other diseases, before the patient appears for treatment. In 109 cases, we found that 20 had had symptoms for less than one year, 67 between one and three years, and 22 over four years. The individual symptoms were as shown in Table 94 on page 630.

It will be seen that a larger proportion of those with pain reported fairly early than of those with urinary symptoms. However, a number of those reporting earliest already had extensive involvement.

As we have seen, prostatic carcinoma may exist without symptoms. When symptoms do appear they are in a majority of cases urinary, and are in no way characteristic. Where pain is the first symptom, we must distinguish between local pain, especially in the bladder, urethra and penis, which is merely the ac-

[1] Young: Annals of Surgery, 1909, l, 1144–1233.
[2] Quoted in the above article.

TABLE 94

Duration of Symptoms in Our 111 Cases of Cancer of the Prostate

Duration.	Difficulty.	Frequency.	Pain, local.	Pain, rectum and perineum.	Pain, groin and testicle.	Pain, legs.	Pain, back.	Pain, suprapubic.
1–6 months..........	10	9	13	4	..	13	9	4
6–11 months.........	4	5	4	1	1	..	2	
12–17 months........	14	12	4	2	3	3	3	2
18–23 months........	3	3	1	..	..	1	2	
24–36 months........	18	22	2	1	1	2	1	2
1½–3 years...........	..	..	..	..	..	..	1	
3–5 years............	4	9	..	2				
6–10 years.	6	7	2	1	..	..	1	
Over 10 years........	2	1	2	..	..	..	1	

TABLE 95

Initial Symptoms in Our First Series of 111 Cases of Cancer of the Prostate

	Cases.	Per cent.
Frequency of urination......................	76	69.3
Difficulty of urination......................	48	43.2
Pain...................................	35	31.5
Retention..............................	4	3.6
Hematuria..............................	4	3.6

The pain was distributed as follows:

	Cases.
Bladder and urethra..	16
Rectum and perineum.......................................	7
Back, sacrum, and gluteal region.............................	6
Legs...	3
Inguinal region and scrotum.................................	2
Hypogastrium...	1

TABLE 96

Initial Symptoms in Cases With or Without Metastases (Bumpus)

	79 cases with metastasis.		283 cases without metastasis.		362 total cases.	
	Number.	Per cent.	Number.	Per cent.	Number.	Per cent.
Frequency and nocturia...	36	45.4	128	41.7	159	43.9
Difficulty of urination.....	13	16.4	92	32.5	105	29.0
Pain....................	27	34.1	34	12.0	61	16.8
No symptoms............	1	1.2	11	3.5	12	3.3
Retention...............	1	1.2	9	3.1	10	2.75
Hematuria...............	..	..	5	1.7	5	1.37
Incontinence............	2	2.5	1	0.35	3	0.82
Pyuria..................	1	1.2	1	0.35	2	0.54
Edema of legs...........	2	2.5	..	..	2	0.54
Weakness...............	..	..	1	0.35	1	0.27
Loss of weight..........	..	..	1	0.35	1	0.27
Enlarged inguinal glands..	1	1.2	..	..	1	0.27

companiment of urinary obstruction or cystitis, and distant pain, as in the legs, hips, back or chest, which is probably due to nerve root involvement by metastases.

The initial symptoms were tabulated by us in 1909 as shown in Table 95, page 630.

It will be seen that in many of these cases two or more symptoms were present at the onset. The usual combination was frequency and difficulty.

Bumpus gives the figures shown in Table 96, page 630, the cases being divided into those in which the x-ray showed metastases and those in which it did not.

In the 27 cases with metastasis where pain was the first symptom, it was distributed as follows:

TABLE 97

	Alone.	Total.
Back	5	14
Thigh	4	11
Chest	2	7
Rectum	2	2
Abdomen	2	2
Thigh and back	5	
Back and chest	3	
Thigh and chest	1	
Thigh, back, and chest	1	
Thigh and inguinal region	1	

It will be seen that the obstructive urinary symptoms inaugurate the great majority of cases. Pain occurs in a much larger proportion of cases with demonstrable metastases (one-third) than of those without (one-eighth), but conversely is absent from two-thirds of the cases with metastasis. Hematuria is a negligible symptom, since it is even less frequent than in benign prostatic hypertrophy, as pointed out by us.

Other cases are recorded in which the first symptoms were a tumor in one of the long bones, an abdominal mass, paraplegia, skin nodules, etc. A number of these cases have come to autopsy from general medical or surgical services without the presence of prostatic carcinoma having been suspected.

As to the occurrence of the various symptoms, we found in 111 cases the figures shown in Table 98, page 632.

In 100 of our cases with extensive involvement, Deming found the symptoms as shown in Table 99, page 632.

From these tables it is seen that the obstructive urinary symptoms predominate. Local pain runs somewhat parallel with the urinary symptoms, and is also not diagnostic. Distant pains, especially in the leg and back, are more suggestive and generally indicate metastasis, as they are more frequent in cases where metastasis can be demonstrated. They are not necessarily associated with metastasis, however, as in many cases where metastases can be demonstrated there has been no pain.

The urinary symptoms, especially frequency and dysuria, are from obstruction, which may be due to (1) carcinomatous stricture of the prostatic urethra, or (2) a coincident benign prostatic hypertrophy. We found in a series carefully studied with the collaboration of J. T. Geraghty, where pathologic material was examined in each case, that there was benign hypertrophy associated with 61 per cent. of the cases of prostatic carcinoma.

TABLE 98

SYMPTOMS IN OUR FIRST SERIES OF 111 CASES OF CANCER OF THE PROSTATE

Urinary symptoms:

Total.

Difficulty, slight 5, moderate 6, severe 28, requiring catheter 22.. 61

Frequency, slight 13, moderate 7, severe 38...................... 58

Complete retention.. 19

Hematuria.. 8

Overflow incontinence..................................... 2

Pain, local:

Total.

Urethra, slight 4, moderate 4, severe 10..................... 18

Penis, slight 3, moderate 4, severe 11....................... 18

Perineum, slight 3, moderate 5, severe 7..................... 15

Bladder, slight 4, moderate 2, severe 9...................... 15

Rectum, slight 2, moderate 0, severe 10..................... 12

Total local pain.. 78

Pain, distant:

Total.

Leg, slight 2, moderate 8, severe 8......................... 18

Thigh, slight 2, moderate 4, severe 8....................... 14

Foot, slight 1, moderate 1, severe 3........................ 5

Total lower limb....................................... 37

Total.

Lumbar, slight 5, moderate 3, severe 7...................... 15

Sacral, slight 2, moderate 2, severe 5....................... 9

Gluteal, slight 0, moderate 4, severe 1...................... 5

Total back.. 29

Total.

Pubic, slight 2, moderate 3, severe 5........................ 10

Hip, slight 2, moderate 3, severe 4......................... 9

Testicle, slight 3, moderate 0, severe 3..................... 6

Groin, slight 1, moderate 1, severe 0....................... 2

Renal colic... 0

Total distant pain..................................... 93

Systemic:

Total.

Loss of weight, slight 7, moderate 11, severe 30.............. 48

TABLE 99

SYMPTOMS IN 100 ADVANCED CASES OF CANCER OF THE PROSTATE

Cases.

Frequency (nycturia 93) 96

Dysuria.. 80

Difficulty:

Small stream.. 87

Dribbling... 76

Hesitancy... 65

Complete retention....................................... 21

Hematuria... 17

Pain in back... 28

Pain in extremities....................................... 22

Loss of weight... 14

Hematuria is infrequent, even in the late stages. Pyuria indicates infection, and therefore usually follows the obstructive symptoms.

Pain in the bladder, urethra, or penis, especially in the form of dysuria, is usually associated with urinary obstruction. Pain in the penis, perineum, and rectum may result from the local growth in the prostate. Pain in the thighs, legs, and buttocks is often due to carcinomatous involvement of or adhesions to nerves in the pelvis. Pain in the scrotum or testis may be referred pain, but when pain is further afield, it is probably due to metastases. Keyes remarks that bilateral sciatica in old men is almost pathognomonic of carcinoma of the prostate.

Loss of weight and strength and anemia are late symptoms. In early cases, and even in those with extensive local symptoms, the strength and nutrition may be maintained perfectly. In the terminal stages a typical picture of malignant cachexia is the rule, though it may be absent in those where uremia or infection intervene earlier to place the patient's life in jeopardy.

Loss of sexual power is not uncommon at the cancer age merely from senility. In 47 cases tabulated by us, the sexual powers were absent in 28, diminished in 9, and normal in 10. In some of the cases where there was no impairment the involvement was extensive. In general, carcinoma affects the sexual powers more than benign hypertrophy. Pain on coitus is rare. We have seen 1 case of priapism due to extensive infiltration of the corpus spongiosum and corpora cavernosa by the carcinoma.

Metastases are usually hidden, but occasionally may cause perceptible tumors. If no other symptoms are present, the appearance of a tumor anywhere in an old man should indicate examination of the prostate. This is especially true in tumors of the bones. In a case of a tumor of the tibia in which amputation was done, there were no symptoms referable to the urogenital tract. Autopsy showed an extensive carcinoma of the prostate.

Edema of the legs or scrotum is a late symptom, and indicates involvement extensive enough to press upon and occlude the veins and lymphatics. We have seen cancer of the prostate in which there was no dysuria, frequency, or pain, with infiltration along the lateral wall of the pelvis so extensive that it caused great swelling of the thigh and leg.

The rectal lumen is invaded very rarely until late in the disease, but the patient may suffer from rectal disturbance due to encroachment of the perirectal tissues. Difficult defecation, constipation, hemorrhoids, pain, and bleeding may occur without ulceration of the mucosa which is rare and late. Stricture of the rectum, with progressively severe symptoms, may occur. These changes are always late and usually terminal; in many cases they do not occur, as is also the case with rectourethral fistula.

In summary, prostatic carcinoma is symptomless at first. When symptoms begin they are those of urinary obstruction in a great majority of cases. Carcinoma of the prostate must therefore be considered in every case of urinary obstruction in men over fifty. Distant pain usually indicates metastasis, but many cases with metastasis have no pain, at least for a long time.

Other Tumors of the Prostate.—As we have seen, mesothelial tumors of the prostate are not confined to any particular age, but are more common, if anything, in youth. Here the first symptoms are practically always those of urinary obstruction, though in a few cases rectal obstruction was in the foreground at the time of onset. The further course is characterized by the more rapid growth of the tumor. Swelling of the perineum is fairly common, especially in children. The mass may be soft and fluctuant, and may resemble an abscess, except that there is no fever. This point is important. Tumor masses presenting in the lower abdomen are common. Symptoms due to metastasis are infrequent.

DIAGNOSIS OF CARCINOMA OF THE PROSTATE

The principal resource in the diagnosis of prostatic carcinoma is the rectal examination. The history of pains in the back and legs (sciatica) and the *x*-ray examination of the bones for evidence of metastases, are sometimes helpful, but the symptoms of urinary obstruction, which usually bring the patient to the physician, are exactly the same as those occurring in cases of benign prostatic hypertrophy. Cystoscopic examination, too, is usually of little aid.

Every male patient above the age of fifty, without any symptoms, may have prostatic carcinoma, and every physical examination made above this age should include a rectal examination. It is only in this way that the early cases can be recognized. In one of our patients (B. U. I. 12,046) a hard nodule was found in the prostate at the age of sixty during a routine medical "survey." He had no symptoms of any kind, felt perfectly well, and was amazed when told that he had cancer and that a radical excision of the prostate and seminal vesicles must be performed. The diagnosis was confirmed and an excellent result obtained.

Patients with carcinoma of the prostate usually consult the physician on account of obstructive symptoms (difficulty, frequency, etc.), pain in the back or legs, or local pain. Hematuria as an initial symptom is rare. Occasionally a bone tumor or a spontaneous fracture is the first manifestation. Since carcinoma is often complicated by benign prostatic hypertrophy this has an important bearing on the obstructive symptoms. Benign hypertrophy complicating an early carcinoma may be responsible for all the obstructive symptoms, while uncomplicated carcinoma usually does not cause obstruction until a rather late stage.

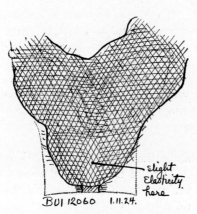

FIG. 416.—Very extensive involvement in a late stage of carcinoma of the prostate. The mass has broken the bounds of the normal structures and fills the entire retrovesical space. The membranous urethra thickened and indurated.

Keeping these facts in mind, one proceeds with the examination. The external genitalia reveal nothing of importance except in certain very late cases, when there may be involvement of the inguinal glands, or carcinomatous infiltration of the bulb and corpora of the penis. The urine also is not characteristic. It may or may not be infected.

On rectal examination, the most important feature is induration. In typical cases this induration is very great, often described as "stony hard," and the prostate is fixed. Extension of this same process to the seminal vesicles or to the intervesicular angle is common, in which case the boundaries between the prostate and the vesicles may be indistinguishable. The membranous urethra is not infrequently involved, when it is broader than normal, indurated, fixed, and its outlines obscured by adhesions (Fig. 416). The rectal wall may be invaded, in which case the rectum is fixed to the prostate. This involvement may extend around the rectum, even surrounding it by a firm, irregular tube of carcinomatous tissue. Ulceration is rare and occurs only in late stages.

A typical, well-advanced case is quite unmistakable. The induration is of extreme firmness, and the surface is very often irregular or even nodular. The prostate is fixed, not only as a result of the carcinomatous growth itself, but of the inflammatory reaction which occurs in the tissues about it. Enlarged, indurated lymph-nodes can sometimes be palpated along the outer side of the seminal vesicles. The membranous urethra is often involved in this reaction and is broadened, fixed, and has its outlines obscured. Extension to the rectal and perirectal tissues is in-

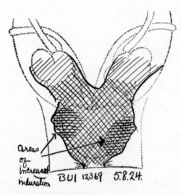

FIG. 417.—Marked involvement of the prostate and seminal vesicles by carcinoma of the prostate. Difficult urination for three years. Note the irregularity of the prostatic outline. Conservative perineal prostatectomy for relief of symptoms. Benign hypertrophy also present.

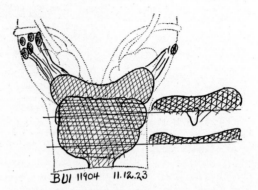

FIG. 418.—Extensive involvement of the prostate and seminal vesicles in carcinoma of the prostate. The seminal vesicles are definitely demarcated from the prostate and slightly less indurated. The membranous urethra is markedly thickened. Definite indurated nodes are felt at the tips of both seminal vesicles. Symptoms of frequency and difficulty for one year. No operation.

dicated by induration and fixation. Characteristic pictures are shown in Figs. 417 to 421.

It is, however, in the less well-advanced cases that real problems of diagnosis arise. These can perhaps be best considered after reviewing a series of cases in

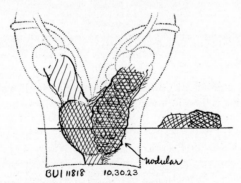

FIG. 419.—Unilateral involvement of the prostate and right seminal vesicle in carcinoma of the prostate. Note the marked nodularity. Symptoms of difficult urination for four years. Punch operation, radium, and x-ray treatment with marked improvement.

which incorrect diagnoses were made. From our series of nearly 2000 cases of prostatectomy, 250 cases of prostatic carcinoma were studied, in all of which microscopic sections were available. In this series there were found 25 cases in which the diagnosis was missed or very doubtful. In 19 of these 25 no suspicion, even, of

malignancy had arisen. Analysis showed that in 7 cases the error was due to the
growth being soft, and lacking entirely the stony induration usually found in

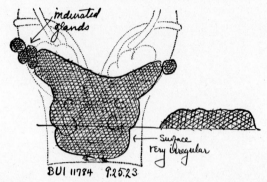

FIG. 420.—Marked involvement of the prostate and seminal vesicles in a case of carcinoma of the
prostate. The membranous urethra is thickened and enlarged, indurated lymph-nodes are felt at
the tips of both seminal vesicles. The intervesicular plateau is very marked. Symptoms of dysuria
for four years. No operation.

carcinoma. In 5 cases induration was present, but the examiners felt that it was
not of sufficient degree to indicate carcinoma. In 5 cases the area of carcinoma was

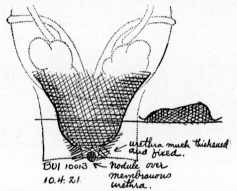

FIG. 421.—Extensive involvement in late stage of carcinoma of the prostate. Involvement of the
seminal vesicles extends further than the finger can reach. The membranous urethra is very markedly
indurated and there is a nodule over it just above the triangular ligament. Symptoms for at least
three years consisting of frequency and pyuria. No operation.

so small that it was missed. In 8 cases the tumor growth was obscured by benign
prostatic hypertrophy. The following table summarizes the findings:

TABLE 100

ANALYSIS OF 25 CASES OF PROSTATIC CARCINOMA WHICH WERE NOT RECOGNIZED

Error due to	Soft type of tumor.	Error in judging induration.	Small size of nodule.	Obscured by benign hypertrophy.	Thin layer over hypertrophy.	Nodule over hypertrophy.	Total.
Diagnosed at operation, suspected before......	1	2	1	0	0	2	6
Diagnosed at operation, unsuspected before....	1	0	0	0	1	1	3
Diagnosed by microscope only	5	3	4	4	0	0	16
Total............	7	5	5	4	1	3	25

Nineteen cases, therefore, of 250 cases of carcinoma of the prostate (7.5 per cent. of the cancer cases operated on, about 1 per cent. of the cases diagnosed hypertrophy) were entirely unsuspected before operation.

The types of growth in prostatic carcinoma giving clinically soft tumors, or at least tumors not characterized by stony hardness, have been fully described in the section on pathology. In 1 case, not necrotic, the tumor was so soft that a diagnosis of abscess was made.

It is probable that some, if not all of those where the induration was misjudged, were slightly less hard than the typical case.

When the area of carcinoma is very small, it cannot, of course, be diagnosed clinically. In some of the cases of this group the neoplasm was only a few millimeters in size.

When benign hypertrophy is present, it may obscure the carcinoma in various ways. 1. If the tumor nodule has arisen in some other place than the posterior lamella (a rare occurrence) it may be completely surrounded by hypertrophic tissue. 2. If the tumor grows in a thin layer in the posterior lamella, it may not be perceptible, owing to the elasticity imparted by the mass of hypertrophic tissue beneath it (Fig. 422). 3. If the tumor grows as a hard nodule in the posterior lamella, it may have a sense of elasticity imparted to it in the same way by the hypertrophied tissue beneath.

Abstracts of some of the typical cases of mistaken diagnosis follow. In view of the great interest of this problem, we have inserted the names of the examiners in each case.

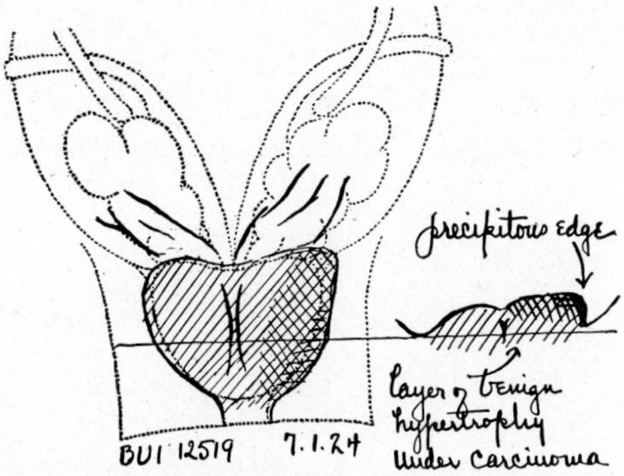

FIG. 422.—Type of rectal finding in prostatic carcinoma which may lead to diagnostic errors. The seminal vesicles and membranous urethra are negative. The prostate is slightly enlarged and elastic, due to benign hypertrophy. Some induration can be felt on the right side due to carcinoma in the posterior lamella, but it does not feel stony hard because of the elastic hypertrophy beneath.

B. U. I. 3245, age fifty-seven. June 11, 1912. Frequency and difficulty of urination for one year. One attack of hematuria. R. U. 0, B. C. 380 c.c. Rectal: Prostate moderately enlarged, both lateral lobes smooth, elastic, rounded, but firmer than normal. Upper end of both lateral lobes slightly indurated. Seminal vesicles negative. A few adhesions, no intervesicular mass. Membranous urethra and rectum negative (Dr. Young). Cystoscopy showed prostatic hypertrophy and a vesical calculus. Perineal prostatectomy, June 14, 1912. Recovery prompt and complete. Unfortunately, the sections from this operation were lost. March 2, 1915, returned for observation, felt perfectly well. Rectal: Prostate a little smaller than normal, no evidence of malignancy (Dr. Young). January 11, 1917, returned with painful and difficult urination. Rectal: Prostate about normal in size, the right lobe a little larger than the left. A few adhesions on the right, none on the left. Left seminal vesicle slightly indurated (Dr. Young). R. U. 100 c.c., B. C. 175 c.c. Cystoscopy showed median and right lateral enlargement. The median portion of the prostate, felt against the cystoscope, was not indurated. Another examiner's rectal: Membranous urethra somewhat adherent. Median furrow obliterated. Right lobe of almost stony hardness, not very irregular, but inelastic and suggesting strongly malignancy (Dr. Howard Cecil). Third rectal: Right lobe slightly indurated and adherent, quite firm, but not stony "and I believe does not suggest malignancy" (Dr. Young). Punch operation, January 19, 1917. Bleeding was persistent, patient shocked. January 20, 1924, suprapubic cystostomy. Death occurred almost immediately afterward. The punch sections showed carcinoma; the infiltrating type of growth. Autopsy showed carcinoma of the prostate and bilateral suppurative pyelonephritis.

Discussion: In this case, the previous prostatectomy had altered the situation. Scar tissue was to be expected. This evidently misled all the examiners but one, though it is evident that while hard, the carcinoma did not show the extreme degree of induration. Cause of error: Mistake in judging induration.

B. U. I. 3396, age seventy-three. October 16, 1912. Difficulty twenty years, frequency one year. Rectal: Prostate enlarged, globular, moderately indurated, not of stony hardness but suggestive. Lateral lobes quite prominent, firm, but not stony. Slight induration of both seminal vesicles (Dr. Young). Perineal prostatectomy November 6, 1912. Nothing suspicious noted at operation. The sections showed adenocarcinoma, with many acini elongated, tubular, and branching, and very little stroma. Metastases developed in three months.

Discussion: While this tumor was microscopically of the soft type, it was firm enough to arouse suspicion in the mind of the examiner. The final decision, however, was in favor of benign hypertrophy. Cause of error: Soft type of neoplasm.

B. U. I. 3713, age seventy-seven. October 18, 1913. Frequency and hesitancy of urination for fifteen years. Rectal: Prostate enlarged, smooth. Median furrow and notch broad and deep. The right lobe is globular, slightly irregular, little firmer than normal in places, but generally elastic. Induration is more toward the apex than the posterior surface, and it is apparently not of stony hardness and compressible. Upper portion of the prostate is soft, few adhesions on each side. Right seminal vesicle is slightly thickened and adherent. The left lobe of the prostate presents a hard nodule near the surface, quite prominent, smooth, compressible, and perhaps has broken through a portion of the capsule of the prostate. Along the inner and upper sides the nodule presents a very precipitous edge. On the outer side it is continuous and shades off into the outer and anterior portion of the prostate which is moderately indurated; the nodule itself is quite hard, but, as mentioned above, is somewhat movable and partly disconnected from the prostate. Upper portion of the left lateral lobe is very slightly irregular, a little firmer than normal, generally elastic. Few adhesions at the upper end. No marked induration of the prostate on the upper side. Membranous urethra and rectum negative, no enlarged glands

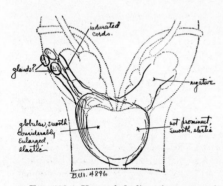

FIG. 423.—Unusual findings in a case of carcinoma of the prostate. Prostate is enlarged, but smooth and elastic. The seminal vesicles are practically negative except for a few indurated nodes at the tip of the left vesicle. Symptoms were frequency, pain in the back and leg, and loss of weight for at least one year. Diagnosis, benign hypertrophy. Prostate proved to be totally involved with the soft type of carcinoma, and bony metastases were discovered later. Died one year after operation.

(Dr. Young). R. U. 30 c.c., B. C. 450 c.c. Operation, October 27, 1913, radical excision of prostate and seminal vesicles. Death occurred shortly afterward. Autopsy showed no carcinoma remaining.

Discussion: In this case there was no real error, as the nodule was suspected, and frozen sections were made of it at operation. Reason for not making positive diagnosis: Small size of nodule.

B. U. I. 4896, age seventy-five. February 15, 1916. Frequency, burning, pain in back and legs for one year. One attack of hematuria, loss of weight. Rectal: Prostate globular and elastic, slightly irregular. Vesicles slightly adherent (Dr. Ernest Watson). Second rectal (Fig. 423): Prostate enlarged, globular, elastic, smooth, no nodules, no areas of marked induration. Right vesicle normal, left enlarged, indurated, and adherent. Enlarged glands felt at tip. "Prostate and vesicles do not suggest carcinoma, but the glands are suspicious" (Dr. Young). Cystoscopy: Enlarged intravesical lobe. Perineal prostatectomy March 20, 1916. On gross section of the specimen, its opacity suggested carcinoma. Sections showed adenocarcinoma, with many acini elongated, tubular, and branching, not much stroma, and some masses of cells due to intra-acinous growth—a type of growth soft clinically.

Discussion: Here, although the question of malignancy was definitely in the examiner's mind, he was misled by the absence of hardness, which was definite and uniform. Cause of error: Soft type of neoplasm.

B. U. I. 5025, age sixty-three. April 6, 1916. Frequency and burning for six months. Rectal: Prostate rounded, smooth and elastic. No areas of induration (Dr. Edwin G. Davis). Second rectal: Prostate not enlarged. Normal in width. Furrow and notch shallow. Lobes possibly a little indurated and adherent, otherwise negative. Seminal vesicles slightly adherent externally, very slightly indurated. Very slight intervesicular thickening. Membranous urethra a little firmer than normal (Dr. Young). R. U. 300 c.c., B. C. 800 c.c. Cystoscopy shows median hypertrophy. Perineal prostatectomy April 26, 1916. Sections showed adenocarcinoma with many acini elongated, tubular, and branching, and a moderate amount of stroma.

Discussion: While we have seen specimens with less stroma than this, it was undoubtedly softer than usual. No suspicion entered the examiner's mind. The thickening of the membranous urethra may have been significant. Cause of error: Soft type of neoplasm.

B. U. I. 5028, age sixty-five. April 5, 1916. Weak stream and hesitancy for six months. Rectal: Prostate broader than normal. Median notch and furrow shallow. Right lobe irregular, presents peculiar induration along the base, edge adherent to pelvic wall. Similar indurated area half-way between base and apex. Induration not stony. Similar area of induration, which is larger, in left lobe at base. Rest of prostate elastic. Seminal vesicles indurated and adherent. Only slight intervesicular thickening. Indurated areas appear to be in substance of prostate, and are, therefore, probably explained by chronic prostatitis (Dr. William A. Frontz). Punch operation May 5, 1916. Sections showed typical adenocarcinoma. Little if any benign hypertrophy.

Discussion: In this case the neoplasm was not of the soft type, but the nodules were somewhat obscured by the benign hypertrophy, losing thereby the sensation of extreme hardness.

B. U. I. 5669, age sixty-eight. January 13, 1917. Pain and weak stream for four years. Rectal: Prostate firm, indurated, adherent, but elastic throughout. Hard, smooth nodule, which is suspicious, at base of left seminal vesicle (Dr J. A. C. Colston). Second rectal: "A phlebolith 8 mm. in diameter external to the lower portion of the left seminal vesicle. Prostate does not suggest malignancy" (Dr. Young). R. U. 125 c.c., B. C. 450 c.c. Cystoscopy shows median and bilateral enlargements. Perineal prostatectomy January 15, 1917. Posterior lamella suspicious, frozen section showed carcinoma. Sections showed benign hypertrophy except in the posterior lamella, where adenocarcinoma, both of the typical sort and with elongated acini, and also infiltrative growth, were found.

Discussion: In this case the type of growth was that characterized by hardness, but it was missed because it overlay, in a thin layer, a large mass of elastic benign hypertrophy.

B. U. I. 7031, age seventy-one. May 13, 1920. Frequency and hesitancy of urination for ten years. Rectal: Prostate distinctly but moderately enlarged. Definitely a case of benign hypertrophy (Dr. John T. Geraghty). Second rectal: Prostate moderately enlarged, furrow and notch shallow. One small nodule about 1 cm. in diameter. No areas of induration. Seminal vesicles somewhat indurated (Dr. Clyde L. Deming). Third rectal: Prostate is enlarged, elastic, somewhat lobular. Indurated area at right upper pole; this, however, is elastic and does not suggest neoplasm (Dr. Geraghty). R. U. 250 c.c. Cystoscopy shows median enlargement. Urine infected. Perineal prostatectomy May 14, 1920. Carcinoma not suspected. The specimen on section showed some suspicious yellow opaque areas. Microscopically, there was adenocarcinoma, with many acini elongated and tubular, moderate amount of stroma, and some invasive growth. Benign hypertrophy also present.

Discussion: The induration was felt, but it was not considered hard enough for cancer. Since the growth was not, microscopically, of a sort which is particularly soft, we must assume that the induration was obscured by the hypertrophy. Cause of error: Obscured by benign hypertrophy, mistake in judging induration.

B. U. I. 9405, age fifty-eight. February 1, 1921. Frequency, difficulty, hesitancy, and burning for three years. R. U. 200 c.c., B. C. 250 c.c. Rectal: Prostate only slightly enlarged. Median furrow and notch present. Lateral lobes rounded, smooth, elastic, no nodules or areas of induration. Membranous urethra normal (Dr. Clyde L. Deming). Second rectal: Prostate slightly larger than normal, firm, smooth, symmetric. Median furrow shallow. No secretion expressed (Dr. Frank H. Rose). Perineal prostatectomy February 9, 1921. Microscopic sections entirely composed of tumor tissue, which is an adenocarcinoma characterized by (1) elongated, tubular, and branching acini, and (2) very small amount of stroma. "This is a rare type of growth which is not hard."

Discussion: In this case the error was due to the type of tumor, which did not cause induration, irregularity, adhesions, fixation, or any of the phenomena by which carcinoma is ordinarily recognized. Cause of error: Soft type of carcinoma.

B. U. I. 9620, age seventy-five. April 20, 1921. Frequency of urination for five months, one attack of complete retention. Rectal: Anal sphincter good tone. The prostate is a little broader than normal, median furrow and notch shallow. Right lobe is slightly irregular in places and slightly indurated and in others moderately indurated and markedly adherent externally, particularly at the upper pole. Near the apex on the right side there is a small nodule, the left lateral lobe of the prostate is smooth, moderately indurated and moderately adherent at the upper end, no nodules. In the median line there is also induration of moderate degree. The right seminal vesicle is not enlarged, it is slightly indurated and slightly adherent externally, left seminal vesicle is definitely enlarged and indurated, the induration being continuous with the prostate and extending upward and outward as far as the finger can reach and markedly adherent along the left lateral wall of the pelvis. Far up, an enlargement and induration, possibly enlarged glands, are felt. In this region the induration is considerable and suggests malignancy. In the region of the prostate the induration is more like that of chronic prostatitis and there is no marked enlargement. Membranous urethra is broader and firmer than normal, the induration being quite marked. No enlarged glands felt on the right side, mass on the left side may be enlarged glands (Dr. Young—Fig. 424). Second rectal: Prostate bulges out toward the rectum. One gets the impression that the posterior lobe is definitely enlarged, indurated, hard. Right lobe a little harder than the left, induration exteds up to seminal vesicle (Dr. Frank H. Rose). Third rectal: (with cystoscope in place) Median portion of prostate greatly increased in thickness, slightly indurated but somewhat compressible. "I do not believe it is malignant" (Dr. Young). Cystoscopy shows collar hypertrophy with numerous clefts. Perineal prostatectomy April 27, 1921. The gross specimen was firm. Frozen section showed carcinoma and radium was applied. Sections showed carcinoma with marked intra-acinous growth, producing large nests of cells, and a moderate amount of stroma. Benign hypertrophy was also present.

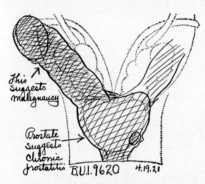

Fig. 424.—Rectal findings in a case in which carcinoma was not definitely diagnosed before operation. The prostate itself is only slightly enlarged and indurated. The left seminal vesicle and the membranous urethra are, however, markedly enlarged and indurated. Sections taken at operation showed carcinoma. Patient living two years after operation, but with pain and dysuria.

Discussion: While not of stony hardness, this tumor was firm enough to arouse suspicion in the minds of the examiners. It belongs to a type which while usually quite hard, may give soft tumors if the stroma is particularly small in amount. Cause of error: Soft type of neoplasm.

Undoubtedly a few of the cases of soft carcinoma and of very small carcinomata will always escape diagnosis. In the rectal examination, however, attention to the following points will minimize errors:

(a) Extensive induration, with adhesions and fixation of the prostate, especially if involving the seminal vesicles, should always cause the examiner to suspect carcinoma, even if the induration is not stony.

(b) Nodules markedly firmer than the surrounding prostate suggest the possibility of carcinoma. Spheroids of hypertrophy may occur in the posterior lamella, but are so rare that such nodules should always suggest carcinoma.

(c) Thickening of the membranous urethra, fixation, and the obscuring of its outlines suggest the inflammatory reaction occurring in carcinoma.

(d) The same is true of similar changes in the intervesicular notch.

(e) Thickening and induration of the lymphatics and lymph-nodes about the tip of the seminal vesicle suggests the possibility of carcinoma.

(f) Examination with finger in rectum and cystoscope in urethra gives a better opportunity to appreciate induration in the posterior portion of the prostate. Of the 25 cases analyzed above, this procedure was omitted in 14, and might have helped to a correct diagnosis if done.

(g) The presence of benign hypertrophy, shown by rectal or cystoscopic examination, in no way excludes carcinoma.

There is nothing characteristic about the prostatic secretion in carcinoma.

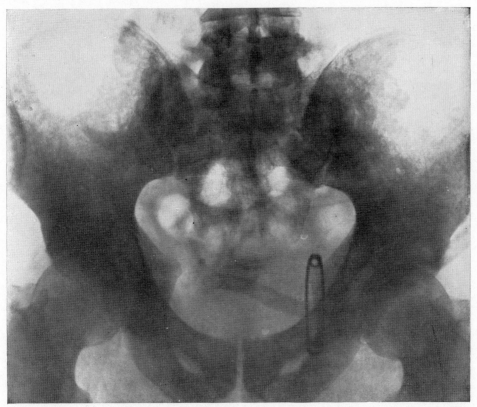

Fig. 425.—x-Ray showing metastatic infiltration of the spine, pelvis, and femora in a case of carcinoma of the prostate. Note that the bone is not eroded, but shows a "wooly" or "spotty" increase in density. J. H. H. x-Ray 110,229.

In all cases where carcinoma is suspected x-ray plates of the bones, especially the vertebræ and pelvis, should be made. Since the metastases are oftener productive than destructive, they are indicated by areas of condensation, usually multiple, small and closely set, giving a peculiar "spottiness" to the picture (Fig. 425).

The cystoscope, while giving little help in the diagnosis of carcinoma, is valuable in doubtful cases in ruling out other conditions, in determining the degree of benign hypertrophy which accompanies the neoplasm, and in detecting other vesical complications (stone, tumor, diverticulum). It also shows intravesical extensions of the neoplasm in the rare cases where they occur. Occasionally such a mass is covered by mucous membrane, which, in conjunction with prostatic induration, makes the diagnosis simple. The mass is sometimes ulcerated, when it is usually indistinguishable from a primary bladder tumor. Indeed it is sometimes quite impossible to say whether we are dealing with a prostatic tumor invading the bladder or a bladder tumor invading the prostate. Such cases are, however, very advanced and well-nigh hopeless from a therapeutic viewpoint.

Occasionally doubt will still remain, and this is especially important in the early cases with small tumors, where radical operation might effect a cure. Diagnosis must then be made at operation and for this purpose the perineal operation has a marked superiority. The prostate is freely exposed, and can be inspected, palpated, or even incised if necessary. If carcinoma is found, the operator is in a position to proceed at once with radical removal.

At operation a markedly vascular and edematous condition of the periprostatic or even perineal tissues may be noted, due to the inflammatory reaction about the neoplasm. In some cases this has aroused suspicion for the first time, even before the prostate was seen. The same reaction may cause the rectum and the layers of Denonvilliers' fascia to be more adherent than usual—this is always suggestive of carcinoma. With the posterior aspect of the prostate freely exposed, palpation can be carried out to better advantage than by rectum and often gives the diagnosis from the irregularity and marked induration. The prostate should not be incised unless necessary to obtain a frozen section. The edges of the incision should then be at once seared with the actual cautery. There is little danger in this procedure, as prostatic carcinoma is not apt to undergo implantation.

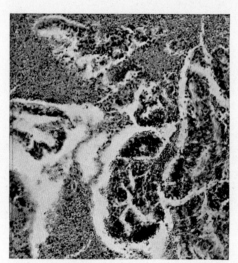

Fig. 426.—Section from a very unusual case of carcinoma of the prostate. There are a few masses of epithelial cells which appear to have generally papillary form, the whole being embedded in a mass of blood-clot and occupying the interior of a cyst within the prostate. The clinical diagnosis was prostatic abscess. B. U. I. 9100.

The following extraordinary case is abstracted here as a matter of interest:

B. U. I. 9100, aged sixty-nine. September 28, 1920. Frequency over three years, small stream for two years, urgency for one year, complete retention for two weeks. No hematuria except after catheterization. Loss of weight, strength, and mental acuity in last two weeks. Urine infected, bacilli, and much pus. Rectal: Immediately on entering the rectum a very large, bulging, fluctuating mass is felt in front and to the left, completely obscuring the region of the prostate and running upward on the left side along the outer wall of the pelvis, obscuring the region of the seminal vesicle. Right seminal vesicle negative. The fluctuating mass which is probably an abscess is very close to the rectal wall and compresses the rectum greatly from in front, and is also very close to the perineum. Rectal wall smooth, no ulcer. Blood urea 0.66 gm. per liter. Operation September 28, 1920, the fluctuating mass incised through the perineum. The fluid contents was not pus, but a reddish-gray pultaceous material. Sections made after embedding it in paraffin showed many papillæ, covered by one or two layers of columnar epithelium, lying in blood-clot, and for the most part uncoalesced (Fig. 426). At one point they had apparently fused, and a few indistinct pseudo-acini were seen. Cystoscopy was impossible, and since the patient was taken home against advice, it is impossible to say whether this was a prostatic carcinoma or a bladder carcinoma (papillary) invading the prostate. In either case the picture was unusual, owing to the presence of the blood-filled cyst.

Certain other conditions may be mistaken for prostatic carcinoma. Chief among these are tuberculosis, chronic prostatitis, and prostatic calculi.

The induration in *tuberculosis* may be indistinguishable from that of carcinoma. The distinction is usually simple, however, by means of other complicating tuberculous lesions, of the kidney, bladder, or epididymis. In the comparatively rare cases where these are absent, and where the patient is of the cancer age, confusion is easy. We have seen two cases in which this error was made.

A case of tuberculosis of one lobe of the prostate, mistakenly diagnosed cancer and subjected to radical operation.

B. U. I. 8150, age sixty-three. September 26, 1919. Family history and personal history negative for tuberculosis, but there had been "attacks of malaria." Increasing frequency for one year, hesitancy for three months, painful urination for two months. No hematuria. Slight loss of weight. Examination of lungs: Increased vocal resonance and vocal fremitus and slightly roughened breath sounds over left lower lobe in back. Rectal: Prostate is very hard and irregular, fixed, adherent at both sides, but more on the left. Some induration of the vesicles. Diagnosis, carcinoma (Dr. J. C. McClelland) Second rectal: Anal sphincter good. The prostate is moderately enlarged. Median furrow and notch obliterated. The right lobe is irregular, somewhat nodular and quite hard, moderately adherent. Induration is not of stony hardness, but it is much harder than seen in ordinary hypertrophy and the prostate is quite tender. The left lobe of the prostate is less enlarged, only slightly irregular, is soft in its anterior and outer portion, considerably indurated in its upper portion, induration being continuous with that on the right side. The right seminal vesicle is apparently negative, not distended, not indurated, very slight adhesions externally. The left seminal vesicle is similar. No enlarged glands felt on either side. The membranous urethra and rectum are negative. There seems to be undoubtedly induration or infiltration of the prostate which has completely invaded or involved the right lateral lobe and extends for a short distance into the upper or inner portion of the left. The appearance is quite different from that usually seen in chronic inflammation or tuberculosis. One must certainly suspect carcinoma and further study should be made (Dr. Young). The patient was also examined by Dr. Geraghty, who concurred in the diagnosis. There was a small discrete nodule in the right epididymis, genitalia otherwise normal. Cystoscopy: R. U. 30 c.c., B. C. 250 c.c. Apparently a general contracture of prostatic urethra. Globular median lobe. No clefts. Cloudy medium obscures vesical mucosa. With finger in rectum and cystoscope in urethra, beak easily felt. Trigone not markedly indurated. Whole course of urethra thicker than normal. Lateral lobes slightly enlarged, thickened, and very hard, but not stony. "There seems to be malignancy present, limited to the prostate." Urine contained moderate amount of pus, with cocci. Radical operation for carcinoma of the prostate, removal of entire prostate, seminal vesicles, ampullæ, and a cuff of bladder about orifice, October 2, 1919. There was a retroperitoneal hemorrhage, and the patient died. Examination of the specimen showed multiple caseous tubercles of the prostate, and autopsy revealed a single caseous tubercle 1 cm. in diameter in the lower pole of the left kidney. No tuberculosis was found in the bladder, ureters, or epididymes, but the seminal vesicles, though not enlarged, showed some tiny tubercles near their bases. The diagnosis was not made at operation because the prostate was purposely not incised until after removal. Careful study of the prostatic secretion might have revealed tubercle bacilli, but it is hard to see how a positive diagnosis could have been made otherwise.

Another case of tuberculosis thought to be carcinoma of the prostate.

B. U. I. 12,212, age seventy-five. February 25, 1924. Increasing frequency for five years, small stream, difficulty, and burning for six months. No hematuria, loss of 15 pounds weight. No family or personal history of tuberculosis. Examination of the lungs negative. Rectal: Prostate markedly symmetrically enlarged, second-degree induration, area of increased firmness on left, which is not stony. Many adhesions on left border. Seminal vesicles not involved

(Dr. Alyea). Second rectal: Prostate very large, smooth, elastic, suggestive of benign hypertrophy at first, except that the right side of the prostate seems to extend into the lower part of the seminal vesicle. No intervesicular plateau of induration. With cystoscope in urethra, very marked thickening. This, with involvement of vesicle, indicates a carcinoma of the posterior portion, and in the center a benign hypertrophy (Dr. Geraghty). Cystoscopy showed intravesical enlargement of median and both lateral lobes. Urine showed moderate amount of pus, *but no bacteria*. Perineal prostatectomy March 5, 1924. An abscess was found in the left lobe. The tissue was thought to be carcinoma until microscopic examination, when it was found to be typical caseous tuberculosis. Strange to say, the convalescence was uneventful, the symptoms were relieved, and the wound healed. The ultimate result remains to be seen.

A case of prostatic enlargement in which hypertrophy, cancer, and tuberculosis were all present.

In another extraordinary case (B. U. I. 7462) a diagnosis of benign hypertrophy of the prostate was made. Rectal: Prostate enlarged, bulges into rectum. Median furrow obliterated. Prostate elastic, no areas of stony hardness. Seminal vesicles palpable but not indurated (Dr. Stump). Second rectal: Prostate enlarged, bulges into rectum. Right lobe more prominent than left, somewhat irregular, quite elastic throughout. Apparently some of the adenomatous spheroids have broken through the capsule. Left lobe also irregular and similar to right, adherent in region of seminal vesicle. Retrovesical area negative (Dr. William A. Frontz). Cystoscopy showed intravesical enlargement, mostly of the median and left lateral lobes. Perineal prostatectomy February 3, 1919. Examination of the specimen showed marked benign hypertrophy, adenocarcinoma of the posterior lamella, which, although in a thin layer, had already begun to invade the lateral lobes, and, in the upper posterior region of the prostate, fibroid tuberculosis. No caseation was seen (see Figs. 141, 407). The fistula persisted for nearly a year, but finally closed entirely. The patient lived for over five years. A few months before death obstruction recurred. Examination showed marked induration rectally, but since the patient died at home, it was not possible to determine whether this was due to carcinoma, tuberculosis, or both.

Painstaking study of the prostatic secretion for tubercle bacilli may make the diagnosis in doubtful cases. When it is otherwise impossible, careful study of the exposed prostate at operation should prevent errors.

Prostatitis is rather less apt than tuberculosis to give induration and adhesions of a degree to simulate carcinoma, but since it is a much more common condition it is of importance. The induration in prostatitis is more apt to be central or distributed indiscriminately through the gland than in carcinoma, but since a few cases of carcinoma do not arise in the posterior lamella this point is not infallible. While the lateral sulci may be obscured by adhesions in prostatitis, the prostate is seldom fixed as firmly as it is in many cases of carcinoma. In our experience prostatitis is not very apt to give rise to confusion. We have seen no instance in which a positive diagnosis of carcinoma was made in a case of prostatitis.

Prostatic calculi simulate carcinoma closely on rectal examination. Very hard, isolated nodules of carcinoma may feel like stones, and vice versa. The entire prostate may feel stony hard on account of multiple calculi. The diagnosis is easily made by the x-ray, or occasionally by eliciting a crepitus on rectal pressure. A few small calculi are sometimes found in cases of carcinoma, but we have never seen an extensive prostatic lithiasis in connection with carcinoma.

TREATMENT OF CARCINOMA OF THE PROSTATE

Radium.—Treatment of cancer of the prostate by means of radium was first introduced by Pasteau and deGrais[1] and Schüller,[2] who reported in 1913

[1] International Congress of Medicine, London, 1913, Section XIV, Urology, Part II, 28, 29.

[2] Ibid., 115–117.

2 cases of cancer of the prostate and bladder in which truly striking results had been obtained by the use of radium introduced into the urethra through an ordinary catheter. This report caused us to procure 100 mgm. of radium for similar work. It soon became evident that for accurate usage much more exact methods would be necessary, and in the shops of the Brady Institute we constructed a series of applicators with which we now treat cases of carcinoma of the prostate and bladder with or without the use of a straight cystoscope. Our instruments are made to carry either one or two tubes of 100 mgm. each of radium (in containers of platinum, 2 mm. thick). For treatment through the rectum or urethra, a simple applicator without cystoscope is used (Figs. 427, 428).

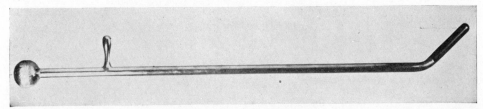

Fig. 427.—Young's rectal or urethral radium applicator carrying one or two tubes of radium, 100 mgm. each, in platinum tubes. The beak is made of silver covered with hard rubber. Note ball at outer end by means of which instrument is fixed in position by clamp attached to table.

With this instrument, the radium is applied through the rectum as follows: With the patient on a cushioned table, lying upon the left side, thighs and legs flexed, the gloved finger is introduced into the rectum, and the prostate is palpated to determine the site of treatment. The applicator, well lubricated, is introduced alongside the finger into the rectum and the convexity of the beak carried to a point at which the application is to be made and accurately placed with the guidance of the finger in the rectum. Slight pressure is made so that the instrument sinks into the rectal mucosa and approaches as closely as possible to the carcinoma. An assist-

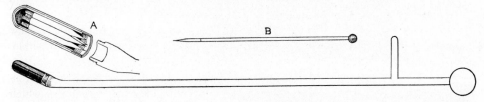

Fig. 428.—Rectal or urethral radium applicator, with hard-rubber cap over silver (A) large enough to contain four needles containing 12½ mgm. radium which may also be used in the treatment of carcinoma of the prostate when attached to staffs (B) and plunged through skin of perineum.

ant then fixes the instrument *in situ* by means of a heavy clamp which is attached to the table on which the patient lies (Figs. 429, 430). The operator then records the application made upon a chart which has been previously made of the region involved. The patient is instructed to keep absolutely still with his body against the back-rest for one hour. As a rule, no difficulty is experienced in carrying this out. In some cases it may be desirable to administer a hypodermic of morphin or to give a large dose of aspirin, but in most cases treatment is borne without such medication.

On the following day the same instrument (sterilized in carbolic acid) is inserted into the urethra until the radium occupies the desired place (as is easily

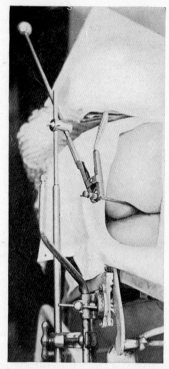

FIG. 429.—Young's rectal radium applicator fixed in place against a certain portion of the tumor mass by clamp attached to table.

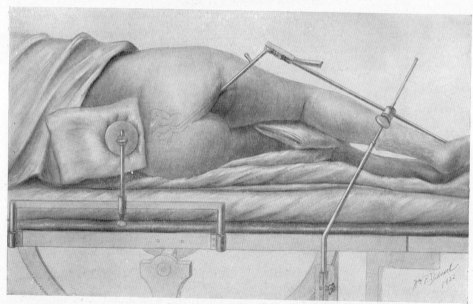

FIG. 430.—Treatment of carcinoma of prostate, vesicles, or bladder by radium applications through rectum with Young's recto-urethral applicator, held in place by clamp attached to table.

determined) and fixed there by the clamp as previously described. On the third day it is usual to make an application through the bladder, the instrument being introduced, the beak turned outward, and the handle elevated so as to bring that portion of the instrument carrying the radium firmly against the mucous membrane of the trigone and thus to approach as closely as possible the retrovesical prolongation of the carcinoma. On the fourth day treatment returns to the rectum and a new site is chosen for the application.

The operator should be careful to have each application at least 5 to 10 mm. distant from any previous application and to record each treatment as accurately as possible on the chart. It is well to skip about and make the treatments as distant from each other as possible. We prefer the use of an instrument which carries 200 mgm. of radium, tandem, in its beak, the advantage being that the danger of overlapping is minimized and the number of treatments reduced.

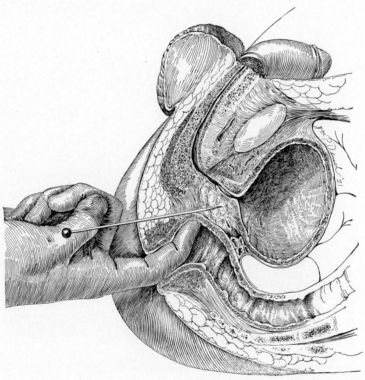

FIG. 431.—Introduction of radium needle into carcinoma of prostate through perineum. Sagittal section to show finger in rectum and position of radium needle.

By means of these instruments and the use of the fixation clamp externally, it has been possible to make these applications accurately to the region desired and to avoid radium burns. We have found it possible in most cases to give from 1800 to 2000 mgm. hours per rectum, 600 to 800 per urethram, and an equal amount through the bladder, with impunity. Before the introduction of these instruments it had not been possible to use radium in such large amounts without producing fearful burns in the rectum. It not infrequently happens that considerable irritation in urethra, rectum, or bladder is produced and in such cases the treatment is at once stopped and deep x-ray therapy begun. After a few days' rest, the patient returns to radium treatment, which should usually alternate as above described, until 3000 to 4000 mgm. hours have been given *in toto*. More than this is usually dangerous. In some cases it is necessary to stop the treatment with less dosage given.

The *local effect of radium* varies very greatly. In some cases there is definite systemic reaction, consisting of depression and general weakness, and occasionally slight nausea and vomiting. The patient may occasionally have a chill. Usually there is little or no reaction and no discomfort is entailed except that caused by the instrument. In some cases, after a few treatments, the patient complains considerably of irritation, and rest, as above described, is advisable. Micturition, as a rule, becomes more difficult for a time, and in some cases complete retention, necessitating a catheter life for a time, comes on. In rare cases normal urination does not

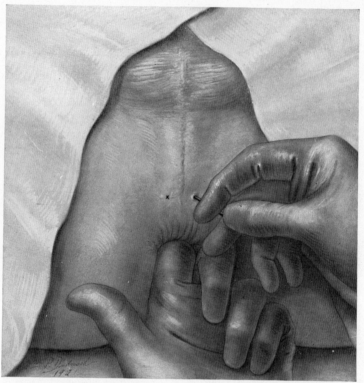

FIG. 432.—Introduction of needles containing radium element through perineum into substance of prostate.   Finger in rectum to show course and position of needle.

return. In most cases, after a period, urination becomes distinctly more satisfactory and it is remarkable how often pain and hematuria disappear completely.

Application of Radium by Means of Needles.—Barringer in 1916, following the work of Douaine, introduced the use of radium needles, which were plunged into the prostate by perineum (Figs. 431–433). These were allowed to stay for prolonged periods and in this way radium was carried directly into the substance of the prostatic tumor. As a rule, from two to four needles, each containing 10 to 25 mgm. of radium element, were introduced at one sitting, and efforts were made to reach the various portions of the prostate. Reports by Bumpus and others of this method of treatment have shown that marked necrosis is apt to occur around

PLATE XV

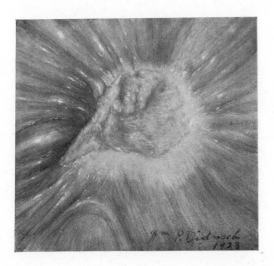

Radium burn of rectum in a case of carcinoma of left lobe of prostate in which 1000 mgh. was given in one week, concentrated over left lobe of prostate. Autopsy two months later: The burn is very deep and surrounded by marked contracture of rectal mucosa. Comment: Radium was applied over much too limited an area, in too large an amount, and in too short a time (B. U. I. 10,871).

the site of the inlying needle and on this account they have advised the use of smaller amounts of radium. We have employed this method in numerous cases.

Radium may also be introduced into the substance of the prostate through a suprapubic wound as carried out by Barringer, Herbst, and others. By means of a catheterizing cystoscope, it may be introduced with a special flexible needle through the urethral mucosa. Barringer has reported cases in which "emanation points" have thus been implanted permanently into the substance of the prostate. We have also introduced radium through the urethra into the prostatic lobes by means of needles passed through our tubular endoscope (Fig. 393).

By means of this instrument it is possible to introduce radium at various places in the median and lateral portions of the prostate and also into tumors which project into the bladder near the vesical orifice.

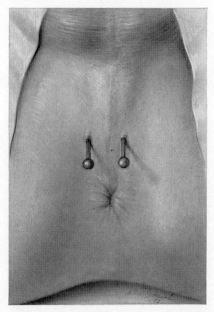

FIG. 433.—Radium treatment of carcinoma of the prostate. One radium needle has been introduced into each half of the prostate through the perineum and under direction of the finger in the rectum. They then remain in place, as shown in the picture, as long as desired.

The Introduction of Radium Through a Perineal Wound into Carcinoma of the Prostate and Vesicles.—In 1922 a patient with carcinoma of the prostate and seminal vesicles, which was a little too extensive for the radical operation, was subjected to radium treatment by the following technic. With the patient in the perineal prostatectomy position and a long tractor in the urethra, the posterior surface of the prostate and seminal vesicles was exposed, as shown in Fig. 434. Examination revealed an involvement of both seminal vesicles, but the cancer did not seem to extend into the tissues beyond. Accordingly, emanation points, each containing 1 millicurie of radium, were inserted into the tissues at intervals of 1 cm., the object being so to fill the entire area invaded by the carcinoma that every portion of it would be within 1 cm. of a tube containing 1 millicurie of radium. As shown in the accompanying illustration (Fig. 435), the "points" were planted thickly into the depths of the prostate and also superficially. In this case, which was published in 1923, really excellent results were obtained, although for a time there was a marked increase in difficulty of urination and even complete retention. Ultimately, normal urination was restored and, on examination one year later, the region of prostate and vesicles, previously invaded by carcinoma, were so soft

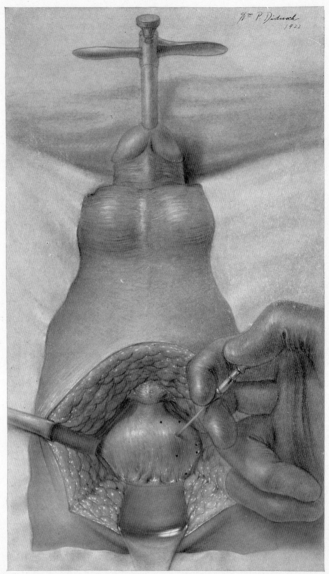

Fig. 434.—Carcinoma of prostate. Introduction of radium element into substance of prostate and seminal vesicles through a perineal exposure. B. U. I. 10,537.

that one would not have been able to detect the fact that carcinoma had ever been present. We believe this method of introducing radium is preferable to the suprapubic route; it is not only possible to introduce it into the prostate with very much greater accuracy, with the proper interval between "points," but also because it is the only way in which radium can be introduced with any accuracy into the carcinomatous invasion of the seminal vesicles and intervening tissues behind the bladder.

Sarcoma of the prostate responds readily to radium and *x*-ray treatment, as shown in Figs. 436 to 440. There is, however, always danger of recurrence or metas-

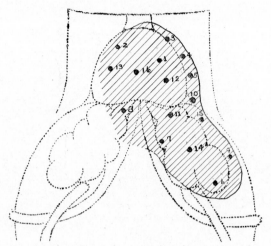

Fig. 435.—Carcinoma of prostate and seminal vesicle. Diagram showing location of radium implantations made at operation. B. U. I. 10,537.

tasis, even when the primary result is favorable. Operation is extremely unsatisfactory; wound implantation with rapid spread often occurs.

Operative Treatment.—(1) *Carcinoma Not Suspected in Cases of Supposed Benign Hypertrophy.*—If, during operation, a markedly indurated area or cut surface suspicious of carcinoma in encountered, diagnosis can usually be made by

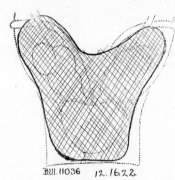

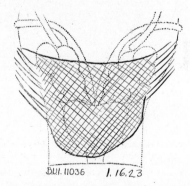

FIG. 436.—Rectal findings in a case diagnosed as sarcoma of the prostate. The vesicles were involved, but the entire growth was very smooth, regular, and not greatly indurated. Patient was under thirty. Urinary obstruction was present.

FIG. 437.—Rectal findings in the same case as that in the preceding diagram after nine doses of deep *x*-ray treatment had been given.

inspection, and if not, by frozen section. If the extent of invasion is not too great, radical operation should be carried out.

(2) *Carcinoma Suspected and Not Extensive.*—After exposure through the perineum inspection should be made for diagnosis and, if verified, the radical operation should be carried out.

(3) *Diagnosis Positive, Extension Not Too Great.*—Radical operation indicated (Fig. 441).

(4) *Diagnosis positive, but extension into seminal vesicles, membranous urethra, or elsewhere too extensive for radical operation,* but yet possible to carry out radium

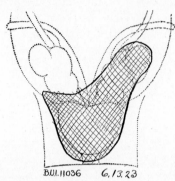

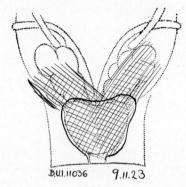

Fig. 438.—Rectal findings in the same case as that in the preceding diagram after 600 milligram-hours of radium and a second course of deep x-ray treatment had been given.

Fig. 439.—Rectal findings in the same case as that in the preceding diagram after further treatment with 1200 milligram-hours of radium.

implantation: In such cases perineal operation with implantation of radium is indicated, and subsequently deep x-ray therapy should be given.

(5) *Diagnosis Positive, Too Extensive for Radical Operation, but Relief of Obstruction or Dysuria Imperative.*—Enucleating prostatectomy may be carried

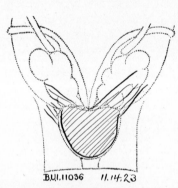

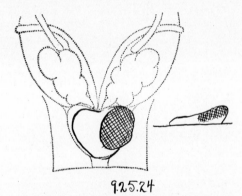

Fig. 440.—Rectal findings in the same case as that in the preceding diagram at the time of discharge and eleven months after the first radium treatments. The prostate had returned to normal size and consistence and the urinary obstruction was relieved.

Fig. 441.—Rectal findings in a case of carcinoma of the prostate suitable for radical operation. Note that the seminal vesicles and membranous urethra are not involved (Judge T.).

out with radium implantation into the walls of the cavity and adjacent involved regions; x-ray subsequently.

(6) *Diagnosis Positive, Too Extensive for Radical Operation, Urination Fairly Easy or Catheter Life Satisfactory.*—Radium treatment with applications through rectum, urethra, and bladder, or implantations through urethra (endoscope) or perineum (puncture) may be carried out, followed by deep x-ray therapy.

(7) *Diagnosis positive, too extensive for radical operation, having been treated*

with radium, onset of increasing obstruction and dysuria, operative relief essential; punch operation, perineal prostatectomy, or suprapubic drainage to relieve obstruction may be employed. Radium implantations through wound may be made simultaneously in the latter two procedures, followed by deep *x*-ray therapy.

Results of Radical Operation for Carcinoma of the Prostate.—This operation has been carried out in 24 cases at our clinic. The technic has been identical with that originally published in 1905 except that since 1917 care has been taken to preserve the anterior pelvic fascia, and not to injure the nerves and blood-vessels in front of it, which supply the region of the external sphincter and triangular ligament, with the object of preventing incontinence.

The ages of these 24 patients were as follows: Under sixty, 4; between sixty and sixty-nine, 17; seventy to seventy-nine, 3. Urinary symptoms have been present a year or less in 5 cases and from two to fifteen years in the others. The principal symptom was frequency of urination in 20 cases. It is interesting to note that difficulty of urination was only present in 10, or 41 per cent.; and hematuria in 6, 25 per cent. Residual urine was not present in 8 cases, 36 per cent., less than 200 c.c., 6; over 200 c.c., 3 cases. Incontinence, 3 cases. Sexual desire was lost or impaired in 6 cases, erections were absent or imperfect in 6 cases, ejaculation was painful in 2 and bloody in 1 case. Eighteen patients, 75 per cent., complained of pain which was located in the glans penis 4, urethra 3, perineum 3, vesical neck 3, back 4, suprapubic region 3. No previous treatment with radium or *x*-ray had been used. All or a portion of the prostate was extremely indurated in every case, and in 12 of stony hardness. In 3 cases the prostate was not enlarged, and in half of the cases it was neither nodular or even irregular of surface. The seminal vesicles were involved (indurated) in only 5 cases. Cystoscopy: Obstruction, impassable by the cystoscope, 4. Lateral lobes enlarged, 6. Median lobe enlarged, 18. Mucous membrane smooth, no ulceration, in all cases. Trigone elevated or hypertrophied, 13. Bladder trabeculated, 13. Intravesical tumor growth, none.

Convalescence: Uneventful, 12; stormy, 2; nausea and vomiting, 5; pyrexia, 2; epididymitis, 3; break down of wound, 2. Perineal fistula closed: Two weeks, 4; three weeks, 2; one month, 4; not recorded, 12; permanent fistula, 1. Catheter drain removed within eight days, 5; ten days, 6; over ten, 2; unrecorded, 11 cases. Postoperative treatment with radium and *x*-ray, 3 cases. Condition on discharge: No pain, 13; pain in bladder, 1; glans, 1; suprapubic, 1; frequency of urination, 5; incontinence, 14. Ultimate results of operation: Obstruction completely relieved, 24, 100 per cent.; perfect urinary control, 10, 49 per cent.; fair control, 4; incontinence by day when walking, 7; complete incontinence, 3, 13 per cent.; persistent perineal urinary fistula, 1. Time followed since operation: Four patients died in the hospital, 16.6 per cent. The cause of death was shock, 1 (autopsy, extensive metastases in peritoneum); septicemia, 1; pyelonephritis, 2. Deaths since leaving hospital, 8; 5 as a result of recurrent carcinoma, 3 local, and 2 metastatic.

The following cases have been examined since discharge and found free from recurrence: B. U. I. 8234, six years; B. U. I. 7774, B. U. I. 10,043, and B. U. I. 10,183, four years; B. U. I. 3715, three years; B. U. I. 930, two years; B. U. I. 3913, B. U. I. 12,046, and B. U. I. 12,519, one year.

Alive and apparently well over three years since operation: B. U. I. 3608, three years; B. U. I. 829, three years; B. U. I. 930, six years; B. U. I. 2156, thirteen years;

B. U. I. 2455, six years; B. U. I. 3659, three years; B. U. I. 3715, eight years; B. U. I. 3913, eight years; B. U. I. 7774, three years; B. U. I. 7539, three years; B. U. I. 10,183, three years, six months. Number of patients operated on three or more years ago, 20; of these, 3 died in hospital; number alive and apparently free from recurrence, three years or over, 14, or 70 per cent. Sixteen cases were operated on five or more years ago. Three died in hospital. Of the remaining 13 cases, 8 lived five years or more (62 per cent.) Comment: The ultimate results compare favorably with those of carcinoma of the breast. If patients could be operated on earlier than our cases, the percentage of cures would be high. The reason of this is that the prostate is a well-encapsulated organ and invasion of surrounding structures occurs late. The chance of cure is therefore good, and if physicians could be persuaded to include rectal palpation in every physical examination, the percentage of early diagnosis could be greatly increased. The small number of cases of complete incontinence recorded is remarkable when we consider the extent of the operation, and the complete removal of the prostate, the internal sphincter, and part of the trigone. And the fact that in the later operations, in which the anterior pelvic fascia and the vessels and nerves supplying the triangular ligament and sphincter are preserved, have been followed by no cases of incontinence is remarkable. That this operation should be applied to all cases in which the carcinoma has not invaded far into the region of the seminal vesicles, has not penetrated the periprostatic fascia nor given metastases, is abundantly proved.

Results of Radium Treatment.—As noted elsewhere, in 1914 we began treatment of cases of certain types of carcinoma with radium. Ten years have now elapsed, and it seems to us appropriate to study all of our cases to determine the results obtained, and to find out as nearly as possible the relative value of the various methods employed. The following study was made by Dr. L. N. Fleming of our staff in an effort to determine the immediate and remote results of the treatment employed, by examinations, and by letters to patients, physicians, etc.

The cases studied comprise 234 patients, all suffering with carcinoma of the prostate and all of whom received radium therapy in some form. In addition, other forms of treatment (operation, etc.) have been employed in various cases.

Ages.—These are shown in the following table:

TABLE 101

Years.	Cases.
41–45	1
46–50	8
51–55	17
56–60	41
61–65	47
66–70	54
71–75	40
76–80	19
81–90	7

The youngest patient was forty-five years of age, with a very rapidly growing and extensive carcinoma of the prostate and seminal vesicles, which ended fatally in a short time. Eight patients were between forty-six and fifty years of age. The great majority of patients were between the ages of fifty-five and seventy-five, although it is interesting to note that 7 patients were over eighty years of age. It is our impression that, as a whole, carcinoma of the prostate has been more virulent in the younger of our patients, and in the older is apt to be more slowly growing and more cirrhotic.

Duration of Symptoms.—One patient, aged forty-five, had symptoms only one month before admission. In this case we found extensive carcinoma of the prostate and seminal vesicles, and the patient lived only nine months.

With increasing age the duration of symptoms before the patients came for treatment was increasingly long. Those between forty-six and fifty averaged only three months' duration of symptoms. Those between fifty-one and fifty-five, nine months; between fifty-six and sixty, eleven months; between fifty-one and sixty-five, fourteen months; between sixty-five and seventy, fifteen months; between seventy-one and seventy-five, twenty-one months; between seventy-six and eighty, three years; between eighty-one and ninety, three years and five months.

In reviewing these statistics of duration it is to be noted at once that the discouraging factor in these cases was that when they arrived for treatment the disease had progressed beyond the possibility of a radical operation, and yet in 66 cases urinary symptoms were present less than one year. It is on account of the fact that prostatic carcinoma is symptomless in its earliest stages that it is so difficult to find cases suitable for a radical operation. These statistics should impress medical men with the great importance of rectal examinations in all men over forty years of age. Certainly it should be a part of every physical examination, and, as a matter of fact, occasional examinations of the urinary tract, including the prostate, are advisable in all men past middle life. We have had 2 cases in which there were absolutely no symptoms in which carcinoma of the prostate was detected in a general survey which was made for symptoms other than urinary.

Symptoms on Admission.—The symptoms are given in the following table:

TABLE 102

	Cases.	Per cent.
Frequency	215	92
Loss of force	173	72
Difficulty	165	69
Hesitancy	158	66
Diminution in size of stream	147	61
Dysuria	168	72
Pain	96	40
Urgency	78	33
Catheter required occasionally	46	19
Catheter required daily	30	12.6
Hemorrhage	28	11.7
Impassable obstruction	5	2.1

A careful study of the cases shows that in 21 (9 per cent.) there were practically no symptoms whatever of urinary obstruction. This is unquestionably a much higher percentage than is seen in a long series of cases of benign prostatic hypertrophy. In fact, in some of the patients, carcinoma was not discovered during a urinary examination. In 2 cases in which there were no symptoms whatever, the carcinoma was discovered during a health survey.

Hemorrhage was an occasional but not very important symptom, as seen in Table 103, page 656.

TABLE 103

	Cases.	Per cent.
Bloody urine	32	12.8
Clots	8	3.2
Occasional hemorrhage	7	2.8
Frequent hemorrhage	1	0.4

As seen here, the presence of blood in the urine or from the urethra after urination is a really very insignificant symptom and nothing like so common as usually stated in the literature. As a matter of fact, hemorrhage as a symptom is less frequent than in hypertrophy of the prostate, as shown elsewhere. Generally speaking, it may be said to be present in about 6 or 7 per cent. of the cases. When we consider that many of these cases came here in the very last stages of the disease from which they died within a few months, the fact that hematuria is an infrequent and unimportant symptom is manifest. Bleeding from the rectum is even much more rare than from the urethra and bears out the fact previously shown of the great infrequence with which the mucous membrane of the rectum is involved in an ulcerated carcinomatous process.

Pain was present in 116 cases (46 per cent.). The location has been tabulated as follows:

TABLE 104

Local pain:	Cases.	Per cent.
Rectum	24	11.0
Bladder	15	6.3
Anterior urethra	12	5.0
Deep urethra	6	2.4
Referred pain:	Cases.	Per cent.
Hips	22	9.2
Legs	11	4.6
Back and lumbar region	6	2.4
Buttocks	6	2.4

As seen here, pain is a much more prominent symptom in carcinoma than in hypertrophy of the prostate. Not only is pain in the urethra, bladder, and perineum far more common, but referred pains to the hips, legs, buttocks, and back are a very suggestive and in some cases a diagnostic symptom. In a good many instances pain has been the one and only symptom which caused the patient to seek relief. This is very seldom the case in benign hypertrophy. Pain associated with urination was also an important symptom, as seen in the following table:

TABLE 105

		Cases.	Per cent.
Beginning urination:	Occasional	1	0.42
	Constant	7	2.8
During urination:	Constant	34	14.2
End urination:	Occasional	1	0.42
	Constant	9	3.6

As seen here pain at the beginning of urination either occasional or occurring at each urination, was present in about 3 per cent. of the cases. Pain during urination at each voiding was present in 14 per cent. of the cases, and in only about 4 per cent. at the end of urination. Here again the percentage of cases with pain is greater than in hypertrophy.

Systemic Effects.—An analysis of the histories shows, symptomatically, evidence of back pressure and renal impairment in 30 cases (12.5 per cent.). These have been tabulated as follows:

TABLE 106

	Cases.	Per cent.
Loss of appetite	14	8.0
Nausea	4	1.6
Vomiting	2	0.8
Headache	2	0.8

This tabulation shows conclusively that there are fewer back pressure effects, and probably, therefore, less serious obstruction to urination as a whole in cases of carcinoma than in prostatic hypertrophy. In some few cases very great renal impairment is shown. Loss of weight is not shown to be very marked in our series of cases.

Condition on Admission.—Seventy patients were found to be very weak (30 per cent.) and in 12 cases the emaciation was pronounced. No cases of marked cachexia were noted, but in many instances the suffering and discomfort were extreme.

Findings on Examination.—Enlargement of prostate:

TABLE 107

	Right lobe.	Per cent.	Left lobe.	Per cent.
Normal in size	1	0.4	0	0
Enlargement: Slight	25	10.5	35	14.7
Moderate	178	74.7	175	73.5
Considerable	19	7.9	24	10

Consistence.—A diagnosis of carcinoma of the prostate has been made very largely on the consistence and character of the surface as found on rectal examination with a gloved finger.

In a study of 234 cases in which adequate rectal examinations are recorded, we find as follows: The induration was present on both sides of the prostate in all but 17 cases. In these 17 cases there were 10 in which the right side alone was involved, in 3 of these associated with induration extending up into the right seminal vesicle; in 7 cases the left lobe alone was involved, in 4 of which induration extended up into the region of left seminal vesicle.

In 217 cases both lobes of the prostate were involved. In 188 of these cases the right seminal vesicle and in 174 the left seminal vesicle was involved. Taking the 234 cases as a whole the induration found on rectal examination was as follows:

TABLE 108

Right lobe:
    First degree—21 cases—hard areas in 3.
    Second degree—52 cases—hard areas in 9.
    Third degree—161 cases—stony hard (all or most) in 107.
Left lobe:
    First degree—7 cases—hard areas in 1.
    Second degree—56 cases—hard areas in 2.
    Third degree—151 cases—hard areas in 70.

The above tabulation gives the distribution of the indurated areas met by the finger of the examiner. There are 10 cases in which the right lobe only was involved, the left lobe and seminal vesicle being normal in size and consistence. Of these 10, the seminal vesicle on that side was involved in but 4 cases. In 7 patients the left lobe only was involved, the right lobe and vesicle being normal. In 7 cases much of the prostate was normal or of only first-degree induration, but there were circumscribed areas of third-degree induration or of extreme hardness. In fact, in 2 cases a diagnosis of carcinoma was possible only after x-ray examination was negative for stone. In these there was an island of cancer surrounded by apparently

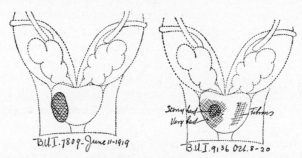

Fig. 442.—Rectal diagrams showing findings in 2 cases with small, circumscribed nodules of carcinoma in the prostate.

normal gland. In these patients the seminal vesicles were soft and not involved. Figure 442 shows clearly the condition on admission.

TABLE 109

Spread of infiltration to adjacent structures:
    Seminal vesicles, right, 191, 70 per cent.; left, 129, 54 per cent.

	Cases.	Per cent.
Membranous urethra	36	15.0
Perivesical	10	4.2
Intravesical	8	3.3
Periprostatic	6	2.4
Rectal wall	5	2.0
Metastases:		
Glands	26	10.9
Palpable	19	8.0
x-Ray	34	14.0

In many of these cases the disease had progressed so far that the patient lived only a few months. The invasion had progressed beyond the limits of the prostate and vesicles in only a small percentage of cases. Particularly striking is the infrequency with which enlarged glands were found, either by rectum or elsewhere, also the comparative infrequency of bony metastases as shown with the x-ray. This figure is based on the total number of cases; 157 cases were x-rayed on admission, and of these, 34 had bony metastases (14 per cent.). This, therefore, represents more nearly the frequency of bony metastases in patients appearing at the clinic.

Non-use of the Cystoscope in Carcinoma of the Prostate.—In practically all cases in this series the diagnosis was made by rectal examination and cystoscopy was not thought necessary. In a few cases it was done, but in the great majority it was not done because of the fact that previous experience had shown that cystoscopy is usually more difficult than in ordinary cases of enlarged prostate. It is impossible, in many cases, to introduce the cystoscope. Its use is almost always followed by marked aggravation of the urinary symptoms. In many cases in which the patient has only a moderate amount of difficulty, being able to void naturally, the use of the cystoscope is followed by complete retention of urine and thereafter a catheter life. Cystoscopy has, therefore, not been done except in cases where it was necessary to make a diagnosis, where symptoms suggesting stones or intravesical tumor were present, or where hemorrhage was so pronounced as to justify cystoscopy with the idea of carrying out fulguration or radium application.

In early cases of carcinoma of the prostate where a radical operation is contemplated after a positive diagnosis of carcinoma is made, the cystoscope is always used in order to study the prostatic orifice and trigone and to be certain that the invasion has not gone beyond the limits of a radical operation.

If cystoscopy is done, examination with finger in rectum and cystoscope in urethra (beak turned downward) is often of great value in determining the thickness and possible invasion of the trigone, and in cases where the diagnosis is uncertain, palpation with the finger against the cystoscope will often reveal induration of the median or lateral lobes which extends downward below the level of the verumontanum and is diagnostic of malignancy.

Treatment.—In almost all cases the disease was considered too far advanced for a radical operation, with certain exceptions which will be noted further on.

Some of the cases were, however, in some respects typical cases for radical operation, but, as a rule, a complicating condition, such as great age, general weakness, diabetes, marked renal impairment, etc., was present to prevent carrying out the radical operation.

The treatment which has been employed in these cases may be divided into twelve classes:

A.[1] *Cases Treated by the Use of Applicators Containing 100 to 200 Milligrams of Radium Element, and Applied Through the Rectum, Urethra, and Bladder.*—At the beginning we first employed an applicator which carried a straight cystoscope, but in a short time found that the cystoscope was of no value in the treatment of carcinoma of the prostate, and devised an applicator with a coudé beak which carried 100 mg. radium element, screened in a platinum capsule. More recently we have employed an instrument carrying two 100-mg. tubes tandem in the beak. This radium was applied by means of a cotted finger in the rectum and held in place with a clamp firmly fixed to the table. At the next treatment the same instrument, properly sterilized, was introduced into the urethra, and at the third treatment it was usually put into the bladder and turned downward so as to reach the carcinoma through the mucous membrane of the trigone. Eighty-two patients have been

[1] In this and succeeding pages the various forms of treatment employed in carcinoma of the prostate are classified as follows:

A = With Young's radium applicator.

B = With radium needles through skin of perineum.

E = External application of massive doses of radium.

F = Deep x-ray therapy.

G = Conservative perineal prostatectomy.

I = Introduction of radium after perineal prostatectomy into remaining prostatic tissues, etc.

treated by this technic. It has not been found advisable to apply the same amount of treatment, or in exactly the same way in every case. In order to determine the therapeutic results, they have been divided as follows:

A-1. *Cases in Which 1400 or Less Milligram-hours (mgh.) of Radium Were Given.*—In this group there are 33 cases. The amount of radium received by the patient in each of these cases was small and quite inadequate, only 11 having received 1000 mgh. or more, and 6 less than 500 mgh. The symptoms present before treatment with radium and the results obtained were as follows:

TABLE 110

Symptoms.	Present in, cases.	Relieved in, cases.
Frequency	27	9
Hesitancy	18	14
Nycturia	24	13
Dribbling	21	11
Dysuria	24	17
Pain in back	9	3
Pain in legs	8	2

Eight had *x*-ray plates taken, and in 2 metastases were found.

Prostate: All were enlarged; 15 stony hard; 7 cases had third-degree induration with stony hard areas; 11 had third-degree induration. As a result of radium applications, in 9 the prostate was changed, all of these showing some degree of softening. The others were apparently not affected. Seminal vesicles: In 26 cases one or both vesicles were involved.

There are 17 cases on which there is no report. Seven patients lived less than one year; 2, one year; 3, two years; 2, three years; 1, five years.

As an example of a good result in this class we cite the following:

B. U. I. 7809, aged forty-seven, admitted June 11, 1919, complaining of frequency of urination, nycturia four times, pain in back and groin, and impotence. Examination showed a nodule about 2 by 3 cm. in size, occupying the larger part of the left lobe of the prostate, and of third-degree induration; rest of prostate and seminal vesicles negative. Cystoscopy: No stricture, no hypertrophy of lateral lobes, median portion very slightly elevated, bladder negative. With

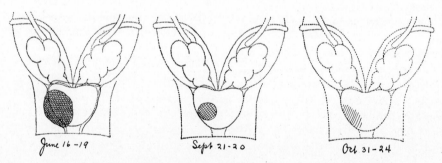

June 16 -19   *Sept 21-20*   *Oct 31-24*

FIG. 443.—Diagrams showing change in carcinoma of prostate treated by radium during a period of over five years. B. U. I. 7809.

finger in rectum and cystoscope in urethra there is moderate induration and slight enlargement of left lateral. Diagnosis, carcinoma of prostate (Young); others disagreed. Radical operation accordingly not advised. Patient was given prostatic massage occasionally for a period of six months. At the end of this time the induration was still present and was stony hard in the left lobe, and it was decided to begin radium treatment. He received 200 mgh. applied to the indurated left lobe through the rectum and 100 mgh. through the urethra. Four months later he returned and the induration of the left lobe was still present, but much smaller, and he was given 300 mgh. by rectum and 200 by urethra. October 31, 1924, no treatment for five years. Urination normal. No pain. Prostate is now about normal in size, right lobe smooth and soft, left slightly indurated and not adherent; seminal vesicles negative; rectum normal and no enlarged glands are felt. The indurated mass in the left lobe has completely disappeared (Fig. 443). November 24, 1924 (letter from doctor) patient is in excellent condition, apparently completely cured.

Comment.—This case is one of early carcinoma involving one lobe of the prostate apparently completely cured by radium—800 mgh.

A-2. *Cases Which Have Received Between 1500 and 2500 Mgh. Radium by Applicator by Rectum, Through Urethra and Bladder.*—Nineteen cases. Ages from forty-five to eighty-one years. Average duration of symptoms, ten months.

The symptoms present before treatment with radium and the results obtained were as follows:

TABLE 111

Symptoms.	Present in, cases.	Relieved in, cases.
Frequency	15	9
Hesitancy	12	8
Nycturia	15	9
Dribbling	12	9
Dysuria	13	7
Pain in back	5	2
Pain in legs	3	1

Eleven had x-ray plates taken, and in 4 metastases were found.

Prostate: Before treatment, in 17 the prostate was enlarged, in 12 stony hard, in 3 of third-degree induration, in 1 there was an area of stony hardness. As a result of treatment, in 18 cases the prostate was changed. In 14 the prostate became much softer, and in 11 cases definitely smaller. Seminal vesicles: In 18 one or both vesicles were involved.

Nine patients lived less than one year; 2 lived one year; 1 lived two years; 1 lived three years; 2 lived or are still living four and one-half years.

The following case is an example of the good results which were obtained:

B. U. I. 6759, aged seventy-five, admitted March 2, 1917, complaining of marked frequency of urination (almost every hour, night and day), dysuria, and dribbling. Rectal examination: Prostate irregular, nodular, considerably enlarged, very hard in places, in others firm on deep pressure, and in others slightly elastic but firm. Invasion of the region between the seminal vesicles present. Cystoscopy: Residual urine, 50 c.c. No intravesical enlargement. Orifice irregular and edematous. With finger in rectum and cystoscope in urethra, there is great increase in thickness and induration of the suburethral portion of the prostate. Diagnosis of malignancy positive (Geraghty). Treatment: Applications of radium through the urethra, bladder, and rectum. April 6th, has now had 700 mgh. per rectum and 200 per urethram. There has been a great improvement in symptoms; voids only once at night and at intervals of six hours during the day. Prostate still markedly indurated in places, but in others much softer. June 1st, six hours of radium during the past week (600 mgh.). Can now retain urine ten hours; prostate much softer. August, 1920, condition excellent, but another course of radium seems advisable. He is to be given 1000 mgh. per rectum, to region of prostate and both seminal vesicles. September 12, 1921, now four and a half years since beginning radium treatment, and one year since last treatment. Patient says for a time there was considerable irritability of rectum and also bladder and urethra with passage of blood-clots. He has, however, entirely recovered, rectum now quite normal, bowel movements regular, voids urine freely. On examination of rectal wall there is contracture or slight stricture. No ulceration. Mucosa smooth. Prostate almost normal in size, only slightly indurated. Seminal vesicles obscured by rectal contracture. No evidence of carcinoma. Patient died of angina pectoris November 17, 1921, four years and eight months after beginning radium treatment; no autopsy. He had an excellent functional result and as noted in the last examination, great change in the prostate and no evidence of carcinoma present..

A-3. *Cases Receiving 2500 Mgh. Radium or More.*—Thirty cases. Ages between fifty-two and eighty-seven years. Average duration of symptoms eleven months. The symptoms present before treatment with radium and the results obtained are as follows:

TABLE 112

Symptoms.	Present in, cases.	Relieved in, cases.
Frequency	24	19
Hesitancy	25	18
Nycturia	26	17
Dribbling	19	18
Dysuria	17	15
Retention	3	1
Pain in back	9	7
Pain in legs	7	3

Twelve had x-ray plates taken, and in 3 metastases were found.

Prostate: Before treatment the prostate was enlarged in 26; and stony hard in 14; 9 had third-degree induration; 3 had third-degree induration with areas of stony hardness. After radium treatment in 29 the prostate was changed: 26 showed definite softening; and in 18 it became definitely smaller. Seminal vesicles: One or both seminal vesicles were involved in 27 cases.

Seven of these patients lived less than one year; 7 lived one year; 5 lived one and one-half years; 2 lived two years; 2 lived three years; 1 lived four years; 1 is living after five years; 1 after six years. In 4 cases there has been no report.

A-B. *Cases Receiving Radium (A) by Rectum, Through Urethra and Bladder, by Young's Applicator, and (B) by Radium Needles Inserted Through Perineum Into Prostate and Vesicles.*—Twenty-three cases. Ages between fifty-four and eighty years. Average duration of symptoms, eight months. The symptoms before treatment and the results obtained are shown in the following table:

TABLE 113

Symptoms.	Present in, cases.	Relieved in, cases.
Frequency	21	19
Hesitancy	17	15
Nycturia	20	18
Dribbling	17	14
Dysuria	19	16
Retention	3	1
Pain in back	8	4
Pain in legs	9	2

Eleven had x-rays taken, and in 5 metastases were found.

Prostate: The condition before treatment was as follows: In 21 cases enlarged; 19 cases hard; in 2 there was third-degree induration containing hard areas; and in 2, third-degree induration. As a result of treatment in 19 cases the prostate was definitely changed; 19 became softer; 15 became definitely smaller. Seminal vesicles: In 21 cases one or both vesicles were involved.

Ten patients lived less than one year; 5 lived one year; 2 lived two years; 1 lived four years. There are 5 in which we have no report.

The following case is an example of very extensive carcinoma of the prostate and seminal vesicles which was rapidly and markedly improved with radium, but not cured.

B. U. I. 9622. C. F. K., age sixty-seven, admitted April 21, 1921 with difficulty and frequency of urination of three years' duration, voiding every half hour. Rectal examination showed extensive carcinoma of the prostate and seminal vesicles (Fig. 444). Cystoscope showed elevated trigone, but no hypertrophy of the prostate. Patient given radium applications, 2100 mgh. by rectum, 500 by urethra, 600 by bladder, and 1000 mgh. (with 4 needles) through perineum—in all, 4200 mgh. Patient improved rapidly under this treatment. Urination became much more free, and on discharge June 22d he voided at intervals of three or four hours and rectal

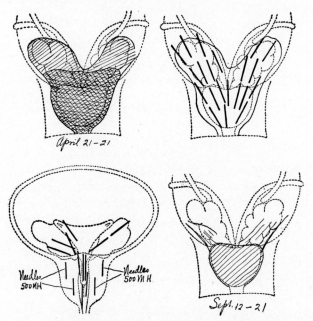

Fig. 444.—Diagrams showing effect of radium treatment on carcinoma of prostate as indicated by rectal findings. Each of the short straight lines indicates the place of application of 100 mg. of radium for one hour; therefore the number of marks multiplied by 100 equals the total milligram-hours given. B. U. I. 9622.

examination showed prostate almost normal in size, only slightly indurated and with only slight adhesions on outer side of each vesicle, as shown in chart. September 12th, no treatment for almost three months. For a time suffered pain in rectum. No mucus or blood. Of late has had no rectal irritation, no pain, and has gained 6 pounds in weight, voids normally at intervals of seven hours. Rectal examination shows prostate a little more prominent than normal, very slight induration along outer side of each vesicle, similar to slight chronic seminal vesiculitis. Rectal wall thickened, mucosa redundant, no ulceration. No enlarged glands.

Examples of good results from the use of a combination of radium applications and needles:

B. U. I. 9362, age sixty-five, admitted December 31, 1920, with difficulty and frequent urination. Examination showed enlargement and marked induration of the prostate and invasion of the lower portion of the left seminal vesicle. Cystoscopy was not done. Diagnosis, carcinoma of the prostate and seminal vesicles. Patient was treated with needles containing radium element inserted through the skin of perineum as follows: January 5, 1921, 2 needles, 20 mg. each, allowed to remain ten hours, totaling 400 mgh. No marked reaction. March 11th, rectal examination shows prostate hard and nodular and induration continues 2 cm. into region of left seminal vesicle. Treatment has produced no marked change. Second radium treatment. Two needles again inserted through perineum, totaling 440 mgh.; also three applications of 100 mgh. each through the rectum, totaling 300 mgh. No further treatment. October 18, 1925, letter: Patient has had no treatment. Urination is quite normal, unnecessary to get up at night, suffers no pain, no hematuria, and sexual powers are normal. General health and weight good. Considers himself cured.

B. U. I. 9788, age fifty-nine, admitted June 22, 1921, complaining of difficulty of urination and catheter life. Examination showed extensive carcinoma of prostate. (See diagram, Fig. 445.) Right lobe moderately enlarged, irregular, extremely hard and adherent, with adhesions

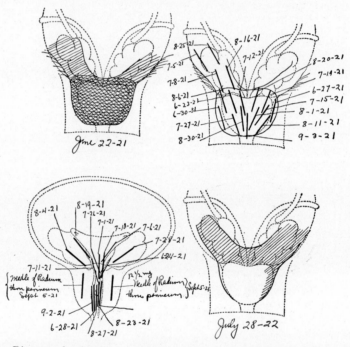

Fig. 445.—Diagrams showing effect of radium treatment on carcinoma of the prostate as indicated by rectal findings. Each of the short straight lines indicates the place of application of 100 mg. of radium for one hour; therefore the number of marks multiplied by 100 equals the total milligram-hours given. The dates are also shown. B. U. I. 9788.

running upward. Left lobe moderately enlarged, irregular, extremely hard, and adherent. Induration extends up into seminal vesicles on both sides for a short distance, upper portions soft. Diagnosis of carcinoma of the prostate positive. Radium treatment begun and applied as shown in chart. Total by rectum 1700 mgh., by urethra 700 mgh., by bladder 800, by perineal needles 500 mgh. Total, 3700 mgh., given between June 22d and August 30th as shown in chart. Progress: September 27, 1921, urination much improved, has given up catheter. Rectal walls smooth, no ulceration. Prostate now about normal in size, slight irregularity and induration. Seminal vesicles negative, very great change. One would not now suspect malignancy. April 27, 1923, has had difficulty of urination and required catheterization for one month. The prostate is enlarged, but smooth and elastic and feels now like small hypertrophy. Moderate induration of seminal vesicles, and rectal wall somewhat thickened from treatment. Diagnosis, prostatic hypertrophy. No evidence of carcinoma, but it is thought wise to give a course of deep x-ray treatments. May 15, 1921, patient has just completed his first course of x-ray treatments, consisting of an erythema dose given over front, sides, and back of pelvis daily for fifteen days.

Duration of each treatment thirty-three minutes, reaction slight. August 16, 1924, report from friend: "Patient is enjoying life and is seen nightly at his club, apparently in good health." Letters not answered.

B. U. I. 9635, age sixty-two, admitted April 27, 1921, with frequency and history of occasional catheter life. Rectal examination: Prostate markedly enlarged, right lobe stony hard, markedly indurated and irregular, very adherent. Left lobe markedly indurated and adherent. Both seminal vesicles involved in the infiltration as shown in the chart (Fig. 446). Enlarged glands are palpable along the pelvic wall. Diagnosis: Extensive carcinoma of prostate and seminal vesicles, right vesicle forming a very large hard mass. Treatment: Radium applications with 100 mg. element applied through rectum, urethra, and bladder. Total 4400 mgh. June 21st, radium needles through perineum totaling about 500 mgh. The result is shown graphically in the accompanying chart (Fig. 446). September 24, 1921, no treatment for three months. Urination normal. Does not get up at night. No pain. Recently had swelling of left leg. Examination showed adenitis in left groin. Prostate about normal in size, only slightly indurated. Seminal vesicles practically negative. Remarkable change as a result of the radium.

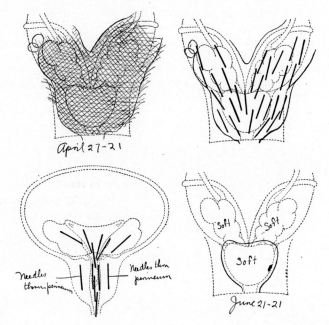

FIG. 446.—Diagrams showing effect of radium treatment on carcinoma of prostate as shown by rectal findings. B. U. I. 9635.

December 2d, patient has just finished one series of deep x-ray treatment. Swelling of leg still present. Glands in groin still enlarged. Urination greatly improved—only twice at night, and normal in day. November 15, 1922, letter from doctor, "Radium treatment has effected a complete cure of his bladder trouble, but I fear he has metastases to the lungs."

A-G-F. *Carcinoma of the Prostate Treated by Radium with Young's Applicator (from 1000 to 5000 Mgh.). Conservative Perineal Prostatectomy and Deep x-Ray (One Series).*—Seven cases. Ages from fifty-nine to seventy-three years. Average duration of symptoms to admission was two years. The symptoms present before treatment with radium and the results obtained are shown in Table 114, page 666.

Six had x-ray plates taken and in 3 metastases were found.

Prostate: Before treatment in all cases was enlarged; in 6 stony hard; and in 2, third-degree induration. After treatment, in all cases the prostate was changed.

TABLE 114

Symptoms.	Present in, cases.	Relieved in, cases.
Frequency	7	4
Hesitancy	6	5
Nycturia	6	5
Dribbling	5	4
Dysuria	5	4
Retention	5	5
Pain in back	4	3
Pain in legs	4	3

In all it became softer, and in 5 cases definitely smaller. Seminal vesicles: In all 7 cases seminal vesicles were involved.

Six cases have been followed completely, and all are dead; 2 lived one year; 3 lived two years; 1 lived five years; 1 not heard from.

The following case is cited as an example of a good result in this class:

B. U. I. 8718, age sixty-four. Symptoms began nine months before admission, with frequency and dysuria, increasing to complete retention. Examination showed enlarged prostate, stony hard, with seminal vesicles and membranous urethra involved. He was given 2100 mgh. and 1 series of deep x-ray. Symptomatically, there was no improvement, although the prostate became much smaller and softer. Then conservative perineal prostatectomy was done. Wound closed in the eleventh week. He gained weight and went on without urinary discomfort and was moderately active until death five years later. There was no autopsy and the cause of death was unknown.

A-F. *Carcinoma of Prostate Treated with 1200 to 4500 mgh. Radium by Young's Applicator and Deep x-Ray.*—Eight cases. Seven cases received one series of deep x-ray, and 1 case two series. Ages from fifty-seven to eighty years. Average duration of symptoms was eleven months. The symptoms present before treatment with radium and the results obtained are as follows:

TABLE 115

Symptoms.	Present in, cases.	Relieved in, cases.
Frequency	8	7
Hesitancy	6	6
Nycturia	6	6
Dribbling	3	3
Dysuria	4	4
Retention	0	0
Pain in back	3	3
Pain in legs	3	2

Six cases had x-ray plates taken, and 1 showed metastases.

Prostate: Before treatment it was enlarged in all cases; in 3 stony hard; and in 5, third-degree induration. After radium treatment, 6 showed softening and decrease in the size of the gland. Seminal vesicles were both involved in 6 cases; in 2, only left involved.

One case is living; 1 not heard from; 2 lived eight months; 2, three years; 2, two years; 1, four years.

B. U. I. 12,752. A. D. E., age sixty-three, admitted August 28, 1924, with marked difficulty and frequency of urination of one year's duration. Examination showed very marked enlargement and great induration of prostate and lower portions of both seminal vesicles, as shown in the accompanying chart (Fig. 447). Diagnosis, carcinoma. Treatment with radium applied by rectum, urethra, and bladder and deep *x*-ray therapy as shown in chart (Fig. 447). He received a course of radium treatment, 3000 mgh. through rectum, urethra, and bladder, as shown in chart, and one series of deep *x*-ray therapy. In a month patient gave up the use of a catheter and urination rapidly improved. He returned for examination on January 21, 1925, at which time he stated that urination was normal, did not have to get up at night to void and urine was sterile. *x*-Ray was negative. On examination prostate was normal in size and con-

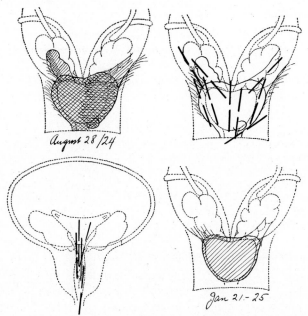

Fig. 447.—Diagrams showing effect of radium treatment on carcinoma of prostate as shown by rectal findings. B. U. I. 12,752.

sistence, only slightly indurated, and there are only slight adhesions and slight induration of the seminal vesicles. One would not have suspected carcinoma at all.

Regardless of this it was thought wise to give him another series of treatments, both with radium through the urethra and rectum and with deep *x*-ray therapy.

A-B-F. *Carcinoma of Prostate Treated by Radium, Radium Needles, and x-Ray.* —Eight cases, ages between fifty and seventy-one years. All had radium by applicator, 600 to 4200 mgh.; and radium needles, 450 to 1000 mgh. Seven cases had one series of deep *x*-ray, and 1 had two series. The symptoms present before treatment with radium and the results obtained are as follows:

TABLE 116

Symptoms.	Present in, cases.	Relieved in, cases.
Frequency	7	5
Hesitancy	6	5
Diminution in size and force	6	5
Nycturia	7	5
Dribbling	4	3
Dysuria	2	2
Retention	2	2
Pain in back	4	2
Pain in legs	3	2

Five cases had x-ray plates, and in 3 metastases were found.

Prostate: Before treatment, enlarged in 8; stony hard in 7; third-degree induration in 1. After radium, in 6 of these cases the prostate became definitely smaller and lost the feel of carcinoma. Seminal vesicles: Both involved in 7; left only in 1.

Three patients are dead, 2 lived at least one year, but have not been heard from since. One is living four years, urination is normal, but he has intestinal symptoms; 1 is living four years, but has not answered letters, and condition is not known; 1 is living six months without urinary symptoms.

A-G. *Carcinoma of the Prostate Treated by Radium Plus Perineal Prostatectomy.*—Twenty-seven cases. Ages from forty-eight to seventy-five years. Average duration of symptoms, eight months. The symptoms present before treatment and the results obtained are as follows:

TABLE 117

Symptoms.	Present in, cases.	Relieved in, cases.
Frequency	22	12
Hesitancy	21	21
Nycturia	20	12
Dribbling	19	12
Dysuria	21	9
Pain in back	9	3
Pain in legs	7	2

Prostate: In 23 cases before treatment it was enlarged; in 11 stony hard; in 8 third-degree induration; in 6, third-degree induration with hard areas. After radium treatment in 7 cases there was softening noted before operation. Seminal vesicles: One or both were involved in 25 cases.

Ten lived less than one year; 6 lived one year; 4 lived two years; 1 lived three years, and 1 lived six years. There are 5 from which we have no report.

A-E. 1. *Carcinoma of the Prostate Treated by Radium per Rectum, Urethra, and Bladder by Young's Applicator and Massive Radium. Average Dose, 700 mgh.*—Five cases. Ages between fifty-five and seventy-eight years. The symptoms present before treatment with radium and the results obtained were as follows:

TABLE 118

Symptoms.	Present in, cases.	Relieved in, cases.
Frequency	5	4
Hesitancy	3	1
Nycturia	2	1
Dribbling	3	1
Dysuria	3	1
Retention	0	0
Pain in back	2	1
Pain in legs	0	0

Prostate: Before treatment in all enlarged; in 4 hard; in 1 third-degree induration. No note of change in gland after radium treatment. Seminal vesicles were involved in all cases.

Two cases lived one year; 2 lived two years; 1 lived three years.

A-E. 2. *Carcinoma of the Prostate Treated by Radium per Rectum, Urethra, and Bladder by Young's Applicator and Massive Radium. Dose, 1500 to 2500 mgh.*—

Four cases. Ages between fifty-seven and eighty years. The symptoms present before treatment with radium and the results obtained are as follows:

TABLE 119

Symptoms.	Present in, cases.	Relieved in, cases.
Frequency	4	3
Hesitancy	2	1
Nycturia	3	1
Dribbling	3	2
Dysuria	3	2
Retention	1	0
Pain in back	1	0
Pain in legs	0	0

No cases were *x*-rayed before treatment.

Prostate was enlarged before treatment in all cases; in 3 hard; and in 1 third-degree induration. After radium treatment the prostate became much softer and smaller in 2 cases. Seminal vesicles were involved in 3 cases.

Two cases lived one year; 1 lived ten years; 1, no report.

A case in which patient lived ten years with carcinoma of the prostate.

B. U. I. 4417. Aged fifty-nine. Admitted June 4, 1915, complaining of difficulty and pain. Suprapubic prostatectomy had been done two months before. Examination of specimen shows carcinoma. On our advice patient was given local treatments with radium through urethra, bladder, and rectum and received 1800 mgh. before admission. Examination showed slightly irregular, indurated prostate, irregular prostatic orifice, marked elevation of trigone. Diagnosis, carcinomatous invasion. Treatment: Applications of radium, 1050 mgh. through trigone and ten hours with 1900 mg. radium applied through perineum and suprapubic region. March 9, 1916, examination shows an induration of moderate degree in the region of the seminal vesicles. Cystoscope shows a marked elevation of the trigone. Radium was applied through trigone 250 mgh., through urethra 250 mgh., and through rectum 250 mgh. June, 1916, urination normal. Condition in seminal vesicles apparently improved. No treatment given. November 30, 1917, invasion in vesicles has extended up on each side. Prostate is a little larger and slightly harder. No treatment given. Patient then had no return of symptoms until July 19, 1919, when hematuria came on. Intermittent recurrences since. In April, 1922 received 200 mgh. radium and four deep *x*-ray treatments. July 25, 1924, urination has become frequent and difficult. Examination shows prostate markedly enlarged, irregular, nodular, and very hard. Lower portions of both seminal vesicles also markedly indurated. The cystoscope shows trigone greatly elevated with irregular growth, but the mucous membrane is intact. No ulceration or tumor. Patient died August 2, 1924 of pneumonia. Autopsy findings showed carcinoma of prostate, bladder, bilateral hydronephrosis with occlusion of left ureter, pyelonephritis, and lobar pneumonia.

Remarks.—The above case is interesting in showing that a patient may live twelve years from onset of symptoms and ten years after positive demonstration of carcinoma in a prostatectomy specimen. It seems probable that radium treatment prolonged his life. The case is also interesting in demonstrating that carcinoma may be present beneath the trigone for ten years without producing ulceration or intravesical growth and also without involving the rectum.

A-E. 3. *Carcinoma of the Prostate Treated by Radium per Rectum, Urethra, and Bladder by Young's Applicator and Massive Radium. Dose, 2500 mgh. and Over.*—Six cases. Ages between fifty and eighty years. Symptoms present before treatment with radium and the results obtained are shown in Table 120, page 670.

x-Rays were taken of 2 cases before treatment, and in 1 metastases were found.

Prostate: Before treatment it was enlarged in 5; stony hard in 4; of third-degree induration in 2. After radium treatment, in 3 cases the prostate became smaller and softer. The seminal vesicles were involved on one or both sides in 5 cases.

TABLE 120

Symptoms.	Present in, cases.	Relieved, in cases.
Frequency	5	3
Hesitancy	5	3
Nycturia	4	2
Dribbling	4	2
Dysuria	5	2
Retention	1	0
Pain in back	2	0
Pain in legs	3	2

One lived two months; 2 lived one year; 1 lived two years; 1 lived five years. No record of 1 case.

Case showing great improvement after radium.   Death six years later of cancer.

B. U. I. 4726.   W. R. S., age seventy-three, admitted November 18, 1918.   Frequency of urination.   Occasional catheter life.   Prostate is considerably enlarged, irregular and of stony hardness.   Both vesicles are invaded.   Patient received radium treatment in four series, totaling 3200 mgh.   He also received massive radiations with large amounts of radium applied through perineum and suprapubic region.   As a result of this treatment there was great improvement. December 3, 1915, patient is already voiding more freely and at longer intervals.   On April 5, 1916 it was noted that urination was much freer and the prostate is now elastic and compressible in places.   January 29, 1920, patient reports great improvement, quite normal.   Urination free and without pain.   No hematuria.   Prostate is still enlarged and very hard.   Additional radium given by rectum and urethra.   Patient died August 20, 1920—cause not stated.   Patient lived six years from onset of symptoms and had been restored from very frequent urination with occasional catheter life to normal urination by radium treatment.

A-G-I.   *Carcinoma of the Prostate Treated by Radium by Applicator to Rectum, Urethra, and Bladder.   Conservative Perineal Prostatectomy and One or Two Capsules Carrying 200 mg. Radium from Six to Twelve Hours.*—Nine cases.   Ages from fifty-five to seventy-eight years.   Average duration of symptoms.   The symptoms present before treatment with radium and the results obtained are as follows:

TABLE 121

Symptoms.	Present in, cases.	Relieved in, cases.
Frequency	8	6
Hesitancy	7	7
Nycturia	9	7
Dribbling	8	5
Retention	5	5
Dysuria	8	4
Pain in back	3	1
Pain in legs	1	0

Three had x-ray plates taken, and in 1 metastases were found.

Prostate: Before treatment, in 9 cases the prostate was enlarged, in 6 stony hard; and in 3, third-degree induration.   One or both seminal vesicles were involved in 7 cases.

One case lived less than one year; 2 lived one year; 2 lived three years; 1 lived four years; 1 lived four and one-half years.   There is 1 case from which we have no report.

Note.—Inasmuch as a core of carcinomatous tissue was removed from the vesical orifice, the results of the radium alone could not be determined.

The following case is an example of fairly successful use of radium before and during prostatectomy for carcinoma:

B. U. I. 7739. C. L. S., age sixty-eight. Admitted May 8, 1919, complaining of complete retention of urine with catheter life. The prostate was enlarged, very hard, and both vesicles were involved. Patient was given applications of radium, 600 mgh. through the rectum and 300 mgh. through the urethra. Perineal prostatectomy was then carried out. Lateral lobes of prostate were enucleated and two tubes of 100 mg. each left in prostatic cavity for six hours (1200 mgh.). Patient was then discharged from the hospital in six weeks, voiding naturally at intervals of four to six hours. October 14, 1922, letter from physician, "I have just examined patient. Condition is excellent. No sign whatever of recurrence, and he has only 1 ounce residual urine." December 12, 1923, patient died as a result of appendicitis. No autopsy obtained.

It can safely be stated that these patients who received radium applications and x-ray in addition to conservative perineal prostatectomy were, as a whole, very greatly benefited by the treatment. In many instances the patients were comfortable as long as they lived.

Résumé of Treatment.—*Radical operation*, with complete removal of prostate, seminal vesicles, and prostatic urethra, according to the technic described in Chapter XVII, is the treatment of choice in all early cases, where there are no demonstrated metastases and the membranous urethra and upper two-thirds of the seminal vesicles are free from involvement. This treatment, unfortunately, is applicable at present in only a small minority of the cases, owing to the failure of early diagnosis. Great stress should be placed on palpation of the prostate in elderly men, with the view of obtaining more cures in carcinoma of the prostate.

Where the carcinoma is so extensive that radical operation is impossible, or metastases have been demonstrated, *radium treatment*, given by rectum, urethra, and bladder by Young's applicators, and preferably supplemented by the embedding of radium needles or emanation seeds in the prostate, is the treatment to be followed. By this means the local growth is inhibited, urinary obstruction usually prevented, and the remainder of the patient's life made comfortable. In some cases the duration of life appears to be decidedly lengthened and it may be that in a few cases cures have been obtained.

Where extensive carcinoma is present and there is urinary obstruction, it is necessary to relieve the obstruction. In some cases, where the renal function is not yet affected, this relief may follow a properly given course of radium treatment. If not, or if the bad condition of the kidneys demands immediate relief, the nature of the obstruction must be studied and a suitable operation performed. Sometimes a punch operation is sufficient, in other cases a perineal operation, with removal of a core of carcinomatous tissue or of benignly hypertrophied lobes, must be carried out. Following such operations healing is favorable and complete relief of urinary obstruction is usually afforded. Radium may be embedded in the remaining prostate at the time of operation.

Where there is great pain from the pressure of metastases upon nerves, deep x-ray treatments often give great relief. It may be that the addition of deep x-ray treatments to radium treatment produces better results in the prostate itself. We feel that this is probably worth trying, although we have not yet had sufficient experience to make definite statements as to its value.

NEOPLASMS OF THE TESTIS AND OTHER SCROTAL CONTENTS
PATHOLOGY

Testis.—Tumors of the testicle are comparatively rare. In the literature they are given as from $\frac{1}{2}$ to 1 per cent. of all tumors. In the records of the Brady Urological Institute there are 25 tumors of the testicle in 12,000 urologic cases, about ⅕ of 1 per cent. Southam and Linell[1] report 38 cases from among 27,000 general hospital admissions, while Hinman finds an average of 0.063 per cent. of male hospital admissions in the literature. Bland-Sutton's statistics showing that the great majority of testicular neoplasms occurred in undescended testes have not been confirmed. Chevassu[2] found 15 undescended testes in 128 cases of tumor (11.7 per cent.). In a series of 117 cases, collected from the literature and the records of the Johns Hopkins Hospital by W. W. Scott, 18 or 15 per cent. were in undescended testes. Of 649 cases collected by Hinman, 12.2 per cent. were in undescended testes. Of the Brady Institute cases, only one was cryptorchid (4 per cent.). At the Manchester Royal Infirmary there were 4 tumors in retained testes (3 abdominal, 1 inguinal) in a period during which 409 operations were performed for cryptorchidism in the same institution.[3] But in 3529 cases of undescended testes collected from the literature by Hinman,[4] there were only 6 tumors (0.017 per cent.). Apparently abdominal testes are more apt to become malignant than those arrested in the inguinal canal and, according to Bulkeley,[5] at least twice as apt to do so as are scrotal testes. Even at that, the proportion would be very small.

Testicular tumors are, in general, more precocious than those of any other organ of the body. It is noteworthy that the average age falls within the period of maximum sexual activity. In Scott's series of 117 cases, the average age was thirty-five years, the youngest twenty months, and the oldest sixty-four years. They are rare below eighteen and over fifty. The largest series that has been collected in infants comprises only 42 cases. Pathologically, these tumors represented all varieties, but the "seminoma" type is much rarer than in adult life.

The following table shows the age incidence in our series:

TABLE 122

Age at onset.	Cases.	Per cent.
?	1	4.2
0–10	1	4.2
10–20	0	0
20–30	3	12.5
30–40	11	45.9
40–50	6	25.0
50–60	0	0
60–70	3	12.5

Testicular tumors are practically always unilateral, and the two sides are affected about equally, with possibly a slight preponderance on the right. In our series of 25 cases, 75 per cent. were on the right side, but this is probably accidental. In Scott's series of 117 cases, 58 were on the right, 49 on the left. In the remainder the side was not noted. Hinman has found 17 cases of bilateral involvement in the entire literature. It is presumed that those were separate tumors, though some of them may have been involvement of the second testis by direct extension.

[1] British Journal of Surgery, 1923, xi, 223–233.
[2] Tumeurs du Testicule, Thèse de Paris, 1909.
[3] British Journal of Surgery, 1923, xi, 223-233.
[4] Cabot's Modern Urology, 1923, i, 580–609.
[5] Surgery, Gynecology, and Obstetrics, 1913, xvii, 703–719.

No definite classification of testicular tumors will be attempted. About half the tumors are definitely teratomatous, and about an equal number are of the type called "seminoma" by Chevassu. The latter are regarded by many (Ribbert, Ewing[1]) as also teratomatous in origin. Other types are very rare.

A few cases of benign *fibroma* and *adenoma* have been reported. The adenomata consist of small masses cf narrow, highly convoluted tubules filled with epithelial cells, and in some places groups of interstitial cells.

A small number of cases has been reported in which an enlargement of the testis was due to a non-malignant hyperplasia, apparently of the *interstitial cells*. These tumors are of very slow growth, and in the one illustrated by Dürck[2] the compressed remains of the seminiferous tubules could be seen throughout. In none of the reported cases has there been any rapid growth or metastasis. Microscopically, one sees masses of polygonal cells resembling normal interstitial cells except for the presence of glycogen and the absence of Reinke's crystals. In the gross, the tumor is ovoid, firm, smooth, and on section brown in color, without necrosis.

We have seen 1 case in an infant of two and one-half years (B. U. I. 11,646) in which the testicle was replaced by a rounded tumor 6 cm. in diameter. On section the tissue was almost white, firm, and perfectly homogeneous. Microscopically, there was a clear structureless hyaline matrix, traversed by a number of moderate sized veins. Radiating from each vein were numerous long, narrow sprouts presenting the typical appearance of embryonal endothelium, including vacuole formation (Figs. 448–450.). There is little doubt that this is a true *endothelioma*, and the observation appears to be unique.

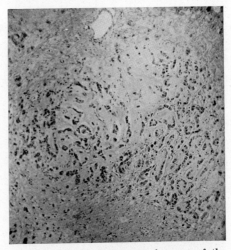

FIG. 448.—A very unusual tumor of the testis in a young child. It consists of small strands of tumor cells embedded in a homogeneous matrix of hyaline appearance. In some places the tumor cells are directly continuous with capillaries. This tumor is probably an embryonal endothelioma. B. U. I. Path. 4774.

Leiomyoma may arise in the epididymis.

Sarcoma is very rare. Southam and Linell picture a tumor diagnosed fibrosarcoma which appears to merit this designation. Hinman accepts 1 case of Sakaguchi, and 3 of Miyata. A truly sarcomatous change in teratoma is seldom if ever seen. The tumor which has commonly been called "sarcoma" in the past is discussed under "Seminoma."

Coming to the common tumors of the testis, we agree with Hinman that the important feature is that there are two principal types: (1) Mixed tumors, usually cystic, and showing tissues arising from more than one germ layer, and (2) tumors composed of one specific type of cell. The first type is undoubtedly to be called teratoma or, preferably, embryoma, and the second type may well be called seminoma, whether we accept the Ribbert-Ewing theory that it is a one-sided de-

[1] Neoplastic Diseases, New York, 1922.

[2] Verhandlungen der Deutschen Pathologischen Gesellschaft, 1907, xi, 130–136.

velopment of teratoma, the Chevassu theory that it is a separate tumor, or, as is perhaps best, remain undecided what it really is.

Seminoma.—This tumor, whatever its pathogenesis, presents a very characteristic picture. The tunica albuginea is distended, but not penetrated by the tumor, and this produces a smooth rounded mass. The outer aspect presents no characteristics of malignancy and the tissues appear normal except for dilated bloodvessels. On section the tumor is grayish white, smooth, and rather opaque. There are not infrequently areas of necrosis with hemorrhage, but these are not as abundant as in embryoma which has undergone malignant degeneration. There are no cysts. Ewing states that the tumor usually begins in the region of the rete testis. As it grows it does not invade the testicular tissue, but pushes it aside. There may be, therefore, a rim of compressed testis just beneath the tunica albuginea, usually thickest on the side opposite the epididymis, but destruction is complete at a fairly early stage and often no remains of the testis are seen. The

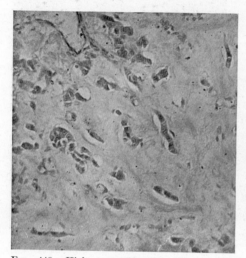
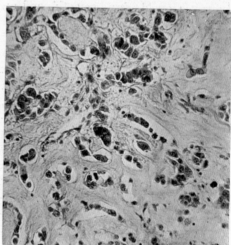

Fig. 449.—Higher magnification of the same tumor. B. U. I. Path. 4774.

Fig. 450.—Higher magnification of the same tumor. B. U. I. Path. 4774.

epididymis may be stretched out over the tumor, but is usually not invaded. The tunica albuginea, in spite of its enlargement, is usually thickened, and confines the tumor everywhere. There may be a moderate degree of hydrocele, usually more marked in the larger tumors, though it may be absent in the largest. The size varies, but may attain that of an adult head.

Microscopically, the tumor is composed of strands and acini of various sizes, separated by connective-tissue trabeculæ which may be thick or thin. This accounts for variations in the consistence of the mass. The trabeculæ are the site of a lymphocytic infiltration, which extends into the alveoli, but is most marked at the margins, adjoining the trabeculæ. Sometimes the tumor cells are broken up into very small strands or groups, in which case the connective tissue is very delicate, and the lymphocytic infiltration appears to be universal. It is in such areas that necrosis supervenes, probably because where the trabeculæ are better developed they carry a better blood-supply. The tumor cells are uniform, with a fairly abundant but very delicate cytoplasm (Figs. 451, 452). The shape is polyhedral, so that the adjacent cells touch at all points. This appearance may be altered in either of two ways: First, the delicate cytoplasm may shrink in areas where the nutrition is poor and necrosis is impending, and, second, in poorly preserved specimens the cytoplasm may shrink down around the nucleus. When this shrinkage occurs, the cells appear to be round, with very scanty cytoplasm, and from this fact has arisen the idea that these tumors are sarcomata. All competent pathologists agree, however, that they are not sarcomata, and that designation should now be abandoned. The nuclei stain rather uniformly with hematoxylin, and are of moderate size, slightly oval, and contain a light chromatin network with one or two nucleoli. Mitoses are seen, but are not frequent.

Ordinarily one sees a uniform picture throughout the tumor, but, unfortunately for the theory that seminoma is an independent entity, one occasionally finds a

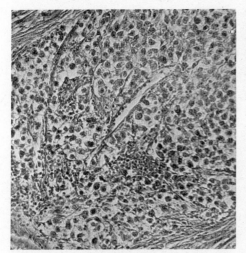 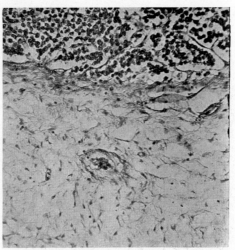

Fig. 451.—Malignant tumor of the testis showing tumor cells arranged in nests, with vesicular nuclei, abundant and very delicate cytoplasm, and round-cell infiltration in the tumor. The nests are inclosed by connective-tissue trabeculæ. This is the type of tumor formerly called sarcoma, now called "seminoma" by the French authors and considered as a form of embryonal carcinoma by Ewing. B. U. I. Path. 3635.

Fig. 452.—In this tumor the cells resemble exactly the cells of seminoma, but the connective-tissue stroma is very edematous and of embryonic type. B. U. I. Path. 3346.

bit of cartilage or a few glands somewhere in the mass. In the same way one occasionally finds a small area of typical seminoma in a cystic embryoma. These two facts comprise the principal reason for believing that seminoma is a form of teratoma, in which this particular type of growth has overgrown all others. This disputed point is interesting, but of little practical importance.

Embryoma (Teratoma).—The external appearance of embryoma (teratoma) is the same as that of seminoma, since it also does not penetrate the tunica albuginea (Fig. 453). On section, however, one sees a much more variegated picture. Usually there are multiple cysts of varying size. There may be islands of cartilage. Malignant degeneration is the rule and, if extensive, it may give rise to large areas of soft, pultaceous tumor, or necrosis may produce a pea-soup-like fluid. Hemorrhage is common. Destruction or replacement of the testis occurs as in seminoma.

Microscopically, the picture is varied. The essential feature is, of course, that tissues from two or three germ layers are present. It is not especially necessary to identify all three layers to be sure that one is dealing with an embryoma, although some insist that this is requisite before the name teratoma can be properly applied. Ordinarily one sees a framework of connective tissue—in some cases embryonic and undifferentiated, in others more developed, with blood-vessels, and smooth and striated muscle. There is some dispute as to whether the blood-vessels are ingrowths from the host, or arise from the teratoma itself. There is frequently carti-

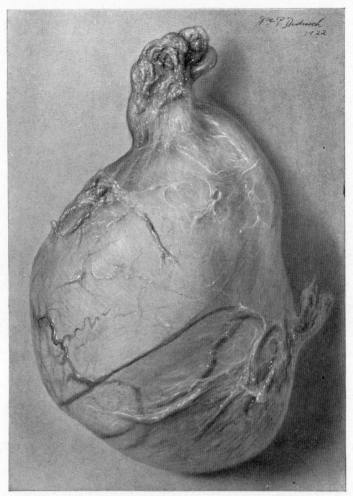

Fig. 453.—Operative removal of malignant tumor of the testis. This picture shows only the scrotal tumor. It was an embryoma with many large cysts and carcinomatous degeneration. B. U. I. 10,862.

lage. The embryonic connective tissue may contain greater or smaller amounts of a gelatinous substance, imparting a myxomatous nature to the growth. A rarer finding is bone. Throughout the tumor are numerous gland-like cavities, which may be collapsed, giving a more solid tumor, or dilated, giving a cystic tumor. The cysts vary in size, and may be as large as 4 or 5 cm. in diameter. The cysts are lined by a layer of epithelium, usually of various types, but occasionally almost uniform throughout the tumor. The character of the epithelium may alter

PLATE XVI

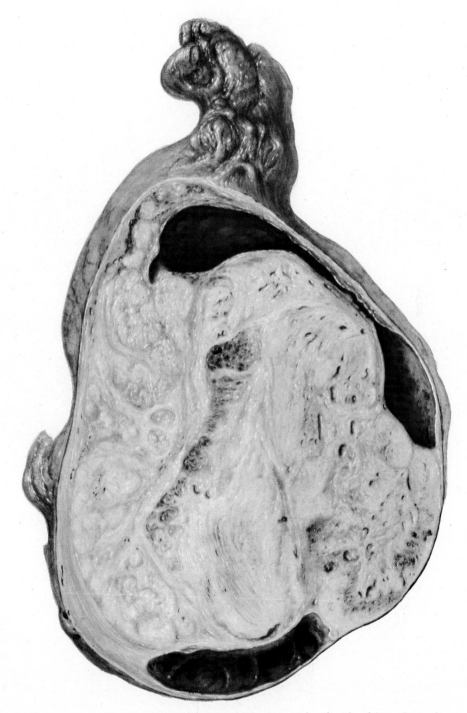

Malignant tumor of testis. The testis is completely destroyed and replaced by embryonal carcinomatous tissue, with necrosis and hemorrhage. Note the hydrocele accompanying the tumor. Large retroperitoneal masses were removed from this case. Death occurred in a few months from metastasis, although autopsy showed no recurrence at the site of the operation (B. U. I. 10,862; B. U. I. Path. 4420).

from point to point even in the same cyst. It may be a simple, rather undifferentiated cuboidal type, cylindric, or stratified. One may see small tubules, recalling embryonic renal tubules. Intestinal epithelium with goblet-cells is common (Fig. 456), also ciliated columnar epithelium, recalling the bronchi, especially where

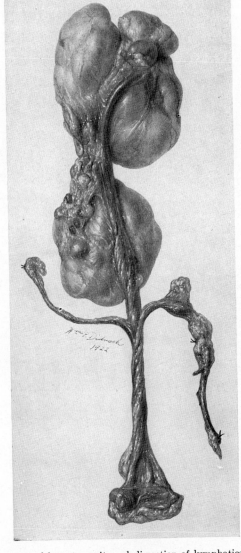

←Metastasis at level of
kidney pedicle.

←Metastasis along aorta.

Gland in pelvis.→

←Glands along iliac vessels

Spermatic vessels
and lymphatics.→

Point of section in groin.→

FIG. 454.—Specimen removed by extraperitoneal dissection of lymphatics and glands. The glands along the aorta formed a carcinomatous mass 4 cm. in diameter and 10 cm. long. Patient died six months later. (Same case as preceding picture.) B. U. I. 10,862.

it is in the neighborhood of cartilage. There may be areas suggestive of liver, pancreas, thyroid, salivary gland, etc. From the ectoderm there may be skin, with hairs (Fig. 457), sweat glands, and sebaceous glands, sometimes teeth. Nervous tissue may be represented by glia or nerve-cells.

The cysts vary greatly in shape. When greatly distended, they approach the

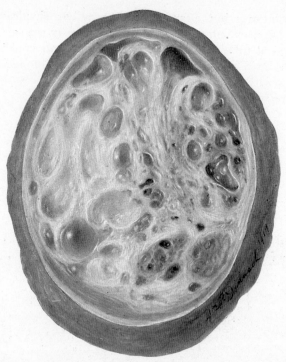

Fig. 455.—Specimen of malignant tumor of the testicle removed at operation. Microscopically this tumor is a cystic embryoma showing a great variety of different tissues from all three germinal layers. The retroperitoneal glands were also removed and the patient has remained entirely well for six years. B. U. I. 7666.

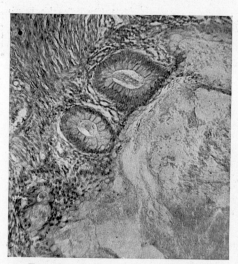

Fig. 456.—Embryoma of the testis which is apparently a true teratoma. The section shows a space lined by columnar epithelium consisting largely of goblet-cells, the space being filled with mucus. The resemblance to intestine is marked. B. U. I. Path. 4235.

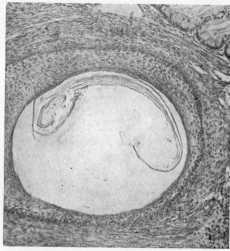

Fig. 457.—Teratomatous embryoma of the testis. In this section there are seen apparently intestinal epithelium like that in the preceding picture and also a typical hair follicle. B. U. I. Path. 4155.

spherical, but at other times they are irregular, elongated, or even multilocular. There may be also masses projecting into the lumina of the cysts, sometimes containing smaller cysts within them, and producing very complicated pictures. The cysts lined by intestinal mucosa contain mucus and are often surrounded by many small, gland-like structures opening into them, recalling the crypts of Lieberkühn.

Very rarely there may be a true dermoid cyst, within which the poles of the embryo can sometimes be identified. The rarity of this finding in the testis is in striking contrast to its comparative frequency in the ovary.

Malignant Degeneration of Embryomata.—Certain cases have been reported in which teratomata were apparently entirely benign. It is very exceptional, however, for malignant degeneration to be absent. The reason for this is not altogether clear. In a few cases a small tumor, stationary in size for years, has suddenly taken on rapid growth. We may suppose that this represents the beginning of the malignant change. In other cases no tumor is noted before rapid malignant growth begins. Probably the benign teratoma is small enough to escape

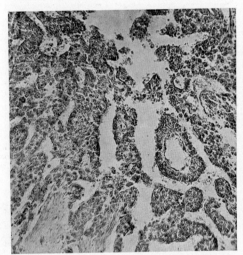

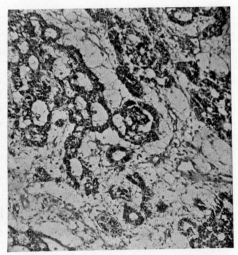

FIG. 458.—This section is from an embryoma (teratoma) of the testis. The portion shown has undergone malignant degeneration which has taken on a form known as the papillary type of embryonal carcinoma. B. U. I. Path. 2245.

FIG. 459.—Another type of embryonal carcinomatous degeneration. Here the tumor cells instead of being papillary are arranged around small lumina and are embedded in a very loose embryonic connective-tissue stroma. B. U. I. Path. 3418.

notice, even though later the purely teratomatous, undegenerated part of it may appear quite large. We may explain this increase in size by some alteration synchronous with the malignant degeneration, and leading to edema, myxomatous infiltration, and distention of the cysts. The malignant change itself is usually carcinomatous. Sarcomatous forms have been described, but are very rare; we have never seen one. The carcinoma is of embryonal type, and the common picture is that of cuboidal or low columnar cells lining innumerable small acini, or covering innumerable small papillæ (Figs, 458, 459). Both glandular and papillary forms may occur in the same case. There are also masses of cells, often containing spaces outlined by a definite palisade-like arrangement of cells. This arrangement, however, may be lacking, in which case the space takes on the appearance of a pseudo-acinus. The nuclei are ovoid, with plentiful chromatin and of medium size. They vary somewhat in size and shape, but giant nuclei are absent, and mitoses are not nearly as frequent as one would expect from the rapid growth. The connective-tissue stroma may be scanty, but, especially in the glandular form, is often abundant though very delicate and of embryonic type. Many proliferating capillaries are seen. Dense trabeculæ do not form. Necrosis is very marked and with it hemorrhage. Sometimes almost the entire tumor is necrotic, with only a thin layer of living cells around the edge.

In spite of the malignancy of these tumors, they are not invasive, and one does not see strands of tumor cells pushing into the tunica albuginea, epididymis, or the remains of the testis. The destruction of the testis apparently results from the pressure of the tumor within the tunica albuginea. In sections taken through the rete, the tubuli recti may be seen surrounded by masses of embryonal carcinoma, but not invaded by it; the edge abutting on the epididmyis is sharp, and there is no tendency to advance into this organ. Extensions to vas, seminal vesicle, or ejacu-

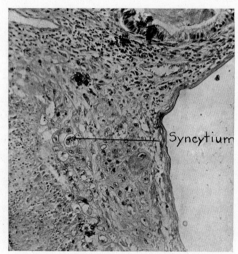

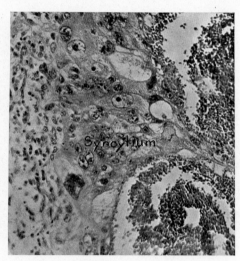

Fig. 460.—Teratomatous embryoma of the testis. In this picture there are seen apparently intestinal epithelium like that in the preceding pictures, a space lined by a very thin flat epithelium or endothelium and a third space filled with blood and lined by a syncytium, the nuclei of which show extreme variation in size and shape. This last picture is known as chorioma or chorio-epithelioma. B. U. I. Path. 4235.

Fig. 461.—Higher magnification of chorio-epithelioma. The character of the nuclei in the syncytium lining the blood spaces is well shown. B. U. I. Path. 4235.

latory ducts are never seen, though the cord may be infiltrated by intralymphatic growth.

When growing in solid acini, these tumor cells often seem to approach the type seen in seminoma, and occasionally one sees areas in a typical embryoma which are indistinguishable from seminoma. This gives reason for Ewing and others to believe that the cell-picture of seminoma represents only a special type of malignant degeneration of embryoma and to include it with "embryonal carcinoma." We prefer to leave this question unsettled. It is of little clinical importance, except for the fact that pure seminoma seems to metastasize a little slower and a little later than the typical malignant embryoma. The difference, however, is so slight that it permits of no distinction as to treatment.

A special form of malignant change is that known as *chorio-epithelioma* (syn-

PLATE XVII

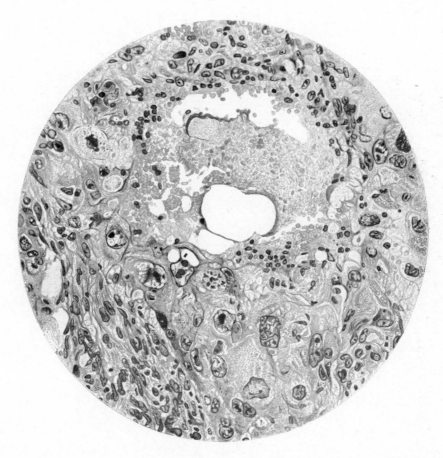

Microscopic drawing of chorio-epithelioma of testis. The syncytium, with its very large irregular nuclei, is shown in direct contact with a blood-filled space (B. U. I. Path. 4235).

cytioma, chorioma[1]). In it one sees tissues similar to those of the chorionic villi, namely, the deeper layer of polygonal cells, or Langhans cells, and the outer layer or syncytium (Figs. 460–462, and Plate XVII). This picture may make up almost the entire tumor, or, more commonly, occur only in a small area. The Langhans cells are polygonal, with ovoid vesicular nuclei and clear cytoplasm. They usually occur in nests near the syncytium, and are not especially striking or characteristic in appearance. The syncytium, however, is very striking. In a pink staining protoplasm are found numbers of nuclei which vary extremely in size, shape, and staining. Some of the large ones, which may be enormous, are almost devoid of chromatin. Mitotic figures may be seen. No cell boundaries can be made out. The syncytium retains its property of invading blood-vessels as do the chorionic villi. As a result one sees it attacking one aspect of a blood-vessel, or, if the process is further advanced and the vessel smaller, a rim of syncytium appears surrounding a blood-filled space. On account of this invasive property the cells of these tumors reach the blood-stream early, metastasis is rapid and extensive, and the chorio-epitheliomata are among the most malignant tumors known. It is probable that small chorio-epitheliomatous areas are somewhat more frequent than supposed. Cooke[2] in 1915 collected 47 cases from the literature.

In a series of 19 cases which we have studied microscopically at the Brady Urological Institute there were 2 showing chorio-epitheliomatous areas. In one case (B. U. I. 9151) a radical operation was done one month after the first appearance of the tumor, and in the other (B. U. I. 10,449) six months after rapid growth began in a tumor which had been present, but quiescent, for seven years. In both the retroperitoneal glands on the side of the testicular tumor were involved

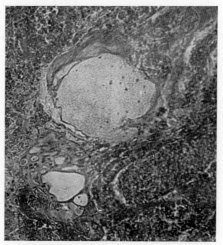

FIG. 462.—An example of chorio-epithelioma. This is a thick section and the structures do not show so well, but the syncytium lining the blood spaces can be seen. B. U. I. Path. 3663.

to an extent forbidding radical removal, as shown at operation. The first case received large doses of radium after the operation, but the metastases continued to grow and death occurred two years after operation. In the second case, the lungs, clear by x-ray before the operation, were studded with at least a hundred nodules from 1 to 2 cm. in diameter four weeks later, and cough, hemoptysis, and pleural pain ensued. Death occurred from asphyxia within a month.

Some cystic tumors in which the epithelial lining is everywhere simple and cuboidal or low columnar have been described, especially by Sakaguchi,[3] as tumors arising from the rete testis. There is considerable doubt about this interpretation, Chevassu feeling that every cystic tumor of the testis is embryomatous.

[1] Carey: Johns Hopkins Hospital Bulletin, 1902, xiii, 268–279, and Frank: Journal of the American Medical Association, 1906, lxvi, 248–256 and 343–350 (Lit.).

[2] Johns Hopkins Hospital Bulletin, 1915, xxvi, 215–221.

[3] Deutsche Zeitschrift für Chirurgie, 1913, cxxv, 294–372 (Lit.).

Occasionally a tumor is composed entirely of the embryonal carcinoma type of cells, and no trace of a pre-existing teratoma can be found. This may represent complete overgrowth and degeneration of the original tumor. Another possible explanation is discussed below.

Tumors in undescended testicles are of the same types as those found in the scrotum. They are, therefore, as stated above, smooth and rounded, usually ovoid. In the inguinal canal they may distend it and remain fixed in the abdominal wall, or project at either end, under the skin or in the peritoneal cavity. When the testis

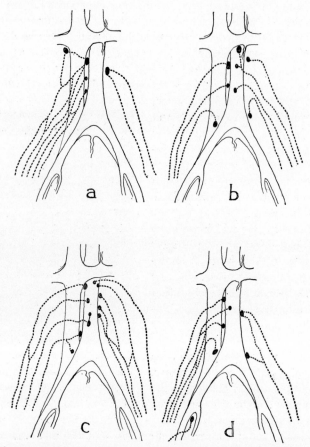

FIG. 463.—Diagram showing four different arrangements of the lymphatics from the testes. Note that those from the right testis pass in front of the vena cava and that lymphatics from either side may drain into nodes in the midline of the aorta, but do not cross to the other side. In *d* is shown a channel crossing the external iliac to drain into one of the external iliac nodes. This is not constant. The channel probably accompanies the vas deferens. Diagram taken from Jamieson and Dobson.

is intra-abdominal, the tumor usually develops a vascular pedicle, and is, therefore, movable. On account of this mobility, and of the fact that the pedicle may be attached anywhere from the pelvis to the renal vessels, there is nothing characteristic about the position of the tumor. It may be felt in the midline or at one side. Attachment to other organs is rare, but since the mass usually attains greater size before being noticed than when in the scrotum, pain and pressure symptoms are more apt to figure in the history.

It is a curious fact that the opposite testis may be atrophic. This occurred in

6 of our cases (25 per cent.) while in only 1 of the remainder was the opposite testis slightly larger than normal.

Metastases.—Most, Cunéo,[1] Jamieson and Dobson,[2] and others have studied the lymphatic drainage of the testicle. It is sharply delimited from that of the scrotum, the vessels passing up through the spermatic cord to terminate in various lymph-nodes which lie along the aorta from the level of the renal vessels to the bifurcation, and occasionally in the pelvis below the bifurcation of aorta and vena cava—nodes of the promontory (Fig. 463).

They vary a good deal in different subjects. They enter always the juxta-aortic nodes of the same side, often some of the pre-aortic or midline nodes, but only exceptionally do channels cross the midline to nodes lying slightly on the farther side (Fig. 464). Thus when dissecting out glands on the right side, in front of the vena cava, the operator may find glands in front of the aorta. The nodes draining the right testis are, in general, somewhat nearer the midline than those draining the left, in accordance with the courses of the respective spermatic veins. All of these nodes are quite small and inconspicuous when not the seat of disease. It is to these regional nodes that tumors of the testicle usually metastasize first, and it

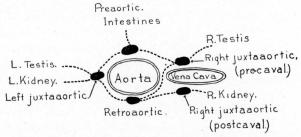

Fig. 464.—This diagram shows the division into groups of retroperitoneal lymph glands. Note that the right juxta-aortic group is divided into anterior and posterior parts by the vena cava. The retro-aortic and retrocaval nodes, however, seldom, if ever receive channels from the testis. Channels from the testes run mostly into the right or left juxta-aortic group, but may sometimes enter the preaortic group.

is for this reason that they are included in the dissection when radical operation is to be performed (Fig. 454). Retroperitoneal metastases may reach enormous size, so that all the other abdominal organs are compressed, the intestine obstructed, and respiration and cardiac action embarrassed. Invasion, however, is rare, even the kidney on the affected side escaping. Growth may occur, however, in the lymphatic vessels of the cord, giving a diffuse induration extending up through the inguinal ring. This is usually fairly late.

Metastasis to the regional lymph-nodes may occur very early, or late, but is usually early. There is no rule for this, and no way in which any prediction of metastasis can be made, except in case chorio-epitheliomatous degeneration is found. We may then feel fairly sure that early metastasis has occurred, and since it is by the blood-stream it is probably generalized. The spread of the disease may be arrested in the regional nodes for a long time. In one case (B. U. I. 10,342) the patient had extensive metastases at the time of admission. Before death the tumors distending the abdomen had a volume almost equal to that of the remainder of the emaciated patient, yet at autopsy not a single metastasis was found any-

[1] Delamère, Poirier, and Cunéo: The Lymphatics, 1904 (London, English translation).
[2] Lancet, 1910, i, 493–495.

where in the body except in the retroperitoneal nodes. In other cases, however, and probably more frequently, the barrier offered by these small nodes is weak, and propagation occurs by way of the thoracic duct, so that the left cervical glands and the lungs are next most commonly affected. Generalized metastasis occurs in the late stages. Metastasis or even extension may occur by way of the blood-vessels, but less commonly. The lungs again would be the point of election. Mac-Callum[1] describes a case in which an unusual form of myxomatous tumor resembling a hydatidiform mole had grown along the spermatic vein into the vena cava, renal veins, kidneys, right heart, etc.

The metastases are in the form of the malignant portion of the tumor, and usually present the same picture. There is perhaps more tendency to grow in solid nests or groups. We have seen a case (B. U. I. 11,522) in which the metastases, of typical embryonal carcinoma, were partially surrounded by a productive tissue reaction with epithelioid and giant cells resembling tuberculosis. Since this was seen only in contact with the tumor cells, it was not thought that it represented a second disease process. In the lungs there is the same tendency as elsewhere to necrosis and hemorrhage, so that hemoptysis is frequent. The large abdominal metastases also usually show softening.

Ordinarily the firm barrier of the tunica albuginea keeps the tumor away from the scrotal lymphatics, which drain into the inguinal nodes. After castration, however, local recurrence in the wound or in the stump of the spermatic cord may be observed, and metastasis to the inguinal nodes is then possible. Owing again to the tunica, extension to the skin and ulceration are rarities, unless the testis be imprudently incised.

Two of our cases are of especial interest in regard to metastasis. In the first (B. U. I. 5473), aged forty-one, the scrotal tumor was the first symptom noted. Castration was done nine months after the onset. Unfortunately the testis is not available, as this operation was done elsewhere before admission. A month after the operation pain and swelling of the abdomen began, accompanied ten weeks later by edema of the legs. Death occurred four months after operation and thirteen months after the onset. At autopsy, metastases in the lungs, liver, peritoneum, vena cava, left renal vein, and portal vein all showed typical embryonal carcinoma, both glandular and papillary. The retroperitoneal mass, however, was a cystic teratoma, of large size, containing hair, teeth, cartilage, etc., and only small areas of malignant degeneration.

The second case (B. U. I. 10,862) was in a man aged thirty-three. Pain and swelling in the scrotum were first noted following an injury. Nine months later radical operation was performed. A mass was found near the junction of the aorta and renal vein, and removed completely (Figs. 453, 454). Death occurred five months after operation, and fourteen months after the onset. At autopsy metastases in the lungs, liver, etc., showed typical embryonal carcinoma, both glandular and papillary. There was no local recurrence. The testicular tumor showed the same type of growth as that seen in the metastases, and a most careful search failed to reveal any cysts or other teratomatous elements. The mass removed from the aorta, however, was cystic, and showed microscopically the various elements of a true teratoma.

Cystic formations in metastases from teratoma have been described, but are

[1] Contributions to the Science of Medicine, by the pupils of William H. Welch, 1900, 497–510.

surely rare.[1] In the second case we would have to assume that the original testicular teratoma giving rise to the metastasis had entirely disappeared. The other possibility is that the retroperitoneal teratoma was primary, but that it had undergone malignant change, and been the source of retrograde metastasis to the testis before manifesting itself elsewhere. If the latter is the true explanation, the cases are of great interest, since we would always have to suspect a retroperitoneal origin for any testicular tumor, and castration alone in such a case would give no hope of cure.

Extension of tumors of other organs to the testis is rare. Occasionally it will be invaded and destroyed in an extensive epithelioma of the scrotum. Malignant tumors of the epididymis and spermatic cord are so rare as to be practically non-existent.

Metastases to the testis are rare, but may occur in any sort of tumor. It is said that they are not uncommon in melanoma, and 2 cases have been reported in epithelioma of the urethra. If the neoplasm is invasive, it will penetrate the tunica albuginea more readily than will the primary testicular tumors.

Case of metastasis to testis from carcinoma within abdomen.

In one of our cases (B. U. I. 7547) the patient, age sixty-six, was well until three weeks before admission. At this time he had a cold and sore throat, with constipation. Following catharsis he had urinary and fecal incontinence. One week before admission, there were suddenly severe pain and partial paralysis of the right leg, with numbness. After admission it appeared that he had noticed a small lump on the right testicle five months previously, which grew very slowly. There was atony of the bladder, with retention and paradoxic incontinence. Orchidectomy was done. While in the hospital there was projectile vomiting without nausea, the incontinence continued, and the patient became drowsy and mentally confused. He died at home six weeks later. The tumor mass involved only a part of the testicle, and had invaded the tunica albuginea sufficiently to produce a number of hard nodules projecting above the surface. Microscopically, it was composed of closely packed cells, with oval vesicular nuclei, arranged in small, indefinite alveoli separated by extremely fine connective-tissue trabeculæ—so fine that they were not apparent at first glance and the tumor appeared quite medullary. There was no lymphocytic infiltration. The testis had not been pushed aside, but was invaded, and remnants of spermatic tubules could be seen throughout the tumor mass. Atypical mitoses were frequent, and there was one area of necrosis. In view of this patient's other symptoms, it is possible, and we believe probable, that this testicular tumor represents a metastasis from a primary growth elsewhere. If it is not a metastasis it is a most unusual type of testicular neoplasm differing in almost all respects from any other we have seen described.

Another similar case follows: B. U. I. 12,201, age thirty-one. Past history negative. Three months before admission slight induration of the umbilicus was noted, to which the patient paid no attention. Four weeks before admission patient accidentally struck his left testis and noticed that it was swollen. Since this occurred immediately he did not attribute the swelling to the accident, but realized that it must have been present before the blow called his attention to it. During the four weeks it increased but slightly in size. On examination patient's general physical condition was excellent, general health in no way effected. There was a subcutaneous induration 2 cm. in diameter at the umbilicus. The left testis measured $2\frac{1}{2}$ x $1\frac{1}{2}$ inches, and was firm and quite tender. The surface was smooth except for a slight boss on the upper inner surface. The enlargement was confined to the testis, the epididymis, vas, and cord being palpable and normal. x-Ray examination showed a marked increase in the width of the mediastinal shadow. The diagnosis was malignant tumor, probably primary in the testis and probably with metastases. In view of the slight uncertainty which existed as to the nature of the mass at the umbilicus, operation was performed, castration being done, and the umbilicus being widely excised. Microscopic examination showed the testis extensively infiltrated with small, round tumor cells con-

[1] Ewing: Neoplastic Diseases, New York, 1922, p. 779; Sternberg: Verhandlungen der Deutschen Pathologischen Gesellschaft, 1904, vii, 105–107; and Hansemann, in the discussion following.

taining numerous mitoses, and which did not push the testis aside, but grew between the tubules, causing them to be widely separated. The subcutaneous tissue at the umbilicus was infiltrated with the same kind of cells. The diagnosis was then changed to malignant tumor of the round-cell sarcoma type, possibly lymphosarcoma. Metastatic nodules soon appeared on the scalp, skin of trunk, and in the opposite testis. x-Ray treatment had a very marked effect on these metastases, causing them to disappear entirely. Patient's general condition remained excellent. At last report, however, further metastatic nodules had appeared and the prognosis is undoubtedly bad. In this case there is much reason to believe that the tumor was not primary in the testis.

Epididymis, Spermatic Cord, and Tunica Vaginalis.—*Cystic tumors* of the epididymis are fairly common and are usually described as due to developmental errors. They are lined by epithelium and the contents usually, though not always, contains spermatozoa. These cysts are fully considered in the chapter on Malformations of the Urogenital Tract.

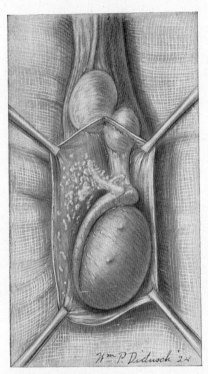

FIG. 465.—Fibroma of spermatic cord and tunica vaginalis, removed by excision. B. U. I. 12,901.

Solid tumors of the epididymis, cord, and testicular tunics, which are rare, are thoroughly taken up by Hinman and Gibson in a recent article[1] where the literature is reviewed.

Tumors of the *spermatic cord* are the commonest and, according to the above authors, account for 90 per cent. of the extratesticular tumors within the scrotum. The greatest number reported have been lipomata. One must distinguish between true lipoma of the cord, which develops from fat normally there, and the lipoma due to the projection through the relaxed inguinal ring of a mass of properitoneal fat. In the latter type the nodule of fat may contain at its center a hernial peritoneal process which, in turn, may contain intestine. Thus the careless amputation of such a lipoma may open the intestine. We have seen a number of such cases. Fibromata are the next most common tumor. They may arise at any point in the cord, but usually at the distal end, and may be in contact with the epididmyis (Fig. 465). In some cases they may be pushed through a relaxed inguinal canal into the abdomen, and when somewhat myxomatous may transmit light. They are usually distinct from the vas and the pampiniform plexus, and they are usually small, but may weigh as much as 1000 grams. Sarcomatous degeneration has been described. We have seen a case (B. U. I. 13,324) in which a firm rounded tumor 2 by $2\frac{1}{2}$ cm. lay in the lower part of the cord. The patient was a student twenty-nine years old. It was easily removed without damaging any other structure, and has not recurred. Microscopically it was a pure fibroma. Hinman and Gibson have collected 19 cases of dermoid cyst or cystic teratomatous tumors of the cord, all apparently benign.

[1] Archives of Surgery, 1924, viii, 100–137 (Lit.).

Other benign tumors of which only a very few cases are reported are myxoma, leiomyoma, and lymphangioma.

No malignant epithelial tumors are on record. Fonteneau in 1908[1] collected 33 cases of sarcoma of the cord, described as spindle-cell sarcoma, myxosarcoma, and fibrosarcoma. Faisant[2] reports a case of malignant teratoma.

In the epididymis a very few cases of lipoma, fibroma, myxoma, and leiomyoma are on record. Eisenstaedt[3] reports a case of fibromyoma, and another in which a tumor proved to be a granulomatous mass occurring as a foreign body reaction to a quantity of paraffin which had been previously injected into the tissues of the cord for some unknown reason.

Four cases of malignant neoplasms of the epididymis diagnosed carcinoma have been reported. Hinman's case showed an unusual picture and may have been an endothelioma. Sarcoma is somewhat commoner, with 10 cases on record. Teratoma may occur in the epididymis, and undergo malignant degeneration. In Ewing's case[4] there were areas of typical "seminoma," although the testis was in no way involved. This case serves Ewing as a strong argument against the origin of "seminoma" from the epithelium of the seminiferous tubules. In Hinman's case the tumor was a pure "seminoma," and the testis was not involved.

In the tunica vaginalis fibroma, lipoma, and rhabdomyoma have occurred. Cases of "adenoma" are reported, but one wonders whether they may not have been granulomata with foreign body phagocytes and giant-cells grouped about cholesterin crystals. We have seen such pictures where the resemblance to an adenomatous growth was at first sight marked. Of malignant growths only sarcoma is reported.

Fibromata may also arise from the tunica albuginea.

If any of these tumors become malignant, they metastasize like tumors of the testis proper to the retroperitoneal glands unless they involve the superficial scrotal tissues, when inguinal metastases may also occur.

Symptoms

Testis.—The symptomatology of testicular tumors is practically limited, in the early stages, to the local enlargement. This is practically always painless, the exceptions often being those cases where the tumor begins, or is first noted, after an injury. In a certain number of cases the tumor is present for a long period, during which it grows only very slowly or not at all. Rapid growth begins after an injury or for no apparent reason. When true malignancy sets in, the alarmingly rapid growth usually sends the patient to the physician fairly early. The small quiescent tumors, presumably benign teratomas, are usually neglected, even by intelligent patients. As we have seen, such a tumor, if found accidentally, should always be removed, since we never know when malignancy and rapid growth will set in. Every enlargement of the scrotal contents is worthy of careful study by the physician, and enlargement of either testicle or epididymis should be viewed with suspicion and, generally, operated upon.

The date of onset will usually be given by the patient as that when rapid growth

[1] Thèse de Bordeaux, 1908 (quoted by Hinman and Gibson).

[2] Lyon Médicale, 1905, cv, 378–380 (quoted by Hinman and Gibson).

[3] Surgery, Gynecology, and Obstetrics, 1923, xxxvii, 361–364.

[4] Neoplastic Diseases, New York, 1922.

began. It is safe to say, however, that, in cases giving a duration of symptoms of over one and one-half or two years, there has been a quiescent period at the beginning. In our series, the duration was as follows:

TABLE 123

DURATION OF SYMPTOMS

0–1 month....... 2 ⎫
1– 3 months..... 3 ⎬ 0–6 months...... 11—45.9 per cent. ⎫
3– 6 months..... 6 ⎭   ⎪
6– 9 months..... 2 ⎫   ⎬ 0–1 year.... 16—66.6 per cent.
9–12 months..... 3 ⎬ 6–12 months..... 5—20.8 per cent. ⎪
1– 2 years....... 3 ⎭   ⎭
2– 3 years....... 1
3– 5 years....... 1   Over 1 year.... 8—33.3 per cent.
5–10 years....... 3

In 1 case, duration seven years, beginning of rapid growth was noted six months before admission.

The initial symptom was as follows:

TABLE 124

	Cases.	Per cent.
Tumor...	23	95.8
Scrotal.............................	22	
Abdominal.........................	1 (undescended)	
Pain, testicular...................................	1	4.2

In the 1 case with initial pain there was injury and the tumor was noted shortly afterward.

At the time of admission symptoms were noted which are shown in Table 125, page 689.

It will be seen that *pain*, absent at first, is not uncommon later on. It is undoubtedly due to the distention of the tunics of the testis and resultant pressure. Loss of weight is also a fairly common symptom. It leads us to suspect that metastasis has occurred, but this is not always the case. Worry is no doubt a factor in the loss of sexual power. *Injury to the testicle* has been stressed by some writers as an important causative factor in testicular tumors. While 7 of our cases had received blows on the testis, one of these had occurred many years before, and the fact that in 70 per cent. there was no such history leads us to believe that usually the blow merely calls attention to a *mass* already present. Abdominal *metastases* may reach a good size before they produce a noticeable tumor, but in some few cases they become apparent before the testicular enlargement is noticed. In these cases we must think of the possibility of the abdominal tumor being primary. In such a case recently seen (not included in the series) a young man noticed some weakness and a "run-down" feeling, with indigestion, a sensation of fulness, and slight swelling of the abdomen. Examination showed extensive abdominal masses, and a moderate sized tumor in the testis which the patient had not noticed. No autopsy was performed. If both testes are in the scrotum, abdominal masses indicate an advanced and inoperable condition.

Interference by metastases with the circulation is indicated by edema of the legs or ascites, again late symptoms. Pressure on the nerves is rare, but there may

TABLE 125

	Cases.	Per cent.
Testicular tumor	24	100
Scrotal	23	
Abdominal	1 (undescended)	
Pain, scrotal	15	62.5
Radiation to groin and hip	3	
Pain, inguinal	2	8.3
Radiation to testis	1	
Pain, abdominal	4	16.6
Lower	1	
Upper	3	
Loin	2	
Pain on intercourse	1	4.2
Pain in leg	2	8.3
Loss of weight	10	41.7
Loss or decrease of sexual power	8	33.3
History of injury to testis	7	29.1
Abdominal tumor	3	12.5
(excluding the undescended testis)		
Edema of legs	2	8.3
Unilateral	1	
Bilateral	1	
Vomiting	2	8.3
Cough	1	4.2
Headache and vertigo	1	4.2
Weakness	1	4.2
Paresis of one leg	1	4.2
Incontinence	1	4.2
Frequency of urination	1	4.2

occasionally be pain or paralysis. Intestinal obstruction or hydronephrosis may occur in late stages. Cough may, of course, have no relation to the testicular tumor, but if cough, expectoration, hemoptysis, and pleural pain supervene in the presence of a testicular enlargement, pulmonary metastasis is strongly to be suspected.

When the testis is undescended, the tumor, of course, appears wherever the testis may be located. Since pain develops late, as in the scrotal cases, the tumor usually attains a considerable size before it is noticed. If directly in the inguinal canal, it may remain fixed in the abdominal wall. If near either end, it may project under the skin or in the peritoneal cavity. If the testis is intra-abdominal, the tumor may be noticed first, or may be ignored until pressure symptoms occur. These may be constipation, vomiting, edema of the legs, etc. In one of our cases (B. U. I. 10,069) there was an acute onset with headache, vertigo, vomiting, and weakness, at which time the patient first noticed a mass in the lower abdomen. Pain in this region began at the same time, and there was loss of 20 pounds in weight during the ensuing month.

The family history is of little importance. In our series only 3 (12.5 per cent.) gave a history of any family malignancy.

The course of the disease is progressive, and usually rapidly so. Sometimes, however, there may be periods of remission in which little if any growth seems to occur. The time of survival of those of our patients who died is shown in Table 126, page 690.

TABLE 126

PATIENTS DYING OF TUMOR OF THE TESTICLE. DURATION OF LIFE

After operation.				After onset.			
0–3 months... 2				1			
3–6 months... 7				1			
6–9 months... 0	0–1 year..... 11			1	0–1 year..... 5		
9–12 months.. 2				2			
1–1½ years.... 2				1			0–2 years 11
1½–2 years.... 2	1–2 years..... 4	0–2 years.... 15		5	1–2 years.... 6		
2–3 years..... 1				1			
3–5 years..... 0				3			
6 years....... 1				0			
7½ years...... 0				1			
12 years...... 0				1[1]			
Total....... 17				1			
				17			

One case, not operated on, with abdominal metastases present, was given x-ray treatment, and survived six months from onset.

[1] In this case, the tumor was small and quiescent for about six and a half years; the patient survived only nine months after rapid growth began.

It will be seen that 11, or about 64 per cent., of those dying lived one year or less after operation. Only one lived over three years. In this case (B. U. I. 2285) the scrotal enlargement was first noticed six years before operation, and death occurred six years after operation, a total duration of twelve years. Metastasis to the spine was demonstrated four years before death.

The average survival after onset, with no allowance for quiescent periods, treatment, or other life-lengthening factors, is only two years, seven months.

Recurrence, local or in the form of metastases, is usually early, but may be occasionally delayed for a long time. In one of Scott's cases it was noted seven years after castration. Mauclaire describes a recurrence "in the scar" eight years after operation. Chevassu comes to the conclusion that recurrence after the third year is very rare, and that, therefore, a four-year cure may be considered as practically definitive.

Epididymis, Spermatic Cord, and Tunica Vaginalis.—The symptoms of tumors of the epididmyis, spermatic cord, and tunica vaginalis are practically always confined to those arising from the local mass.

DIAGNOSIS

Testis.—Owing to the rapid course and bad prognosis of neoplasm of the testis early diagnosis is imperative if we are to expect favorable results, even from radical treatment.

The diagnosis depends principally upon *local palpation*. In the typical case the testis is symmetrically enlarged, so that in general terms the scrotal tumefaction is smooth and ovoid. On inspection the condition of the scrotal skin depends on the size of the tumor. After a certain size is reached, the skin becomes smooth and tensely stretched. Large veins may be seen through it. There is usually some slight redness, which in only a very few cases reaches a degree suggestive of inflammation. Edema of the subcutaneous tissue is rare, and so is ulceration. On palpating the spermatic cord, it is found to be normal or only slightly indurated. In a few late cases it may be enlarged and infiltrated with tumor growth. If the pulsations of the spermatic artery can be plainly felt, it indicates that the artery is enlarged, and points toward neoplasm. The vas is usually quite normal. The epididymis may usually be felt, and is normal except that in large tumors it is stretched out over the surface and appears longer, flatter, and more adherent than normal. Sometimes it is difficult to make out the epididymis on the surface of the huge tumor masses, particularly if the testicle is rotated. In very large growths the epididymis may be so attenuated that it is not palpable. Ordinarily, however, it affords the most valuable aid to diagnosis, as once it is outlined, one may be sure that the enlargement involves the testis proper. The tumefied testis itself is enlarged, ovoid, smooth. The size may vary from scarcely above normal to a foot in diameter. The consistence is usually firm, and uniformly so, due to the tension within the tunica albuginea. Occasionally one may make out fluctuating areas due to necrosis with liquefaction. Sometimes there are large bosses on the tumor, but seldom small, hard nodulations. The tumor has a heavy, solid feel, and does not transmit light. Chevassu describes cases of very myxomatous tumors which transmit light, but these are rare. The skin moves freely over the tumor, and there are no adhesions, ulcers, or sinuses.

The presence of *hydrocele* is the most frequent obstacle to thorough palpation, and since it is often present with tumor, makes the transmission of light of little importance. Heydenreich describes a case where the hydrocele accompanying a tumor contained 10 liters of fluid. Hydrocele, however, will not infrequently still allow palpation of the epididymis, so that we may rule out tuberculosis. In very doubtful cases it may be permissible to tap the hydrocele in order to palpate the testis. One should select a place where the wall is obviously thin and not attached to the testis, and keep the needle point away from it. It is better, however, not to tap at all, certainly not when no light is transmitted. If the hydrocele is not tense, it may be possible to make out the enlarged testis within it, and sometimes on transillumination one may see a shadow in one part of the hydrocele larger than any that could be cast by the normal testis. It is of no use to try to distinguish before operation the various types of testicular neoplasm. One caution should be observed: always palpate with the utmost gentleness to avoid forcing bits of tumor into the blood or lymph-channels.

The principal lesions which may give rise to confusion in neoplasm of the scrotal testis are syphilis, hydrocele, hematocele, spermatocele, and tuberculosis.

Gumma of the testis does not attain the large size of some tumors, but otherwise is often very difficult to distinguish. We have seen a gummatous testicle with a hydrocele covered by a very thick, hard sac, which was 4 by 5 inches in size. It is painless, firm, and spares the epididymis like neoplasm; is more apt to ulcerate than neoplasm, but this is usually late. A Wassermann test should always be done, but one must be cautious in drawing conclusions from it. If the Wassermann is negative, syphilis is probably not present. If the Wassermann is positive, tumor is not at all excluded, since it may occur in the syphilitic as in the non-syphilitic individual. A therapeutic test, including an intensive course of arsphenamin and potassium iodid, may be given, but should not be kept up for over a week if no diminution in the growth is observed. If doubt remains, operation should be performed without hesitation, since even if there is no tumor, the removal of a gummatous testis can do no harm.

Hydrocele also may be present with or without tumor. Its relationship with tumor has already been considered. In some cases without tumor it may be impossible to make a positive diagnosis. This is usually in tense hydroceles, with thickened walls or opaque contents which prevent the transmission of light. The thickening may be due to inflammation or hemorrhage. We have seen one case in which the inner surface of the tunica vaginalis was beset with a number of plaques about 5 mm. in thickness, composed of a granulomatous mass of cells, largely lymphocytic, and a number of foreign body giant-cells distributed about cholesterin crystals deposited through the mass. The fluid in the sac contained large quantities of the same crystals, making it opaque, and giving it a characteristic shimmering appearance like "eau-de-vie de Dantzig." Inflammation is especially apt to follow repeated tappings. Simple hydrocele often has an equatorial constriction seldom seen in the hydrocele of malignancy. Since operation is the treatment of choice in hydrocele, one will be able to see the testis and make a definite diagnosis. If for any reason paracentesis is substituted, one should never neglect to make the most careful palpation immediately after the fluid has been evacuated.

Hematocele produces a picture closely resembling neoplasm. As Sebileau and Descomps[1] justly remark, hematocele is much rarer than testicular tumor, so that in case of doubt, it is better from all points of view to make the diagnosis of cancer rather than hematocele. The differences in form, consistence, and surface characteristics do not allow of a distinction. The testis may be entirely lost in a hematocele—depending largely on the extent to which the tunica vaginalis surrounds the testis—and when this is the case the resemblance to neoplasm is close. If the tip of the globus major of the epididymis, or a paradidymal cyst, can be palpated and proves to be movable, it is evidence that the cavity of the tunica vaginalis is empty, and points toward tumor. Exploration alone makes the diagnosis certain.

Spermatocele is usually present in the form of a small movable cyst in or attached to the globus major of the epididymis, but sometimes it is indistinguishable from hydrocele, if large. Light is often not transmitted. Usually the tumor is small enough so that the testis can be palpated separately.

Tuberculosis seldom gives rise to confusion, and then only when the testis is extensively involved, and fused into one mass with the epididymis. Hinman reports a case of this kind, in which there was little tendency to caseation, and in which the mass resembled neoplasm even after removal and incision. A coexistent hydrocele may make the separation of the epididymis and testis by palpation difficult. Usually, however, the irregular, nodular character of the growth, most marked in the epididymis, is diagnostic. Rectal examination is of especial value in this connection. While testicular neoplasm never induces any change in the prostate or vesicles, tuberculosis of the epididmyis, as we have shown elsewhere, is, in a great majority of cases, associated with induration and irregularity of these organs. In fairly early stages tuberculosis (and also other infections) involves the epididymis, whereas tumors and gummata usually involve only the testis, even in late stages.

Scrotal elephantiasis should cause no confusion. The doughy consistence of the tumefaction and the thickening of the skin are characteristic.

General examination of the patient is undertaken with the view of discovering whether *metastases* are present. The spermatic cord should be palpated as far as

[1] Nouveau Traité de Chirurgie, par le Dentu et Delbet, vol. xxxii, Maladies des Organes Génitaux de l'Homme, Paris, 1916.

possible at the time the genital examination is done. By following the vas toward the testis one can usually locate the globus minor and then the rest of the epididymis. Palpation of the abdomen may show masses if the retroperitoneal involvement is great enough. These masses are fixed, not tender, smooth and rounded. Multiple bosses are sometimes observed. In late cases fluctuation may be made out. In early cases it is impossible to feel masses which may already be of considerable size, for example, 3 to 5 cm. in diameter. It is possible that the x-ray in conjunction with pneumoperitoneum might be useful here. This lack in our diagnostic procedures emphasizes the importance of the radical operation. Hinman reports a four-year cure in a case where good sized masses were removed from the retroperitoneal area.

Since generalized metastases have no special affinity for bone, it is only in the chest that the x-ray is usually of assistance (Fig. 466). *Multiple tumor nodules in the lungs in a man below forty-five are almost pathognomonic of testicular neoplasm.*

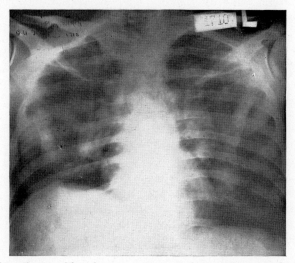

Fig. 466.—Chest plate of case with pulmonary metastases from malignant embryoma of testis. B. U. I. x-Ray 1710.

This fact is of importance when the testis is undescended. Metastases in the skin, cervical lymph-nodes, etc., will be apparent.

Where diagnosis is impossible without *exploration*, there should be no delay. If the testis is the seat of a tumefaction, the cord should be at once clamped, ligated, divided with a cautery, and the mass removed and sectioned. The examination should be thorough, and facilities for a frozen section should be at hand. We have seen a case in which a longitudinal incision, made in the operating room, showed a smooth, perfectly homogeneous surface and the lesion was thought to be a neoplasm. Subsequent cuts showed the testis to be riddled with the typical serpiginous caseated areas of gumma; by a curious coincidence the first cut had just avoided all of them.

Neoplasm of the Undescended Testis.—The most important sign in this condition is the absence of a testis from the scrotum. If this is so, and there is a tumor in the abdomen, testicular neoplasm must always be suspected. If the abdominal tumor is smooth, rounded, not tender, and mobile, the suspicion becomes almost a certainty. The position of the tumor is not characteristic. In our case (B. U. I. 10,069) it was in the midline, ovoid, about 8 inches in long diameter, which lay parallel to the long axis of the body, and resembled exactly in position and shape a greatly distended bladder. In this case the cord was probably somewhat prolapsed into the inguinal canal, as a very small, indefinite mass, which the patient said gave a testicular feel, could be palpated in the uppermost part of the scrotum. There was, therefore, the possibility of an atropic testis. The vascular pedicle (spermatic vessels) was later found to be attached close to the internal inguinal ring.

Renal tumors are ruled out by cystoscopic examination and pyelography. In the case of any tumor, laparotomy is always indicated, at which time the exact diagnosis will appear. Retroperitoneal tumors are fixed and usually located high up.

If the testicular ectopia is inguinal, the mass may resemble an incarcerated hernia. Here again the empty scrotum assists us. The history and manner of onset will give clues, with steady increase in size and in favor of neoplasm.

One should remember that undescended testes may also be the seat of gumma and tuberculosis.

Spermatic Cord, Epididymis, and Tunica Vaginalis.—The diagnosis of tumors of the cord and epididymis is difficult, since they are usually mistaken for more common lesions such as hydrocele or spermatocele. If in the upper part of the cord, they may simulate hernia closely, even to being reducible into the abdomen. Tuberculosis and syphilis (gumma) may rarely cause masses in this region. Careful local examination will usually disclose, if the tumor is not too large, whether it is solid or cystic, whether it extends into the inguinal canal, and whether it is joined to the vas deferens, pampiniform plexus, or epididymis. Epididymal tumors are usually mistaken for tuberculous epididymitis. The final diagnosis usually remains to be made at the time of operation, when the same careful search for malignancy should be carried out as in the case of tumors of the testis.

TREATMENT

Testis.—The treatment of tumors of the testis is not very satisfactory, as can be seen by reference to Tables 127–131. Since practically all tumors of the testis are malignant, the mode of treatment has to be based on this assumption, since one is seldom, if ever, able to say that a given tumor is surely benign.

The different methods of treatment that have been proposed are: Castration, radical operation, radiant treatment with radium or x-ray, and the injection of such substances as Beebe's autolysin, Coley's serum, etc. We feel strongly that in any disease as serious and fatal as these malignant tumors of the testis are, one should leave no stone unturned in the effort to secure a good result. For this reason we believe that a radical operation should be done whenever possible and as early as possible, provided no distant metastasis can be demonstrated. This conclusion is fortified by our observation of certain fatal cases in which, although the tumor growth was very extensive, it had extended nowhere beyond the regional lymph area. It is undoubtedly true that in some such cases there is a definite period during which metastases are present in the retroperitoneal glands, but have not yet reached any other part of the body, when the radical operation will effect a cure which could not be accomplished by castration alone. On the other hand, it is equally true that sometimes latent metastases, which are not demonstrable, already exist before operation, and any form of treatment is practically hopeless. In one such case the radical operation was successful and complete, and at the time of autopsy, several months later, while most of the organs of the body contained metastases, there was no recurrence whatever at the site of the operation.

The *radical operation* for tumor of the testis involves the removal of the testis, epididymis, most of the vas deferens, spermatic cord, spermatic vessels, retroperitoneal lymph-nodes on the affected side from the brim of the pelvis to the renal vessels, and the connective tissue, fat, etc., surrounding these structures and carrying the lymphatic channels. One approaches the retroperitoneal area extraperitoneally, rolling the peritoneum, with its contents, forward, and obtaining in this way an excellent exposure, including the aorta and vena cava. This operation is fully described in Chapter XIX. In view of the magnitude of the operation, it is extraordinary how little shock is involved, how low the operative mortality, and how readily the patients usually recover. The results of our series of 8 cases are given in Table 129.

Castration, according to our view, should be reserved for those cases where the general condition of the patient does not permit radical operation, or for very advanced cases with ulcerating growths which demand palliative treatment.

Treatment with radium and x-ray has not been particularly successful in malignant tumors of the testis. We do not feel that there is, as yet, sufficient justification for substituting radiant therapy for operative treatment. Postoperative radiation may, however, be carried out with the idea of doing everything possible to improve the bad prognosis in these cases. Radium will undoubtedly cause regression of the tumor masses for a time in some cases, but we have never observed a permanent effect.

Incision or puncture of malignant testicular tumors should be avoided at all costs.

Spermatic Cord, Epididymis, and Tunica Vaginalis.—The treatment of tumors of these organs is usually by simple excision, since they, in contradistinction to tumors of the testis itself, are but seldom malignant. If the cyst or tumor involves the epididymis extensively, it is usually advisable to perform epididymectomy, since simple removal of the tumor would undoubtedly destroy the function of the epididymis. In addition, if even a small part of the wall of cystic tumors is left in place, there may be recurrence. When the tumor, however, is pedunculated or definitely demarcated from the unaffected portion of the epididymis, it may be removed by simple excision or resection without epididymectomy.

Tumors of the tunica vaginalis can practically always be removed by simple excision. The remains of the tunica vaginalis are usually sewed back as in the operation for hydrocele. In operating upon tumors of the spermatic cord the principal precaution to observe is to dissect them out with great care to preserve the blood-supply of the testis.

Tables 127 and 128, page 696, give the clinical data and results in 117 cases of tumor of the testicle at the Johns Hopkins Hospital.

TABLE 127

ANALYSIS OF 117 CASES OF TUMOR OF TESTIS

Number of cases from literature and Johns Hopkins Hospital records...... 117
Number of cases in undescended testicle............................... 18, or 15 per cent.
Left testis involved.. 49, or 41.8 per cent.
Right testis involved.. 58, or 49.5 per cent.
Side of primary growth not given..................................... 10
Average age at onset... 35 years
Oldest age at onset.. 64 years
Youngest age at onset.. 20 months
Swelling alone the initial symptom................................... 79, or 67.5 per cent.
Swelling and pain the initial symptoms............................... 14, or 12 per cent.
Initial sign or symptom not given.................................... 24
Number of cases operated upon.. 108
Average duration before operation.................................... 12 months
Number of radical operations reported................................ 12
Abdominal metastasis occurred in..................................... 66 cases
In 30 cases average time after operation before recurrence or abdominal
    metastasis... 7.3 months
Number of cases well one year or more after operation................ 15, or 13.5 per cent.

TABLE 128

ANALYSIS OF CASES OF PATIENTS LIVING OVER ONE YEAR

Number of years well.	Number of cases.	Operation.
11	1	Castration
8	1	Castration
7	1	Castration
6	2	Castration / Radical
5	3	Radical / Radical / Castration
4	1	Castration
3½	1	Radical
3	2	Castration / Castration
2	1	Castration
1	2	Castration / Radical

The following tables show the results in our series of 25 cases of tumor of the testis at the Brady Urological Institute:

TABLE 129

Radical Operation, 8 Cases

B. U. I.			Pathologic findings.	Result.	Metastases.
4106	H.		No metastasis found.	Dead in 1 year.	Metastases in abdomen.
9142	L.		"Apparently metastasis" sections lost.	L. and W. 9 years.	
7666	C.		No metastases found.	L. and W. 4½ years.	
9151	M.		Metastasis + at renal vein. Large.	Dead in 2 years.	Metastasis abdomen, lung.
10,449	S.		Metastasis + at renal vein, large, not removed.	Dead in 3 months.	Metastasis lungs.
10,862	F.		Teratoma, retroperitoneal.	Dead in 5 months.	Metastasis, lungs, liver, etc.
11,522	M.		Small metastasis +.	L. and W. 1 year.	
11,062	M.		Metastasis (?) at promontory. None in section.	L. and W. 1 year.	
Total....... 8			Metastasis 5; none 3.	L. and W. 4 (9, 4½, 1, 1 years), 50 per cent. Dead, 4, 50 per cent. Of living, 3 apparently had regional metastasis, 1 did not. Of dead, 3 apparently had regional metastasis, 1 did not.	

TABLE 130

Castration, 16 Cases

B. U. I.			Result.	Metastases.
641	P.		Dead, 1 year, 9 months.	Metastases, abdomen.
2052	Y.		L. and W., 11 years, 9 months.	
2285	M.		Dead, 6 years.	Metastasis to spine.
4750	T.		Dead, 3 weeks.	Embolus (?) metastasis abdomen.
5473	D.		Dead, 4 months.	Metastasis (?)—teratoma—retroperitoneal.
7547	W.		Dead, 1½ months.	Metastasis, cerebral (?).
7589	G.		Dead, 5 months.	"Recurrence" local (?) abdominal (?)
8032	D.		Dead, 1½ years.	Local recurrence.
8447	L.		Dead, 10 months.	Metastasis lungs, liver, abdomen.
8577	P.		Dead, 1 year, 3 months.	Metastases lungs.
9517	S.		Dead, 3 months.	Metastases, abdomen.
10,069	S.		L. and W., 1 year, 10 months.	(Undescended).
10,320	W.		Dead, 4 months.	After intestinal operation, no metastases found.
10,342	J.		Dead, 10 months.	Metastases, abdominal.
10,623	H.		Dead, 5 months.	?
11,609	H.		L. and W., 2 years, 6 months.	
11,646	X.		L. and W., 6 months.	None found, probably benign tumor.
Total....... 17			L. and W., 4 (11¾, 2½, 1¾ years, 6 months), 23.5 per cent. Dead 13, 81 per cent. 12 died of metastasis or recurrence, 1 of intercurrent disease 4 months after operation, no metastasis found. Only one patient, who lived 11 years, may be said to be cured by the operation of castration.	

Other treatment was given as follows:

TABLE 131

POSTOPERATIVE TREATMENT

	Castration.			Radical.			No operation.		
	Dead.	Living.	Total.	Dead.	Living.	Total.	Dead.	Living.	Total.
x-Ray................	2	0	2	1	1	2	1	0	1
Radium..............	3	1	4	2	0	2	0	0	0
x-Ray and radium.....	2	0	2	0	0	0	0	0	0
Beebe's autolysin......	0	0	0	1	0	1	0	0	0
Total..............	7	1	8	4	1	5	1	0	1

NEOPLASMS OF THE PENIS AND SCROTUM

PATHOLOGY

Penis.—The penis may be the site of any of the various skin diseases, and some of these may produce masses simulating tumors. Nodules may occur on the penis in multiple neurofibromatosis (Von Recklinghausen's disease).

BENIGN TUMORS.—*Cysts* of various kinds are seen. Ordinary sebaceous cysts (wens), single or multiple, are occasionally found under the skin. Mucous cysts, lined with mucous membrane, are found at various points, and are probably derived from urethral glands. A rather specialized kind occurs in connection with the preputial cavity, due to imperfect splitting of the preputial process in the embryo. They are commonest near the frenum, and are usually seen in infants. Further details are given in the chapter on Malformations of the Urogenital Tract. True dermoid cysts occur, although rare. They are usually found at some point along the raphé.

Lipomata, myomata, and *fibromata* are rare.

Vascular tumors are occasionally seen. Aneurysm of a penile vessel may occur. *Venous varices* in a slightly developed form are common, but in only a few reported instances have they been large enough to give any trouble. They are usually *in the prepuce* or *on the dorsum of the shaft,* but may involve the glans. There is a legend that enlarged veins of the penis prevent perfect erection by receiving all the blood, but there is little evidence in favor of this view. Reclus[1] removed such a varix to improve erections. Lymph varices are rare, and usually occur near the coronary sulcus on the dorsal surface—the point where the dorsal lymphatic channels begin.

Cavernous hemangiomata are rare, and are usually seen on the glans or at the meatus. Kroll[2] reports a case in which the tumor involved one-half the glans and 2 cm. of the urethra, and gave rise to profuse hemorrhage. The appearance, as described, recalls that of some of the vascular caruncles seen in women. Microscopically, the picture was typical of hemangioma. Where in contact with erectile tissue, no direct connection was apparent, but there was no fibrous capsule.

[1] Quoted by Legueu and Michon, Maladies de la vessie et du penis, Nouveau Traité de Chirurgie, Le Dentu and Delbet, Paris, 1912, xxx, 312.

[2] Medizinische Klinik, 1922, xvii (i), 564–566.

In a case seen by us (B. U. I. 7829) the hemangioma was very extensive, involving also the scrotum and internal surfaces of the thighs, and extending deep into the femoral muscles. The scrotal and penile masses, and superficial portions of those on the legs were removed, but it was impossible to reach the deeper extensions (Figs. 467–470).

In regard to warts (verrucæ) and papillomata the same remarks apply as in the case of the urethra (q. v.). Most of these growths occur in individuals with phimosis, or with long foreskins which are seldom retracted for purposes of cleanliness. Since inflammation is an important factor, we have the same confusion with polypoid or condylomatous excrescences which may simulate or precede true

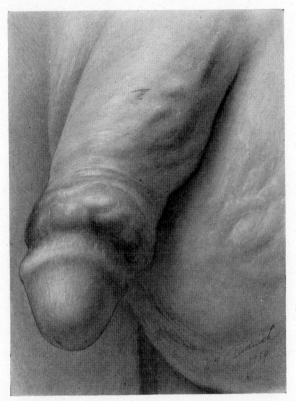

Fig. 467.—Extensive hemangioma of penis and scrotum. B. U. I. 7829.

epithelial new growths. Indeed, there is little to be said concerning the gross appearances of these lesions which is very helpful. Only when definite papillæ of goodly length, or perhaps branched, can be isolated, is the diagnosis of papilloma certain.

Under the microscope, however, we are on firmer ground, and here the papilliform structure should not be mistaken. The papillæ are covered with a stratified epithelium, usually with horny layer (Fig. 472), but this may be absent, due to maceration.

The epithelial overgrowth may assume this papillary form, with little change below the original skin level, or it may consist of a hypertrophy of the normal dermal papillæ, with increase in size, and marked enlargement and lengthening of the interpapillary processes. This is the picture of the true wart, and it may be combined with that of a more definitely papillomatous process. While there is usually an accompanying mononuclear infiltration of the subjacent tissues, the connective-tissue reaction is much in the background compared with the condylomata. Not infrequently, with closely packed papillæ and large masses of epithelial cells dipping down between the papillæ, these "papillary warts" present a bizarre picture, where it is easy to imagine a malignant change beginning. This transition will be discussed further in the succeeding paragraphs.

These benign epithelial growths may spread until they cover large areas. In extreme cases they spring from the entire glans and inner surface of the prepuce,

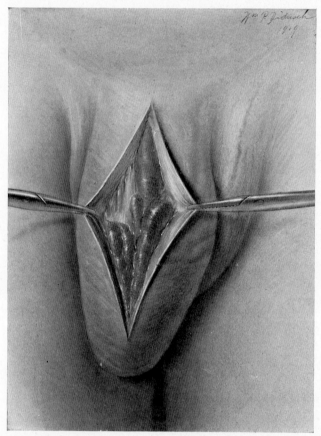

FIG. 468.—Hemangioma of penis and scrotum. Preliminary exposure of tumor. B. U. I. 7829.

producing a large cauliflower-like mass. The usual point of origin is in or near the coronary sulcus. There may be associated growths of similar nature in the fossa navicularis or pendulous urethra. Only rarely do these lesions occur in those of cleanly habits, or where a successful circumcision has been done.

In a small number of these warty epithelial growths the keratinization is much increased, so that a true cutaneous horn is produced. Such horns are usually located on the glans, and may be single or multiple. If the horn is removed without excising the skin the horn-forming tendency persists in the underlying growth, and it is re-formed. Malignant changes may occur in these horny warts, but they may remain benign for long periods. We have seen a case (B. U. I. 2551) in which there were two horns, symmetrically placed one on each side of the meatus.

MALIGNANT TUMORS.—Malignant neoplasms of the penis include carcinoma (epithelioma) and sarcoma, a small number of cases described as "endothelioma" and "melanoma," the nature of which is not altogether certain, and a very few cases of teratoma.

Carcinoma is by far the most frequent, and among the cases studied personally and in the literature, we have found no cases not properly designated as epithelioma. Indeed, the common cancer of the penis is identical with cutaneous epithelioma

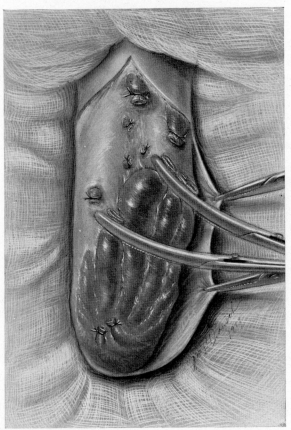

FIG. 469.—Hemangioma of penis and scrotum. Ligation and excision of hemangioma. B. U. I. 7829.

as found elsewhere on the body, and cannot be said to have any specific characteristics of its own.

Carcinoma of the penis is commonly stated to account for from 1 to 3 per cent. of all malignant tumors, but this estimate seems to us too high. It is based on the figures of Paget, von Winiwarter, and Billroth, dating from a period when fewer malignant growths were recognized than at present. Andrews[1] found 0.79 per cent. of carcinoma of the penis among 7881 malignant tumors. In the Brady Urological Institute series there are 35 carcinomata of the penis among 12,500 urologic cases. During the same period about 500 vesical neoplasms and about 600 car-

[1] Quoted by Barney, Massachusetts General Hospital Publications, 1908, ii, 275–305.

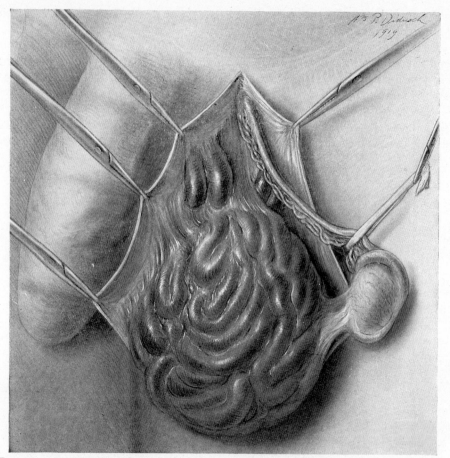

Fig. 470.—Hemangioma of scrotum. Separation of tumor from testicle and cord. B. U. I. 7829.

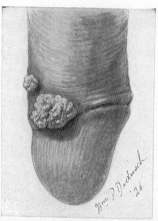

Fig. 471.—Benign papillomata or venereal warts in the coronary sulcus. In this case the growths are larger than usually seen.

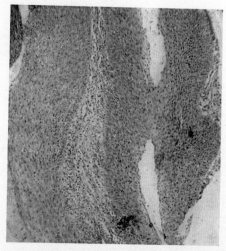

Fig. 472.—Benign papilloma of the penis. This section is from a case of many years standing which showed elsewhere beginning malignant changes. B. U. I. Path. 4128.

cinomata of the prostate were seen, and even malignant tumors of the kidney were more numerous (43 cases).

Epithelioma of the penis is quite precocious, and many cases occur before the "cancer age." Kaufmann,[1] in a series of 227 cases, found it most frequent in the sixth decade (50–60). In Küttner's collection of 562 cases, Barney's series of 100 cases, Schreiner and Kress[2] series of 18 cases, and our series of 35 cases the ages are as follows:

TABLE 132

Age.	B. U. I.		Age.	Barney.	Schreiner and Kress.	Küttner.
25–30.........	1	1	21–30	1	1	24
31–35......... 36–40.........	4⎱ 2⎰	6	31–40	14	2	51
41–45......... 46–50.........	8⎱ 4⎰	12	41–50	25	5	131
51–55......... 56–60.........	4⎱ 5⎰	9	51–60	20	5	169
61–65......... 66–70.........	1⎱ 3⎰	4	61–70	24	4	124
71–75......... 76–80.........	0⎱ 2⎰	2	71–80	13	1	58
?.............	1	1	81–90	3		
Totals......		35	..	100	18	562
Average age.......... 47.6			..	56.02		

While our shorter series seems to show an earlier age incidence than any of the older series, which is probably accidental, yet it is evident from all statistics that many cases are seen under forty.

A great many antecedent circumstances have been discussed as causative factors in carcinoma of the penis. Chief among them are phimosis, chronic urethral discharges, ulcers or scars of previous ulcers, papillomata of the glans, trauma, and contact with malignant growths in the vulva, vagina, or cervix of the conjugal partner. It is very difficult to evaluate properly the importance of these factors.

Phimosis is generally considered as predisposing to carcinoma. All writers remark upon the freedom of circumcised Jews and Mohammedans from the disease, Küttner[3] alone presenting evidence to the contrary. He learned by correspondence with Djemil Pasha of the Military Medical School at Constantinople that in five years 4 operations had been carried out there for carcinoma of the penis in Mohammedans. Djemil further stated that in two series of 100 genital operations, there were 3 carcinomata of the penis in the circumcised group and only 2 in the uncircumcised group. It is conceivable, from these figures, that Jews enjoy a racial immunity, and that early circumcision may have no effect whatever in preventing cancer of the penis. Barney, Demarquay, and others have noted a very high proportion of phimosis among the cases of cancer they have studied. Schreiner and Kress found a history of phimosis in only 1 of their 18 cases. In our series of 35 cases phimosis had been present at some time in 16, but this statement must

[1] Deutsche Chirurgie, 1886, l, a.

[2] Journal of Radiology, 1921, ii, No. 9, 31–39.

[3] Beiträge zur Klinischen Chirurgie, 1900, xxvi, 1–79.

be qualified. In at least 3 of these circumcision had been performed many years before, in 1 case thirty-four years. In some others—the exact number cannot be given—the phimosis had developed as a result of induration or edema due to the cancerous growth. We may conclude then that an unretractable or adherent prepuce should be removed—the prophylaxis of cancer being only one of the reasons therefor—but that circumcision does not necessarily prevent cancer. Some of the circumcisions followed by cancer may have been incomplete, but it is impossible to give statistics on this point.

Chronic urethral discharges undoubtedly increase the irritation in case of phimosis, but otherwise are of little moment. No investigator has found a relationship between a history of gonorrhea and the development of cancer. In our series of 35, 18 had had gonorrhea, and the remainder denied it.

A number of cases is reported in which the cancer began in the scar of an old healed venereal or traumatic ulcer. In 2 of our cases this history is definite, and Barney describes 2 similar cases. Where ulcers are in existence at the time the cancer begins, we are usually unable to state the exact date of the inception of malignant growth. There are undoubtedly cases where an ulcer has existed for many years before there was any evidence of cancer. One of our cases falls in this class, and will be discussed fully in a subsequent paragraph.

The long-continued presence of papillomata or polypoid vegetations undoubtedly predisposes to cancer, as we shall see that microscopically all stages of beginning malignancy can be found in these growths. This change is so common and has been so frequently reported that no extensive discussion is necessary at this point.

Trauma plays a small rôle in the reported cases of penile carcinoma excepting possibly that associated with circumcision. Küttner reports a cancer occurring in the scar of a crushing injury to the glans sustained in childhood. In many cases (4 in our series) the wound of a circumcision operation has failed to heal and has ultimately become frankly carcinomatous. It should be remembered, however, that many of these cases are circumcised comparatively late in life, and we may presume that often something—a mass, an increased discharge, tenderness, etc., has decided the patient to submit to the operation, and that, therefore, not infrequently the cancer is already present at the time the circumcision is done. This was true in at least 2 of our 4 cases with this history.

It is also impossible to attach much importance to contact with malignant growths of the female genitalia, although it is true that this history was present in 1 of our cases. Barney found only 9 cases in the entire literature in which there was a question of contagion, while there are constantly many examples of its failure to take place.

In one family in which the wife had carcinoma of the uterus, with a purulent discharge, the husband had a marked chronic urethritis with the staphylococcus present in large numbers, but no tumor.

Epithelioma of the penis bears a definite relationship to pre-existing benign lesions. It is impossible in many cases to say just what this is, as the history may be deficient, and the tumor seen only in an advanced stage. Where a good history is obtained, however, in cases where a retractible prepuce has enabled the patient to see the original lesion, we find that it begins, (1) as a wart-like excrescence; (2) as a flat, plaque-like, often ulcerated growth, or (3) as a very superficial, weeping erosion. The wart-like excrescence may be single or, less often, multiple, or in the form of a papillary outgrowth. In a few cases the tendency is entirely to grow outward, producing a cauliflower-like mass with no induration at its base, in others very little projects above the surface, while a deep induration is present from the beginning. Most cases show combinations of these two tendencies, recalling the picture in infiltrating papillary carcinoma of the bladder. The gross appearance results from these tendencies, with the addition of ulceration which is common in all epitheliomata.

The flat, plaque-like growth, when seen in an early stage, may not be ulcerated, and is often whitish, with some desquamation. Schuchardt spoke of this as "psoriasis preputialis." We have seen a flat growth which was not white, but reddened, with an irregular surface and only small, very superficial erosions. Under the microscope one saw the epithelium growing downward in long, irregular strands, in many of which small epithelial pearls had formed. The basement membrane was lacking at some points. Surrounding the neoplastic cells everywhere was an intense round-cell infiltration. Much importance probably attaches to this infiltration, as, according to Murphy, it represents the active efforts of the body to combat the cancerous growth. Some pathologists feel that when the epithelial cells have nowhere passed beyond the zone of lymphatic infiltration, we are justified in speaking of the lesion as a "precancerous" one, and in believing that no metastasis has as yet taken place. The picture here described is good evidence that epithelioma often begins without wart or other projecting lesion.

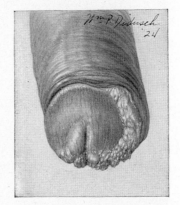

FIG. 473.—Papilloma of the penis. The papillæ shown here are of the benign type, but at the base of the lesion malignant changes were found by the microscope after removal. B. U. I. Path. 4128. (See Fig. 472.)

The erosions, excoriations, or raw patches are possibly early stages of the above process. Too few have been seen to allow any statement as to the amount of induration present, and we have no sections of them.

The site of the primary lesion may be on the glans or on the inner surface of the prepuce, the relative frequency being about equal for each. Other sites are very rare. In advanced growths both glans and prepuce are usually involved, so that it is impossible to tell where the growth started.

The appearance of the established tumor depends on the tendency toward outward growth. Usually this is well marked, so that cauliflower-like masses of various sizes are produced. The surface is sometimes well preserved, but more often ulceration is present, frequently a crater-like central excavation. The appearance varies from time to time as new growth or necrosis has the upper hand. In some cases the edge is not lobulated, but slightly elevated and very hard; the base of the ulcer is also hard. In early growths induration may be slight, and the edge not more raised than in a chancre or other genital ulcer, as that the diagnosis is difficult. As the process advances, proliferation may constantly produce new fungating masses, but necrosis eventually overtakes them all, so that the penis is gradually destroyed as the tumor creeps nearer its base.

Microscopically, the growths present the typical picture of epithelioma, with

VOL. I—45

irregular, invasive strands of neoplastic cells pushing in all directions. When cut across, these strands appear as rounded nests of cells. In some cases epidermization is marked, the inner cells of the strand large, hydropic, with pyknotic nuclei and intercellular fibrillæ, while here and there are epithelial pearls (Fig. 474), into the center of which the keratinized epidermal cells are desquamated. These pearls may be very large and resemble small dermoid cysts. This picture is known as *squamous-cell* epithelioma or epidermoid carcinoma. In other cases the pearl formation is abortive and the desquamated cells show only granular degeneration and no epidermization. This is an intermediate form. Still other cases show no pearl formation whatever, all the cells resembling those of the basal layer of the skin. This is known as *basal-cell* epithelioma (Fig. 475). It is doubtful whether there is anything very specific about these distinctions, as we have seen cases in which the penile growth was apparently basal-celled, while the inguinal metastases were of the squamous type. If sections are taken at the edge of the ulcer, one may see the transition between normal skin and the cancerous growth (Fig. 475). In only a few cases is definite papillary structure observed projecting above the skin level, but when present there is fusion of the papillæ and invasion of the pedicles as in other papillary carcinomata. In the depths, however the appearance is no different from that of the non-papillary epithelioma. One cannot, therefore, tell by observing the type of cell in a tumor whether it has the tendency to form papillæ and push out above the surface or not. We have never personally observed a basal-cell epithelioma of the penis which was papillary.

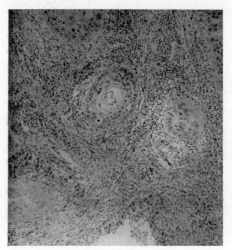

Fig. 474.—Typical picture of squamous-celled epithelioma of the penis. In this case the masses of tumor cells are surrounded by a well-marked inflammatory reaction, with round-cell infiltration, which indicates that the organism is still resisting the spread of the neoplasm. B. U. I. Path. 3570.

Küttner states that he has observed pictures which convince him that the carcinomatous processes grow through preformed lymphatic channels; a matter of some interest but little practical importance. When in contact with erectile tissue, the first growth, according to the above author, is into the trabeculæ, the invasion of the blood sinuses themselves being secondary. The sinuses are, however, invaded, as we have observed repeatedly, and filled with cancer nests, so that one may see areas in which the original architecture of the erectile tissue is entirely preserved, all the spaces being packed with cancer (Fig. 476). We have not observed the intratrabecular growth. With the erectile tissue sinuses filled with cancer, it is remarkable that blood-stream metastasis is not more common in penile epithelioma. Küttner explains this by saying that the cancer masses push the endothelium ahead of them and so never come in direct contact with the blood. This is apparently sometimes the case, but we do not believe that it is always true, as we have studied sections in which the cancer cells were undoubtedly in direct contact with the blood, without endothelial investment. Barney believes that internal metastases are more common than is usually stated (15 per cent. of the deaths in his series).

So few cases of gland formation in tumors of the penis (*adenocarcinoma*) are reported that it is not necessary to make a special grouping therefor.[1] All have been of the glans or prepuce. Waldeyer suggested an origin from the sebaceous glands of the preputial cavity.

Extension in epithelioma of the penis takes place by way of the erectile tissue and along the lymphatics. In our series there is a beautiful example of lymphatic extension. A cross-section of the entire penis shows the urethra, corpus spongiosum, and corpora cavernosa normal, while under the skin of the dorsum are three lymphatic channels each containing a process of tumor cells filling its lumen. The glans is first invaded, the heavy tunic of the cavernous bodies protecting them for a time. Eventually the corpora cavernosa are attacked, and may be invaded from

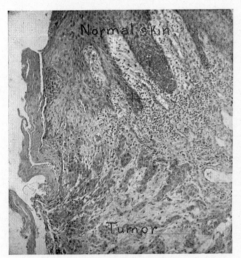

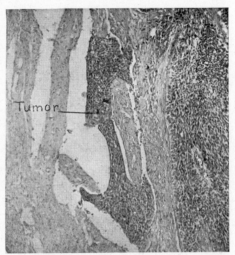

FIG. 475.—The edge of an epithelioma of the penis showing, above, normal skin, and, below, the transition from this into an invasive form of epithelioma. Since there is no epidermization this tumor would be known as basal-celled epithelioma. B. U. I. Path. 3948.

FIG. 476.—Invasion of the sinuses of the corpus cavernosum by epithelioma of the penis. Note that the tumor cells grow only in spaces distending them, but not invading the trabeculæ. B. U. I. Path. 4901.

end to end, though the growth advances slowly. The growth does not, as a rule, send out long single processes in the corpora, and Küttner concludes from his studies that *amputation 2 cm. proximal to the border of palpable induration is always sufficient.* The corpus spongiosum is spared to the last when the tumor involves the entire cross-section of the penis. This, no doubt, explains why urinary obstruction is so rare. In late stages the penis is destroyed, the crura of the penis and the bulb infiltrated, and the scrotum and abdominal wall involved by the ulcer. Perineum, prostate, and bladder may rarely be invaded. Extension along the urethra ahead of the main growth is, for some unexplained reason, extremely rare.

In earlier stages a retractible prepuce may become phimotic from edema or infiltration. In such case, or if there has been a congenital phimosis, the prepuce may apparently be invaded by extension across the preputial cavity. It is eventu-

[1] Demarquay: Maladies Chirurgicales du Penis, Paris, 1877. Waldeyer: Archiv für Klinische Chirurgie, 1870, xii, 849–855. Buday: Archiv für Klinische Chirurgie, 1895, xlix, 101–110.

ally ulcerated, and tumor masses often appear through holes in the prepuce separate from the original orifice. A few instances have been reported which are apparently implantations on the inner surfaces of the thighs or the anterior surface of the scrotum.

Metastasis from epithelioma of the penis is most frequent and earliest by way of the lymphatics. The anatomy of the lymph-channels is, therefore, of great importance in planning radical operations. Our knowledge of this anatomy depends upon the work of Zeissl and Horowitz,[1] Küttner,[2] Cunéo and Marcille,[3] and Bruhns,[4]

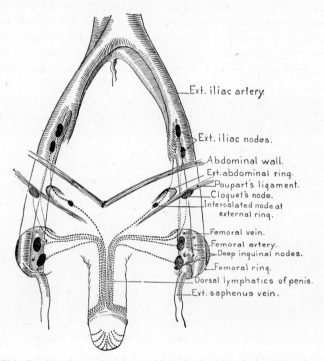

Fig. 477.—This diagram shows the course of lymphatic channels from the glans penis, prepuce, and integument of the distal portion of the penis. The channels run around the coronary sulcus to the midline where they turn upward to form the dorsal lymphatics. They may lie at some distance from the midline. At the base of the penis they turn right and left and may be divided unequally between the two sides. Those which terminate in the inguinofemoral nodes empty into the deep glands, and it is, therefore, necessary in operations to clean out the femoral triangle clear down to the artery and vein. Others do not terminate here, but pass upward through the femoral ring to empty into external iliac nodes. One fairly constant channel passes through the inguinal canal with an intercalated node at the external ring to empty into an external iliac node. Complete dissection of the femoral triangle, therefore, does not absolutely ensure against metastasis.

all at least twenty years old. It is to be hoped that new contributions to this subject may be made.

The following brief résumé may be given: The collecting trunks from the penis and urethra (Fig. 477) run circumferentially around the penis, those from the glans in the coronary sulcus, the others at intervals along the shaft. On the dorsum of the penis they join to form a number of longitudinal channels, the dorsal lymphatics, which are usually near the midline, but may lie a good distance laterally

[1] Wiener Klinische Wochenschrift, 1890, iii, 388 (Gesellschaft der Ärtze in Wien).

[2] Beiträge zur Klinische Chirurgie, 1900, xxvi, 1–79.

[3] The Lymphatics (Delamere, Poirier, and Cunéo), 1904 (London, English translation).

[4] Archiv für Anatomie und Physiologie, Anatomische Abteilung, 1900, 281–294.

thereto. These channels anastomose somewhat, but, in general, those from the penile skin and prepuce, glans, and penile urethra remain distinct and make three separate groups, which follow quite different paths after passing the root of the penis: 1. The channels from prepuce, frenum, and penile skin turn to right and left and run to the inguinal glands, mostly the upper medial nodes of the superficial layer, but a few to the deep nodes close to the femoral vessels. There may be one or two tiny intercepting nodes just at the base of the penis. 2. The channels from the glans anastomose to form a small plexus in front of the symphysis. From this plexus channels go (a) to the inguinal nodes, mostly the deep ones—Cunéo believes that no channels from the glans go to the superficial inguinal nodes—(b) through the crural canal under Poupart's ligament to the external iliac nodes, and (c) a constant channel, usually single, lying under the spermatic cord and passing through the inguinal canal to enter an external iliac node. There may be a small intercalated node at the external inguinal ring. 3. The channels from the urethra go (a) to the deep inguinal glands (few); (b) the iliac glands via the femoral canal; (c) by a single channel passing over the symphysis between the insertions of the recti abdominales and then laterally along the inner surface of the abdominal wall to the external iliac or internal epigastric nodes; (d) by anastomotic channels along the dorsal vein of the penis to join under the symphysis the channels from the membranous urethra, which are drained by the pudic and prevesical channels into the internal iliac (hypogastric) group of nodes. (See also Fig. 399.)

While it is common to see metastases in the inguinal glands, intrapelvic masses are by no means rare, and one can see from the above synopsis how they may occur even in the absence of inguinal involvement. Such cases are reported. These considerations are important in connection with the operative technic, and will be referred to again in the section on Treatment.

While lymphatic metastasis is not, as a rule, rapid, it is practically always farther advanced than the local extension. Thus a case with infiltration of the corpora as far as the base of the penis is almost certain to have wide-spread metastases.

Since the ulcerated tumor is always infected, the regional glands may be enlarged by the inflammatory process, indistinguishable clinically from metastasis. In Barney's series 75 per cent. showed enlarged glands, while of those which were removed and examined, 40 per cent. were not cancerous. In other cases enlarged inguinal glands have returned to normal after simple amputation.

Microscopically, the metastases resemble the original tumor, though, as we have stated, pearl formation may be marked in the metastases when it is absent or abortive in the primary growth. Sometimes these pearls become very large and are filled with semifluid débris, so that the enlarged lymph-nodes appear as cystic bodies, which may rupture and spread malignant cells over the wound if not carefully handled (Fig. 478). Eventually the growth passes beyond the lymph-node, involving subcutaneous tissue, skin, and other adjacent tissues, with external ulceration. Even before this, inflammatory reaction produces fibrosis and infiltration of the connective tissue, so that the affected glands are matted firmly together.

When generalized metastasis occurs, any organ may be affected. There is no special site of predilection, except possibly the liver. The frequency with which generalized metastasis occurs is somewhat uncertain, especially in the earlier stages. It is generally believed to be infrequent and late, and we have found no reason to doubt this conclusion. Barney found a generalized metastasis in 15 per cent. of the cases in which he had complete data, but a number of late and terminal stages were included.

Melanoma of the penis has been recorded in a few instances. Payr[1] has described and beautifully illustrated a case. This neoplasm arises from the chromatophores of the skin, and since there is some doubt as to whether they arise from the epithelium or the mesothelium, the tumor is sometimes called melanocarcinoma and sometimes melanosarcoma. These cells are the pigment-producing cells of the skin, and in tumors they retain this power, so that the growths are marked by a black color. In the gross they further differ from epithelioma in being beneath the skin and in being non-ulcerative. The skin is thinned out, stretched over the tumor, and semitransparent, so that the characteristic color can be seen through it. Later there may be superficial erosions on the most prominent parts of the tu-

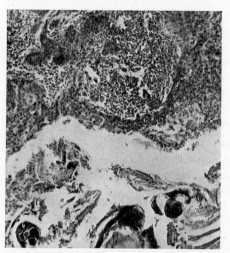

Fig. 478.—Metastasis of epithelioma of the penis to an inguinal lymph-node. The tumor is squamous-celled and it will be seen that epidermization and desquamation have produced a good sized cyst which is really an exaggerated epithelial pearl. B. U. I. Path. 3948.

mor. The nodules may become multiple. The usual site of origin is on the glans. Metastases occur by the lymph or blood-channels and, as frequently seen in melanotic tumors, are apt to be in the skin. They retain the black color of the primary tumor.

Endothelioma of the penis has been described a number of times. Joelson has collected 9 cases.[2] This tumor usually arises as an induration of the shaft of the penis, involving the corpora. While it may be localized at first, the induration usually soon becomes diffuse, producing a priapism. On section the sinuses of the erectile tissue are filled with masses of tumor cells, which have been assumed to arise from the endothelium lining the spaces. Borrmann[3] has seen such a specimen which made him believe that the tumor was really a carcinoma beginning in the penile urethra and invading the corpora. He raises the question of whether all so-called endothelioma of the penis do not arise in this way.

Mesothelial tumors of the penis are principally sarcomata. Joelson has recently collected 17 cases of round-cell, spindle-cell, and mixed-cell sarcoma and fibrosarcoma. The microscopic pathology is sufficiently indicated by these names. Of these 17, 13 originated in the corpora cavernousa, only 3 in the glans, and in 1 case the origin was not stated. While involving the erectile tissue, they differ from the so-called endotheliomata in producing a definite rounded nodule, which remains demarcated from the remainder of the penis, and does not go on to diffuse infiltration. Ulceration occurs eventually. Metastasis is slow, but we are unable to make definite statements as to how it occurs.

A very few *teratomata of the penis* have been reported.

[1] Deutsche Zeitschrift für Chirurgie, 1899, liii, 221–235.
[2] Surgery, Gynecology, and Obstetrics, 1924, xxxviii, 150–158.
[3] Lubarsch and Ostertag: Ergebnisse von Allgemeinen Pathologie, 1902, vii, 833.

The penis may be involved *secondarily*, the principal tumors concerned being carcinoma of the urethra and prostate. Carcinoma of the penile urethra is certain to invade the tissues of the penis before it has advanced very far. In the case described by Culver and Foster[1] the whole shaft of the penis was indurated. Carcinoma of the prostate often invades the walls of the membranous urethra, presumably through the lymphatics, and less frequently pushes on into the bulb. When this occurs, the erectile tissue is invaded, the sinuses being filled with tumor cells, just as in epithelioma of the glans, but in the reverse direction. At the base of the penis the process may break into the corpora cavernosa and eventually produce a carcinomatous priapism. We have seen one such case.

Scrotum.—Tumors of the scrotal contents (testis, epididymis, cord, and testicular tunics) have already been considered, so that this section concerns only tumors arising from the scrotal skin, dartos, and connective tissue.

BENIGN TUMORS.—Cysts of the scrotum are infrequent, but cannot be considered as great rarities. They may be congenital, in which case they may be dermoid or mucous, and are found along the raphé. Mermet[2] reports cases in which a row of cysts extended along the entire scrotal raphé. Congenital cysts of the perineum, when large, may push into the scrotum and seem to be scrotal, as in a case of Johnson.[3] Further discussion will be found in the section on Malformations of the Urogenital Tract.

Sebaceous cysts are not uncommon on the scrotum. Certain cysts, as the one described by Churchman,[4] are apparently due to the presence of an old hematocele. The fluid has a brownish color due to the altered hemoglobin.

Other tumors described as multilocular serous cysts are apparently lymphangiomata.

Hemangiomata are rare. Venous varices—independent of varicocele—may develop. Sebileau and Descomps[5] mention a case of cirsoid aneurysm. There have been 2 cases in our clinic in which the varices involved the scrotum, the penis, and the inner surface of the thigh (Figs. 467, 479).

Lipomata of the scrotum are also rare. In structure they offer no points of differentiation from other lipomata, but must be carefully distinguished from those of the spermatic cord.

Many of these benign tumors, especially the congenital ones, may show a marked increase at the time of puberty.

MALIGNANT TUMORS.—*Epithelioma of the scrotum* is the most important tumor of the scrotum, although much less common than carcinoma of the penis, at least in this country. In 12,500 cases at the Brady Urological Institute, there have been 2 cases of epithelioma of the scrotum. In the same period 35 cancers of the penis were seen. In England, on the other hand, 30 cases of scrotal cancer appeared at the Manchester Royal Infirmary in five years, during which period there were only 25 cases of cancer of the penis.[6] The reason for this marked difference is not obvious.

Epithelioma of the scrotum was formerly known as chimney-sweep's cancer,

---

[1] Surgery, Gynecology, and Obstetrics, 1923, xxxvi, 473–479.

[2] Bulletin de la Societe d'Anatomie de Paris, 1894, 69th year, 3d series, viii, No. 1, p. 53.

[3] Journal of Urology, 1923, x, 295–310.

[4] Johns Hopkins Hospital Bulletin, 1905, xvi, 264.

[5] Nouveau Traité de Chirurgie, Le Dentu and Delbet, 1916, xxxii (Maladies des Organes Génitaux de l'Homme).

[6] Wilson: Quoted by Morley, Lancet, 1911, clxxxi, 1545–1548.

from the observation that persons engaged in this occupation were particularly liable to it. The assumption was that the soot, volatilized tar, etc., in the chimneys, coming in contact with the thin skin of the scrotum, provided the etiologic moment for the cancer. It is different to estimate the accuracy of the observation, and further observations cannot be made, since chimneys are now usually swept in a way that does not require the sweep to enter them.

Although tar derivatives have been observed to produce malignant epithelial growths in animals under certain experimental conditions, it is not exactly apparent why the substances mentioned should affect in human beings only the scrotum

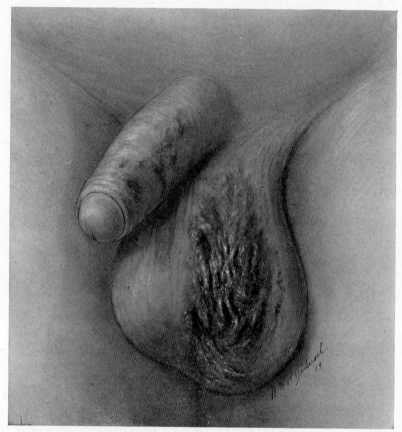

FIG. 479.—Hemangioma of penis and scrotum. B. U. I. 8231.

and not the penis. With the idea that volatile organic products are especially apt to cause irritation ending in cancer, it has been stated that firemen, foundry workers, and paraffin workers were also especially subject to this disease. But, according to Sebileau and Descomps, mule drivers and piano movers are equally susceptible, so that there is little reason to lay much stress on this etiologic theory, which is largely of historic interest.

Pathologically, the lesion is a cutaneous epithelioma, similar to those arising elsewhere.

It may begin as a small, wart-like excrescence, or as a flat plaque. Ulceration is early. Preceding papillomatous tumors or warts occur on the scrotum as they do on the penis and were formerly called "soot-warts."[1] The tumor itself may be proliferative, with cauliflower-like masses, or destructive, with a flat, indurated edge surrounding an ulcer (rodent ulcer type).

Microscopically, one sees typical epithelioma, which may be of the squamous-cell or basal-cell type, exactly similar to the pictures described in the paragraphs on epithelioma of the penis.

Like all epitheliomata, the tumors are of slow growth, and tend to involve the deeper tissues late. This is probably due to the fact that the testis and its adnexa have a completely separate system of lymphatics, which do not anastomose with those of the superficial layers. The penis, perineum, and lower abdomen may be involved in late stages, and eventually the testis and spermatic cord.

Metastasis of scrotal epithelioma occurs mainly by the lymphatic channels. The lymph area has been best studied by Morley.[2] According to him, there is a

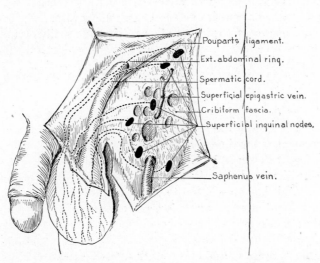

FIG. 480.—Diagram of the lymphatic drainage of the scrotum. There are about six main trunks, as a rule. Note that the anterior ones run well up on the base of the penis. None pass under the spermatic cord. All drain into the superficial inguinofemoral nodes. None pass through into the deep nodes or the iliac nodes. It is, therefore, not necessary in removing these glands to do a deep dissection of the femoral triangle.

fine-meshed network of lymph capillaries covering the entire scrotum, and lying beneath the skin and external to the dartos. This network anastomoses freely with similar superficial networks on the penis, thighs, and perineum, and the two halves of the scrotum anastomose freely. Collecting channels of larger size drain the lymph from this network, and dip down so that they run internal to the dartos (Fig. 480). The collecting channels anastomose with one another on the same side to a slight degree, but not with those of the opposite half of the scrotum, of the penis, or of any other region. There are ten to fifteen trunks on each side. The most medially placed of those on the anterior surface run up along the side of the root of the penis. They then turn laterally, running above Poupart's ligament, across the spermatic cord, and either above or beneath the superficial epigastric vein, to drop finally below Poupart's ligament and enter some of the uppermost and most external

[1] Curling: Diseases of the Testis, American Edition, Philadelphia, 1856.
[2] Lancet, 1911, ii, 1545–1548.

of the superficial inguinal nodes—occasionally only an inch or so below the anterior superior spine. The groups from the lateral and posterior surfaces of the scrotum turn laterally at the base of the scrotum without running on the penis, cross to the thigh below Poupart's ligament, and empty into any of the superficial inguinal nodes, even the lowest and farthest out. Channels run both over and under the saphenous vein. Channels from the posterior median part of the scrotum may run across under the spermatic cord. In over thirty-five injections Morley never saw a channel pass the inguinal nodes to empty into the iliac group, as frequently happens with channels from the glans penis. Primary lymphatic metastases, therefore, can occur only in the inguinal glands, unless some aberrant channel be present.

Generalized metastasis may occur in later stages. We have no statistics on its frequence.

Melanoma of the scrotum has been reported a very few times. It resembles in all respects melanotic tumors appearing elsewhere in the skin.

Sarcoma of the scrotum appears also to be extremely rare.

Teratoma has been reported; it is another rarity. It usually occurs in the raphé, and appears to have certain relations with the other congenital tumors. It may undergo malignant degeneration.

SYMPTOMS

Penis.—*Benign tumors of the penis* cause few symptoms aside from the local mass. Urination is seldom interefered with. The congenital cystic tumors may undergo enlargement at the time of puberty. Any tumor of the penis, if of sufficient size, may interfere with coitus, but it is surprising what obstacles patients will overcome in this direction. Angiomatous tumors may give rise to hemorrhage, which may be severe. This has no relation to urination, but may be precipitated by an erection. The patient is usually able to see the source of the blood.

Papillomata are usually painless, though they may be tender and cause dyspareunia. When congenital phimosis is present, the only symptom may be a purulent discharge from the preputial cavity until such time as the masses have reached a large size, when a general enlargement of the head of the penis will be noticed.

Cutaneous horns of the glans, when large, become tender as the result of trauma, and interfere with coitus.

Epithelioma of the penis is often painless, but may be very tender in some cases. The patients frequently complain of itching, even in the early stages. Pain may be accentuated by erection.

If a benign tumor precedes the cancer, no alteration in the symptoms may be noted until an intractable ulceration appears. This is the cardinal symptom of cancer of the penis, and usually has as its result a series of variegated and unsuccessful local treatments which the patient undergoes before the proper diagnosis is made.

There is usually no interference with urination. Only 2 of our 35 patients made this complaint, and in 1 of them the tumor arose as a nodule just at the meatus. Hemorrhage may occur, but is usually slight.

When congenital phimosis is present, the lesion may not be noted for a long time. These patients are usually accustomed to a certain amount of discharge from the preputial cavity, and suspect nothing until it becomes very profuse and foul-smelling, or until an easily palpable nodule appears beneath the preputial skin.

With the beginning of ulceration, enlargement of the inguinal glands is common, due to the inevitable infection. Later metastatic enlargement may be added to the inflammatory enlargement. There may be pain and fever, and occasionally abscess occurs.

In later stages there is a large, spreading destructive ulcer with the foul smell associated with malignancy or other necrotic conditions. Loss of weight and strength is usually delayed, and may be absent even when metastases are extensive. There may be slight fever.

Inguinal *metastases* may interfere with locomotion when extensive. They may ulcerate into the femoral vessels, causing fatal hemorrhage. Scrotal edema may occur. Iliac metastases may press upon veins and sacral nerve roots, just as do those from prostatic cancer, and may cause neuralgic or sciatic pains of great severity, edema of the leg, or paralysis.

In general, it is remarkable how long patients ordinarily neglect cancer of the penis. This is not altogether due to negligence, as men of all classes have the idea that if they consult a physician, amputation will be recommended, and they will, therefore, endure almost anything to retain even the pathologic organ as long as possible. It is extraordinary to learn that some with large, necrotic ulcers still perform coitus. As in other diseases, it is pain that is most effective in bringing the patient to seek treatment. We have seen one individual with a large fungous mass involving most of the glans, who stated frankly that he had had the lesion for twelve years, and would not even then have come to the hospital if it had not begun to be painful. The growth was papillary, with only a beginning malignant change.

The course of the disease is slow. Since we often do not know the exact date when the malignant change occurred, it is difficult to give exact figures. The duration is usually, however, a matter of two to four years, and Barney mentions 1 case still living eleven years after the diagnosis had been made, although no operation had been performed, and the growth had advanced steadily.

Scrotum.—The symptoms of *benign tumors of the scrotum* are those caused by the local enlargement. As stated above, congenital cysts may enlarge at puberty, and bring the patient for treatment at that time. Varices and angiomata may give rise to hemorrhage. There is usually no interference with urination or with the sexual function.

Epithelioma of the scrotum causes no symptoms at first except possibly some itching about the small primary lesion. Ulceration is early, and there may be a discharge of serum. Hemorrhage may occur from the ulcerated surface. Pain is uncommon in the earlier stages, but may be present. Metastasis causes inguinal masses, suppuration, or pain. Internal metastases give symptoms according to their location. Secondary lymphatic metastasis to the iliac nodes is not uncommon, when sciatic pains may occur as in penile and prostatic carcinoma. The ulceration is infected, so that inguinal buboes may be present, even in the absence of metastasis. It is often difficult or impossible to say whether the palpably enlarged glands are cancerous.

DIAGNOSIS

Penis.—*Benign tumors* of the penis, excepting papillomata, present no difficulty in diagnosis. By palpation one can determine whether they are connected with the urethra or corpora. Cystic tumors are usually recognizable by palpation, and it is only these which are apt to be connected with the urethra. Only very infrequently will any confusion with malignant growths be possible, in which case a biopsy is permissible, the operator being ready to carry out radical excision if necessary. If the meatus is involved, the extent of the tumor (angioma, papilloma, etc.) within the urethra should be determined by endoscopy.

Papillomatous growths, on the other hand, must always be considered as potentially malignant, even when the patient is under forty. This suspicion is increased by any induration at the base, or a marked tendency to ulceration. If the papillary character is not obvious, condylomatous lesions come into question, and syphilis must be considered. A Wassermann test and a short period of intensive treatment will usually clear up this point. One should watch carefully the response to local treatment and, if it is delayed, further diagnostic efforts must be made, of which the most certain is a biopsy.

Epithelioma of the penis is difficult to diagnose in its early stages. In our series the initial lesions—according to the statements of the patients—were as follows:

TABLE 133

	Pimple.	Flat ulcer.	Papilloma.	Black spot.
Glans..............	7	6	1	1
Prepuce............	5	8	0	0

In 5 cases the original appearance was not known, as it had been concealed beneath a congenital phimosis. As to phimosis, 11 of our 35 cases had had congenital phimosis, but in 5 of these circumcision had been done before the appearance of the cancer. In 3 others circumcision was done in the early stages of the disease, and the wound never healed. In 14 phimosis was absent, in 2 phimosis had occurred during the course of the disease from edema or infiltration, and in 8 information as to the presence or absence of phimosis was lacking.

Trauma, except possibly that of circumcision, does not figure in our series. In 2 cases the epithelioma appeared in the scar of an old ulcer, and in 1 case there was a history of contact with a carcinomatous cervix uteri in the year preceding the onset.

That a benign wart-like lesion can exist for a long time before malignant changes occur is indicated by 8 cases in which the onset dated back from five to fifteen years. In the remainder the duration was as follows: Two to five years, 8 cases; one to two years, 6 cases; six months to one year, 6 cases; none to six months, 5 cases. In 1 case the duration was not stated, and 1 other patient, a colored man with phimosis, stated that he had had sores on his penis "all his life."

It is safe to say that every penile wart or ulceration which is resistant to treatment should be suspected of malignancy. Other lesions coming into question are especially granuloma inguinale, syphilis, either chancre or gumma, and tuberculosis. Lesions of granuloma inguinale may be found on the penis, and are usually distinguished from cancer by the absence of deep induration, but the diagnosis may be very difficult. A few injections of tartar emetic will usually bring about resolution of these lesions. Syphilis often shows induration comparable to that of epithelioma, and may, therefore, resemble closely the flat ulcerated type. The therapeutic test, best with the arsenicals and flumerin, is useful. Tuberculosis of the penis is rare, but is usually extremely resistant to treatment. It may advance slowly, destroy tissue, and have an indurated edge and base like epithelioma. It may occur in the absence of demonstrable tuberculous lesions in the urogenital tract or elsewhere. If other tuberculosis is present, the diagnosis will be suggested, but if not, a biopsy is the only recourse. Even this may be indecisive, as the microscopic picture in skin tuberculosis is often ambiguous. Actinomycosis and other mycotic lesions, as well as leprosy, may occur, but are very rare in this country.

Apparently cancer may rarely develop in neglected syphilitic lesions, and probably also from chancroids. This is another reason for believing that an unhealed genital ulcer is always a danger point. In the few which seem to resist all forms of treatment, we must make sure that no malignancy is present, and be on the watch for its appearance.

In the small warts and flat plaques, ulcerated or not, induration will sometimes be slight or absent. In such cases the malignant change may be only beginning, as described in the section on Pathology. To be safe, however, such lesions must be treated as if frankly cancerous.

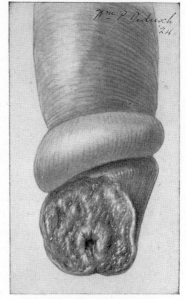

In short, in doubtful cases a biopsy alone will enable us to come to a decision. One hesitates to cut into malignant growths, but apparently no ill effects are to be expected in epithelioma of the penis, especially if operation is done immediately afterward. The segment must be removed with the knife, as the cautery too often sears the entire block, making the section useless. The segment should be generous, and cut carefully to include the most suspicious parts of the lesion and, if possible, the adjacent skin edge. Too often a small block shows only a cellular infiltration, where the subsequent history proves that the lesion must have been carcinomatous. After excising the block the wound should be burned with the cautery.

In later growths the proliferative masses characteristic of the fungating type leave no room for doubt (Fig. 482). In these, as well as in the flatter type, with thickened, everted edges, the tissue itself has a characteristic ap-

FIG. 481.—Carcinoma of penis. A flat, erosive ulcer involving the glans and eroding away the urinary meatus. There is also an inflammatory paraphimosis.

pearance. When carefully cleaned of exudate, it is opaque and whitish in appearance, variegated by little granular projections of the same sort of tissue, or by red dots, representing the vascular cores of the greatly hypertrophied dermal papillæ. When either of these appearances is pronounced, in an ulcerated lesion with indurated base, a definite diagnosis can be made at once.

When phimosis, congenital or acquired, is present, one must lay bare the lesion. A dorsal slit is the usual procedure, and is probably quite justified. It is possible, however, to avoid this by inserting through the preputial orifice the smallest size of child's cystoscope, with which, if a current of water is kept flowing through the preputial cavity under enough pressure to distend it, an excellent view can be obtained. We were able to confirm a diagnosis of cancer in a case by this method. An excellent magnified view of a malignant ulcer was obtained.

Enlargement of the inguinal glands gives no idea as to the presence of metastasis, since numerous cases are reported in which such enlargements subsided completely after simple amputation. In one of our series (B. U. I. 6942) the inguinal regions were occupied by immense, firm, matted, and adherent glands. The penile growth was advanced, and amputation was done simply as a palliative measure, since it was thought that metastasis was too extensive for radical treatment. The inguinal masses soon disappeared, and the patient is alive, well, and at work daily, over six years after operation. Sections of the penile growth showed squamous-cell epithelioma, with invasion of the erectile tissue.

Pain in the back, sciatic pain, or edema of the legs probably indicate deep lymphatic metastases in the iliac nodes. These metastases do not show in the x-ray, since they do not ordinarily involve the bone. The liver should always be carefully examined, as it is one of the favored sites of metastasis.

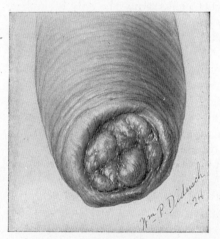

Fig. 482.—Carcinoma of the penis. Proliferative type of growth with fungous masses protruding from within the preputial cavity.

A permanent induration of the corpora of the penis suggests neoplastic infiltration, though it may be caused by thrombosis in the erectile tissue, which is rare. If no tumor is visible on the glans or elsewhere on the surface, rectal and endoscopic examinations should be done to rule out carcinoma of the prostate and carcinoma of the urethra, either of which may invade the corpora. If from the prostate, the corpus spongiosum may be free in the pendulous portion. Thrombosis is usually accompanied by great pain, tenderness, and fever. If no other source is found, the tumor known as endothelioma is to be suspected, and if exploration is done one should be prepared for radical operation if necessary.

Sarcoma, according to the literature, is oftenest a circumscribed nodule, which ulcerates late. If seen early, the diagnosis may be doubtful, and is best made by exploratory operation with a tourniquet about the root of the penis. We have seen a case in which a very distinguished pathologist returned a diagnosis of sarcoma from excised tissue, which afterward proved to be syphilitic.

Scrotum.—*Benign tumors of the scrotum* present few difficulties of diagnosis. The most important point is to palpate carefully for any connection with the testicle, epididymis, cord, or urethra. If there is any connection with the urethra, endoscopy should be done. Urethral diverticula sometimes appear as scrotal tumors, but can be emptied by pressure, the urine flowing from the meatus. Peri-urethral inflammations and abscesses are distinguished by pain, tenderness, and fever.

Epithelioma of the scrotum is also quite easy to diagnose, as a rule. The observations made as to the gross appearance of epitheliomata of the penis apply here also, and here also the difficulties arise only in early cases. Scrotal ulcers may be, as on the penis, granuloma inguinale, syphilis, and tuberculosis. In case doubt persists, biopsy is justified.

Unfortunately the diagnosis is frequently late in epithelioma, both of the penis and scrotum. This can be avoided by keeping in mind the various forms of primary lesion described above, and by suspecting carcinoma in every genital ulcer which is unusually resistant to treatment, especially if there is the slightest induration.

TREATMENT

Penis.—*Benign tumors of the penis* should be removed. Warts and papillomata are easily destroyed by fulguration. If large, the possibility of malignancy should be excluded by the means already described. Cysts, hemangiomata, etc., are excised.

Epithelioma.—Radical operation should be carried out wherever possible. For a number of years we have followed a technic which is described at length in another chapter (see Vol. II, page 648). The principle upon which this operation is based is that the entire lymphatic area from the tumor on the penis to the fat and glands in the groin should be removed in one piece. It has been our practice to start externally near the anterior superior spine and remove the entire mass of fat and glands in each groin, two operators working from above downward simultaneously and meeting in the suprapubic region. From there the dissection extends downward, hugging the symphysis pubis and cleaning out the space between the root of the penis and the symphysis pubis and upper portion of the triangular ligament, the excision extending through the fascias to the tunica of the corpora cavernosa at its root. The entire mass is carried downward, thus removing all the structures from around the corpora cavernosa until a point is reached at which amputation is to be done. In this dissection the glands of the femoral canal and in the upper part of the scrotum are also removed with their overlying fat. In this way the most complete possible radical operation is carried out as is described in detail elsewhere.

The results obtained by this operation have been most satisfactory. In 16 cases in which the complete radical operation was done, 2 have not been followed, 2 are living but not well (followed nine and six months), 5 are dead, and 7 are well (seven, five, five, three, two and one-half, one and one-half, and one years). As many of these cases came with extensive long-standing ulcerative carcinoma of the penis present and palpably enlarged glands in both groins, the results obtained are really quite remarkable.

The radical operation should be carried out even where the glands are definitely involved in both groins because there is a chance of cure as shown by our statistics. Even where a complete cure is not obtained, the carcinomatous mass in the groin and penis is removed and local recurrences may not occur or, at any rate, are less extensive and distressing than when the glands are not removed. In very extensive cases with metastases manifest beyond the groins the radical operation is not indicated, particularly if the patient is in bad condition. One may then have to be satisfied with a simple amputation of the penis to remove the sloughing tumor mass.

The use of radium and x-ray has been very unsatisfactory in our hands. No case has been cured, and cases which are early and most favorable for a radical cure have been allowed to develop metastasis. It is indeed strange that the ray treatment is so unsatisfactory in these tumors which are so superficial and easily reached for intensive treatment, but such is the experience of other clinics.

Total emasculation and other very extensive excisions of the external genito-urinary tract have, we believe, little to recommend them. We have never had recurrences in the scrotal contents after a satisfactory radical operation, as above described, and such mutilation as castration adds immensely to the unhappiness of the patient as well as his discomfort. Castration has been urged in the past on the plea that impotence and lack of desire would result and the mental condition of the patient become more tranquil. This was based on the assumption that amputation of the penis would practically preclude coitus; as a matter of fact, even though amputation be fairly extensive, the line of excision being at the base of the penis and within 2 cm. of the symphysis pubis when exposed at operation, nevertheless erection occurs and intercourse is not infrequently possible and quite satisfactory. We have been amazed to find that many of these patients report libido, erections, and ejaculations quite satisfactory. The greatly shortened length does not seem to interfere with the accomplishment of ejaculations. On this account it is evident that castration should not be carried out, certainly in view of the fact that the line of lymphatics does not extend toward the scrotum, but away from it.

Transplantation of the urethra into the perineum is not, we believe, necessary or satisfactory. Urination is thus made much more bothersome. As the carcinoma generally involves the glans and corpora cavernosa very much more than the urethra, when Buck's fascia and the tunica albuginea covering them have been freely exposed, it is generally safe to save at least 1 inch more of the urethra than the corpora and thus bring the urinary meatus into a good position in front of the scrotum with a small cone-like elevation of skin around it so that the urinary stream does not run down the scrotum, but flows clear. By means of an obliquely cut or slit urethra stricture is prevented, but should this occur it may be dilated or a silver tube or quill may be provided to conduct the urinary stream clear of the scrotum.

A complete study of our cases shows the following results:

TABLE 134

Operated upon, 28.

    Radical operation,[1] apparently complete, 16.

        Well, 7 (seven, five, five, three, two and a half, one and a half, one and a quarter years).

        Dead, 5 (two and two-third years, eight, four, one, "few," months).

        Living, but not well, 2 (nine, six months).

    Radical operation, obviously incomplete, 2.

        Dead, 2 (eight months, "soon after operation").

    Amputation of penis only, 8.

        Well, 1 (six years).

        Dead, 1 (three years).

        Discharged with metastasis or recurrence, 2.

        Not followed, 4.

    Local excision of tumor and separate removal of inguinal glands, 2.

        Dead, 1 (four months).

        Not followed, 1.

[1] By the radical operation we mean amputation of the penis and wide removal of the inguinal lymph-bearing area.

Not operated on, 7.
  Refused operation, not followed, 2.
  Inoperable, 3.
  Incomplete data, 2.
Summarizing the cases treated by operation, we have:
  Well, 8.
  Dead, 8.
  Not followed, 7.
  Discharged with metastasis or recurrence, 2.
  Result doubtful, 3.
      1. Seven months, healed, but has "pyelitis," and general condition is "poor."
      2. Two months "improving."
      3. Three years, died of "paralysis, much benefited by the operation."
We have had no good results from radium treatment.

Scrotum.—The treatment of tumors of the scrotum offers little complication. Warts and papillomata may be fulgurated, other tumors are to be excised. Epithelioma should receive radical treatment, with excision of the inguinal glands, as described in Chapter XIX.

VOL. I—46